Ophthalmic Ultrasonography

Documenta Ophthalmologica Proceedings Series volume 38

Editor H. E. Henkes

1984 **Dr W. JUNK PUBLISHERS**
a member of the KLUWER ACADEMIC PUBLISHERS GROUP
THE HAGUE / BOSTON / LANCASTER

Ophthalmic Ultrasonography

Proceedings of the 9th SIDUO Congress, Leeds, U.K.

July 20–23, 1982

Edited by Jeffrey S. Hillman and Malcolm M. Le May

1984 **Dr W. JUNK PUBLISHERS**
a member of the KLUWER ACADEMIC PUBLISHERS GROUP
THE HAGUE / BOSTON / LANCASTER

Distributors

for the United States and Canada: Kluwer Boston, Inc., 190 Old Derby Street, Hingham, MA 02043, USA
for all other countries: Kluwer Academic Publishers Group, Distribution Center, P.O.Box 322, 3300 AH Dordrecht, The Netherlands

Library of Congress Cataloging in Publication Data

SIDUO. Congress (9th : 1982: Leeds, West Yorkshire)
Ophthalmic ultrasonography.

(Documenta ophthalmologica. Proceedings series ; v. 38)
Includes index.
1. Ultrasonics in ophthalmology--Congresses.
I. Hillman, Jeffrey S. II. Le May, Malcolm M.
III. Title. IV. Series. [DNLM: 1. Eye diseases--Diagnosis--Congresses. 2. Ultrasonics--Diagnostic use --Congresses. W3 DO637 v.38 / WW 143 S569 1982o]
RE79.U4S5 1982 617.7'1543 83-13612

ISBN-13: 978-94-009-7280-3 e-ISBN-13: 978-94-009-7278-0
DOI: 10.1007/978-94-009-7278-0

Copyright

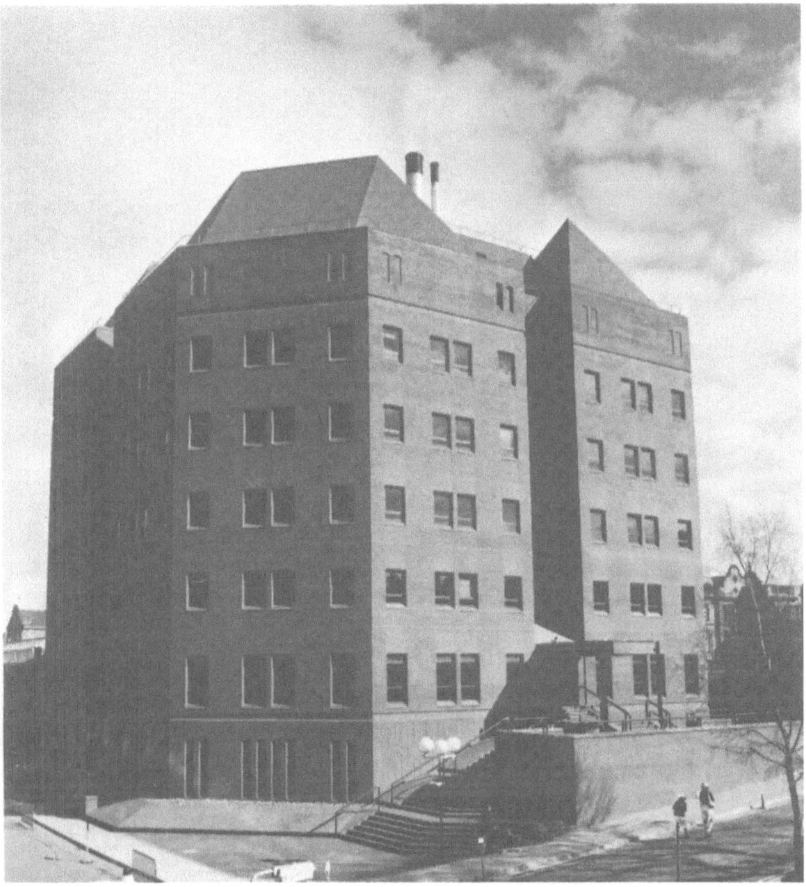

CLINICAL SCIENCES BUILDING, St. JAMES'S UNIVERSITY HOSPITAL, LEEDS.
Photograph by University of Leeds Audio-Visual Service.

CONTENTS

PART ONE: THE EYE

1. Intraocular tumours

2. Vitreo-retinal pathology

3. Other intraocular pathology

4. Biometry for lens implantation

5. Clinical biometry

PART TWO: THE ORBIT

1. Orbital tumours

2. Optic nerve and muscles

3. Miscellaneous

PART THREE: PHYSICS & TECHNIQUES

ULTRASOUND IN THE MANAGEMENT OF INTRAOCULAR TUMOURS

(With particular reference to their local resection)

WALLACE S. FOULDS
(Glasgow, Scotland)

Hon. President of the Congress

Until recently the standard treatment for all intraocular malignant tumours was excision of the eye. In the case of retinoblastoma, increasing use of radiotherapy and of chemotherapy has led to a much more conservative approach to these problems. In the case of the commonest intraocular tumour in adults, the malignant melanoma of the choroid, a somewhat similar situation has arisen. Not only has it been suggested that excision of the eye is without benefit as regards survival, but that enucleation may actually worsen the prognosis for life by dissemination of tumour cells during the surgical procedure (1). As a result, many eyes which were enucleated are now left *in situ*. This more conservative approach to the management of intraocular malignancy has made accurate diagnosis and follow-up even more important than heretofore and in both aspects ultrasound has a crucial role to play.

In relation to retinoblastoma, clinical diagnosis is rarely in doubt, although difficulty may occasionally be experienced in cases of persistent hyperplastic primary vitreous and retrolental fibroplasia. As you all know characteristically a retinoblastoma apart from showing a solid and not a cystic appearance on ultrasonography, usually shows high density echoes from the scattered calcification which is a feature of these tumours, while persistent hyperplastic primary vitreous and retrolental fibroplasia show the characteristic retrolental mass often accompanied by retinal detachment.

Retinoblastoma can usually be diagnosed on Ophthalmoscopy, for the tumour is pink and not white which differentiates it from many of the other conditions which may on occasion mimic this malignancy. Even in the best of hands, a mistake can however be made. In a recent patient presenting with a retinal mass, the lesion appeared pink and clinically was highly suspicious of retinoblastoma with a solid tumour close to the optic nerve head (Fig. 1). Ultrasound confirmed the presence of a solid epiretinal tumour near the optic disc (Fig. 2). Enucleation was decided upon because of proximity of the tumour to the optic nerve head. Histologically however, the enucleated globe showed a benign astrocytoma (Fig. 3), and in retrospect, more attention to the ultrasonic appearances might well have obviated enucleation of this eye.

When we come to malignant melanoma of the choroid, it is known that overall, up to 20% of eyes removed for suspected melanoma turn out on

Hillman, J. S./Le May, M. M. (eds.) Ophthalmic Ultrasonography

ISBN 978-94-009-7280-3

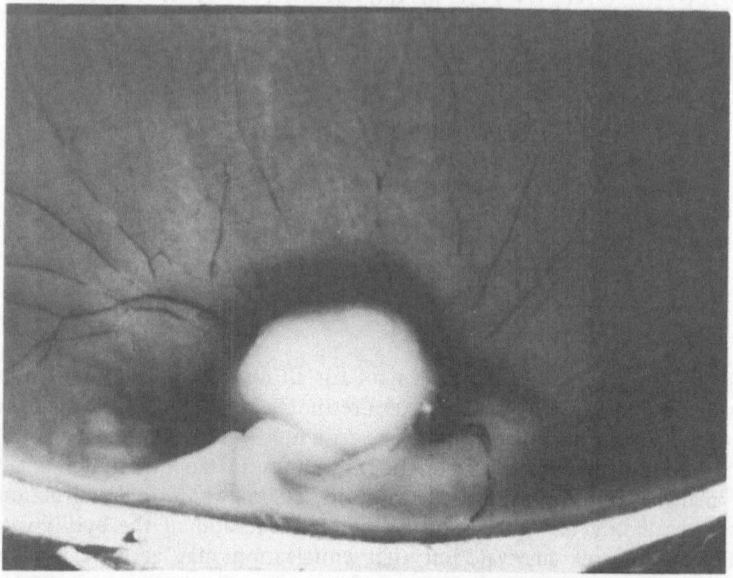

Fig. 1. **Macropathological photograph of an infant's eye removed for suspected retinoblastoma. There is a tumour in the posterior fundus close to the optic nerve head.**

histopathological examination not to have such a tumour (2, 3). The commonest differential diagnosis is disciform degeneration which may of course occur in the non-macular retina and clinically present as a large mass.

In centres using the full range of diagnostic techniques, the number of eyes wrongly removed should be small (4). When one considers the information available from binocular indirect ophthalmoscopy, trans-illumination, 32P uptake, fluorescein angiography, infra-red photography, red-free photography and ultrasound, it is surprising that any mistake in diagnosis should be made at all. Difficulties however, do arise. Thus some melanomas may be cystic and mimic anterior choroidal detachment, while equally choroidal detachments may mimic melanoma. In general, there is little difficulty in differentiating a peripheral melanoma from a choroidal detachment on ultrasound, the echo-free interior of the choroidal detachment being in marked contrast to the solid nature of the melanoma. Even using ultrasound however, there may occasionally be difficulties in the differentiation. An illustrative patient is a woman in her late fifties who presented with a smooth apparently cystic lesion in the anterior choroid and ciliary body (Fig. 4). The lesion trans-illuminated freely (Fig. 5) and the initial ultrasound picture confirmed the cystic nature of the lesion. Further scans however, showed in addition a solid underlying tumour consistent with a diagnosis of melanoma

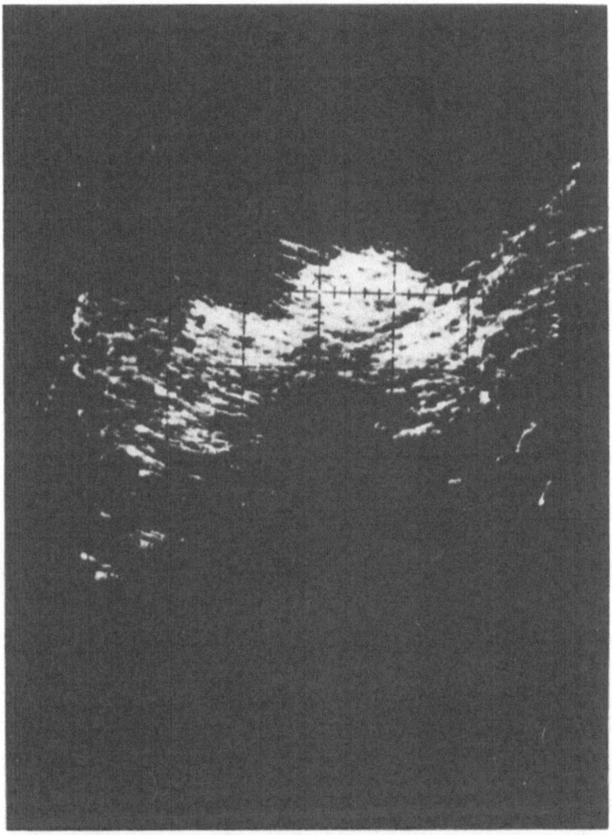

Fig. 2. Ultrasound appearances of the posterior pole of the eye illustrated in Figure 1. There is a solid epiretinal mass.

(Fig. 6). The patient eventually underwent a local choroidectomy, and the histology revealed an epitheloid celled malignant melanoma.

When a melanoma is complicated by haemorrhage, the diagnosis again may present clinical difficulties. In many cases in which there is vitreous haemorrhage, ultrasound can quite unequivocally confirm the presence of an underlying tumour. In a recent case, what was clinically a malignant melanoma overlying the optic disc in an eye with no perception of light was complicated by a choroidal haemorrhage, so that the appearances on ultrasound were not at all typical with a large echo-free zone within the mass, making the diagnosis of sub-pigment epithelial haemorrhage likely, and suggesting that the lesion itself might be a peripapillary disciform degeneration. Fluorescein angiography was equivocal and the situation of the tumour made testing with 32P impossible. Some three months later, when the sub-pigment epithelial

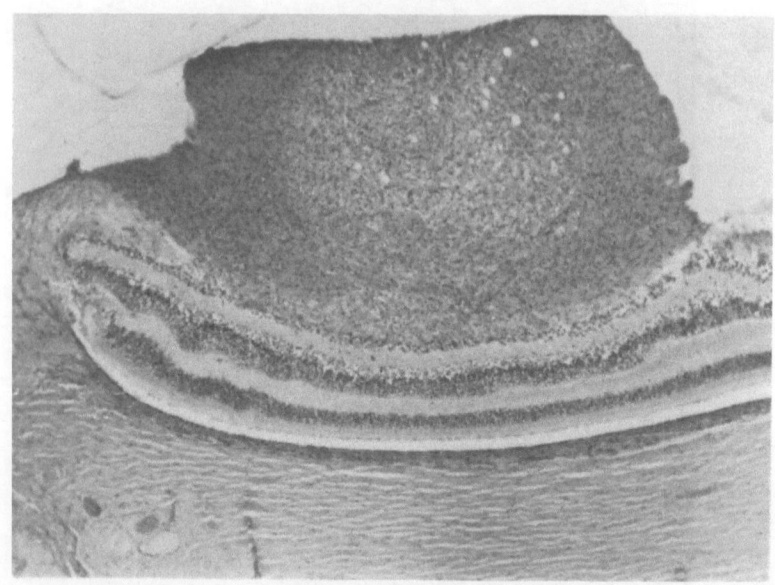

Fig. 3. Histological appearance of the lesion illustrated in Figures 1 and 2. The tumour is a benign astrocytoma.

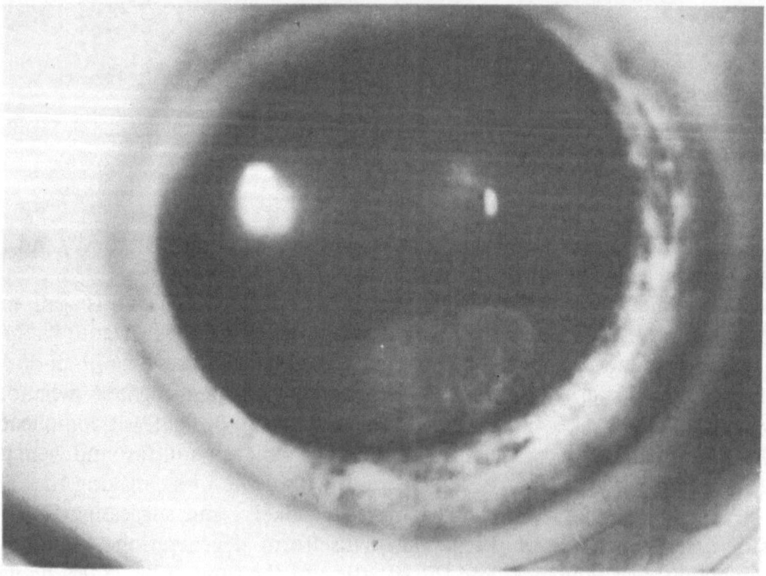

Fig. 4. Clinical appearance of a lesion in which the differential diagnosis lay between anterior choroidal detachment or melanoma.

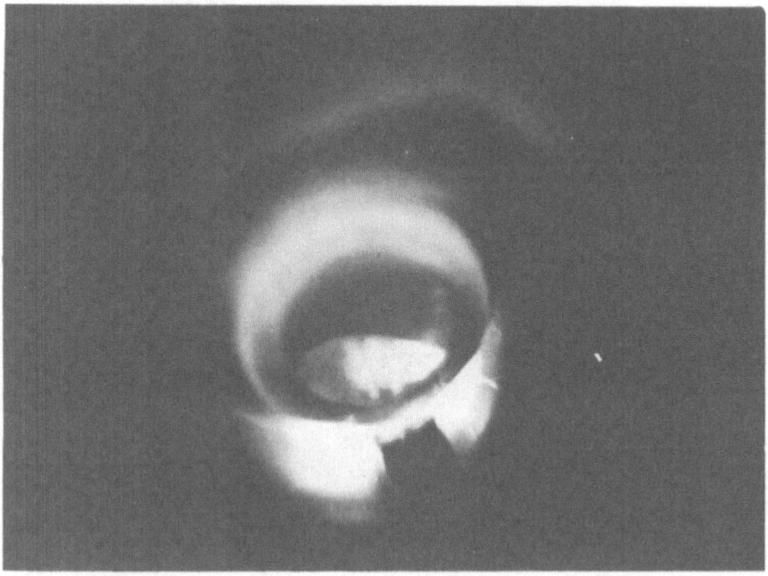

Fig. 5. The same lesion as in Figure 4 to show that it transilluminated freely.

blood had absorbed not only the clinical picture, but also the appearance on ultrasound showed the characteristics of a malignant melanoma confirmed by pathological examination of the excised eye.

A rather rare diagnostic difficulty is the osseus choristoma. Such a lesion may present as a mass in the peripapillary fundus, and may be hyper-fluorescent on fluorescein angiography (Fig. 7). Ultrasound or CAT scan will reveal the dense intralesional calcification which is characteristic of this abnormality (Fig. 8).

The current vogue for observing melanomas of the choroid rather than carrying out enucleation or other therapy has given ultrasound a very important role in their management, as the only modality likely to show evidence of extraocular spread at an early stage, as illustrated by the following case. The patient was a middle-aged woman who had a relatively small, but posteriorly situated tumour which had been kept under observation for some two years. Ultrasound revealed the unexpected presence of an extraocular extension posteriorly which was indeed somewhat larger than the intraocular tumour. This patient underwent exenteration.

When it comes to treatment of melanoma by relatively conservative methods of therapy such as photocoagulation or radiation, the use of radioactive plaques, either 60 Cobalt (5), or 106 Ruthenium/Rhodium (6), or in some centres radiation using high energy protons, the value of ultrasound is largely that of a diagnostic aid, although serial ultrasound measurements may give an indication of response to therapy. Not so however, when the possibility of local excision is entertained, for not only has ultrasound a valuable role in

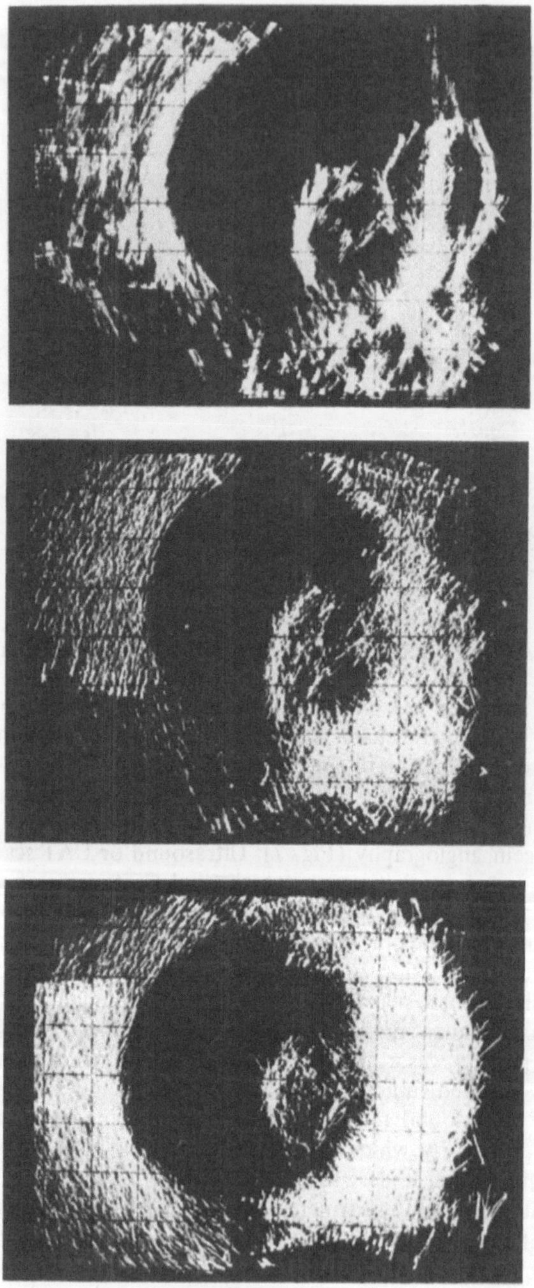

Fig. 6. Ultrasonic appearance of the lesion illustrated in Figures 4 and 5. In the initial cut (a) the cystic nature of the lesion was confirmed. In subsequent cuts (b, c) a solid underlying mass was demonstrated which proved to be a malignant melanoma.

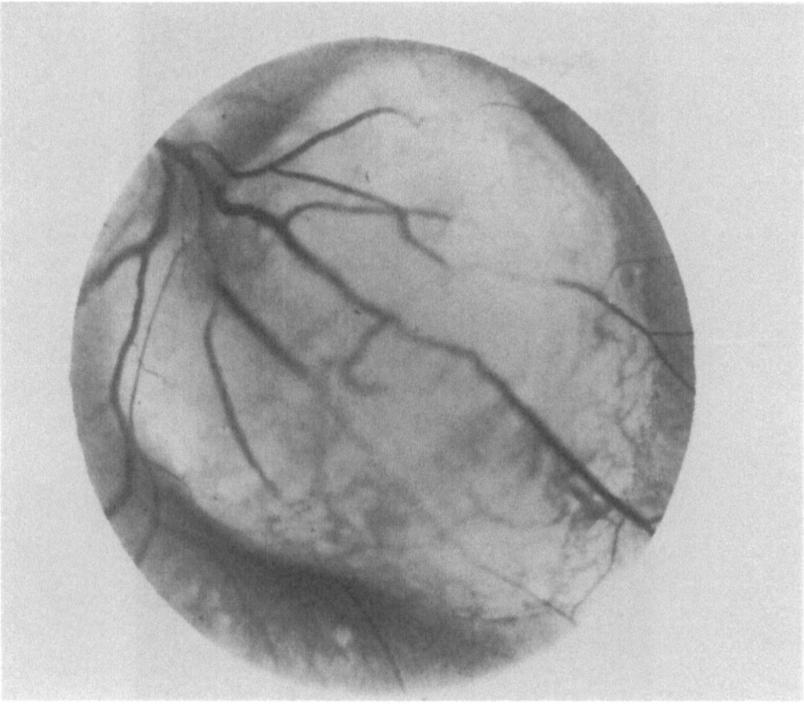

Fig. 7. Clinical picture of the eye of a patient presenting with an osseus choristoma (courtesy of Dr. S. Murray).

making the diagnosis, but a supremely important role in indicating the exact size and position of the tumour and alerting the surgeon pre-operatively to the possibility of extraocular extension.

In general, the information obtained by ultrasound is more reliable for tumours in the posterior choroid than for tumours in the anterior choroid or iris, although even in the iris, ultrasound can prove useful on occasion. In a recently seen young man, both irides showed an abnormal appearance with ectropion uveae and dye leakage on fluorescein angiography (Fig. 9). Intraocular pressure was slightly raised in the right eye, and the possibility of the iris naevus syndrome was considered as a diagnosis (7). Ultrasonic examination of the left iris however (Fig. 10), showed a solid mass behind the iris, and local iridocyclectomy confirmed the presence of an iris melanoma.

Unfortunately, the ultrasonic imaging of tumours in the anterior choroid and ciliary body is less good than of those more posteriorly situated, and exact measurements are difficult to make. Nevertheless, an estimate of how far back is the posterior limit of an anteriorly situated tumour is always useful in planning local excision.

A frequent problem when considering whether tumours are suitable for

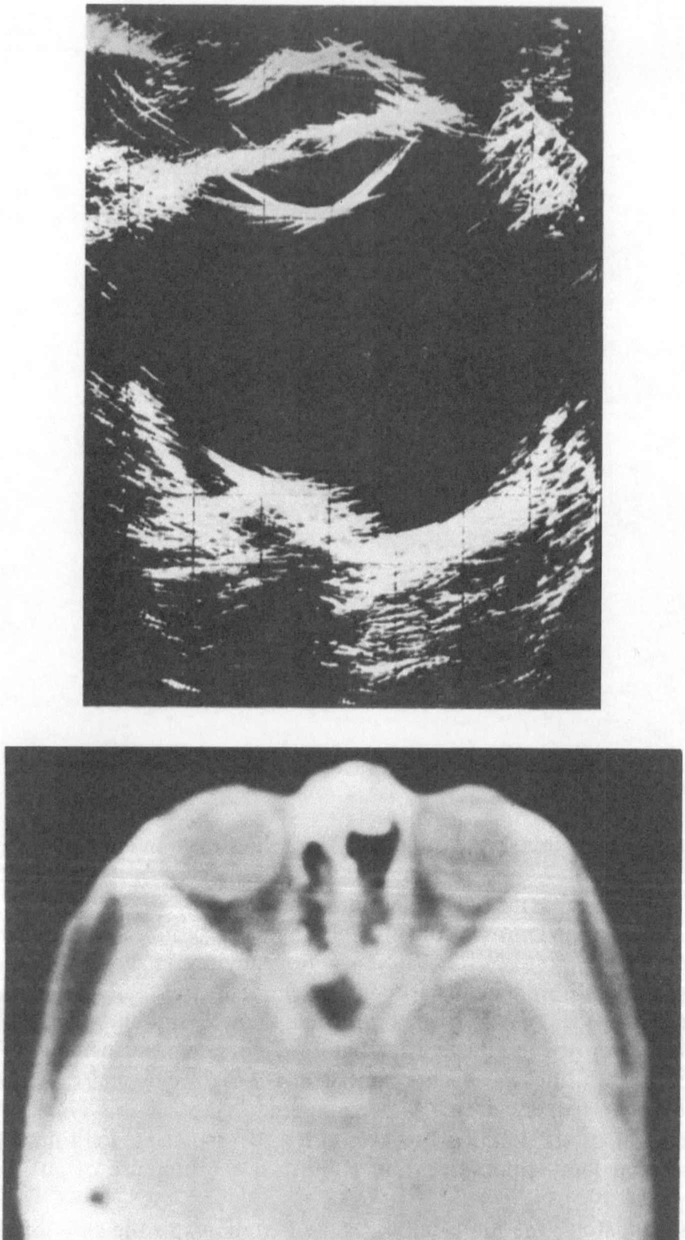

Fig. 8. Ultrasound appearance (a) and CT scan (b) of the lesion illustrated in Figure 7. Ultrasound shows the high density associated with intralesional calcification and 'shadowing' of the deeper tissues. CT scan showed two calcified lesions, one in the fundus oculi and the other in the optic nerve.

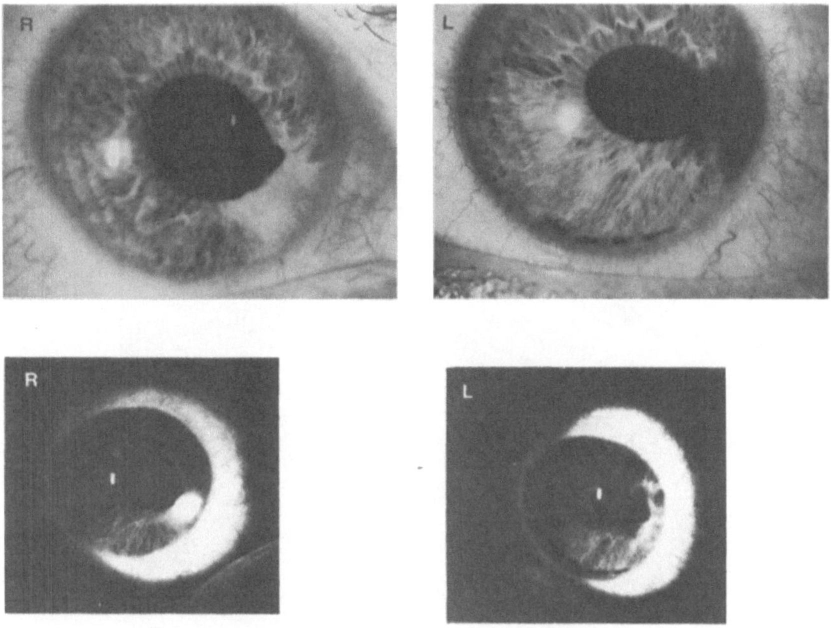

Fig. 9. Clinical appearance (a) and fluorescein iridogram (b) of both eyes of a patient with the presumed iris naevus syndrome.

local excision is whether the base of the tumour is smaller than the apparent size of the lesion. Not infrequently, what appears to be a very large choroidal melanoma has a relatively small base on ultrasound enabling local excision to be carried out without too much technical difficulty.

Extraocular extension poses its own particular problems for local excision. My own technique for local excision of choroidal tumours has been to expose the tumour via a lamellar scleral dissection, removing the deeper layers of sclera with the tumour. Obviously, an extra-scleral extension necessitates modification of this technique, usually by the necessity to perform a full thickness sclerectomy at the site of extension and replacement of the defect either by a full thickness scleral homograft or preferably by a partial thickness augograft from an uninvolved area of the same eye.

For me ultrasound is a most important parameter in the assessment of patients being considered for local excision of choroidal melanomas, and I thought you might find it interesting to see a short film on the surgical technique I use (Fig. 11). The patient in question came from Leeds, and pre-operatively had a typical melanoma of the choroid in an only eye. The tumour was some 12 mm. in diameter and situated in the inferior fundus just over one disc diameter from the macula. After exposure via a large fornix based lamellar scleral flap the tumour was dissected free from the underlying retina and removed without difficulty, haemorrhage being prevented by controlled systemic hypotension. The intact retina, which was not adherent to the tumour acted as a barrier to intravitreal fibroblastic

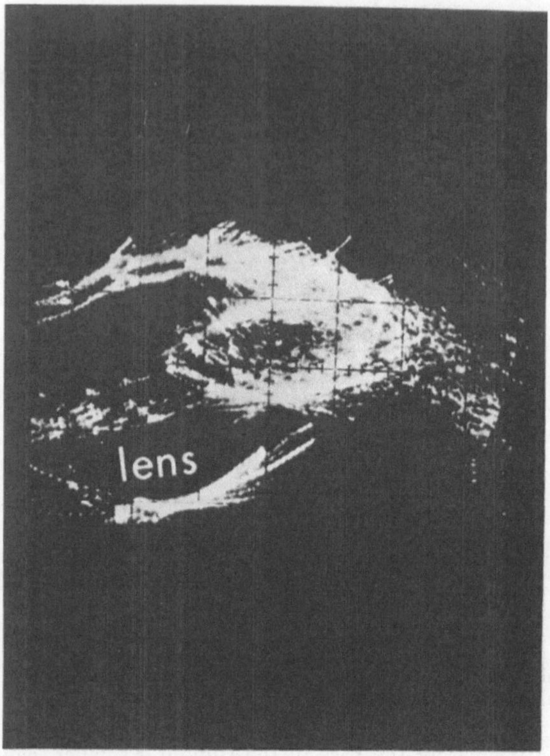

Fig. 10. **Ultrasonic appearance of the left eye of the patient illustrated in Figure 9 to show a solid mass behind the left iris which proved to be a melanoma.**

invasion and post-operatively the patient retained 6/12 vision and good reading acuity.

An interesting sidelight on local excision of choroidal tumours is whether a large lamellar dissection leads to staphyloma. In practice, the opposite appears to be the case, for although some patients, after a half thickness resection of sclera retain a normal outline of the globe (Fig. 12), in others, the affected area of sclera is flattened and shortened rather than ectatic.

One complication of local excision which occurs in a small number of cases, and which may be picked up early by the use of ultrasound is traction retinal detachment. The complication commonly follows post-operative haemorrhage and may be prevented by an adequate vitrectomy in those cases in which choroidectomy is combined with cyclectomy, for it has been my experience that intraocular haemorrhage is rare after local resection of tumours located entirely within the choroid, even if the resection has been complicated by a full thickness retinal break.

Previously if during resection of a choroidal tumour, a full thickness break occurred it has been my practice to apply an indent to the sclera to

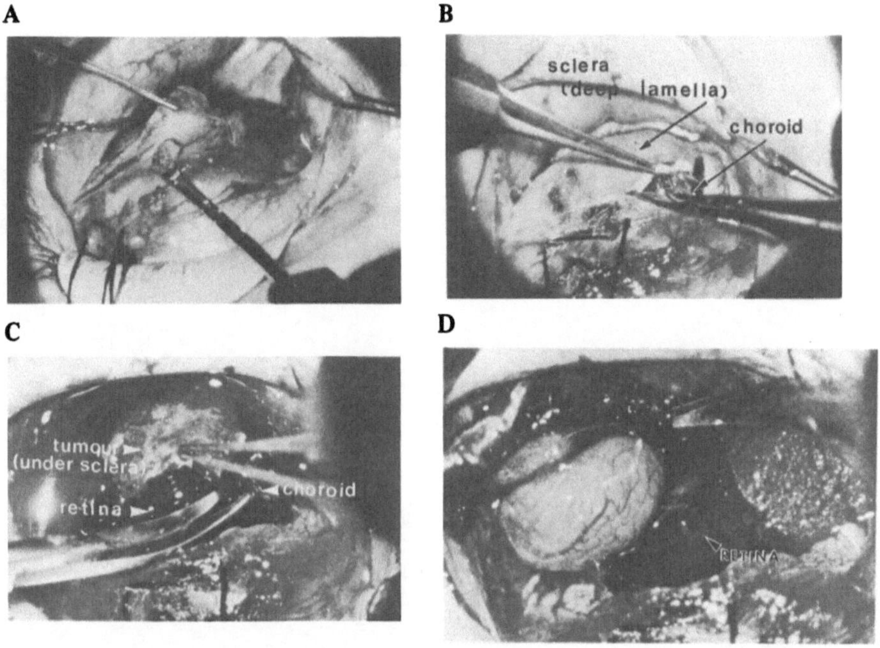

Fig. 11. Four stills taken from 16 mm. movie film to illustrate the technique of local choroidectomy.
a) Development of half thickness scleral flap.
b) Exposure of area of choroid containing tumour.
c) Incision of choroid around tumour.
d) Dissection of tumour from retina prior to its removal.

prevent retinal detachment, but for various reasons, I have recently thought that provided there is bare half thickness sclera below the retinal break, such a procedure may not be necessary. This approach received support from the behaviour of the retina in a recent case with a large posteriorly placed melanoma, who developed a full thickness retinal break during the tumour resection. In this case no indent was used nor cryotherapy or photocoagulation and subsequently the retina remained flat.

The use of ultrasound and other diagnostic parameters has enabled me to locally resect around 60 intraocular melanomas over the past 12 years and the technique has been used with increasing frequency during the last few years. An examination of the results relating to patients with choroidal tumours treated this way until March of this year shows that overall these have been very satisfactory (Tables 1 and 2).

Without doubt ultrasound has proved of inestimable value in the preoperative and post-operative assessment of patients undergoing local iridocyclectomy or choroidectomy and without it development of the techniques of local excision outlined in this address would have been much more difficult if not impossible.

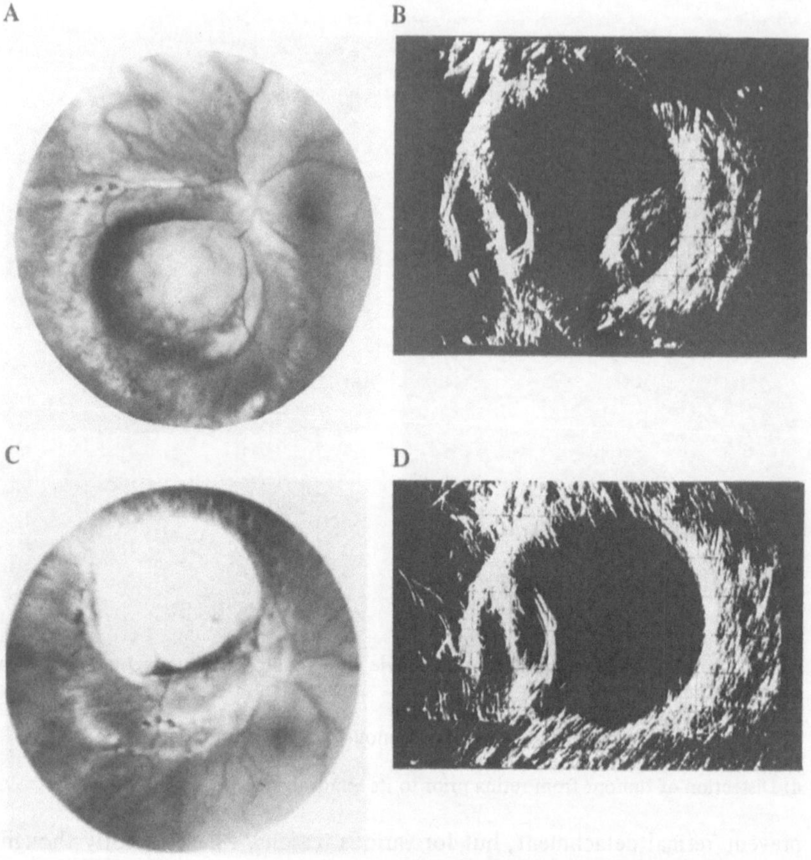

Fig. 12. Pre-operative clinical and ultrasound appearance (a, b) of a patient who subsequently underwent local resection of a posteriorly placed choroidal melanoma. The post-operative appearance (c, d) showed a posteriorly placed choroidal coloboma and on ultrasound a normal outline of the globe.

Table 1. Summary of results of local resection of choroidal tumours

Total cases	42
Cosmetically Satisfactory Eye	36 (86%)
Useful Sight (6/60 or better)	29 (69%)
Orbital Recurrence	0
Enucleation for Intraocular Recurrence	2)
	) (16%)
Enucleation for Other Reason	5)
Tumour Related Deaths	3
(March 1982)	

Table 2. Summary of visual results after local resection of choroidal tumours

6/6 – 6/12	11 (26%)
6/18 – 6/60	8 (19%)
CF (+ good field)	8 (19%)
HM – PL	7 (17%)
NPL (or enucleated)	8 (19%)

ACKNOWLEDGEMENTS

I should like to thank the many Ophthalmologists throughout the United Kingdom and elsewhere who have referred patients for consideration of local resection of choroidal and ciliary body tumours. I am particularly indebted to Dr. M. LeMay, who carried out the ultrasound examination on these patients, Professor W. R. Lee for histopathological reports, Mrs. A. Currie for photographic assistance and Miss O. M. Rankin for secretarial help.

REFERENCES

1. Zimmerman, L. E., McLean, I. W., and Foster, W. D.: Statistical analysis of follow up data concerning uveal melanomas and the influence of enucleation. Ophthalmology (Rochester) 87, 557–564 (1980).
2. Ferry, A. P.: Lesions mistaken for malignant melanoma of the posterior uvea. A clinico pathologic analysis of 100 cases with ophthalmoscopally visible lesions. Arch. Ophthalmol., 72, 463–469, (1964).
3. Badtke, G., Tost, M., and Lohse, K.: Zur differential diagnose intraokularer tumoren, in: Krebs probleme in der Augenheilkunde, Fenke Stuttgart, (1965).
4. Blodi, F. C. and Roy, P. E.: The misdiagnosed choroidal melanoma. Canad J. Ophthalmol. 2, 209–201 (1967).
5. Stallard, H. B.: Malignant melanoma of the choroid treated with radioactive applicators, Trans. Ophthal. Soc. U.K. 79, 373–392 (1959).
6. Lommatsch, P. K.: Experiences in the treatment of malignant melanoma of the choroid with 106 Ru/106 Rh Beta Ray applicators. Trans. Ophthal. Soc. U.K. 93, 119– (1973).
7. Cogan, D. G., and Reese, A. B.: A syndrome of iris nodules ectopic descemets membrane and unilateral glaucoma. Documenta Ophthalmologica 26, 424–433 (1969).

Author's address:
Tennent Institute of Ophthalmology
University of Glasgow
Western Infirmary
Glasgow G11 6NT
UK

ECHOGRAPHIC DIAGNOSIS OF LARGE CHOROIDAL MELANOMAS

RONALD L. GREEN
(*Los Angeles, USA*)

INTRODUCTION

The use of standardized echography for the diagnosis of choroidal melanomas has been well established. Using this technique several authors have reported very high degrees of accuracy in differentiating choroidal melanomas from other types of tumours (Ossoinig et al. 1975; Hodes and Choromokos. 1977; Fuller et al. 1979). These reports have included tumors ranging from 1.7 mm to 16 mm in thickness. The classical echographic criteria using the standardized A-scan include the presence of 1) a solid lesion (maximal high surface spikes showing no after movement), 2) a regular internal structure, 3) low to medium reflectivity (10 to 60% spike height), and 4) internal vascularity. An additional important criterion using the B-scan is a mushroom or collar button shape of the tumor. (Coleman et al. 1974)

Large melanomas differ somewhat from the established classical criteria stated above. The diagnosis of very small melanomas is the most difficult. In general, larger tumors are easier to differentiate, both clinically and echographically; however, when a tumor becomes very large the diagnosis can again become more difficult. This study reports the echographic features of 11 large melanomas that were examined consecutively over a 10 month period. These tumors all had a maximum elevation ranging from 8 to 16.5 mm.

MATERIALS AND METHODS

All patients were examined with the Kretz 7200 MA Standardized A-scan using an 8 MHz probe. In addition, the patients were examined with a contact B-scan, either the Sonometrics Ocuscan 400 or the Xenotec Ultrascan, both of which use a 10 MHz probe.

RESULTS

In general, the internal structure of a melanoma has a regular appearance with low to medium reflectivity. In our series, 9 of the 11 tumors showed moderate irregularity of the internal structure, most evident in the superficial portions (Fig. 1). Although the tumors were predominantly of low to medium

Hillman, J. S./Le May, M. M. (eds.) Ophthalmic Ultrasonography
©1983, Dr W. Junk Publishers, The Hague/Boston/Lancaster
ISBN 978-94-009-7280-3

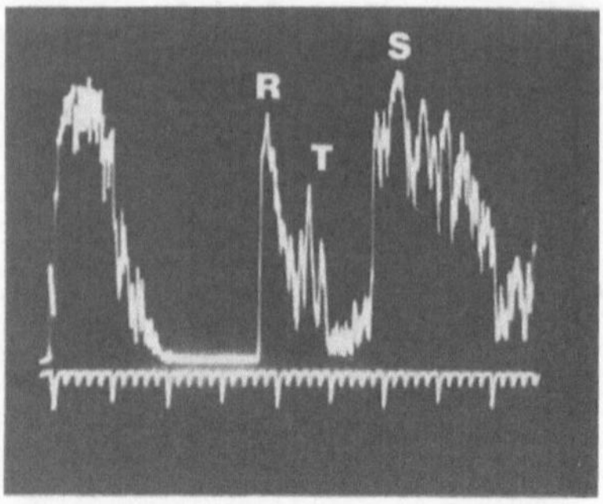

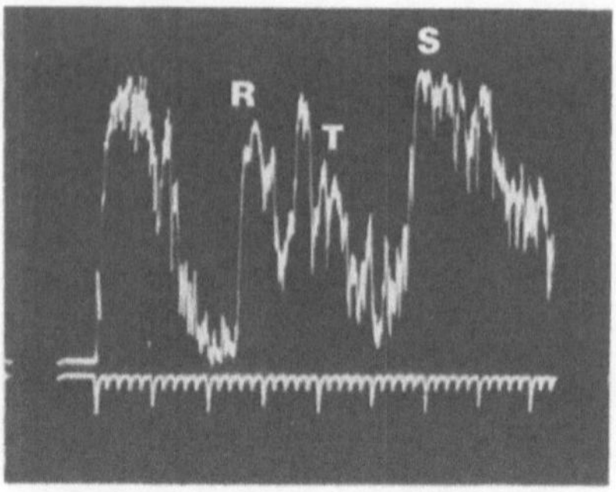

Fig. 1. A-scan echogram of 2 highly elevated choroidal melanomas. Both echograms show a moderately irregular structure of the internal tumor spikes. R = surface spikes indicating the surface of the retina and the tumor; T = tumor signals; S = scleral spikes.

spike height, it was not unusual to see medium to high spikes from the more superficial aspects.

Ten of the eleven cases showed a significant angle Kappa: the angle Kappa being the angle produced by the baseline and a line through the top or the center of the echo spikes (excluding the surface spike) (Ossoinig et al. 1975). The steeper the angle the more significant the sound attenuation produced by the tumor. The majority of our cases showed an angle of 50° or steeper at tissue sensitivity (Fig. 2). Although the angle can vary to some extent in different sound-beam directions we considered only the maximum angle. The one tumor that did not show a significant angle Kappa was of very low reflectivity, even in the superficial portions. In this one case however, the angle may have been larger had we measured it at a higher system sensitivity.

Vascularity of the tumor, indicated by fast spontaneous movement of the internal spikes (Fig. 3), was present in 100% of the cases; this is clearly more than reported in series involving tumors of all sizes (Ossoinig et al. 1975; Fuller et al. 1979).

Seven of the eleven tumors showed a surface spike at tissue sensitivity of less than 90% spike height, although most published examples of choroidal melanomas show a maximal 100% high tumor surface spike. By demonstrating this 100% spike, the examiner knows that the beam is perpendicular to the surface of the tumor. In larger tumors, however, the very steep convex surface may reflect some of the returning echo away from the probe, thereby preventing a 100% high spike (Fig. 4).

Seven of the eleven tumors showed some evidence on B-scan of mushrooming, indicative of a break in Bruch's membrane. In some cases, this mushroom or collar button appearance was not seen in all acoustic sections through the tumor, but could be demonstrated in only 1 or 2 sections. (Fig. 5).

COMMENTS

The criteria for the diagnosis of choroidal melanomas using standardized A-scan echography have been established by several authors. These include

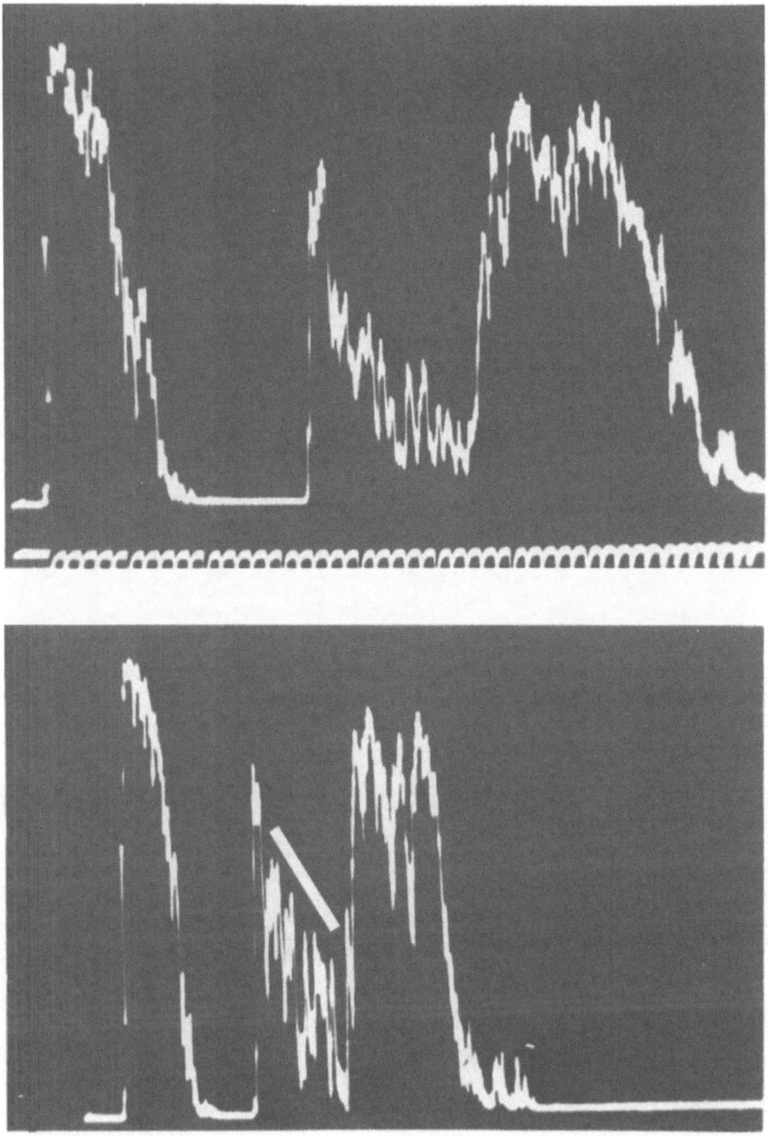

Fig. 2. A-scan echogram of a choroidal melanoma at (a) globe expansion and at (b) orbit expansion. The angle Kappa should be determined at orbital expansion.

1) a solid mass lesion as indicated by a nonmobile maximally high tumor surface spike, 2) low to medium reflectivity, 3) regular internal structure, 4) vascularity. B-scan criteria have included a mushroom shaped appearance, which indicates a break in Bruch's membrane. Our series indicates that slightly different criteria may be required for large melanomas, specifically tumors of a maximum elevation of 8 mm or greater.

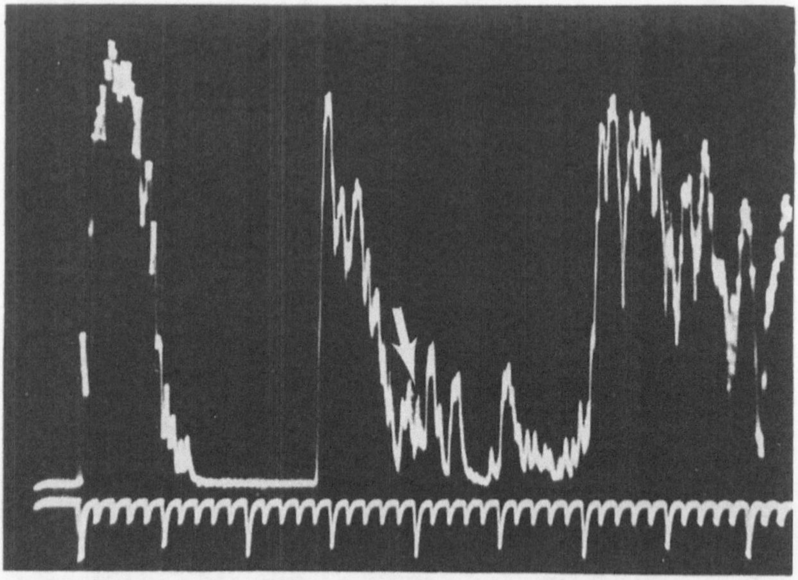

Fig. 3. A-scan echogram of large choroidal melanoma. The arrow indicates a blurred signal which represents fast spontaneous vascular movement during the actual examination.

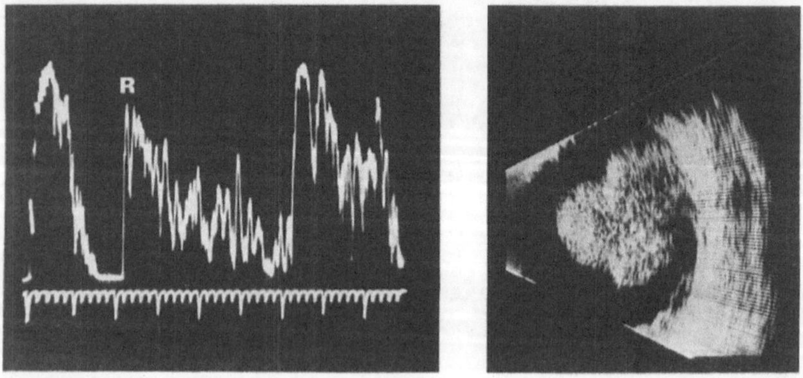

Fig. 4. A-scan and B-scan from large highly elevated choroidal melanoma; a) the surface spike (R) is less than 100% on the A-scan; (b) this is due to the convex surface of the tumor which is demonstrated on the B-scan.

Although the reflectivity of larger melanomas is predominantly low to medium, we have found that the internal structure may not be as regular as those of smaller tumors. Medium to high reflective spikes may be noted in a somewhat irregular pattern in the more superficial portions of the tumor. This appears to be due to engorged blood vessels and areas of necrosis, which

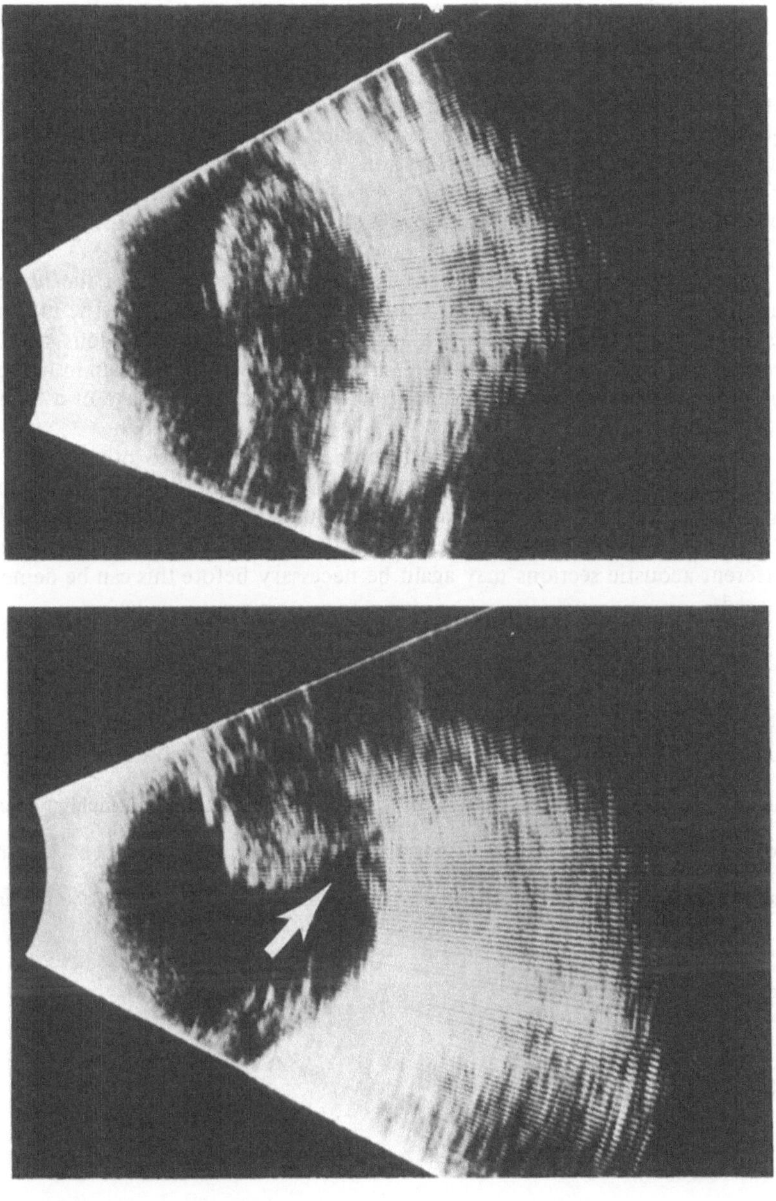

Fig. 5. **B-scan echograms from a large choroidal melanoma; a) the top echogram does not show evidence of mushrooming; b) the echogram on the bottom is a section through the edge of the tumor and demonstrates the mushroom appearance (arrow).**

tend to occur more frequently in larger tumors. A very important feature that we found, however, is that the great majority of tumors showed a significant angle Kappa. Although these tumors have shown high and somewhat irregular spikes in the superficial portions, they consistently show lower spikes in the deeper portions.

Large tumors may not demonstrate a 100% high surface spike at tissue sensitivity when using the standardized A-scan. This should not be misread by the examiner when he attempts to place the beam perpendicular to the tumor surface at its maximum elevation. It is important to scan the surface of the tumor with the A-scan and, by demonstrating the highest surface spike possible, the examiner can satisfy himself that the beam is in a perpendicular direction.

Vascularity was a very consistent finding in our series. All of the tumors showed vascularity, as evidenced by spontaneous movement of the internal spikes. As this vascularity may not be noticed in all acoustic sections, careful screening of the tumor is necessary as this can be a very useful sign in helping to differentiate a choroidal melanoma from a large hemorrhage or a highly elevated metastatic lesion.

It has been pointed out that melanomas, in contrast to other types of choroidal tumors, have a tendency to break through Bruch's membrane, thereby producing a mushroom appearance with the B-scan. This also can be a very important sign when present. However, careful screening of many different acoustic sections may again be necessary before this can be demonstrated.

REFERENCES

Coleman, D. J., Abramson, D. A., Jack, R. L., and Franzer, L. A. Ultrasonic diagnosis of tumors of the choroid. Arch. Ophthalmol. 91:344–354 (1974).

Fuller, D. F., Snyder, W. B., Hutton, W. L. and Vaiser, A. Ultrasonographic features of choroidal malignant melanomas. Arch Ophthalmol. 97:465–1472 (1979).

Hodes, B. L. and Choromokos, E. Standardized A-scan echographic diagnosis of choroidal malignant melanomas. Arch. Ophthalmol. 95:593–597 (1977).

Ossoinig, K. C., Bigar, F. and Kaefring, S. L. Malignant melanomas of the choroid and ciliary body. Bibl. Ophthalmol. 83:141–154 (1975).

Author's address:
Department of Ophthalmology
University of Southern California
Estelle Doheny Eye Foundation
Los Angeles, CA 90033
USA

SPECTRUM OF MANIFESTATIONS OF METASTATIC MALIGNANT MELANOMA

B. M. KERMAN and M. L. FINDL
(*Los Angeles, USA*)

INTRODUCTION

Malignant melanoma is a neoplasm having its origin in pigmented cells of the skin and uveal tract. Both cutaneous and ocular melanoma share a tendency to metastasize to the liver, lungs, gastrointestinal tract, skin, heart, bone, central nervous system, and lymph nodes (Noyes, 1978). The incidence of metastatic melanoma to the globe and orbit is quite low (Ferry, 1972, Font et al. 1967), although one study suggests that in patients with disseminated cutaneous melanoma, the incidence of ocular metastases may be 33% (Fishman et al. 1976). Although the ultrasonographic characteristics of primary choroidal malignant melanoma have been well described (Coleman et al. 1974, Ossoinig, 1974), there is little information in the literature regarding the appearance on ultrasound of metastatic melanoma to the globe or orbit. This paper presents the clinical and ultrasonographic characteristics of five cases of metastatic malignant melanoma.

CASE REPORTS

Case 1. a 33 year old male with known metastatic cutaneous malignant melanoma presented in March, 1979 with pain in the right eye. On ultrasonographic examination, a mass was noted in the infero-nasal posterior right orbit. The internal echo characteristics consisted of low internal reflectivity with marked spontaneous spike motion (Fig. 1). Paraocular examination showed that the lesion was well outlined with its posterior border 28 mm deep in the orbit (Fig. 2). Ultrasonographic diagnosis was skin melanoma metastatic to the orbit.

Case 2. a 32 year old female was referred for ultrasonography in July, 1980 with the diagnosis of metastatic melanoma to both orbits. In 1978, she had a malignant cutaneous melanoma removed from her right cheek with concurrent radical neck dissection. In April, 1980, recurrent nodular tumors were noted on the skin of the face. Ocular examination revealed palpable masses in the left upper eyelid and in the right lower eyelid. Exophthalmometry readings were 24.5 mm OD and 22.0 mm OS. Ultrasonography was performed on both orbits. The right orbit showed a low reflective well

Hillman, J. S./Le May, M. M. (eds.) Ophthalmic Ultrasonography
©1983, Dr W. Junk Publishers, The Hague/Boston/Lancaster
ISBN 978-94-009-7280-3

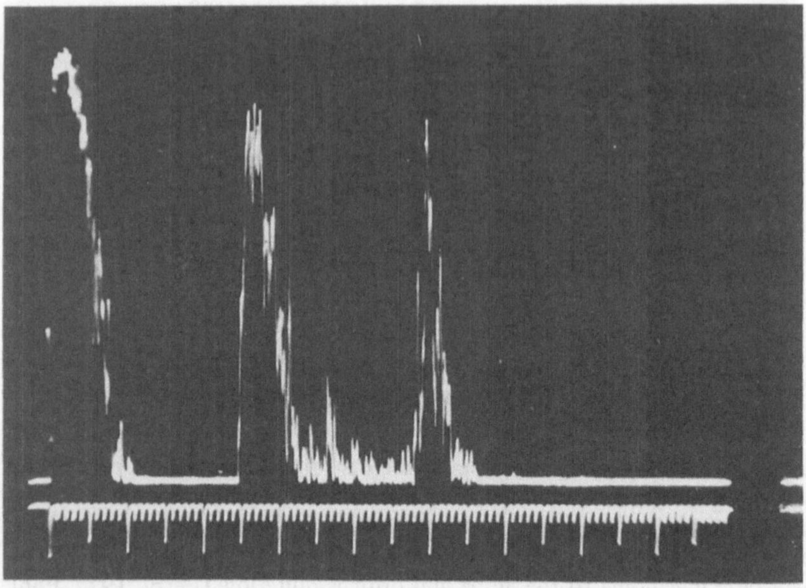

Fig. 1. Case 1: Transocular orbital ultrasonogram showing low internal reflectivity.

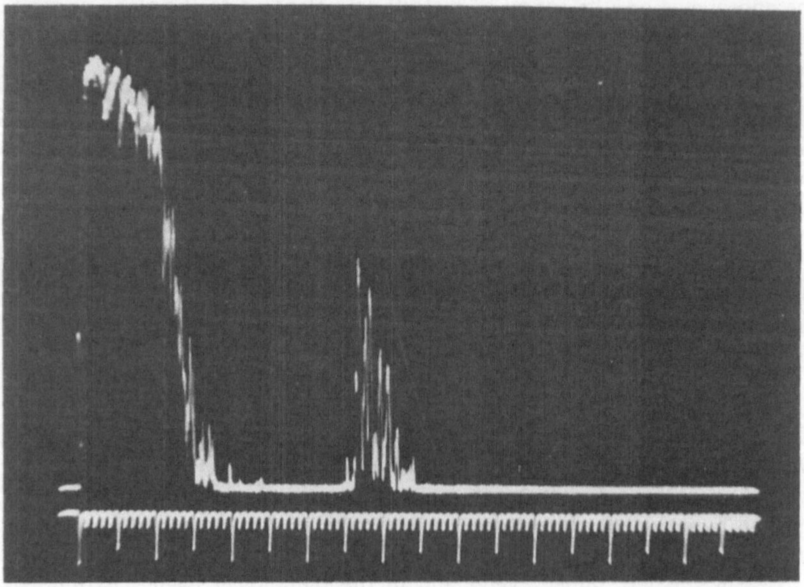

Fig. 2. Case 1: Paraocular orbital ultrasonogram, showing well outlined posterior border.

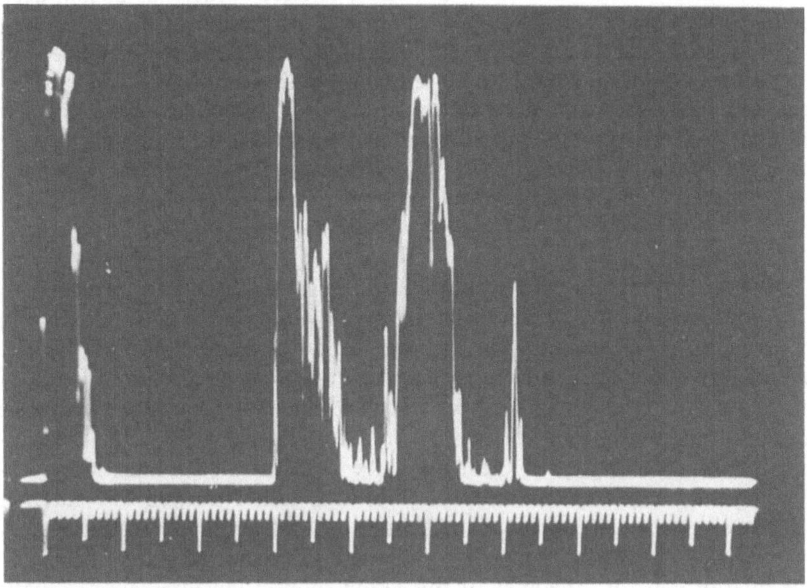

Fig. 3. Case 2: Transocular orbital ultrasonogram OD.

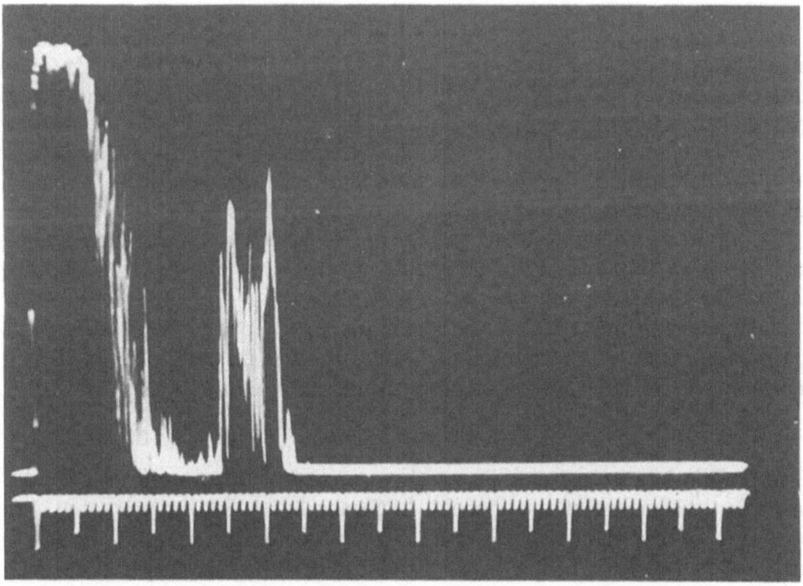

Fig. 4. Case 2: Paraocular orbital ultrasonogram OD.

outlined mass, 15 mm in thickness whose posterior border was 25 mm deep in the orbit (Fig. 3, 4). The left orbit showed two lesions. One was located supero-nasally, was 11 mm wide, and had its posterior border 26 mm deep in the orbit. The second was infero-temporal, was 4 mm wide, and had its posterior border 16 mm deep in the orbit. Both lesions consisted of low internal reflectivity. The supero-nasal mass was poorly outlined, and the infero-temporal mass was diffusely infiltrating. Ultrasonographic diagnosis was bilateral orbital metastases from skin melanoma.

Case 3. a 33 year old male with a known diagnosis of cutaneous malignant melanoma since 1979 presented in October, 1981 with lesions on the skin of the face, scalp, trunk, groin and legs. He noted blurred vision in his left eye in September 1981, and five weeks later, he developed blurred vision in his right eye. Ocular examination revealed bilateral conjunctival chemosis and injection and bilateral ocular mass lesions with secondary retinal detachments. Ultrasonography of the right globe demonstrated a mass lesion extending inferiorly from the optic nerve. This lesion showed low internal reflectivity, marked spontaneous spike motion, and an inferior retinal detachment (Fig. 5, 6). Ultrasonography of the left globe showed a mass located at the inferior equator. The apex of this lesion showed low internal reflectivity with moderate spontaneous spike motion. However, the base of the lesion showed high internal reflectivity. An inferior retinal detachment was present. Ultrasonographic diagnosis was skin melanoma metastatic to the choroid in both eyes with secondary retinal detachments.

Case 4. a 39 year old female with Down's Syndrome was examined clinically in February, 1979 and found to have vision of no light perception, glaucoma and chemosis in her right eye. Ultrasonography at an outside facility suggested intraocular and orbital tumor in the right eye. Ultrasonography at UCLA demonstrated only a disorganized phthisical eye with no intraocular structures identified. The eye was enucleated and was found to contain a necrotic malignant melanoma with extraocular extension. In November, 1981, clinical examination of the left eye suggested a choroidal malignant melanoma in this eye. Ultrasonography of the left eye revealed a dome shaped lesion in the superior equatorial globe (Fig. 7). The internal echo characteristics consisted of low to medium internal reflectivity with moderate spontaneous spike motion. Ultrasonographic diagnosis was malignant melanoma of the left choroid, possibly metastatic from the right choroid.

Case 5. The left eye of a 67 year old woman was enucleated in 1978 for malignant melanoma of the choroid. In September 1980, she presented with proptosis of the right eye. Ultrasonography demonstrated a low reflective mass lesion posterior to the globe, involving the infero-nasal posterior orbit (Fig. 8). The lesion was 21 mm in greatest thickness. The lesion consisted of very low internal reflectivity with trace spontaneous spike motion. Ultra-

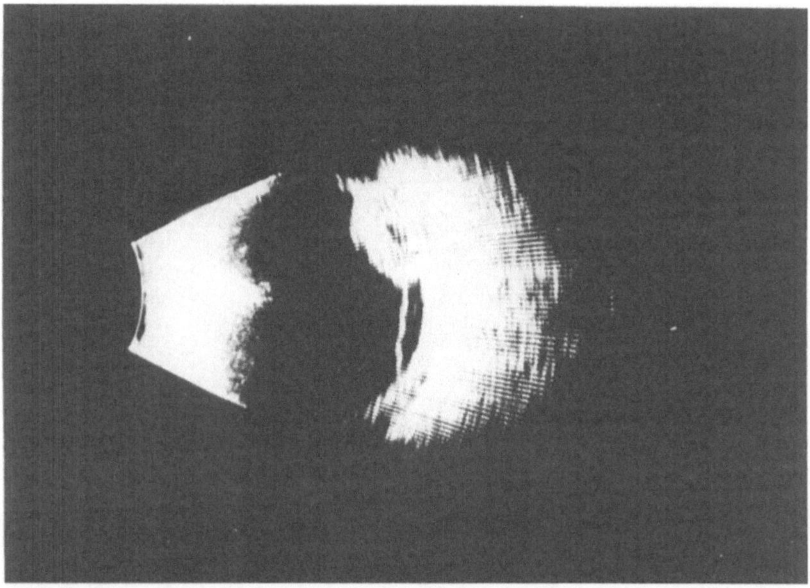

Fig. 5. Case 3: Ocular B-scan ultrasonogram showing elevated mass lesion with adjacent retinal detachment.

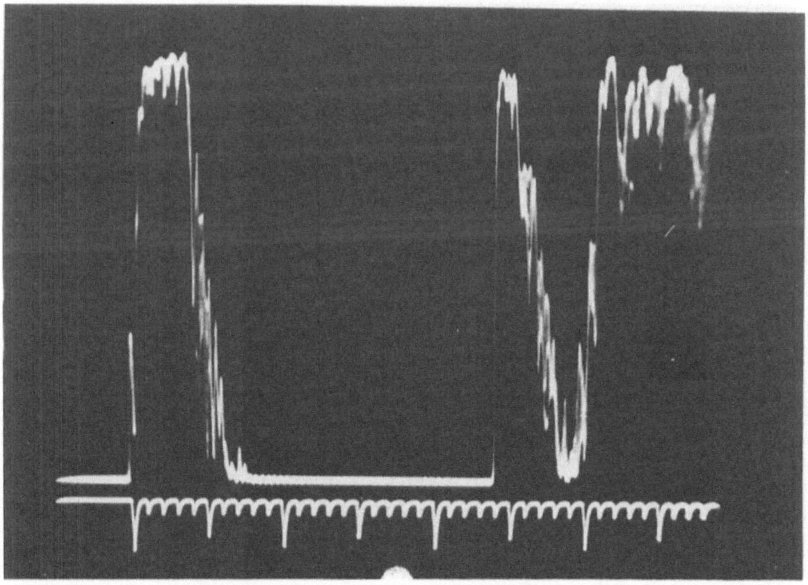

Fig. 6. Case 3: Ocular A-scan ultrasonogram showing low internal reflectivity within the mass lesion.

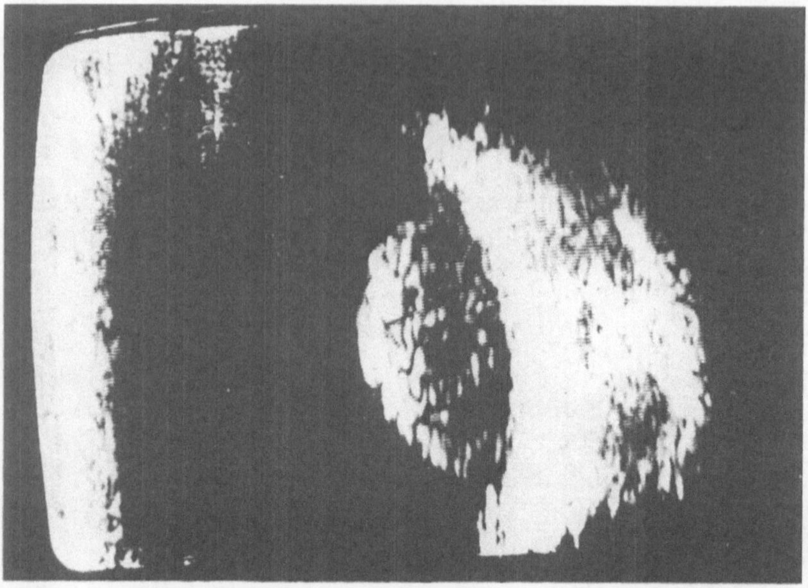

Fig. 7. Case 4: B-scan ocular ultrasonogram OS showing dome shaped mass lesion.

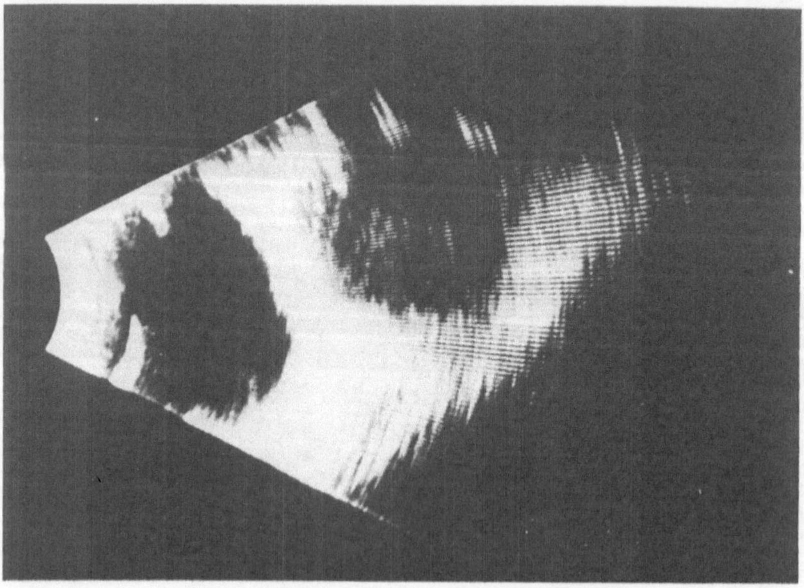

Fig. 8. Case 5: Orbital B-scan ultrasonogram OS, showing low reflective mass lesion posterior to globe, causing slight indentation of globe.

sonographic diagnosis was malignant melanoma of the right orbit metastatic from the left choroid. Hepatic ultrasound was performed and showed hepatomegaly and multiple defects consistent with metastatic tumor. Needle biopsy of the liver demonstrated metastatic malignant melanoma.

DISCUSSION

This paper has demonstrated the ultrasonographic characteristics of three cases of malignant melanoma metastatic to the orbit and two cases of malignant melanoma metastatic to the globe. In two of the orbital cases and one ocular case, the metastases were from cutaneous melanoma. In one orbital case and one ocular case, the metastases were from choroidal melanoma. Since no histopathology studies are available for any of the presumed metastatic tumors, there is a question as to whether they truly represent metastases or whether they represent new primary tumors. All patients with the exception of Case 4 showed metastases to other parts of the body. It would not seem logical in the presence of known metastatic disease to postulate that the ocular and orbital lesions represented new primary tumors. Additionally, primary orbital melanoma is an exceedingly rare tumor. (Coppeto et al. 1978). In Case 4 however, there is the possibility that the melanoma in the left eye might represent a second primary tumor, rather than a metastasis. Statistical calculations, however, suggest that this is an exceedingly rare event (Shammas et al. 1977).
masatal, 1977)

All tumors demonstrated low internal reflectivity and internal spontaneous spike motion, basically the same ultrasonographic characteristics as have been described for primary malignant melanoma of the choroid. This was true regardless of the location of the tumor (ocular and orbital) or the primary site (skin or choroid). Most likely, the ultrasonographic characteristics of these tumors is dependent on the internal arrangement of the cells within the tumor. Both the globe and orbit are relatively confined spaces with rich vascular supply. These characteristics may allow metastatic lesions to grow as solid cellular masses, richly vascularized by small blood vessels. The lack of large stagnant blood vessels, internal septae, and large areas of necrosis alternating with areas of viable tumor cells explains the low internal reflectivity and internal spontaneous spike motion seen within these lesions.

REFERENCES

1. Coleman, D. J.; Abramson, D. H.; Jack, R. L.; Franzen, L. A. Ultrasonic diagnosis of tumors of the choroid. Arch. Ophthalmol. 91:344 (1974).
2. Coppeto, J. R.; Jaffe, R.; Gillies, C. G. Primary orbital melanoma. Arch. Ophthalmol. 96:2255 (1978).
3. Ferry, A. P. Primary malignant melanoma of the skin metastatic to the eye. Am. J. Ophthalmol. 74:12 (1972).
4. Fishman, M. L.; Tomaszewsky, M. M.; Kuwabara, T. Malignant melanoma of the skin metastatic to the eye. Frequency in autopsy series. Arch. Ophthalmol. 94:1309 (1976).
5. Font, R. L.; Naumann, G.; Zimmerman, L. E. Primary malignant melanoma of the skin metastatic to the eye and orbit. Am. J. Ophthalmol. 63:738 (1967).

6. Noyes, W. E. Cutaneous melanoma and its relation to melanoma of the uveal tract. Surv. Ophthalmol. 23:143 (1978).
7. Ossoinig, K. C. Preoperative differential diagnosis of tumors with echography III. Diagnosis of intraocular tumors. Current Concepts in Ophthalmol., F. C. Blodi (Ed). St Louis: Mosby, 4: 296 (1974).
8. Shammas, H. F.; Watzke, R. C. Bilateral choroidal melanomas. Arch. Ophthalmol. 95:617 (1977)

Authors' address:
UCLA Department of Ophthalmology
Jules Stein Eye Institute
800 Westwood Plaza
Los Angeles, CA 90024
USA

AN ANALYSIS OF 30 CASES OF PROVEN MALIGNANT MELANOMA OF THE CHOROID; ULTRASONOGRAPHIC AND HISTOLOGICAL FINDINGS

J. L. NOBLE and I. B. MARSH
(Manchester, England)

INTRODUCTION

The value of ultrasound in the evaluation of intra-ocular tumours is well documented. Reports of large numbers of cases by Coleman, Ossoinig and other authors reveal approximately 95% accuracy when this method of investigation is included in the diagnosis of malignant melanoma of the choroid. The typical features of this tumour on both A- and B-Scan ultrasound examination are well established.

We felt it would be interesting to determine the accuracy of ultrasound examination using the Kretz A Scan and Bronson-Turner B Scan machines in the diagnosis of scleral infiltration and extra-scleral extensions.

This paper is therefore a retrospective analysis of 30 cases of histologically proven malignant melanoma of the choroid, where an attempt was made at the time of the ultrasound examination to detect evidence of scleral infiltration and/or extra-scleral extension.

On A-Scan examination Ossoinig has stated that scleral infiltration should be suspected when a graduated upwards step is seen at the posterior surface of the tumor. Evidence of scleral infiltration on B-Scan is not so clear cut. Choroidal excavation is not infrequently seen on B-Scan, and a subjective opinion as to whether this extends beyond choroid and into sclera has to be made. Evidence of massive extra-scleral extension is by contrast easily detected on B-Scan.

RESULTS

The age of the patients at presentation varied from 20–85 years with a peak incidence of 60–69 years. (Table 1). The sexes were almost equally affected. Symptoms were mainly of less than 6 months duration. (Table 2).

SYMPTOMS	Number of Patients
1 Asymptomatic	11
2 Sudden decrease of visual acuity	3
3 Pain	1
4 Blurring of vision	19

Hillman, J. S./Le May, M. M. (eds.) Ophthalmic Ultrasonography
©1983, Dr W. Junk Publishers, The Hague/Boston/Lancaster
ISBN 978-94-009-7280-3

Table 1

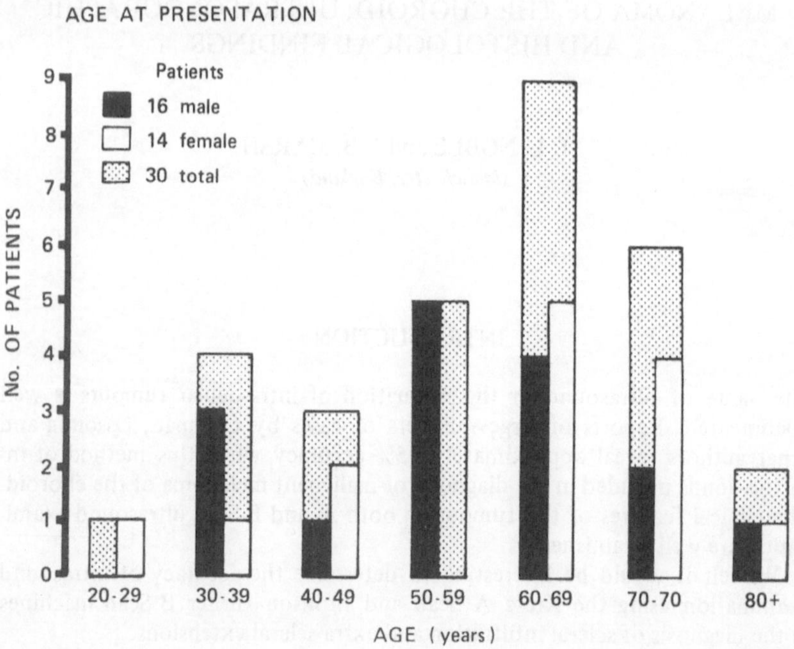

Table 2

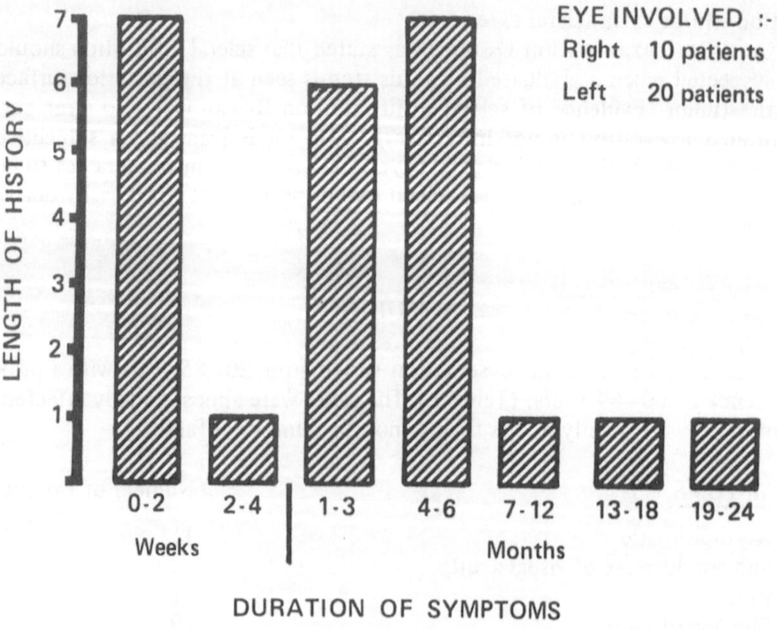

<u>Signs</u>		Number of Patients
A Visual Acuity	6/6 – 6/12	10
	6/18 – 6/24	1
	6/36 or less	19

B Other Clinical Signs	Number of Patients
1 Solid Detachment	26
2 Pigment cells (a) Vitreous	3
(b) Anterior chamber	2
(c) Corneal endothelium	1
3 Lens opacities related to melanoma	3
4 Vitreous haemorrhage	3

On ultrasound examination the reflectivity of the tumours was seen to vary between 10–60%. (Table 3). Scleral infiltration was suspected in 16 patients but in no case was evidence of extra-scleral extension seen.

On histological examination the tumors were graded in terms of malignancy as follows:-

	Number of Patients
Low to intermediate	6
Intermediate	21
Rapidly growing	3

Scleral infiltration was seen histologically in 14 patients, and 4 patients showed evidence of extra-scleral extension.

The results were then correlated for scleral infiltration and extra-scleral extension as follows:-

	Number of Patients
Ultrasound positive Pathology positive	9 – one extra-scleral extension
Ultrasound positive Pathology negative	7
Ultrasound negative Pathology positive	5 – three extra-scleral extensions

Examples of the findings on ultrasound examination can be seen.

At histology, scleral infiltration was seen to be microscopic in nature in most instances, with a few pigmented cells seen lying between the scleral lamellae. In only one case of extra-scleral extension was the mass of significant size. (> 1.5 mm).

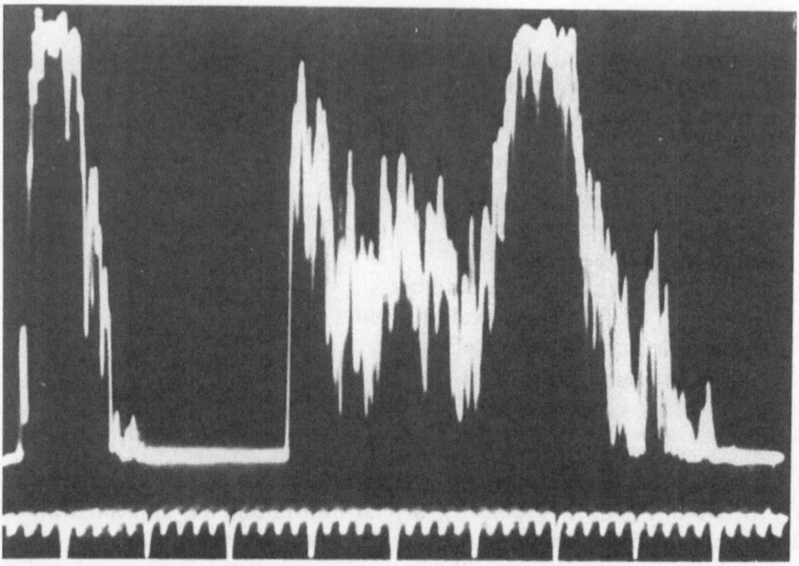

Fig. 1. Patient 1. Ultrasound positive. Pathology negative.

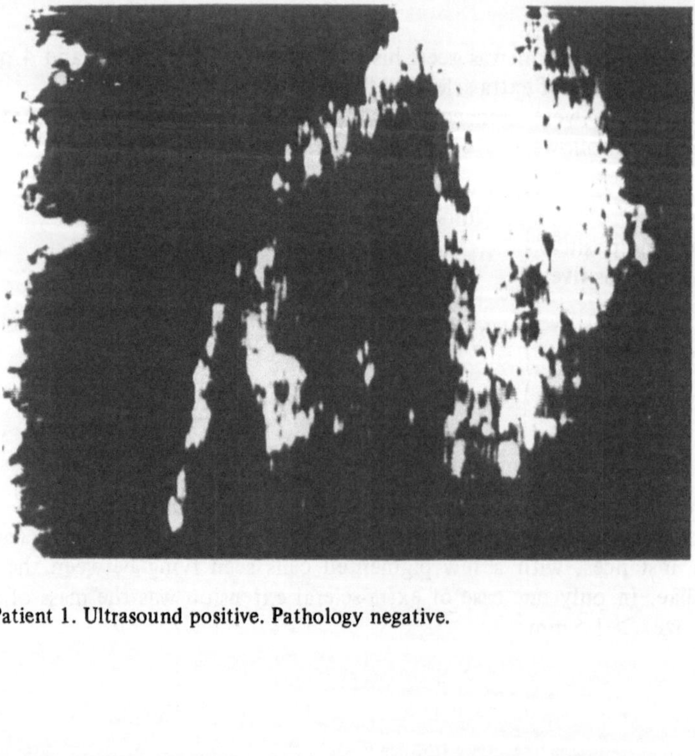

Fig. 2. Patient 1. Ultrasound positive. Pathology negative.

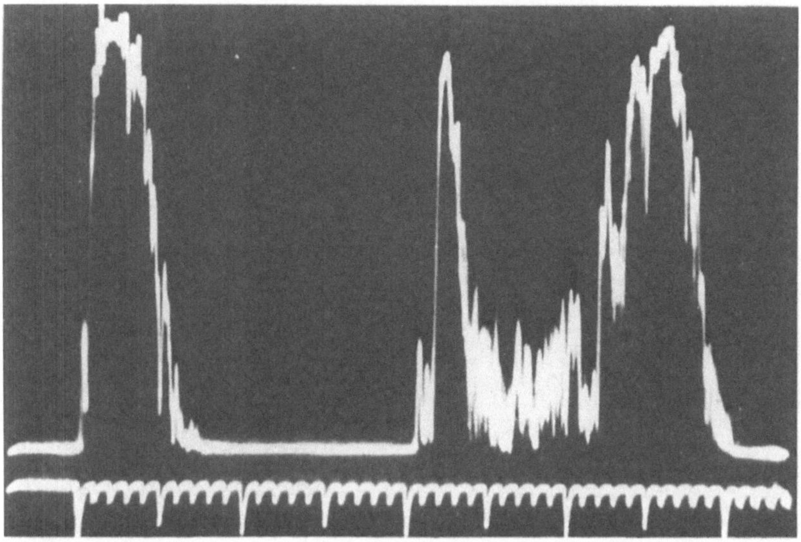

Fig. 3. Patient 2. Ultrasound positive. Pathology positive.

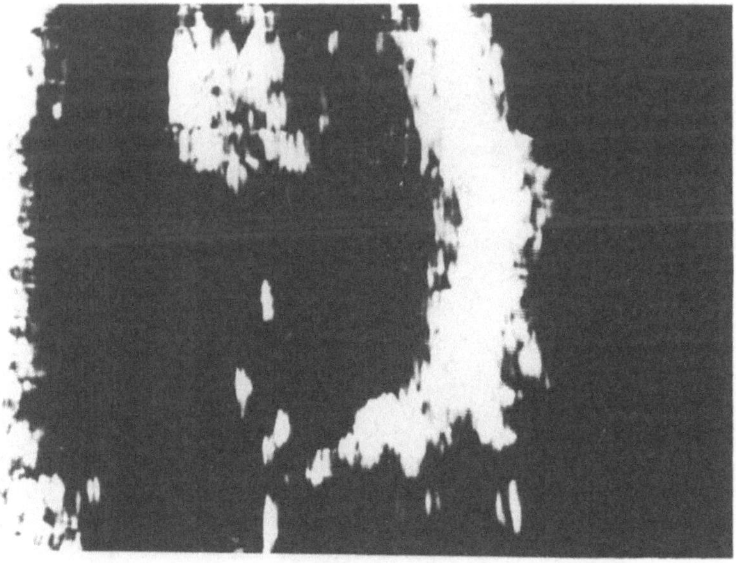

Fig. 4. Patient 2. Ultrasound positive. Pathology positive

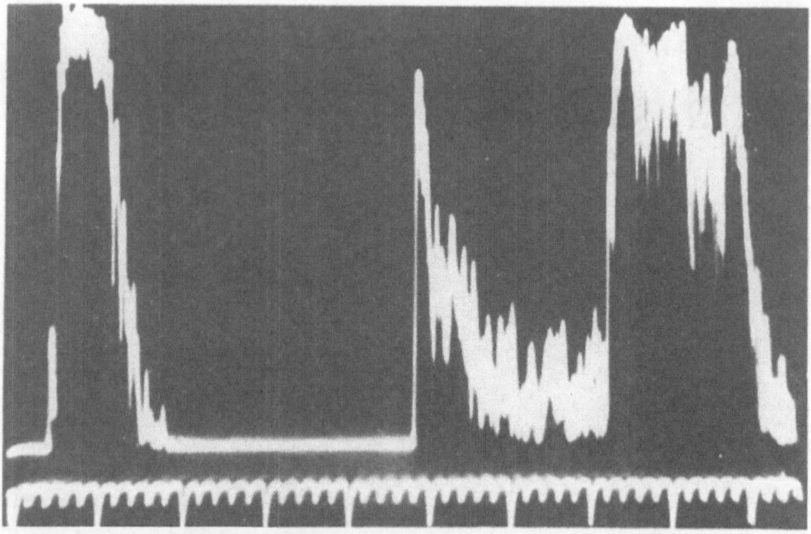

Fig. 5. Patient 3. Ultrasound negative. Pathology positive.

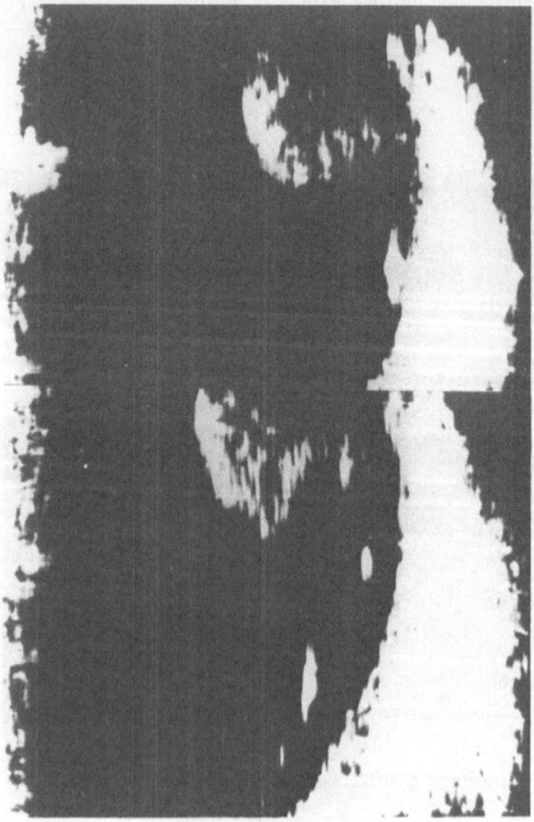

Fig. 6. Patient 3. Ultrasound negative. Pathology positive.

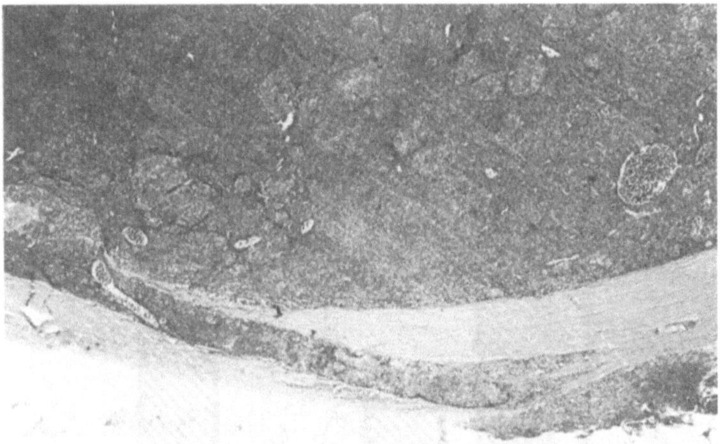
Fig. 7.

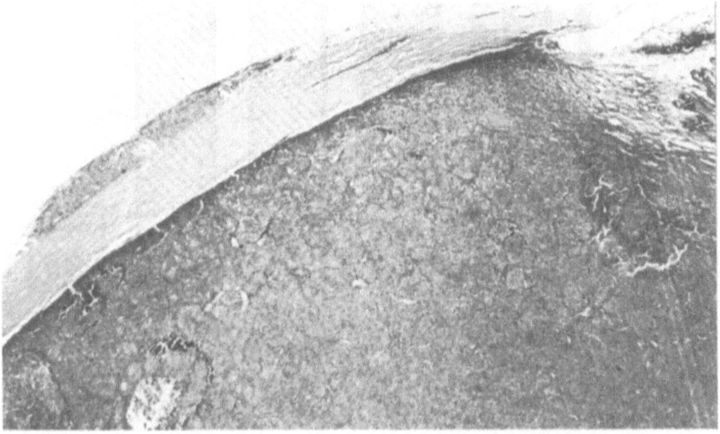
Fig. 8.

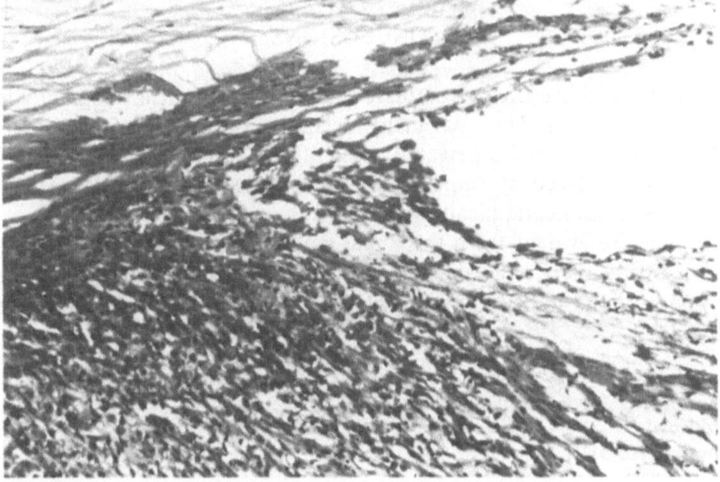
Fig. 9.

Table 3.

ULTRASONOGRAPHIC FINDINGS I

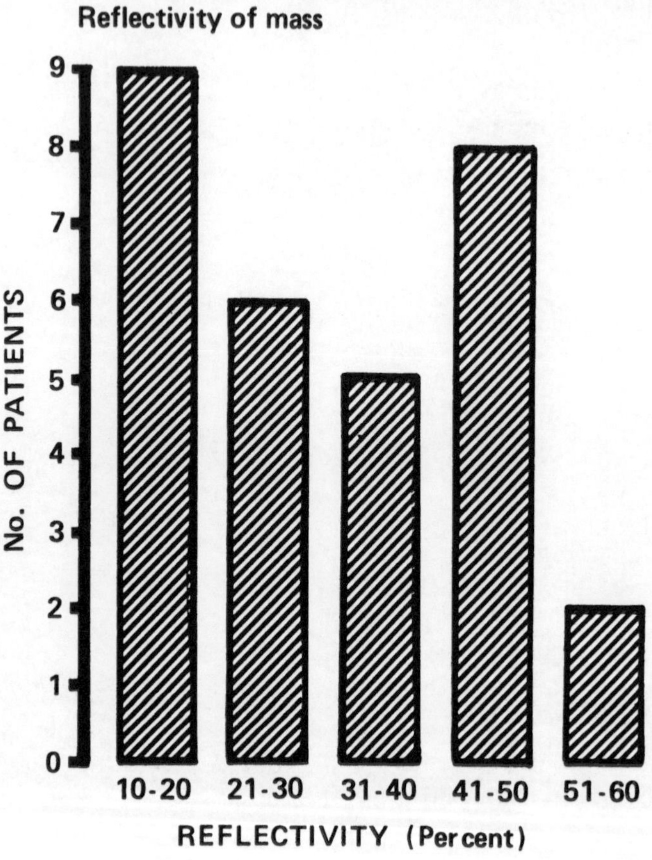

CONCLUSIONS

In our paper we have tried to evaluate the accuracy of ultrasonography in the diagnosis of local spread of malignant melanoma of the choroid. In order that scleral infiltration may be detected, a significant amount of the scleral thickness must be replaced by tumour. Extra-scleral extension must exceed 1.5–2 mm to be ultrasonographically visible.

It is therfore evident from this small study, that whilst ultrasound examination is a valuable and accurate method of diagnosing malignant melanoma of the choroid, its ability to detect scleral invasion and extra-scleral extension is limited.

Authors' address:
Manchester Royal Eye Hospital
Oxford Road
Manchester M13 9WH
UK

ULTRASONOGRAPHIC CHARACTERISTICS IN PREDICTION OF CELL TYPE IN CHOROIDAL MALIGNANT MELANOMA

M. L. FINDL, K. ZAKKA, B. M. KERMAN and R. Y. FOOS
(Los Angeles, USA)

INTRODUCTION

Ultrasonography has been demonstrated to be an effective tool in the diagnosis of malignant melanoma of the choroid and ciliary body. The diagnostic criteria for this tumor have been described by several authors. By applying the parameters of internal reflectivity, spontaneous spike motion, orbital shadowing, choroidal excavation, and internal hollowing accuracy of up to 96% has been claimed (Coleman et al. 1974, Ossoinig, 1974).

Recent studies of malignant melanoma of the choroid and ciliary body based on multivariate analysis have attempted to determine which tumor characteristics best predict mortality. The factors which have been shown to be of importance in this prediction are cell type, greatest single dimension, extraocular extension and mitotic activity (McLean et al. 1977).

Because cell type is a major prognostic factor it would be of obvious importance to predict the cell type of a specific tumor prior to definitive therapy. The primary objective of this study was to determine if cell type and other histopathological criteria could be determined ultrasonographically.

MATERIALS AND METHODS

All patients examined at the Ophthalmic Ultrasound Laboratory of the Jules Stein Eye Institute between the dates of March, 1976 and September, 1978 who had the ultrasonographic diagnosis of malignant melanoma of the choroid or ciliary body were reviewed. Histopathological data were available on 33 of these patients. These 33 eyes form the basis of this study.

Independent observers working in double blind fashion evaluated the ultrasonographic and histopathologic characteristics of these tumors. Ultrasonographic criteria evaluated were internal spike height (graded from 0–100%) (Fig. 1), spontaneous spike motion (graded from 0–4), lesion elevation, orbital shadowing and choroidal excavation. Histopathologic criteria assessed were cell type (graded as spindle, mixed or epithelioid), pigmentation (rated from 0–5) (Fig. 2) and number and extent of blood vessels (graded 0–4). Correlations were then performed between the ultrasonographic and histopathologic parameters, as displayed in Table 1.

Hillman, J. S./Le May, M. M. (eds.) Ophthalmic Ultrasonography
© 1983, Dr W. Junk Publishers, The Hague/Boston/Lancaster
ISBN 978-94-009-7280-3

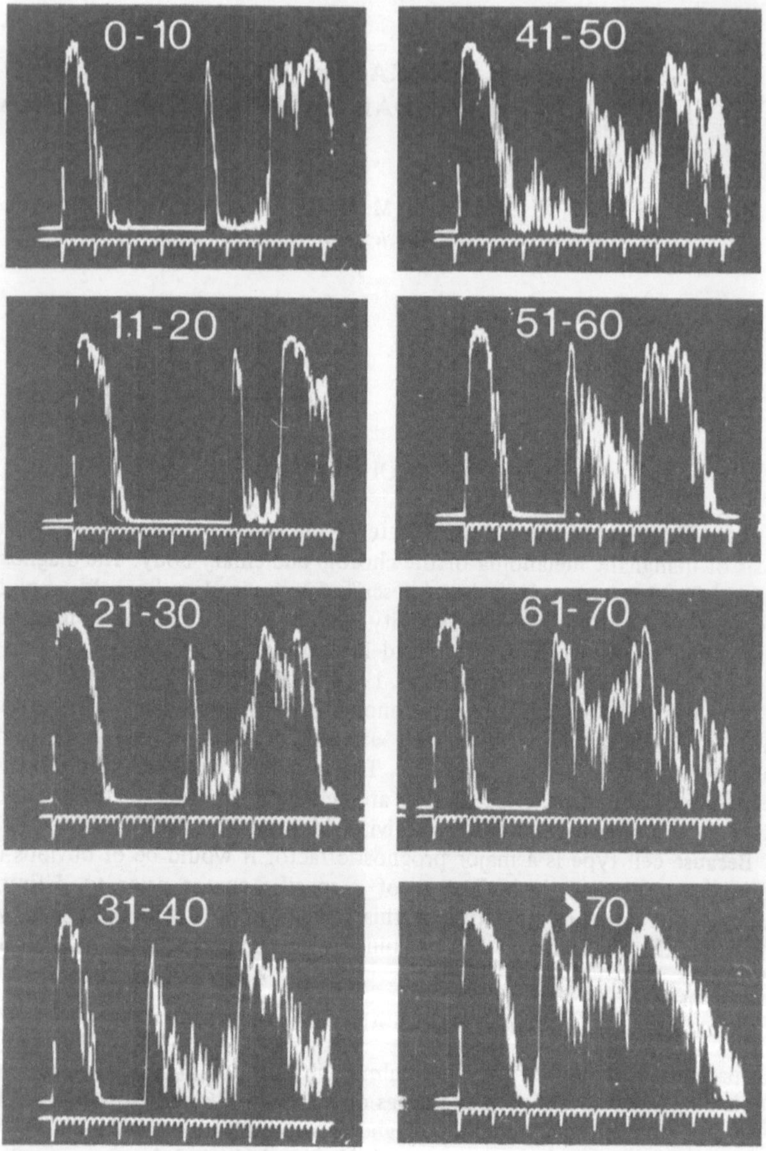

Fig. 1. Representation of internal echo spike height, expressed as a percentage of maximal possible echo signal display height.

RESULTS

Figures 3 and 4 show the distribution of the echo spike height patterns for the histopathologic cell type classifications of spindle cell, mixed cell and epithelioid cell tumors[1]. These figures demonstrate that the distribution

[1] Since there were only two pure epithelioid cell tumors these were combined with the mixed cell tumors for analysis.

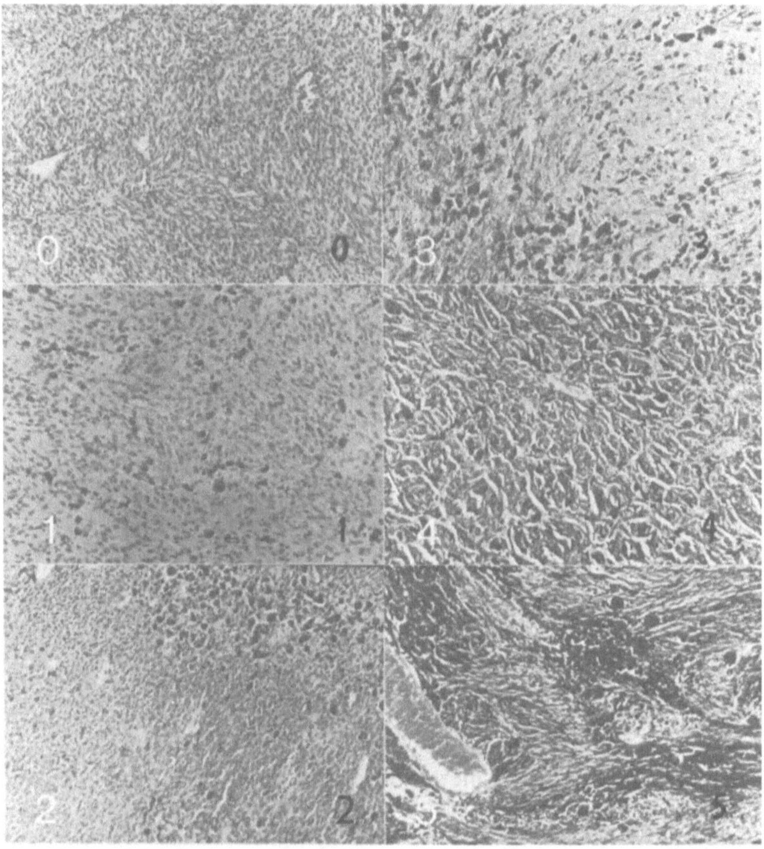

Fig. 2. Gradations of amount of tumor pigmentation, expressed as 0–5.

Table 1. Correlations performed between ultrasonographic and histopathologic characteristics

ULTRASOUND		HISTOPATHOLOGY
INTERNAL REFLECTIVITY	⟷	CELL TYPE
CHOROIDAL EXCAVATION	⟷	CELL TYPE
ORBITAL SHADOWING	⟷	CELL TYPE
VASCULARITY	⟷	VASCULARITY
INTERNAL REFLECTIVITY	⟷	PIGMENTATION

of the reflectivity is independent of histopathologic cell type ($p > 0.10$).

9/15 (60%) of the spindle cell tumors and 5/14 (35%) of the mixed and epithelioid cell tumors showed orbital shadowing. Choroidal excavation was demonstrated in 3/15 (20%) spindle cell lesions and 4/14 (28.5%) mixed and

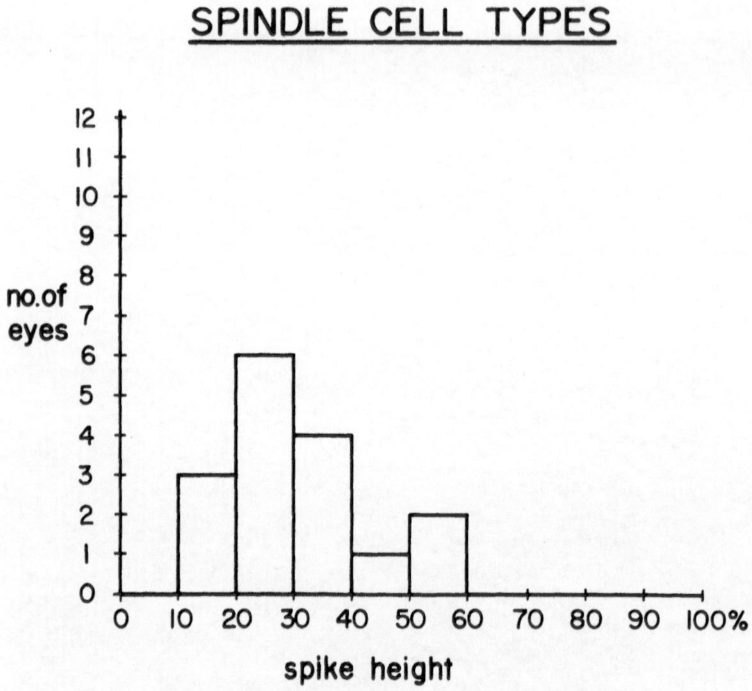

Fig. 3. Distribution of internal echo spike height for spindle cell tumors.

epithelioid cell tumors. Ultrasonographic evidence for vascularity as manifested by spontaneous spike motion was detected in 13/16 (81.3%) spindle cell lesions and 12/17 (70.6%) of the mixed and epithelioid group. None of these differences was found to be statistically significant. Additionally, there was no correlation between internal reflectivity (echo spike height) and pigmentation. Nor did ultrasonographic spontaneous spike motion correlate with extent and number of blood vessels histopathologically.

DISCUSSION

Current management of malignant melanoma of the choroid includes enucleation, external irradiation, cobalt plaque, photocoagulation, and observation. Indeed, many choroidal malignant melanomas can be safely observed without significant threat of loss of life. If these tumors are to continue to be managed conservatively, optimal patient management would dictate classification of these lesions into low or high mortality risk groups. Several studies suggest that the following factors would place the patient into risk categories: cell type, greatest single dimension, extraocular extension, and mitotic activity. This study was initiated in an attempt to determine the effectiveness of ultrasound in the prediction of cell type and other histopathologic features (McLean et al. 1977, Shammas et al. 1977).

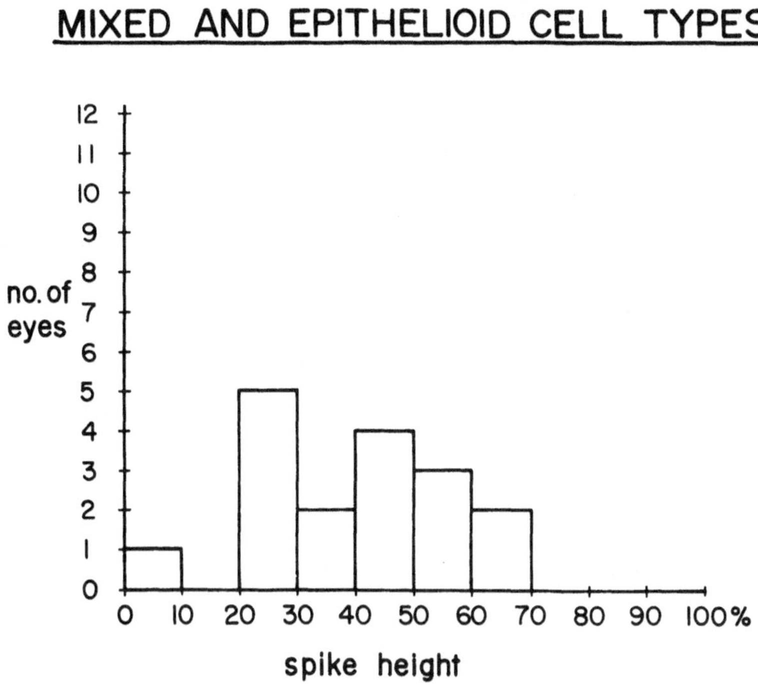

Fig. 4. Distribution of internal echo spike height for mixed and epithelioid cell tumors.

We found that there was no significant correlation between histopathologic cell type and ultrasound echo spike height, choroidal excavation orbital shadowing and spontaneous spike motion. The presence of spontaneous spike motion did not prove to be statistically significant in the prediction of number and extent of blood vessels. Ultrasonographically spontaneous spike movement is an evaluation of the presence of blood flow. This blood flow is usually in small blood vessels in the base of the tumor. The vessels seen histopathologically were generally large, dilated vessels in which blood flow was probably stagnant. Some authors suggest that pigmentation is related to mortality. Pigmentation was histopathologically evaluated for this reason but ultrasonographically the pigment granules are themselves too small to form significant reflective surfaces. Therefore, there was no statistically significant correlation between internal reflectivity and pigmentation.

CONCLUSIONS

The internal reflectivity on quantitative A-scan of spindle cell malignant melanoma is similar to the internal reflectivity of mixed and epithelioid cell malignant melanoma. Therefore, cell type cannot be differentiated by internal spike height. There is no correlation between ultrasonographic internal reflectivity and degree of pigmentation seen histopathologically. The number and extent of blood vessels seen on histopathology did not correlate with the amount of spontaneous spike motion seen ultrasonographically.

REFERENCES

Coleman, D. J.; Abramson, D. H.; Jack, R. L.; Franzen, L. A. Ultrasonic diagnosis of tumors of the choroid. Arch. Ophthalmol. 91:344 (1974).

Davidorf, F. H.; Lang, J. R. The natural history of malignant melanoma of the choroid: small vs large tumors. Tr. Am. Acad. Ophthal. & Otol. 79:310 (1975).

McLean, I. W.; Foster, W. D.; Zimmerman, L. E. Prognostic factors in small malignant melanomas of the choroid and ciliary body. Arch. Ophthalmol. 95:48 (1977).

Ossoinig, K. C. Preoperative differential diagnosis of tumors with echography III. Diagnosis of intraocular tumors. *Current Concepts in Ophthal.*, F. C. Blodi (Ed). St. Louis: Mosby, 4:296 (1974).

Shammas, H. F.; Blodi, F. C. Prognostic factors in choroidal and ciliary body melanomas. Arch. Ophthalmol. 95:63 (1977).

Authors' address:
ULCA Department of Ophthalmology
Jules Stein Eye Institute
800 Westwood Plaza
Los Angeles, CA 90024
USA

ECHOGRAPHIC PATTERN EVALUATION OF EYES WITH CHOROID MELANOMA FOR CORNEAL GRAFT UTILIZATION

A. LOFFREDO, G. CENNAMO, A. DE LELLIS, A. SAMMARTINO and A. DEL PRETE
(Naples, Italy)

ABSTRACT

It is well known that in clinical practice the corneae from eyes enucleated for malignant melanoma of posterior choroid are usually utilized for corneal grafting. This research refers to cases of posterior melanomas which extended anteriorly, in which the utilization of the corneae for grafting was doubtful. Echographic study of the tumour and of the surrounding tissues was useful in detecting: 1) the infiltration of tissues; 2) the Bruch's membrane breaking; 3) the vitreous changes, characterized by its high reflectivity.

All these conditions were accompanied the presence of tumour cells in the aqueous humour and so the echographic findings may advise against the use of the corneae from such melanomas for grafting.

Some recent studies by Hanselmayer and Roll (1980) have demonstrated by histological and ultrastructural methods the diffusion routes of malignant melanoma of the choroid into the cornea. Such researches demonstrated that when the tumour has infiltrated the ciliary body and the root of the iris, there may be some tumour cells among the deep corneal layers. Also the surface of the endothelium of the peripheral cornea is sometimes covered or flatly substituted by neoplastic cells. In these stages there may also be some free cells in the aqueous humour. On the other hand it is known that the use of the cornea removed from an eye suffering from malignant melanoma for keratoplasty is allowed only when there is a very posterior localization of the tumour. Indeed, we have observed the presence of tumour cells in the aqueous humour when malignant melanoma, even if located very posteriorly had broken through Bruch's membrane.

This observation induced us to study which parameters allow corneal utilization from eyes with melanoma. The need for the present research arose from the difficulty in obtaining corneae for keratoplasty in our country and from the observation that in cases of vacularized opacities of the cornea, the immediate utilization of corneal graft from enucleated eyes had given the best clinical results even in cases in which a keratoprosthesis seemed to be the only surgical procedure.

Hillman, J. S./Le May, M. M. (eds.) Ophthalmic Ultrasonography
©1983, Dr W. Junk Publishers, The Hague/Boston/Lancaster
ISBN 978-94-009-7280-3

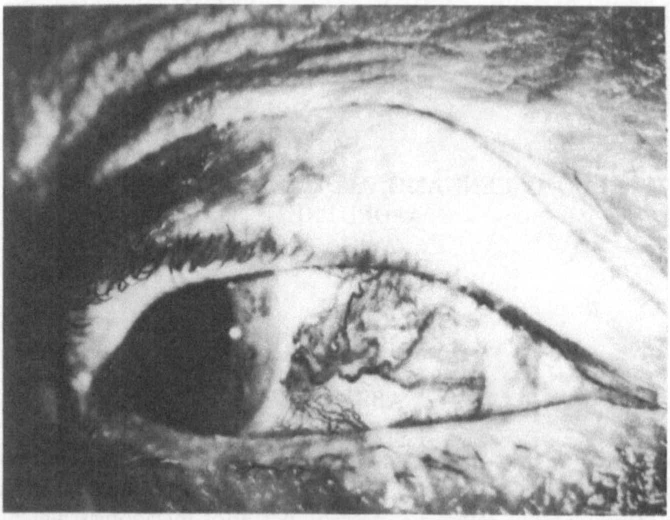

Fig. 1. Dilation of episcleral vessels.

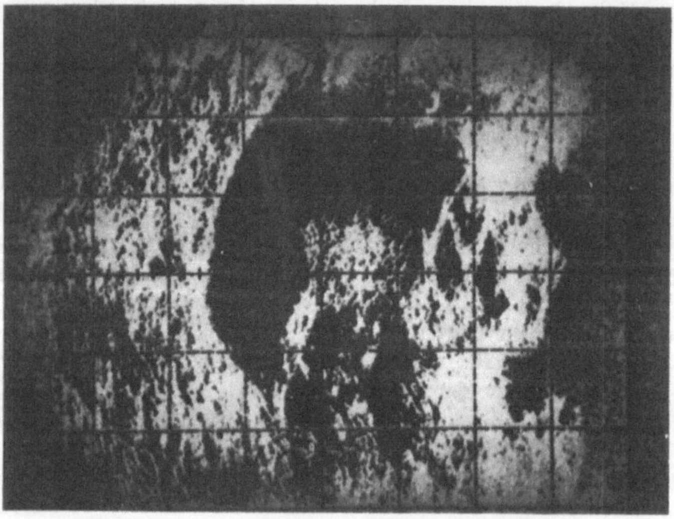

Fig. 2. Melanoma in eye with opacities of the lens and vitreous (B. scan).

Our experience concerns 32 cases of eye melanoma for which there was doubt about the eventual use of the corneae for keroplasty. We considered the clinical and ultrasonographic parameters to establish the viability of the cornea.

Clinical parameters were: the dilation of episcleral vesses (Fig. 1); the topography of the tumour and in some cases tissue infiltration, but these

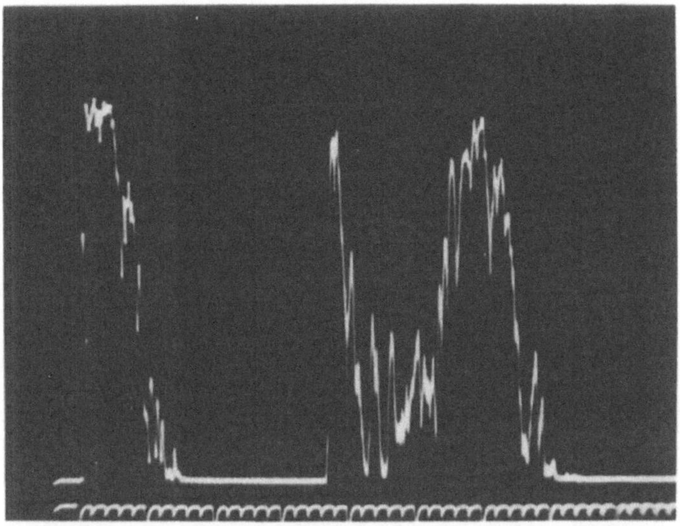

Fig. 3. Standardized A-scan echography of malignant melanoma.

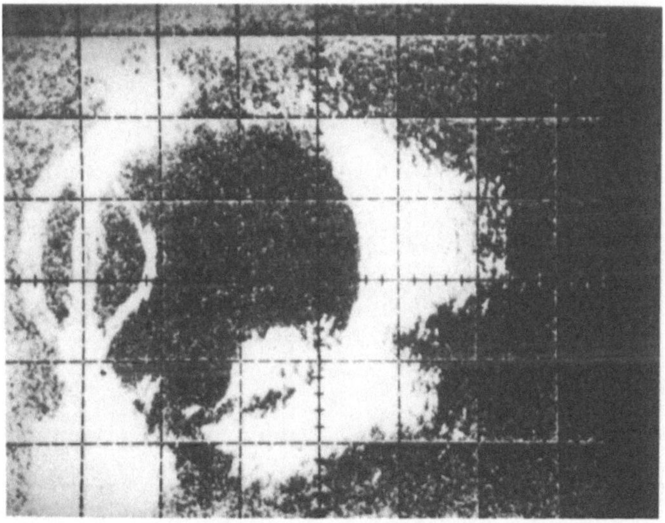

Fig. 4. B-scan representation of malignant melanoma.

characters generally are not evident when there are opacities of the lens and of the vitreous (Fig. 2).

Ultrasonographic parameters shown by standardized A-scan echography and B-scan were: the exact location, the extention, the breaking of Bruch's membrane (Fig. 3–4) by the tumour and the infiltration of the sclera and of the optic nerve (Fig. 5–6).

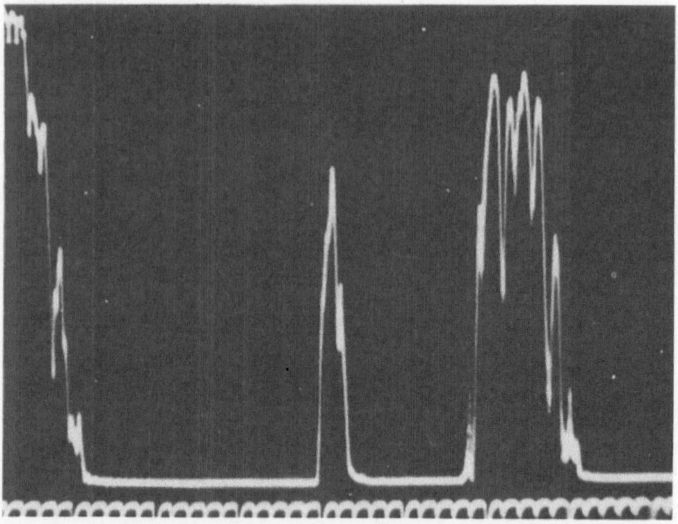

Fig. 5. Standardized A scan Echography of malignant melanoma not invasive for the sclera.

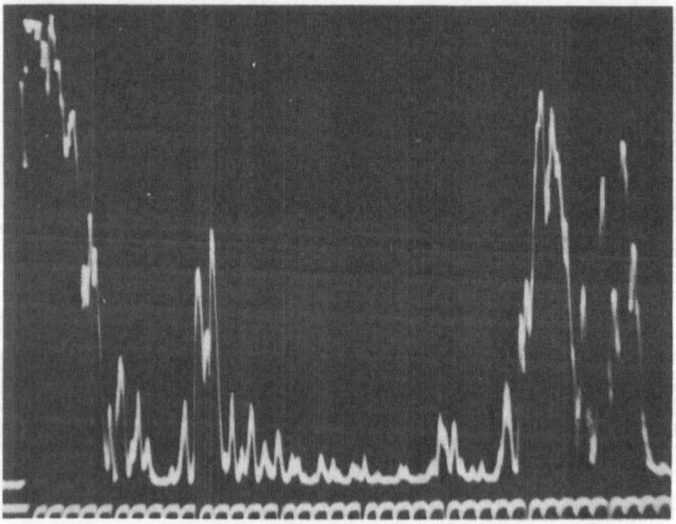

Fig. 6. Standardized A scan Echography of malignant melanoma invasive for the sclera.

The breaking of Bruch's membrane gives a characteristic mushroom appearance on B-Scan representation while the scleral or the optic nerve infiltration (Figs. 7–8) is better visualized by standardized A-Scan echography.

Another important parameter to be considered is the vitreous unhomogeneity well shown by A-scan echography. This latter condition was associated

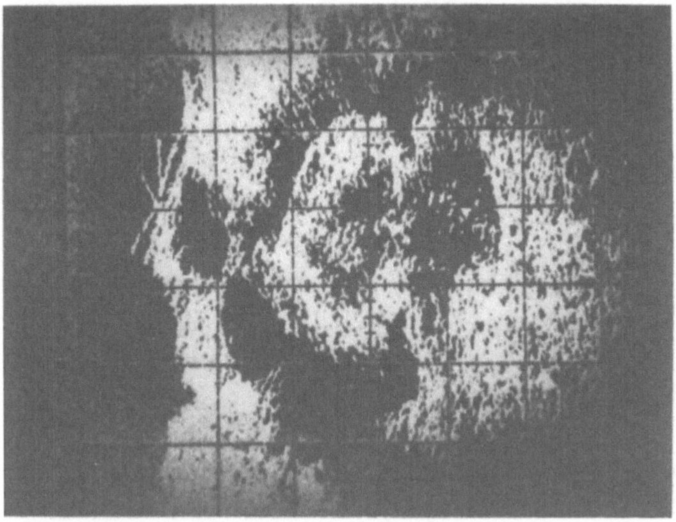

Fig. 7. B scan representation of Bruch's membrane breaking by malignant melnoma.

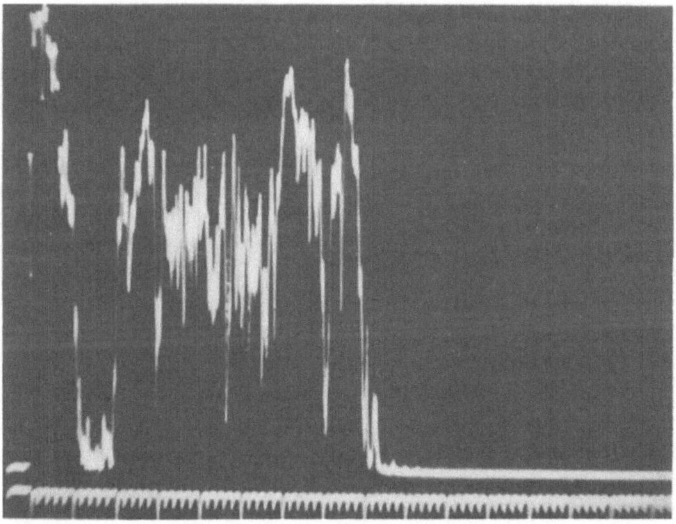

Fig. 8. Standardized A scan Echography showing the optic nerve infiltration by Malignant Melanoma.

in our research with the presence of tumour cells in the aqueous humour in about 5 our of 9 cases (Fig. 9). All these cases showed the breaking of Bruch's membrane or the infiltration of the ciliary body and/or the iris root.

In conclusion our research states that not all the eyes with melanoma of

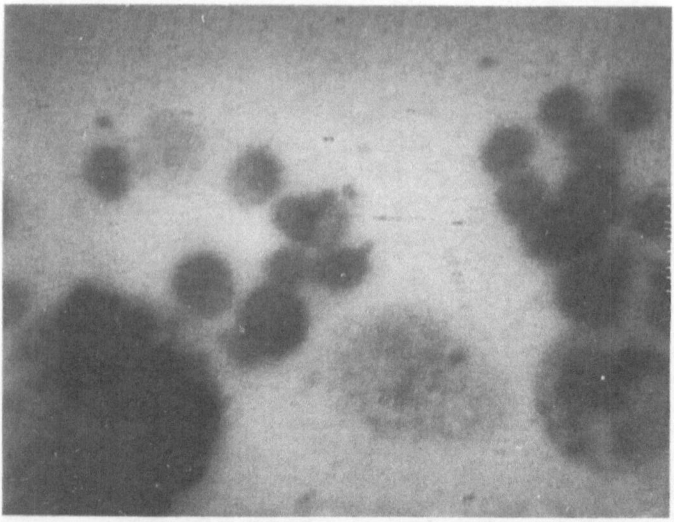

Fig. 9. Tumour cells in the aqueous humour in a case of malignant melanoma breaking through Bruck's membrane.

the posterior segment are suitable corneal donors for keratoplasty. On the other hand not all the eyes with melanoma are to be enucleated.

Clinical examination appears to be insufficient for determining in which cases the eye is to be enucleated and which of the enucleated eyes are possible corneal donors.

The echographic examination gives data that is impossible to have from clinical observation alone especially in cases of lens and vitreous opacities. In fact, the echography permits a decision regarding the availability of corneae from eyes enucleated for malignant melanoma in providing us some features such as:

(a) the breaking of Bruch's membrane
(b) The infiltration of the sclera of the ciliary body and of the iris root
(c) The vitreous changes and its unhomogeneity.

These conditions in our research are associated with the presence of tumour cells in the aqueous humour in a high percentage of cases. On the contrary the infiltration of the posterior sclera and of the optic nerve appears to be less unfavourable because of the absence of tumour cells in the aqueous humour in three of the studied cases.

REFERENCES

Coleman, D. J., Lizzi, F. L., Jack R. L.: Ultrasonography of the eye and orbit. Lea and Febiger, Philadelphia. 1977.

Gallenga R., Bellone G., Gallenga P. E., Pasquarelli A.: Ultrasonografia clinica dell'occhio e dell'orbita. L111 Congresso SOI, Malta, 1971.

Hanselmayer H., Roll P.: Electron microscopic study of the cornea in melanoma of the uvea. The cornea in health and disease, VIth Congress of European Society of Ophthalmology, Royal Society of Medicine International Congress and Symposium Series No. 40, published Jointly by Academic Press Inc. (London) Ltd., and the Royal Society of Medicine.

Ossoinig K. C., Bigar F., Kaefring S. L.: Malignant Melanoma of the choroid and ciliary body A differential diagnosis in clinical echography. Ultrasonography in Ophthalmology. Bibl. Ophthalmologica No 83. S. Karger 1975. 141–154.

Ossoinig K. C.: Standardized Echography: Basic Principles, Clinical Application, and Results. Reprinted from: International Ophthalmology clinics. Ophthalmic ultrasonography: Comparative Techniques. Winter 1979, Vol. 19, No. 4. Published by Little, Brown, and Company, Boston Massachussetts.

Author's address:
Istituto di Clinica Oculistica
II Facolta di Medicina e Chirvrgia
Universita degli Studi,
80131 Naples
Italy

A- AND B- MODE ULTRASOUND BIOMETRY IN THE PROTON BEAM IRRADIATION OF UVEAL MELANOMAS

PETER L. LOU and EVANGELOS GRAGOUDAS
(*Boston, USA*)

ABSTRACT

Ultrasound biometry data were used for a treatment planning computer program that allows three-dimensional viewing of the eye containing a uveal melanoma. This program enables one to select an orientation of the eye relative to the path of the proton beam which best covers the tumor while avoiding important ocular structures.

During the follow-up period ranging from four to twenty-seven months after proton beam irradiation, 36/50 (72%) eyes showed a decrease, 10/50 (20%) showed no change, and 4/50 (8%) showed a transient increase in height. 20/50 (40%) eyes showed a choroidal excavation, 10/50 (20%) showed retinal detachment.

INTRODUCTION

The management of malignant melanoma of the uveal tract is currently in a state of flux, largely as a result of recent suggestions that enucleation of such tumors may actually promote metastases (Zimmerman and McLean, 1979; Zimmerman, McLean and Foster, 1978, 1980). Alternative therapies which seek to destroy tumor cells without decreasing vision or potentiating metastasis have been suggested. They include photocoagulation (Vogel, 1972; Meyer-Schwickerath and Vogel, 1977), radioactive plaques (Bedford, 1970; MacFaul, 1977), full-thickness eye wall resection (Peyman and Raichand, 1979), and charged particle irradiation (Gragoudas, Goitein et al., 1982; Char, Castro et al., 1980).

Charged particle irradiation such as protons and helium ions have several advantages over other modalities of therapy in the management of uveal melanomas. These are based exclusively on their physical characteristics – namely minimal scatter, tissue sparing at the entry site, increased dose at the end of the range and a sharp dose fall off at the end of the beam – which are ideal for highly localized dose distributions. Thus, a uniform dosage can be delivered throughout the tumor with minimal irradiation to the surrounding tissues.

Hillman, J. S./Le May, M. M. (eds.) Ophthalmic Ultrasonography

ISBN 978-94-009-7280-3

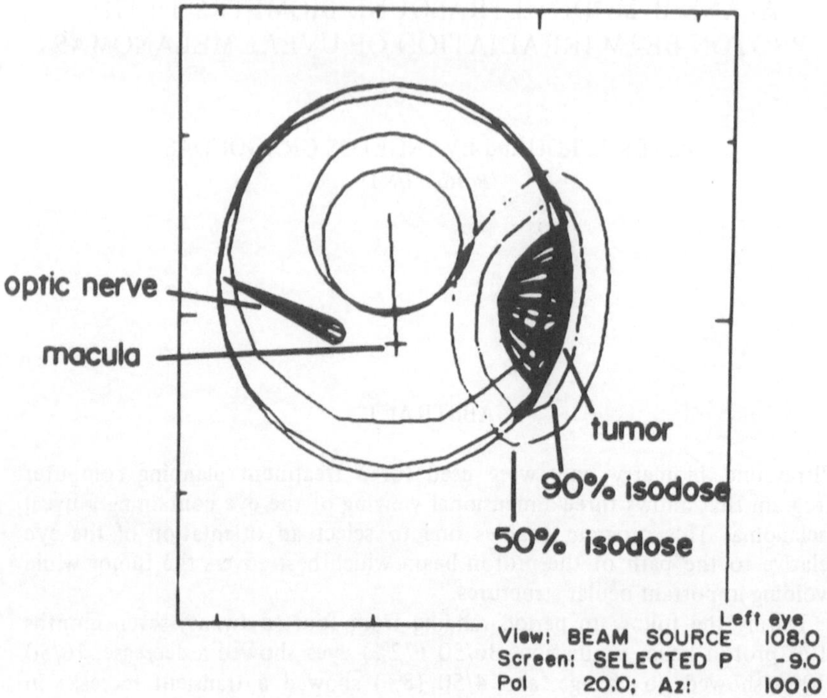

Fig. 1. Computer simulation of proton beam's eye view of the patient's eye. The dotted lines are the aperture edge and constitute the 90% and 50% isodose contours.

This paper describes the use of A- and B- mode ultrasound biometry to a treatment planning computer program which provides a three dimensional, close to real time viewing of the eye containing a uveal melanoma. This program enables one to choose an orientation of the eye relative to the path of the proton beam which best covers the tumor while avoiding important ocular structures. The use of biometry in monitoring tumor height regression after proton treatment is also described.

METHODS

Fifty patients with uveal melanomas of various sizes were treated. The patient selection criteria have been described previously (Gragoudas, Goitein et al., 1982). Axial length measurements were obtained by A-scan biometry, using a Sonometrics Ophthalmoscan 200 immersion water bath system, at 1550 m/s tissue velocity. Tumor height was obtained by measurement of the greatest perpendicular distance between the dome of the elevated retina and the base

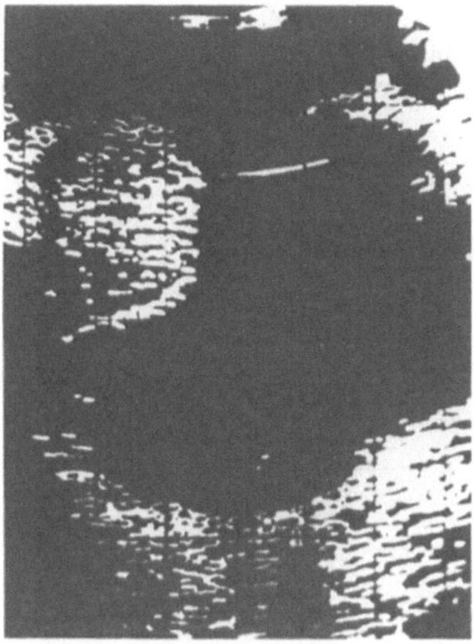

Fig. 2. B- mode display of an eye containing a uveal melanoma (left) and the same eye six months after proton beam irradiation (right), showing near total regression of the tumor mass.

of the choroidal tumor on storage B-scan display, and correcting for the magnification factor.

The biometry values thus obtained, along with radiographic coordinates given by four tantalum rings sutured to the sclera to outline the edges of the tumor, were incorporated into a treatment planning computer program. This program treats the eye as a sphere and displays the important ocular structures (lens, macula, optic disc), the tumor and the position of the tantalum rings. The direction of gaze can be manipulated in real time to determine the optimal orientation of the eye relative to the beam that best covers the tumor and avoids critical normal structures (Fig. 1).

Each patient received a dose of either 7000 or 9000 rads, in five equal fractions over a period of eight to nine days. Ultrasound biometry was repeated at specific time intervals after treatment to measure regression of the tumor mass. The follow-up period ranged from four to twenty-seven months.

RESULTS

The age, sex, and eye involvement of fifty patients are listed in Table 1. As can be seen, most uveal melanomas occurred between the fifth and seventh decades of life, although the range included one patient fifteen years of age. There was no significant sex or age predilection.

Tumors were divided into small, medium, and large sizes, depending on whether they were less than 2 mm, 2 mm to 5 mm, or greater than 5 mm in

Table 1. Age, sex, and involved eye

Characteristics		Number of Patients	Percent of Patients
Age (years):	10–19	1	2
	20–29	3	6
	30–39	4	8
	40–49	6	12
	50–59	16	32
	60–69	16	32
	70–79	3	6
	80–89	1	2
	Total	50	100
Sex:	M	23	46
	F	27	54
	Total	50	100
Involved Eye:	Right	28	56
	Left	22	44
	Total	50	100

Table 2. Size and location of tumors

Size	Posterior Segment	(%)	Ciliary Body	(%)	Total	(%)
Small	4	(8)	0	(0)	4	(8)
Medium	17	(34)	2	(4)	19	(38)
Large	18	(36)	9	(18)	27	(54)
Total	39	(78)	11	(22)	50	(100)

height by ultrasound biometry. In this series there were more large and medium size melanomas than small tumors (Table 2).

Choroidal excavation was present in 40% of all melanomas. Although it was found in all tumor sizes, it occurred mainly in the medium and large tumors. The figures were 4%, 18%, and 18% respectively for small, medium, and large tumors (Table 3).

Retinal detachment was not observed with small tumors. But its incidence increased with tumor size, from 4% with medium tumors to 16% with large tumors (Table 3).

During a follow-up period ranging from four to twenty-seven months after proton beam irradiation, 72% of the tumors showed a decrease in size regardless of their initial height. Twenty per cent of the tumors showed no change in size, and 8% showed a slight increase in height. This increase was temporary, and did not persist for more than twelve months after irradiation. Regression did not appear to relate to tumor size, since both small and large tumors occasionally showed dramatic regression.

Table 3. Incidence of choroidal excavation and retinal detachment

Size	Choroidal Excavation	(%)	Retinal Detachment	(%)
Small	2	(4)	0	(0)
Medium	9	(18)	2	(4)
Large	9	(18)	8	(16)
Total	20	(40)	10	(20)

Table 4. Tumor size and regression pattern

Size	Decrease in Size	(%)	No Change	(%)	Increase in Size	(%)
Small	2	(4)	1	(2)	0	
Medium	15	(30)	4	(8)	2	(4)
Large	19	(38)	5	(10)	2	(4)
Total	36	(72)	10	(20)	4	(8)

CONCLUSIONS

Ultrasound biometry has provided useful information to an interactive, three-dimensional treatment planning computer program developed for the treatment of uveal melanomas. The program enables us to select the best direction of gaze relative to the path of the proton beam and to determine the extent to which vital ocular structures are irradiated.

Our findings of 40% incidence of choroidal excavation compares favorably with a quoted figure of 42% by Coleman and co-workers (1974).

Eight per cent of the treated tumors showed an increase in height following treatment but this was transient; none of the tumors with more than a year's follow-up demonstrated increase in height. This led us to speculate that proton beam treatment might cause a temporary swelling of uveal tissues, giving a false impression of continued tumor growth. Longer follow-up period had shown that regression after proton beam irradiation is a relatively slow process and the effects of radiation could be observed in some cases more than a year after treatment.

ACKNOWLEDGEMENT

The authors acknowledge the contributions of the Harvard Cyclotron Staff and the Staff of Radiation Medicine, Massachusetts General Hospital in the treatment of these patients.

REFERENCES

Bedford, M. A. The use and abuse of cobalt plaques in the treatment of choroidal malignant melanomata. Trans. Ophthalmol. Soc. UK 93:139 (1970).

Char, D. H., Castro, J. R., Quivey, J. M., et al. Helium ion charged particle therapy for

choroidal melanoma. Ophthalmology 87:565 (1980).
Coleman, D. J., Abramson, D. J., Jack, R. L., Franzen, L. A. Ultrasonic diagnosis of tumors of the choroid. Arch Ophthalmol. 91:344 (1974).
Gragoudas, E. S., Goitein, M., Verhey, L. et al. Proton beam irradiation. Ophthalmology 87:571 (1980).
Gragoudas, E. S., Goitein, M., Verhey, L. et al. Proton beam irradiation of uveal melanomas. Arch. Ophthalmol. 100:928 (1982).
MacFaul, P. A. Local radiotherapy in the treatment of malignant melanoma of the choroid. Trans. Ophthalmol. Soc. UK 97:421 (1977).
Meyer-Schwickerath, G., Vogel, M. Treatment of malignant melanomas of the choroid by photocoagulation. Trans. Ophthalmol. Soc. UK 97:416 (1977).
Peyman, G. A., Raichand, M. Full-thickness eye wall resection of choroidal neoplasms. Ophthalmology 86:1024 (1979).
Vogel, M. H. Treatment of malignant choroidal melanomas with photocoagulation: Evaluation of a ten year follow-up data. Am. J. Ophthalmol. 74:1 (1972).
Zimmerman, L. E., McLean, I. W. An evaluation of enucleation in the management of uveal melanomas. Am. J. Ophthalmol. 87:741 (1979).
Zimmerman, L. E., McLean, I. W., Foster, W. D. Does enucleation of the eye containing a malignant melanoma prevent or accelerate the dissemination of tumor cells? Brit. J. Ophthalmol. 62:420 (1978).
Zimmerman, L. E., McLean, I. W., Foster, W. D. Statistical analysis of follow-up data concerning uveal melanomas, and the influence of enucleation. Ophthalmology 87:557 (1980).

Authors' address:
75 Blossom Court
Boston, MA 02114
USA

ECHOGRAPHIC MODIFICATIONS OF THE CHOROID IN ITS TUMOURS AND PSEUDO-TUMOURS

JACQUES POUJOL and MICHEL LE ROY
(Paris, France)

SUMMARY

This paper reports the results in a recent series of about 150 eyes in patients with suspected choroidal melanomas, metastatic tumours, hemangiomas or pseudo-tumours where the diagnosis, established with B-scan, was checked by histology after enucleation or by follow-up over at least two years in cases of choroidal hemangioma or pseudo-tumour.

Three kinds of modifications were observed with contact B-scan, using different instruments:
- choroidal excavation,
- choroidal infiltration,
- choroidal detachment.

The appearance of each modification is described and its diagnostic value is discussed.

The echographic appearance of the normal choroid and of its pathological changes has become better known over the past few years due to improvements in B mode echographic techniques (Coleman et al., 1972, Poujol 1978 and 1980). A more precise diagnosis of choroidal tumours and a better differential diagnosis of pseudo-tumours is now possible.

MATERIAL AND METHODS

This paper concerns about 150 eyes in patients referred over the past few years for suspected intra-ocular tumours. The diagnosis was made in B-scan and verified either histologically after enucleation or by follow-up of at least two years in cases where the diagnosis was hemangioma or pseudo-tumour. The instruments used were: the BRONSON-TURNER unit, the EO2 and recently the TRISCAN from BIOPHYSIC MEDICAL and, occasionally, the SONOMETRICS OCUSCAN.

RESULTS

The tumour itself, whether benign or malignant, develops as a mass adjoining the choroid. We will not discuss here the characteristics of this mass.

Hillman, J.S./Le May, M.M. (eds.) Ophthalmic Ultrasonography

ISBN 978-94-009-7280-3

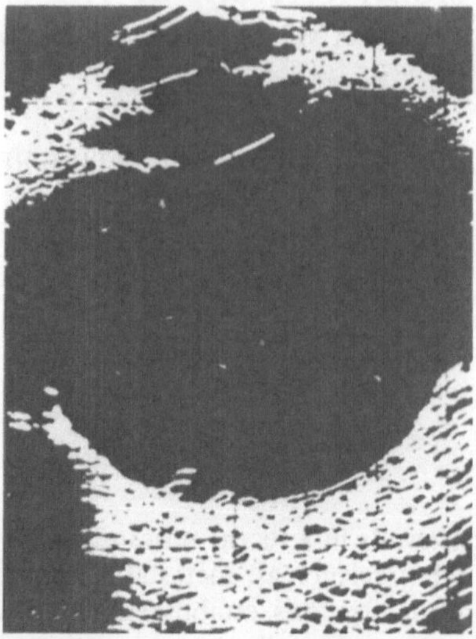

Fig. 1. **Typical choroidal excavation in a medium size malignant melanoma. The choroidal excavation (between arrows) extends to the width of the tumour.**

Three types of modification can be observed in the choroid itself: excavation, infiltration and detachment.

Choroidal excavation was described as being an indication of the presence of a choroidal tumour by Coleman in 1972. In fact, Purnell had published a picture of this in 1967 but had at that time assumed that it was an artefact.

Excavation (Figure 1 and 2) was found in nearly 80% of our true tumour cases but also in more than 20% of the pseudo-tumours, (Poujol et al., 1981). In one particular case of choroidal tuberculoma (Figure 3) the image had disappeared completely after two months' treatment. In the tumour group, although this phenomenon is observed as often in melanomas as in metastatic tumours of the choroid, it was not found once in choroidal hemangiomas. Lastly, although the contrary has been suggested, excavation is observed in melanomas of the ciliary body although it is more difficult to visualise in contact B mode, due to the very anterior position of these tumours.

Choroidal infiltration is seen as a thickening of this membrane often accompanied by hyper-reflectivity. It can be observed in certain flat and large choroidal metastases, angiomas and in choroidal localization of certain general diseases such as leukemia (Figure 4).

Spontaneous choroidal detachment often resembles a choroidal tumour through the ophthalmoscope. B scan echographic diagnosis differentiates, amongst other signs, the appearance of the angle of junction of the choroid with the ocular wall (Figure 5), which is very different from the one seen

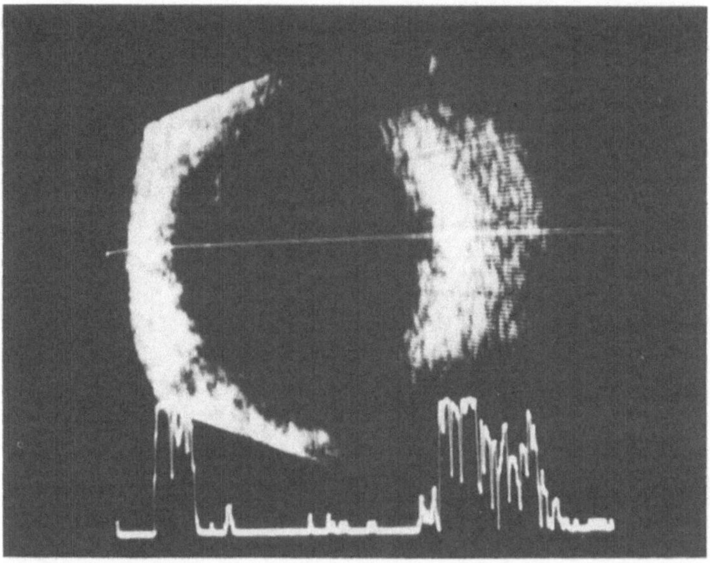

Fig. 2. Choroidal excavation in a flat melanoma. In such a case, the choroidal excavation is the only echographic sign indicating that the lesion could be a melonoma.

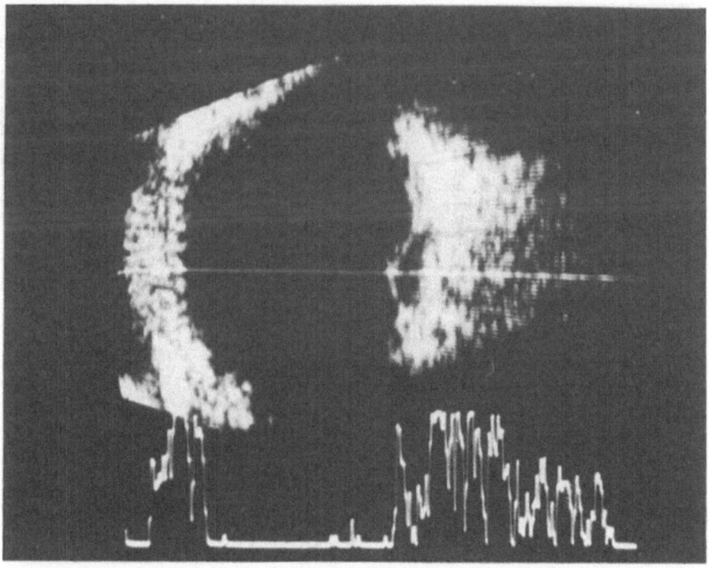

Fig. 3. Choroidal tuberculoma. The echographic picture is highly suggestive of a small melanoma with typical choroidal excavation.

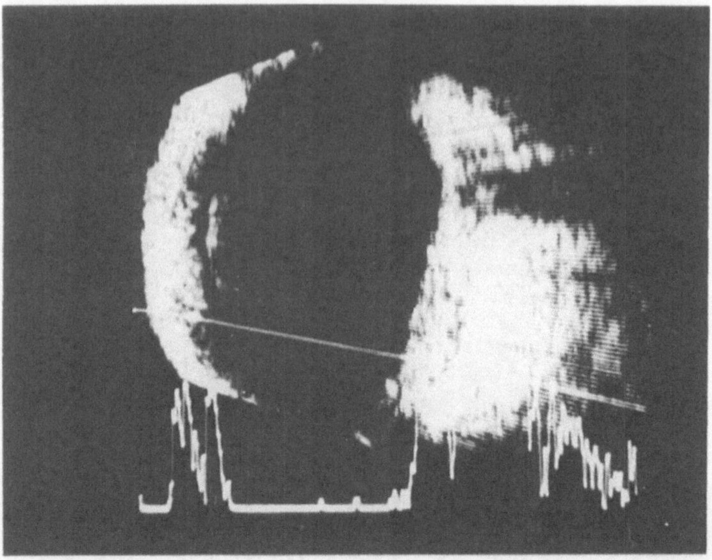

Fig. 4. Choroidal infiltration in a case of lymphocytic leukemia. The infiltration is localized at the posterior pole of the eye and the choroidal thickening there is approximately 6 mm.

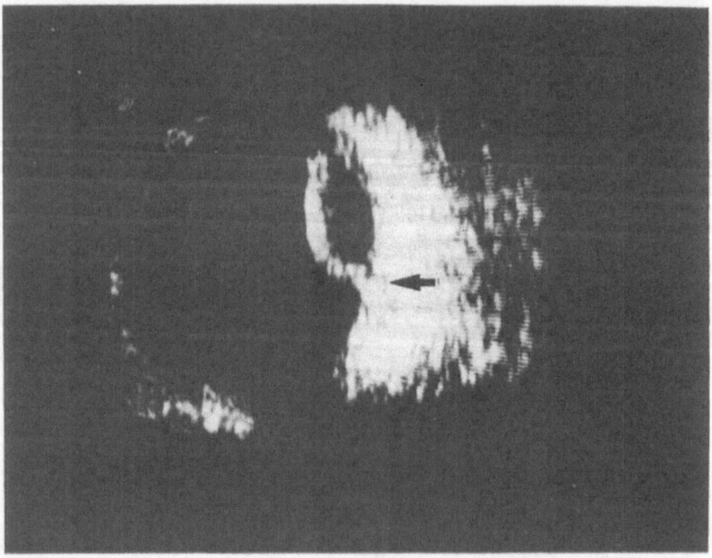

Fig. 5. Spontaneous choroidal detachment. Such a detachment mimics a melanoma but the angle of junction of the choroid with the ocular wall (arrow) is characteristic of a choroidal detachment.

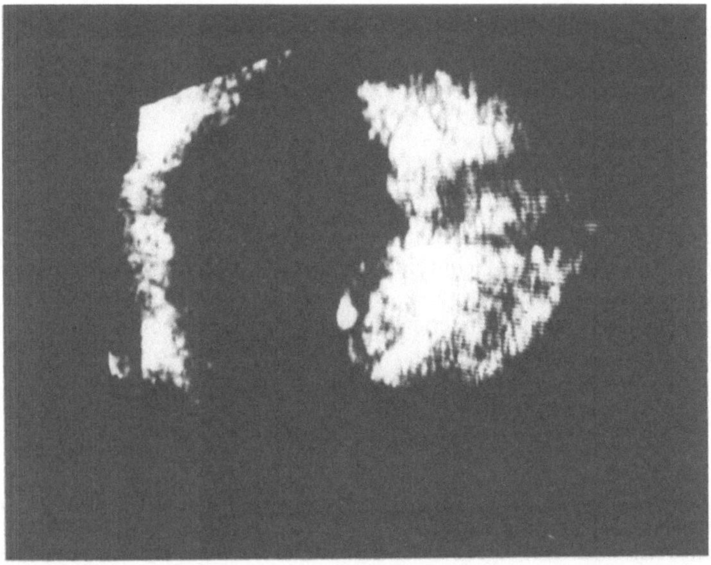

Fig. 6. Hematoma of the posterior pole of the eye. This dark swelling resembled a tumour, but the thickened choroid is clearly visible inside the swelling.

with a tumorous choroidal excavation (Poujol 1981). This detachment was due, as in most of our cases, to a thrombosis of a vortex vein.

DISCUSSION

Choroidal excavation is observed with a regularity which depends on the type of equipment used. It is with a bistable system that it was described and we easily observed its presence with such a system (EO2). It is not as easy to see with the BRONSON-TURNER machine. A unit with grey scale (TRISCAN) shows this phenomenon with the most regularity, providing that the settings of the gain and contrast are sufficiently low to avoid saturation.

The excavation is sometimes only observed along a limited portion of the choroid and seems to correspond perfectly to the narrow implantation of a tumour.

The origin of this excavation certainly seems to be due, as Coleman suggested in 1972, to the replacement of choroidal tissue which is vascular and highly echogenic with tissue which is less echogenic. This does not however imply that the tissue is tumorous and choroidal excavation can be observed with many pseudo-tumours, especially when inflammatory tissue is present, as in our case of choroidal tuberculoma (Figure 3). It is therefore a non-specific indication. However, it must be emphasised that if the choroid is present behind a swelling, such a swelling does not have a tumourous origin (Figure 6).

Choroidal infiltration is often difficult to distinguish from simple choroidal thickening of different origin (Poujol 1980).

The origin of a choroidal detachment is easy to recognise if it follows ocular surgery. It is less easy to recognise if the detachment is spontaneous and hemorrhagic, which is where echography is most useful.

CONCLUSION

An echographic B-scan study of the choroid provides a great deal of information in the diagnosis of choroidal tumours, expecially those which show little swelling or cover a small area, but there is no pathognomonic sign of a true tumour. However, it is practically certain that no tumour is present if the choroid is visible behind a swelling.

REFERENCES

Coleman, D. J.: Reliability of ocular and orbital diagnosis with B-scan ultrasound. Am. J. Ophthalmol. 73: 501–516 (1972).

Coleman, D. J., Abramson, D. H., Jack, R. L. & al. Utrasonic Diagnosis of tumours of the choroid. Arch. Ophthalmol. 91: 344–354 (1974).

Brachet, A., Peyre, C., Poujol, J. & al. Les décollements spontanés de la choroide. Bull. Soc. Ophthalmol. France, 3: 249–253 (1981).

Fuller, D. G., Snyder, W. B., Hutton, W. L. & al. Ultrasonographic features of choroidal malignant melanomas. Arch. Ophthalmol., 97: 1465–1472 (1979).

Poujol, J.: Intraocular tumours. In: 'Handbood of Clinical Ultrasound', de Vlieger, M. & al, edit, Wiley & Sons, New York, 86: 863–874 (1978).

Poujol, J.: Ultrasonographic measurement and clinical value of choroidal thickening. 2nd Meeting of the World Federation for Ultrasound in Medicine and Biology, Miyazaki, Japan; July 1979. In: 'Ultrasound in Medicine and Biology', T. Wagai & R. Omoto, edit., Excerpta Medica, pp. 101–105 (1980).

Poujol, J.: Aspects échographique de l'angle de raccordemant à la paroi oculaire dans le décollement choroidien (A characteristic sign of choroidal detachment – the appearance of the angle of junction with the ocular wall). In: 'Ultrasonography in Ophthalmology 8'. Proceedings of the SIDUO VIII Symposium, Nijmegen 1980, J. M. Thijssen & A. M. Verbeek, edit. Junk, Den Haag, pp. 265–267 (1981).

Poujol, J., Le Roy, M., Toufic, N.: Reliability of B-scan differentiation between choroidal tumours and pseudo-tumours. In: 'Recent advances in Ultrasound Diagnosis 3'. Proceedings of the 4th European Congress on Ultrasonics in Medicine, Dubrovnik, May 1981. A. Kurjak & A. Kratochwil, edit., Excerpta Medica, Amsterdam, pp. 511–513 (1981).

Purnell, E. W.: Intensity Modulated (B-Scan) Ultrasonography. In: 'Ultrasonics in Ophthalmology', Goldberg, R. E. and Sarin, L. K., edit. W. B. Saunders Company, Philadelphia, pp. 102–123 (1967).

Author's address:
Laboratoire d'Echographie
Centre National d'Ophtalmologie des Quinze-Vingts
28 rue de Charenton
75012 Paris
France

EXPERIMENTAL IMITATIONS OF THE LESS PROMINENT LESIONS OF THE FUNDUS AND THEIR ECHOGRAPHIC ANALYSIS

V. DORN
(Zagreb, Yugoslavia)

INTRODUCTION

The ultrasonic differentiation of less prominent lesions of the fundus of the eye (small retinal or vitreal detachments, subretinal exudation, haemorrhage, minimally elevated or flat neoplasmas etc.) is often limited.

The greatest difficulties are found in exploring prominences at resolution limits. Flat prominences with smooth borders produce echograms in which it is very difficult to find all characteristics (Mazzeo and Scorrano 1979) for echographic diagnosis. With very thin lesions, some criteria are not easily applied as there is less attenuation in the tumour and the dimensions are close to the resolving power of the echoscope (Dadd, et al. 1975). Problems in diagnosis of thin or less prominent lesions in vitreo-retinal pathology (Oksala 1977, Coleman, et al. 1977, Schroeder 1978), retinal/intraretinal (Hillman and Ridgway 1975) and subretinal space (Ossoinig 1972, Ossoinig, et al. 1975, Till and Hauff 1981) have also been mentioned.

Stimulated by the clinical problem we tried to imitate such lesions experimentally and to determinate the elevation which can be differentiated by means of standardized echography.

MATERIAL AND METHODS

Our postulates required: (2) On the animal (porcine) eye globes to make measurable pathological lesions, (b) to make them structurally similar to ocular pathology and (c) to make them accessible to examination .

We used both fresh human blood (possibility of exact application by means of tuberculin syringe, formation of coagulum and, as the most important, biologic, cellular composition of the blood) and paraffin oil (border parafin oil/water, oil viscosity).

a. The imitations of pathological structures in porcine eye globes by application of fresh human blood

The lesion was produced as follows. A small, 1–1.5 mm, linear scleral incision was made behind the equator, near to the posterior pole with a Graefe knife.

Hillman, J.S./Le May, M.M. (eds.) Ophthalmic Ultrasonography

ISBN 978-94-009-7280-3

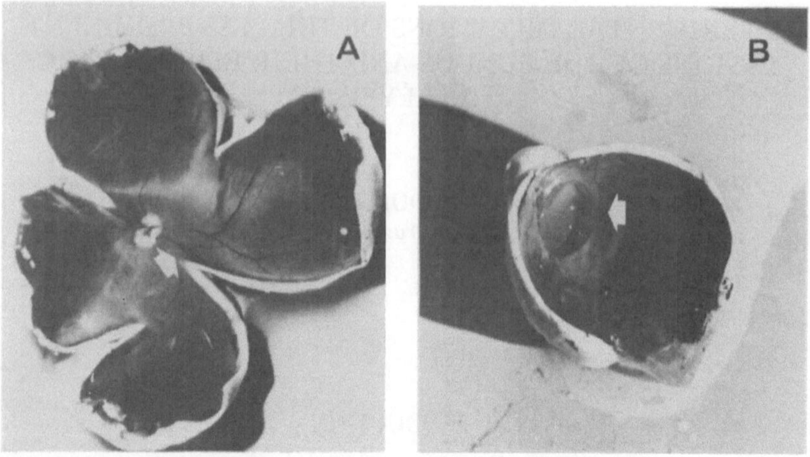

Fig. 1. **The imitations of pathological structures in porcine eye-balls: A. Application of the blood. Arrow indicates the flat subretinal lesion. B. Application of the paraffin oil. Arrow indicates the appearance of the vitreoretinal lesion.**

0.03, 0.05, 0.1 and 0.2 ml of the recent human blood was injected subretinally using a fine needle and tuberculin syringe. The resultant small or large haematoma was subretinal (Figure 1A). The scleral incision was closed immediately with cautery. Volumes of less than 0.05 ml showed a tendency to leak out.

b. The imitation of pathological structures in porcine eye globes by application of paraffin oil

The lesions with paraffin oil were made with an identical procedure. Liquid Paraffin (Pharmacopoea Iug.III.P-040) was used. The lesser volumes of paraffin oil, leaked from the scleral incision, and we therefore used 0.2 and 0.3 ml. The appearance of the vitreoretinal lesion in a dissected eye-ball is shown in Figure 1B.

Standardized A-scan equipment (7200 MA Kretztechnik with the NM 8/5 K probe) was used. Tissue sensitivity was 65 dB. Topographic echography, distal and proximal echo, detected the lesion and referred us to the best probe position for measurements. By reducing the system sensitivity we analysed the lesion displayed on the screen, its reflectivity, dB readings for retinal, intermediate, scleral and other echo signals. A series of photographs were taken of the lesions displayed (e.g. Figure 2 and Figure 3) and the readings for prominence and selectivity limits were measured.

RESULTS

The imitations of pathological structures by application of the blood presented comparatively the affections of the retinochoroid, cellular-infiltrative

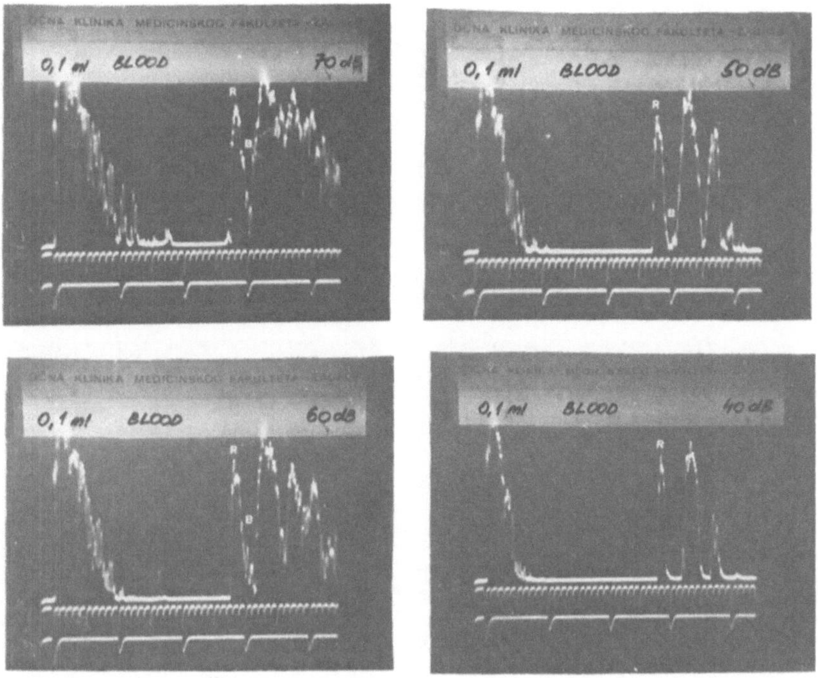

Fig. 2. Series of A-scan echograms of the lesion made of injected blood retroretinally. R = retina, B = blood.

subretinal processes and circulatory vascular affections of the vitroretinal border. The application of the paraffin oil suggested the pictures of vitreal detachment, serous retinal detachment, retinoschisis, vitreal membranes, vitreal syneresis and similarly.

The examinations of flat lesions originating from the applied blood showed that in prominence of 2.0–2.5 μs the intermediate echoes from the blood can be evaluated (Figure 4). Table 1 demonstrates the results of the experiments with the blood. The minimal prominence of the lesion made from paraffin oil to be evaluated amounted to 3.5 μs. Table 2 demonstrates the results of the experiments with paraffin oil.

DISCUSSION AND CONCLUSIONS

A-scan differential diagnostic criteria for small lesions in retinal space (Hillman & Ridgway 1975, Ossoinig 1972) and in subretinal space (serous fluid, subretinal haemorrhage, melanoma, metastatic carcinoma, haemangioma, naevi, disciform degeneration, Coats' disease) are previously established (Ossoinig 1972, Ossoinig, et al. 1975, Till & Hauff 1981). Additional characteristics in B-scan display were described by Coleman and co-authors (1977). Schroeder's (1978) contribution to diagnostic criteria showed the practical

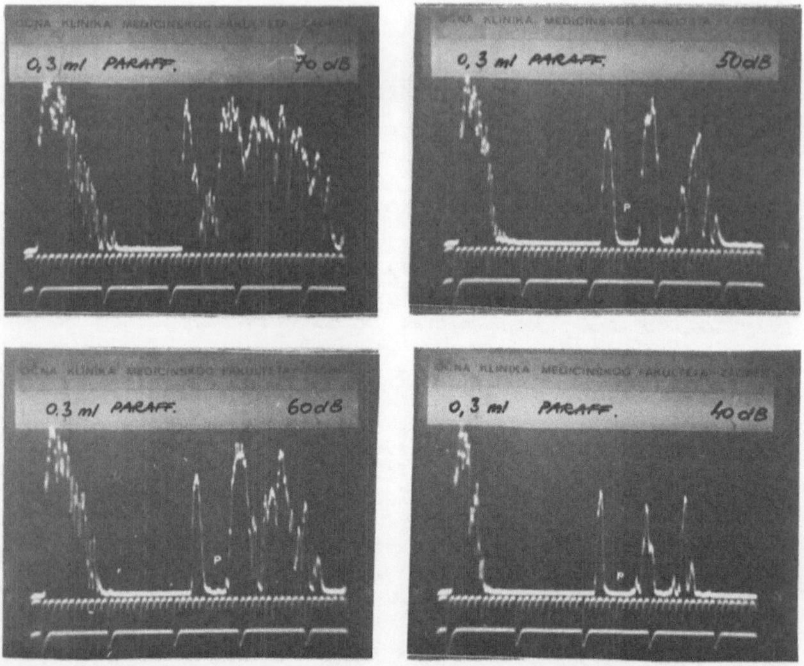

Fig. 3. Series of A-scan echograms of the lesion made of paraffin oil (P). Acoustic silent, homogeneous medium.

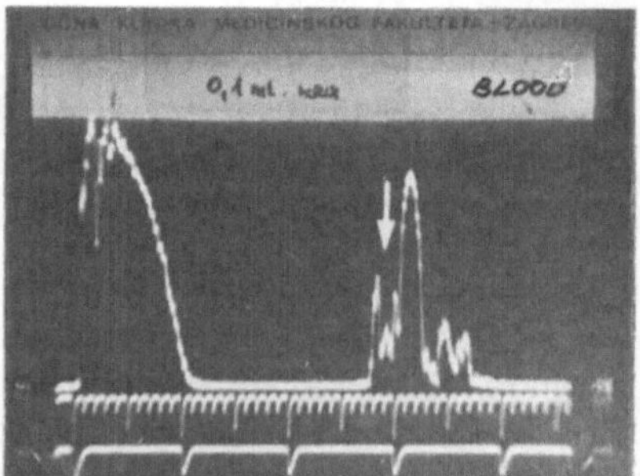

Fig. 4. Example of minimal lesion thickness to be evaluated. Prominence 2 μs. Arrow indicates echo signals of subretinal blood.

Table 1. Application of the recent human blood

Applied volume	Eyeball labeled	Prominence μs	Scleral echo reference	Retinal echo reference	Intermediate blood echoes
0.03 ml	P.V.K	2.0–2.5	16 dB	35 dB	63 dB
0.05 ml	P.IV.K	2.5	18 dB	40 dB	63 dB
0.1 ml	P.1.K.	3.5	13 dB	34 dB	66 dB
	P.2.K	2.5–3.0	14 dB	34 dB	66 dB
	P.4.K	2.5–3.0	18 dB	36 dB	66 dB
	P.5.K	2.5–3.0	20 dB	36 dB	63 dB
	P.III.K	4.0	22 dB	50 dB	65 dB
0.2 ml	P.II.K	8.0	13 dB	20 dB	68 dB
	P.VI.K	6.0	22 dB	46 dB	66 dB
	P.3.K	3.5–4.0	18 dB	34 dB	60 dB

Table 2. Application of the paraffin oil

Applied volume	Eyeball labeled	Prominence μs	Scleral echo reference	Retinal echo reference
0.2 ml	P.2.P	3.5	12 dB	42 dB
	P.3.P	4.0	22 dB	30 dB
	P.4.P	3.5	18 dB	34 dB
0.3 ml	P.VII.P	8.0	20 dB	35 dB
	P.VIII.P	9.0	25 dB	40 dB
	P.1.P	6.0	18 dB	34 dB

value of use of a contact B-scanner in small lesions of vitreal, vitreoretinal and subretinal space.

According to Ossoinig's experience the lesions of the ocular fundus must be elevated at least 0.75 mm to be detected and must be of more than 1.5 mm thickness to be differentiated with echography. (Ossoinig 1972, Ossoinig, et al. 1975, Till & Hauff 1981). Less prominent lesions of the fundus such as very flat retinal or subretinal haemorrhages or naevi, cannot be distinguished from correspondingly flat normal structures (Ossoinig 1972). Using B-mode lesions causing more than 1 mm of elevation can be demonstrated and under optimal conditions, tumors causing only 0.5 mm of elevation can be depicted (Coleman, et al. 1977). According to Oksala (1977) subretinal space must be sufficiently high (⩾2 mm) for its acoustic properties to be examined by ultrasound. Echography also requires a certain minimum tissue thickness in order to diagnose this tissue (Till & Hauff 1981). Summarizing the above mentioned data and our experimental work it can be concluded:

The echographic evaluation of the less prominent lesions of the fundus is limited both in relation to their size or position and by resolving power of ultrasonic equipment.

Minimal lesion thickness to be evaluated is equal to or greater than 2 μs.

Very small or flat lesions with borderline echographic criteria require careful follow up examinations and documentation as safe control of growth change.

REFERENCES

Coleman, D. J., Lizzi, F., Jack, R. L.: Ultrasonography of the Eye and Orbit. Philadelphia, Lea & Febiger (1977).

Dadd, M. J., Hughes, H. L., Kossoff, G.: Ultrasonic Characteristics of Choroidal Melanoma. Bibl. Ophthal. 83: 155 (1975).

Hillman, J. S., Ridgway, A. E. A.: Retinoschisis and Retinal Detachment. An Ultrasonic Comparison. Bibl. Ophthal. 83: 63 (1975).

Mazzeo, V., Scorrano, R.: Our Echographic Experience about Choroidal Melanomas. In: Diagnostica Ultrasonica in Ophthalmologia (Gernet H., ed.) Münster, R. A. Remy Verlag (1979) p. 119.

Oksala, A.; Ultrasonic Findings in the Vitreous Space in Patients with Detachment of the Retina. Albrecht v. Graefes Arch. klin. exp. Ophthalmol. 202: 197 (1977).

Ossoinig, K. C.: Clinical echo-ophthalmography. In: Current Concepts in Ophthalmology III, (F. C. Blodi, ed.), St. Louis, Mosby (1972) p. 101.

Ossoinig, K. C., Bigar, F. & Kaefring, S. L.: Malignant Melanoma of the Choroid and Ciliary Body. Bibl. Ophthal. 83: 141 (1975).

Schroeder, W.: Topographische Diagnostik am hinteren Augenabschnitt mit der Kontakt-B-Bildechographie. Albrecht v. Graefes Arch. klin. exp. Ophthalmol. 207: 61 (1978).

Till, P., Hauff, W.: Differential diagnostic results of clinical echography in intraocular tumors. In: Docum. Ophthal. Proc. Series, Vol. 29 (J. M. Thijssen & A. M. Verbeek, eds.) The Hague, Junk (1981) p. 91.

Author's address:
University Eye Clinic
Kišpatićeva 12
YU-41000 Zagreb
Yugoslavia

ECHOGRAPHY AND CARDIO-GREEN^{R} ANGIOGRAPHY IN EIGHT CASES OF CHOROIDAL HAEMANGIOMAS

V. MAZZEO, A. GIOVANNINI*, L. RAVALLI and G. COSTANTINI*
(Ferrara and Bologna, Italy)*

SUMMARY

During the past years we examined eight cases of choroidal haemangiomas, some of them belonging to patients with Sturge-Weber syndrome. All underwent echographic examination with standardized A-scan, simultaneous A-B scan, contact B-scan and fluorescein angiography. All but one also took a Cardio-green^{R} angiography. Some differential diagnoses are also reported.

INTRODUCTION

Choroidal haemangioma (C.H.) is quite a rare tumour. Recently two papers have been published dealing with clinical pictures of 6 and 10 cases respectively (Goes and Benozzi 1980, Bonnet 1981).

The purpose of this paper is to describe the ultrasonographic and indocyanine green infrared color angiographic features of 8 cases we have examined over the past five years. Some differential diagnoses are also considered.

MATERIALS AND METHODS

8 patients were referred to the University Eye Clinics of Ferrara and Bologna to confirm the clinical diagnosis or suspicion of C.H.

The clinical pictures are summarized in Table 1.

Seven were male and one female. The youngest of the group being a 20 year old woman. It must be noted that the two youngest patients also showed facial angiomatous manifestation and therefore belong to a Sturge-Weber Syndrome (Case no. 1 and 3). 3 tumours were located around the disc superiorly, 1 was supero-temporally a little further away from the disc, 1 was situated between the disc and the macula, 2 were temporal and 1 was inferior to the macula.

The prominence measured by means of echo (see below) ranged between 1.6 and 5.8 mm. The follow-up lasted between 56 and 13 months.

Only one case (no. 4) had a satellite serous retinal detachment while another showed something like a serous bulge over the top of the mass (no. 1).

Hillman, J.S./Le May, M.M. (eds.) Ophthalmic Ultrasonography
© 1983, Dr W. Junk Publishers, The Hague/Boston/Lancaster
ISBN 978-94-009-7280-3

Table 1

	Name	Sex	Age	Side	Prominence by echo (mm)	Location	Visus	Others manif.	Follow-up months	Increase
1	S.S.	F	21	R	3.73	Nasal near the disc	0.1	+	24	±
2	A.E.	M	42	R	5.81	Temporal to the macula	0.02	—	56	+
3	T.G.	M	32	R	2.90	Between macula and papilla	0.6	+	24	±
4	P.F.	M	47	L	3.57	Temporal to the macula	0.04	—	48	—
5	T.S.	M	45	R	3.22	Superior near the disc	0.02	—	48	—
6	P.G.	M	55	L	3.32	Supero nasal near the disc	1	—	24	—
7	C.G.	M	41	L	4.15	Supero nasal	0.5/0.6	—	56	+
8	P.M.	M	58	L	1.66	Inferior to the macula	0.1	—	13	—

All patients underwent normal clinical examinations including fluorescein angiography.

Indocyanine green infrared colour angiography (Cardio-green^{R} angiography) was performed according a simple technique (Buffet, et al., 1979) suitably modified (Giovannini 1981). In short an infrared color Kodak Ektachrome film IE 135–20 was used, the film speed varying from 50 to 100 ASA according to the radiation emitted by the light source. An average yellow filter was placed in front of the light sources and camera stopping the light radiation of wavelength shorter than 500 nm. The Xenon lamp (300 W/S) of the retinograph was used as the source of infrared radiation. The best results were obtained without using high intensities (number 50 on the flash power unit).

A-scan echography was performed using the Kretztechnik 7200 MA, the probe was 8 MHz unfocused. The echographic A-scan technique was the one described by Ossoinig (1974). The significant echo-pattern is: solid lesion, sharply rising anterior echo, very high internal reflectivity (85–100%) and regular internal structure (Ossoinig, et al., 1975).

Both contact and immersion B-scan techniques were performed with a Sonometrics Ophthalmoscan 200 using probes of different frequencies from 10 to 20 MHz. The immersion technique has been widely described by Coleman, Lizzi and Jack (1977). The contact technique by Bronson et al., (1976) and Coleman et al., (1979). C.H. is described as a low, dome shaped, strongly reflective mass usually at the posterior pole. There is no hollowness or acoustic shadowing. The radio frequency (RF) signal appears to be high and regular.

RESULTS

Cardio-green^{R} angiography was positive in all performed cases. Green staining of the tumour mass increased progressively from the early arterial phase to the very late venous phase when the dye had already disappeared from the retinal and normal vessels (Figure 1).

These characteristics allow us to differentiate C.H. from any other kind of tumour (Bonnet, et al., 1976 a–b). This phenomenon is due to the characteristics of the dye, which has a very high molecular weight (775) and is almost completely bound to the plasmatic proteins (98%). Consequently the dye does not leak from choroidal vessel walls but concentrates itself in the very large vascular channels of C.H.

The A-scan echo traces were all characteristic showing very high internal reflectivity (Figure 2). No attenuation following the Poujol technique (1981) nor spontaneous movements were found. Once the tumoral area had been found while performing immersion simultaneous A- and B-scan, a technique suggested by Coleman et al. (1977) was used. This consists in lowering the sensitivity or increasing the probe frequency in order to show the internal tissue texture and the very high reflectivity (Figure 3). In this way a dense structure was seen. Using this technique it was much easier to see the retina and the tumour edge when they are not already separated. Something like a

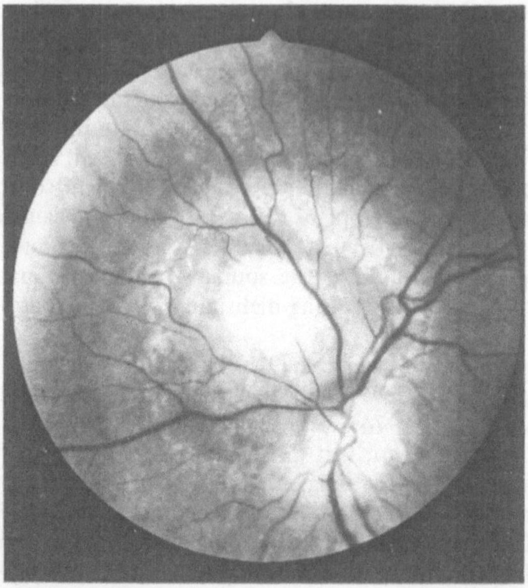

Fig. 1. Indocyanine green infrared colour angiography. Choroidal Haemangioma stains diffusely and intensively green.

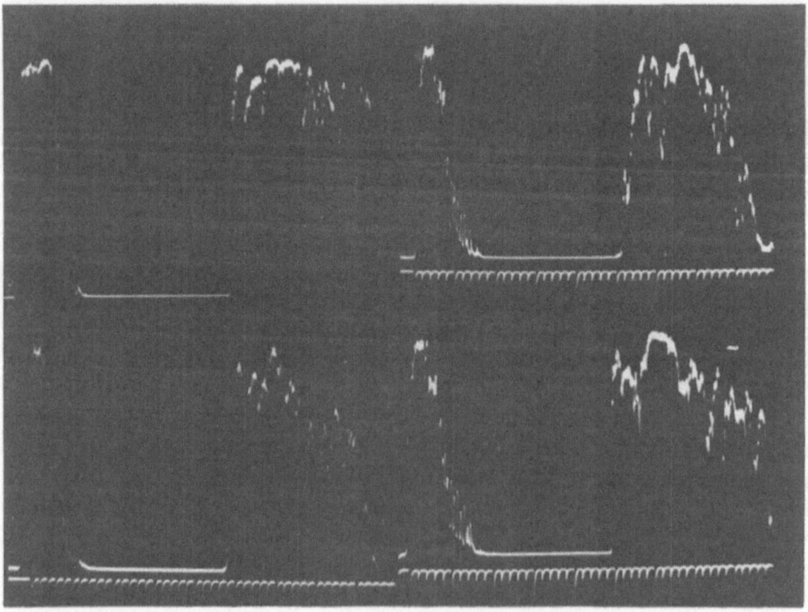

Fig. 2. A-scan echograms from four different Choroidal Haemangiomas. Very high internal reflectivity at tissue sensitivity is to be noted.

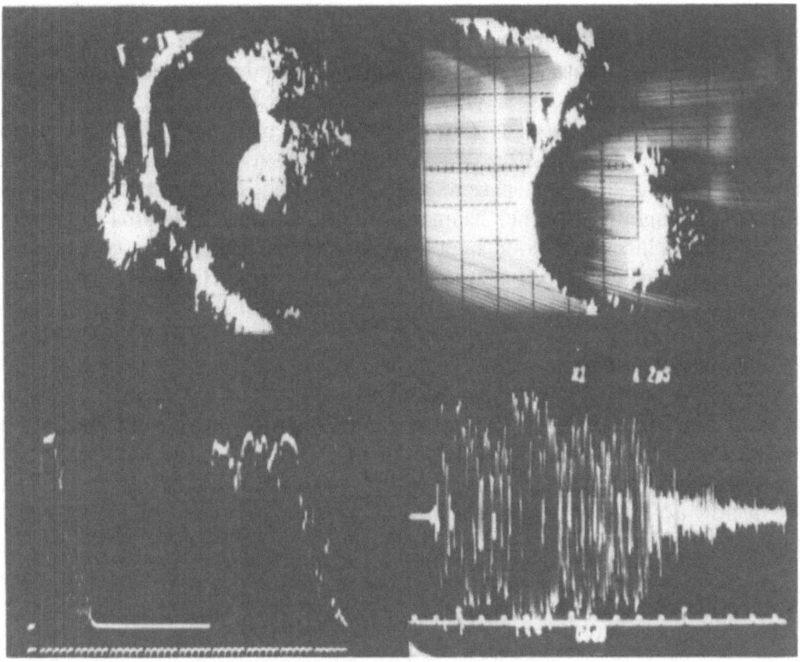

Fig. 3. Choroidal Haemangioma. Top left (immersion B-scan, 10 MHz): a high reflective dome shaped mass is found. Top right (gray scale immersion B-scan, 15 MHz): the tumoral area is still very high reflective. Bottom left (A-scan echo trace at tissue sensitivity): reflectivity around 100%. Bottom right (Radio Frequency signal): retina and tumour are visibly separated. Regular internal structure, wide spaced echoes and slow decay slope are shown.

choroidal excavation or acoustic vacuole was also seen but acoustic shadowing was never demonstrated. The RF signal was checked every time but was not always as regular as may be seen in the picture. To measure the prominence both the A-scans 'linear' and 'special amplification' were used. In the absence of any other evidence an average sound velocity of 1660 m/sec was chosen (Trier and Otto 1981). In the two cases followed-up for longer period, the tumours had nearly doubled in thickness, while the two belonging to the Sturge-Weber Syndome showed a slight but manifest increase in comparison to the others.

DIFFERENTIAL DIAGNOSIS

When the differential diagnosis is to be made choroidal melanoma must first be excluded (Mazzeo, et al., 1981). Looking at the pathognomonic echopattern of choroidal malignant melanoma, a low internal reflectivity is almost invariably present and most easily appreciated on the RF signal. There are however many other lesions which show very high internal reflectivity, the most important being metastatic tumours (Mazzeo, et al., 1980). Carcinomatous metastases also show many other clinical features similar to C.H.: location at the posterior pole, flat or slightly domed shape, very low serous detachment in the early stages, yellow or white in colour.

It must be emphasized that metastases are more frequent than haemangiomas. When therefore a very high reflective solid mass is discovered at the posterior pole in a patient with no history of neoplasma, the first differential diagnosis is either haemangioma or metastasis. In this case indocyanine green infrared colour angiography can differentiate the two lesions. Conditions which can echographically simulate a C.H. have been found mostly in sub-retinal organization (such as longstanding haemorrages), disciform degeneration and inflammatory forms characterized by oedema (Rochels and Reis 1980).

One of the most puzzling cases dealt with was that of a young woman with an exudative choroiditis. In this case a very high reflective solid area and a localized shallow serous retinal detachment were seen at the posterior pole. The lesion disappeared completely within a month (Mazzeo, et al., 1981). The follow-up of a case is extremely important in order to evaluate the behaviour of a lesion and so clarify the diagnosis.

CONCLUSIONS

Although Goes and Benozzi (1981) describe C.H. showing medium reflectivity, very high reflectivity seems to be the pathognomic feature of this kind of neoplasm.

In the literature melanomas or metastases are often reported as having atypical structures and atypical reflectivities thus creating problems in their differential diagnosis. No case report has been found dealing with C.H. showing low reflectivity. In case no. 8, which was the flattest lesion, the echography was very uncertain, a follow-up would have helped us. Cardiogreen[R] angiography however solved the problem. For this reason indocyanine green colour infrared angiography seems to be the most reliable technique to confirm the clinical and echographic diagnosis of choroidal cavernous haemangioma.

REFERENCES

Bonnet, M.: 'Cavernous hemangioma of the choroid. Clinical review of 10 cases.' Ophthalmologica (Basel), 182: 113 (1981).

Bonnet, M. and Habozit, F.: 'Diagnostic angiographique des tumeurs primitives de la choroide'. Conf. Lyon. Ophtal. 130: 1 (1976).

Bonnet, M., Habozit, F., Tuaillon, J., and Magnard, G.: 'Fait anatomoclinique: hemangiome caverneux de la choroide'. Arch. Ophtal (Paris) 36: 703 (1976).

Bronson, N. R., Fisher, Y. L., Pickering, N. C., and Trayner, E. M.: 'Ophthalmic B-scan ultrasonography for the clinician'. Inc. Westport Conn., Intercontinental Publication (1976).

Buffet, J. M., Bacin, F., and Audouin, M. C.: 'Une technique simple d'angiographie en infra rouge au vert d'indocyanine'. Bul. Soc. Ophtal. France 79: 209 (1979).

Coleman, D. J., Dallow, R. L., and Smith, M. E.: 'A combined system of contact A-scan and B-scan'. In: Ophthalmic Ultrasonography: Comparative techniques. (R. L. Dallow ed.) Int. Ophthal. Clin. 19, 211 (1979).
Coleman, D. J., Lizzi, F. L. and Jack, R. L.: 'Ultrasonography of the eye and orbit'. Philadelphia, Lea and Febiger (1977).
Giovannini, A.: 'Diagnostica angiografica dell'emangioma della coroide'. Proceedings LXI S.O.I. Cong. Roma, 1981. In press.
Goes, F., and Benozzi, J.: 'Ultrasonographic aid in the diagnosis of choroidal hemangioma'. Bull. Soc. Belge Ophthal. 191: 97 (1980).
Mazzeo, V., Ravalli, L., and Pistocchi, F.: 'L'ecografia nei tumori del bulbo oculare'. In; Clinica dei tumori dell'occhio e dell'orbita (A. Rossi ed.). Relazione al LXI Cong. S.O.I., Roma (1981) p. 187.
Mazzeo, V., Scorrano, R., Gallenga, P. E., and Rossi, A.: 'Echographic pattern of choroidal metastatic tumors'. In: Current Concepts on Ultrasound. (P. E. Gallenga, P. Zulli, C. Colagrande, F. A. Catizone eds.) Roma, Novappia (1980) p. 67.
Ossoinig, K. C.: 'Quantitative echography. The bases of tissue differentiation'. J. Clin. Ultrasound 2: 33 (1974).
Ossoinig, K. C., Bigar, F., and Kaefring, S. L.: 'Malignant melanoma of the choroid and ciliary body. A differential diagnosis in clinical echography. In: Ultrasonography in Ophthalmology (J. Francois, F. Goes eds.) Ophthal. no. 83, Basel, Karger, (1975), p. 141.
Poujol, J.: 'Echographie en ophthalmologie'. Paris, Masson (1981).
Rochels, R., and Reis, G.: 'Echographie bei skleritis posterior'. Klin. MBL. Augenheilk. 177: 611 (1980).
Trier, H. G., and Otto, K. J.: 'The accuracy of A-Mode echography in the evaluation of intraocular tumor growth'. In: Recent Advances in Ultrasound Diagnosis 3. (A. Kurjak, A. Kratochwil eds.). Amsterdam, Excerpta Medica (1981) p. 506.

Authors' address:
Clinica Oculistica
Università di Ferrara
corso Giovecca, 203
I-44100 Ferrara
Italy

LOW REFLECTIVE CHOROIDAL METASTATIC TUMOR

D. DORO, G. B. MOSCHINI and P. CARDIN
(Padua, Italy)

ABSTRACT

Standardised A-scan echography of a non-pigmented choroidal tumor showed low reflective subretinal echoes in the left eye of a 49 year-old man. The retinal fluorescein angiography was inconclusive. The highly positive CEA titre prompted us to extensive radiological and biopsy investigations which revealed a primary follicular thyroid carcinoma and multiple brain and bone metastases. The post mortem histological examination of the choroidal metastases showed a tissue pattern which accounts for the melanoma-like acoustic reflectivity.

To our knowledge only seventeen cases of orbital and ocular metastases from thyroid carcinoma have been reported in the literature; the orbit and the ocular globe were respectively involved in 11 and 4 cases (Ferry et al., 1974, Offret et al., 1979, Slamovits et al., 1979); in two cases the exact location was not specified clearly. As carcinomas generally metastatise to the globe, the preferential orbital rather than ocular spread can be explained by a probable lymphatic channel connection between the thyroid and the orbit as suggested by Kriss (1970) in a study using radioisotope lymphography.

We thought it interesting to report a case of choroidal metastasis from thyroid carcinoma not only because of its rarity but mostly because of the peculiar echographic and histological characteristics.

CASE REPORT

A 49 year-old man who complained of a dark veil in front of the right eye visited our Clinic in Padua in August 1980. Funduscopy showed a white-yellow choroidal mass, six dioptres high extending from the posterior pole to the equatorial upper temporal region (about three disc diameters) surrounded by an area of gray orange-dotted retina. No other pathological features were found in the right eye and the examination of the left eye was negative. Visual acuity was 20/20 in both eyes. Standardised A-scan echography of the right eye (Kretztechnik 7200 MA equipment, 8 MHz probe) at

Hillman, J.S./Le May, M.M. (eds.) Ophthalmic Ultrasonography

ISBN 978-94-009-7280-3

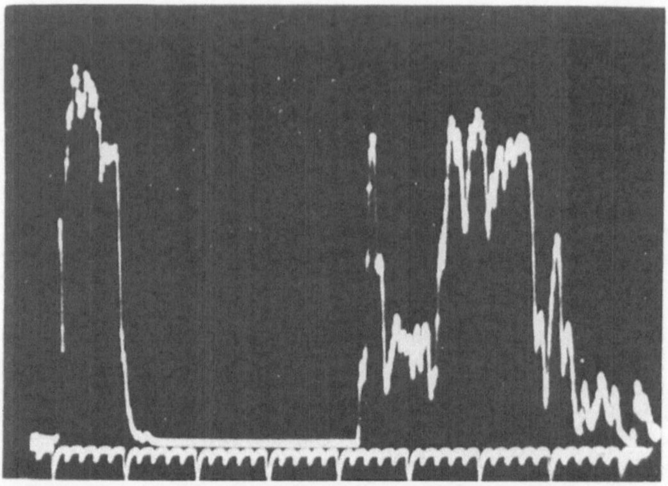

Fig. 1. Echogram showing low reflective subretinal echoes, very low angle kappa and choroidal infiltration.

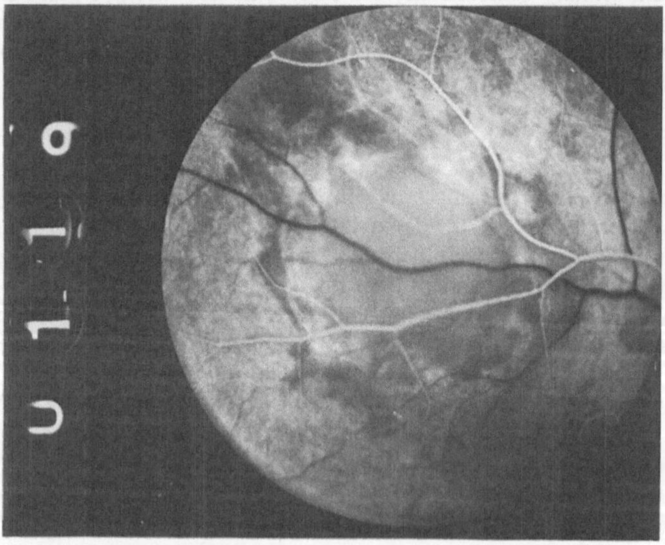

Fig. 2. Patched hyperfluorescence at the periphery of the choroidal mass and central hypofluorescent area in the arterial phase of retinal fluorescein angiography.

tissue sensitivity revealed low reflective (about 35% of the scleral spike) subretinal echoes, very low angle kappa, minimal spontaneous movements and choroidal infiltration (Figure 1).

Retinal fluorescein angiography of the choroidal mass in the arterial phase showed a patched hyperfluorescence at the periphery of the lesion whereas an area of hypofluorescence was evident centrally (Figure 2).

An increase of fluorescence was noted in the arterovenous phase even if areas of hypofluorescence persisted. In the late phases the whole lesion was homogeneously hyperfluorescent. The retinal vessel overlying the tumor were not dilated or tortuous and pathological vessels could not be detected in any phase.

As both A-scan echography and fluorescein angiography were not conclusive as to the diagnosis of either metastatic tumor or non-pigmented choroidal melanoma, an assay of the plasma carcinoembryonic antigen (CEA) level was performed. A value of 160 ng/ml was found (normal value 0–5 ng/ml). This highly positive value was highly suggestive of a metastatic problem (Smith 1979).

Routine blood tests and chest X rays were normal, digestive tract X rays demonstrated duodenal ulcer.

Neurological and urological examinations were negative. Surprisingly brain CAT Scan showed large high-low density areas in the right frontal, parietal and cerebellar lobe, and a low density area in the left upper parietal lobe. These findings were consistent with metastatic lesions.

A biopsy of the right thyroid lobe, which showed increased uptake of ^{131}I led us to the histological diagnosis of primitive follicular thyroid carcinoma.

In the following months the choroidal mass extended as far as the macula and the optic disk and eventually a serous retinal detachment around the tumor appeared. The examination of the right eye had always been negative.

This patient also had multiple bone metastases, and died seven months after the choroidal mass was found. The post-mortem histological examination of the right eye showed a thickened choroid which was diffusely infiltrated (Figure 3); in some areas typical follicolar structure could be observed; the tumor cells were large and polygonal and had giant nuclei; the interstitial tissue was scanty.

These findings enabled us to make a diagnosis of choroidal metastasis from poorly differentiated thyroid carcinoma.

DISCUSSION

The dense cellular distribution and the lack of fibrous bands in the choroidal metastasis account for the low reflectivity subretinal echoes. It is well known that as a rule choroidal metastasis from carcinoma are characterized by irregular high reflective (above 80%) echoes due to broad fibrous septa infiltrating tumor cells. However we must stress that densely cellular choroidal metastasis characterized by low reflective echoes were found in seminoma (Freyler et al., 1977), lung microcytoma (Verbeek 1980) and uterine carcinoma (Mazzeo et al., 1980). It is evident that low reflective choroidal metastases echographically mimic choroidal melanoma.

As Ossoinig pointed out recently (1982), the echographic features of choroidal melanoma 'type one' are low reflectivity and very low or no angle kappa. So in our patient it was just not possible to make a clear diagnosis by A-scan technique but a CEA titre assay and extensive radiological and biopsy investigation were needed to solve our clinical case.

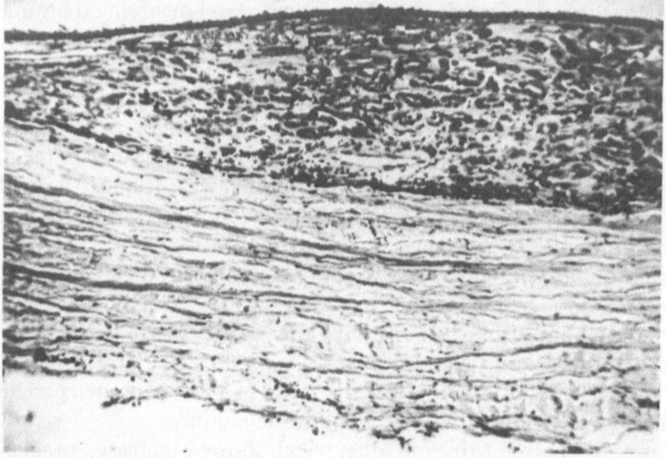

Fig. 3. Histological section (hematoxylin-eosin X40) of sclera and choroid diffusely infiltrated by tumor cells. The interstitial tissue is scanty.

REFERENCES

Ferry, A. P., and Font, R. L.: Carcinoma metastatic to the eye and orbit. A clinicopathologic study of 227 cases. Arch. Ophthalmol. 92: 276 (1974).

Freyler, H., Egerer, I.: Ecography and Histological Studies in Various Eye Conditions. Arch. Ophthalmol. 95: 1387 (1977).

Kriss, J. P.: Radioisotopic thyroidolymphography in patients with Graves' disease. J. of Clin. Endocrinology and Metabolism. 31: 315 (1970).

Ossoinig, K. C.: Ultrasound Investigation in Ophthalmology 5th int. Course Erice Italy (1982).

Mazzeo V., Scorrano, R., Gallenga, P. E., Rossi, A.: Echographic pattern of choroidal metastatic tumors. In Current Concepts on Ultrasound. Gallenga P. E. et al., eds. Roma, Novappia (1980).

Offret, H., Saraux, H., Dhermy, P., Fichet, D., Jagueux, M.: Metastase oculaire révélatrice d'un microcarcinome du corps thyroide. J. Fr. Ophthalmol. 2: 445 (1979).

Slamovits, T. L., Mondzelewski, J. P., Kennerdell, J. S.: Thyroid carcinoma metastatic to the globe. Br. J. Ophthalmol. 63: 169 (1979).

Smith, J. L.: Neuro-ophthalmolgy Focus 1980 Masson Publ. New York, U.S.A. (1979).

Verbeek, A. M.: A choroidal oat-cell metastasis mimicking choroidal melanoma. In Ultrasonography in Ophthalmology. V. M. Thijssen and A. M. Verbeek eds., Docum. Ophthal. Proc. Series, Vol. 29; Junk, Den Haag (1981).

Author's address:
Istituto di Clinica Oculistica dell'
Universita di Padova
1-35100
Padova
Italy

ULTRASONOGRAPHIC AID IN THE DIAGNOSIS OF RETINOBLASTOMA-SUSPECTED CASES

F. GOES
(Ghent, Belgium)

We recently examined two cases of leucocoria which posed a difficult differential diagnosis problem. The first case, Manuela B, a 2.5 year old girl was referred because of an extensive retinal detachment in the temporal region of the left eye. The retina had a yellowish colour and some small minor vascular anomalies could be seen at the edge of the lesion. Ultrasound examination demonstrated a retinal detachment echo in the temporal (4.0 μs) and inferior region (6.0 μs) (Figure 1). This echo was followed by a 2.0 μs broad complex with a high reflectivity (50–85%), a rather irregular structure and low absorption. A repeat examination two months later showed a more elevated retinal detachment (8 μs). Neither ultrasound nor fluorography could exclude the possibility of a tumour mass and CT examination remained negative. Enucleation was performed because of blindness of the eye and enlargement of the detachment. Histology showed an exudative retinopathy (Coat's disease) with a subretinal mass composed of fibrous tissue, cholesterol, macrophages, giant cells and a large amount of calcification.

The second case, Bonnie M, a 4 month old boy, was referred with the diagnosis of disseminated histiocytosis X. In addition to the typical skin lesions this child also had thrombocytopenia and hepatomegaly. Fundoscopy showed the presence of a whitish mass in the temporal region of the right eye. Ultrasound examination showed in the temporal and posterior region a solid elevated mass of 8 μs to 11 μs with very high reflectivity (75–100%) and irregularly spaced higher and lower spikes over the first 5 μs and lower internal reflectivity (25%) over the prescleral zone (Figure 2). The eye length was normal and symmetrical being 17.95 mm right eye and 18.20 mm left eye. With this ultrasound picture a diagnosis of retinoblastoma was made, although the association of retinoblastoma and histiocytosis disease is unknown in the literature. The histology confirmed the diagnosis.

In leucocoria one must always exclude the possibility of retinoblastoma which is the most common intraocular malignancy, occuring in approximately 1:15000 live births (Shields and Augsburger, 1981) and one must try to separate these tumours from the congenital malformations (P.H.P.V., Coats' disease and Reese dysplasia), from retrolental fibroplasia and from inflammatory (pseudoglioma) and traumatic (haemorrhage) conditions. We had occasion to examine 122 leucocoria eyes in 83 children. Tumour was

Hillman, J.S./Le May, M.M. (eds.) Ophthalmic Ultrasonography

ISBN 978-94-009-7280-3

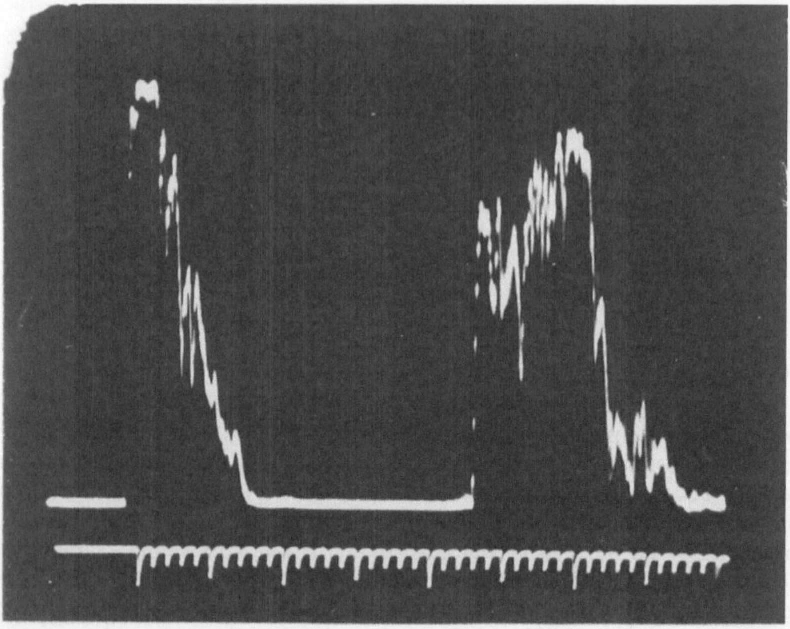

Fig. 1. A scan ultrasound of clinical suspected lesion.

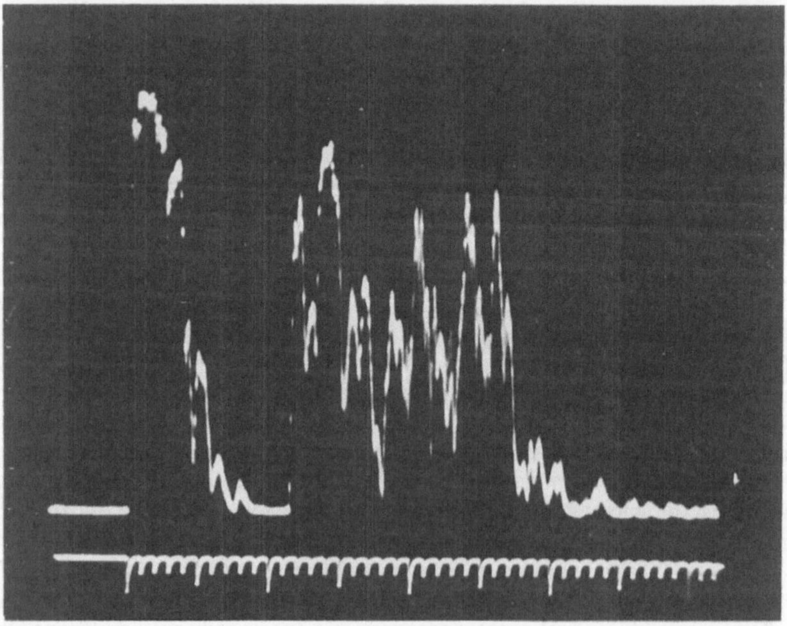

Fig. 2. A Scan of retinoblastoma in Abt. letterer-Siwe disease demonstrating high reflectivity.

Table 1. Clinical associated signs in 33 congenital cataract cases

Congenital Cataract		
N:	33 eyes – 21 children	
Age:	1 month – 10 year	
		< 6 months 57%
		< 1 year 67%
E.R.G.:	normal 65%	
	absent 17%	
Cornea:	≤ 9 24%	
	≤ 10 52%	
Length:	↓↓ 18%	
	↓ 21%	
	nl 45%	
	↑ 15%	

Table 2. Clinical associated signs in 34 R.L.F. cases

Retrolental Fibroplasia (R.L.F.)		
34 eyes:	19 children	
bilateral:	89%	
prematurity:	2–4 months	
weight:	< 1.5 kg in > 70%	
age:	(4 months–9 years)	
		< 6 months 11/6
		< 1 year 17/9
E.R.G.:	absent 21/26	
Cornea;	≤ 10 26%	
	≤ 11 50%	
Length:	↓ 62%	
	(↓↓ in 34%)	
	↑ 15%	

suspected in all cases and all were examined by A-Scan ultrasound. This paper reviews our findings.

Congenital cataract was diagnosed in 33 eyes of 21 children (12 bilateral cases) and the clinical findings are summarised in Table 1. A shortening of the eye was present in 13 cases (39%) and significant microcornea was present in more than half (52%) of these eyes. Ultrasound examination rarely revealed abnormalities in the posterior eye segment (2 retinal detachment, 1 minor vitreous alteration).

Retrolental fibroplasia was diagnosed in 34 eyes of 19 children (Table 2) and nine children (17 cases) were younger than one year. Microcornea was present in 50% of the cases and eye-length was reduced in 62%. Anterior synechiae were present in 9 eyes and ERG was absent in most of the cases. Ultrasound showed a retinal detachment in 21 eyes (62%). Also there was important vitreous organisation (> 40% reflectivity) in 9 eyes and less pronounced alteration in 25 eyes (Figure 3).

Retinoblastoma was present in 19 children in whom we examined 29 eyes. Ten children (16 cases) were younger than one year. Eye-length measurement

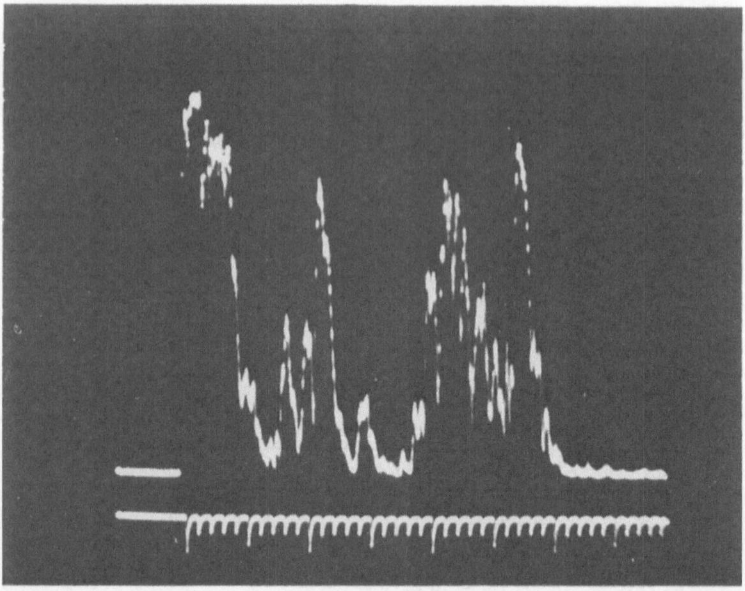

Fig. 3. A Scan of RLF showing retinal detachment and medium-amplitude vitreous organization.

was carried out in 10 eyes and the axial length was found to be normal in 8 eyes, slightly elongated (1 mm) in one and slightly shortened (1.5 mm) in another case. The eye-length differences between the affected and the non-affected eye in the same subject ranged from − 0.8 mm to + 1.1 mm. Ultrasound examination always showed typical high internal reflectivity of the tumour (75 and 100%) but it could not differentiate between tumour and pseudotumour in one case. Important signs of necrosis and calcification were nearly always present. The intraocular tension was usually normal and microcornea was never present.

The ultrasound picture of a retinoblastoma depends on the internal structure and on the extent of the tumour. According to Ossoinig et al., (1981) two criteria remain valid for the ultrasound diagnosis:

(1) *Extremely high reflectivity* (80–100% spike height at tissue sensitivity) caused by calcium deposits producing a chain of high overloaded spikes (Figure 4).

(2) *Shadowing* caused by the sound absorption of the tumour so that the underlying scleral wall echo becomes much weaker (Figure 5).

These two main criteria are only valuable in case of significant calcification which is present in over 90% of retinoblastomas (Ossoinig et al., 1981). Neither rosette formation nor vessels in the tumour can produce such strong echoes. This was confirmed by Basta et al., (1981) who found a close correlation between tumour calcification and A-scan reflectivity and it is also illustrated in our series where we had at least absence of rosette formation in 3 cases but where the same typical high reflective echogram was obtained.

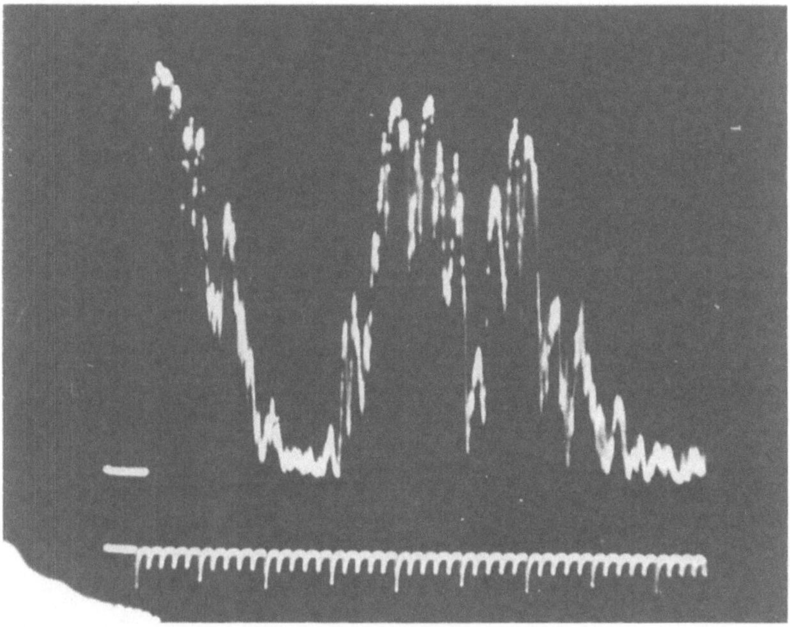

Fig. 4. A Scan of retinoblastoma showing high internal reflectivity in a tumour without rosette formation.

We also had one retinoblastoma case with very low internal reflectivity in which the histological report stressed the absence of tumour calcification. According to former authors (Gitter et al., 1968, Rochels and Nover, 1979) microphthalmia almost certainly excludes a retinoblastoma but Ossoinig et al., (1981) mentioned shortening of the eye-length of 1 mm in most of their retinoblastoma cases. In our series we found no statistically important eye-length changes but we feel that more biometric studies should be done in leucocoria cases.

Persistent hyperplastic primary vitreous was diagnosed in 9 unilateral cases. The patients age at the time of examination was always less than 12 months (Table 3) and a normal corneal diameter was only present in two cases. Eyelength measurements were performed in 8 eyes and an important shortening (− 3 mm) was found in two eyes and moderate shortening (− 0.5 and − 1.5 mm) was found in a further two eyes. Ultrasound examination showed the presence of a retinal detachment in 3 cases: in addition, some low-amplitude echoes could be demonstrated in the anterior vitreous (Figure 6).

Inflammatory pseudoglioma was diagnosed in 8 unilateral cases. Only 2 children were younger than one year (Table 4). Microcornea was present in only one case (10.5 mm) and the eye-length was normal in 5 cases and reduced in one case (− 2.3 mm). The anterior segment was shortened in 3 cases

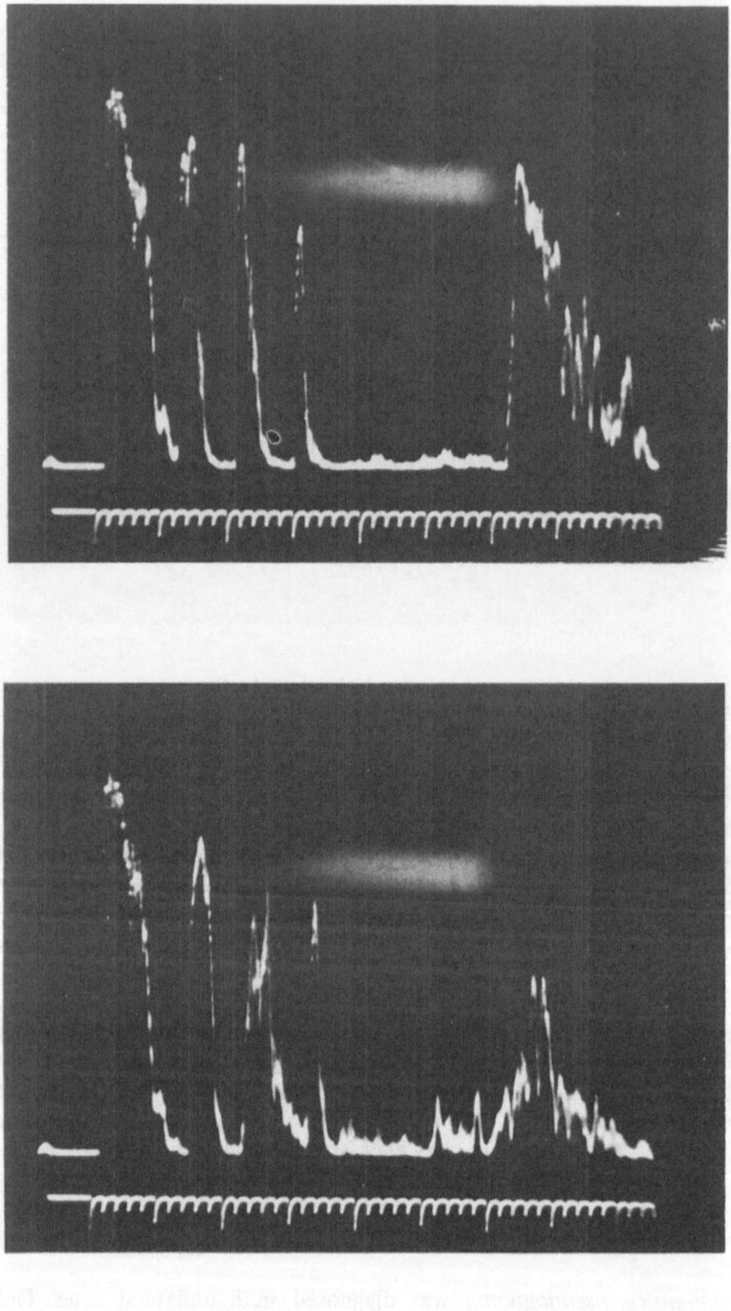

Fig. 5. A Scan of retinoblastoma showing sound absorption demonstrating lower scleral wall-echo in affected (down) eye compared to normal axial echogram in the non-affected eye.

Table 3. Clinical associated signs in P.H.P.V.

Persistant Hyperplastic Primary Vitreous (P.H.P.V.)		
	N	: 9 eyes
Age	< 6 months	: 55%
	< 1 year	: 100%
Cornea	⩽ 9	: 11%
	⩽ 10	: 33%
	nl	: 22%
E.R.G.	nl	: 11%
	absent	: 44%
L	: ↑	: 1/8
	↓	: 4/8

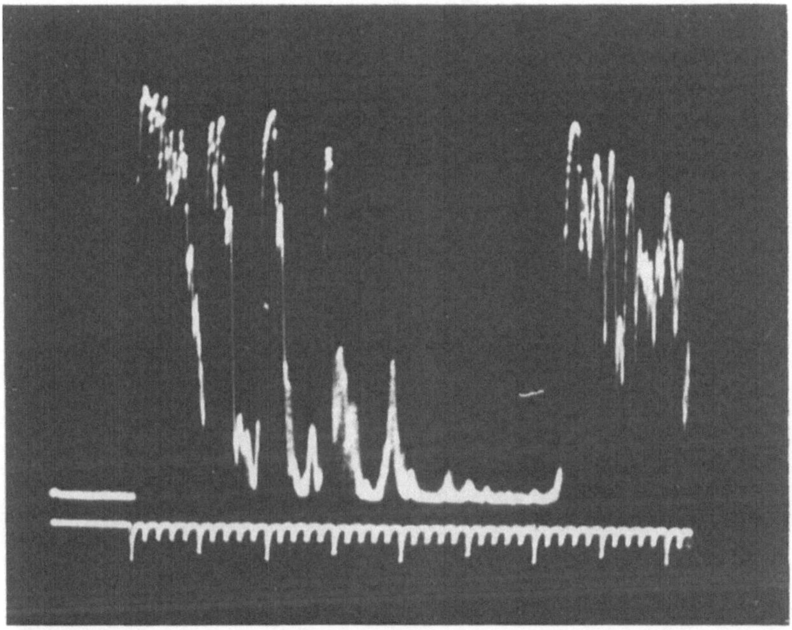

Fig. 6. A Scan of P.H.P.V. showing low-amplitude retrolental echoes.

(twice ↓↓) and in all cases posterior synechiae were present. Ultrasonography demonstrated a retinal detachment in 3 cases. Vitreous alterations were always present but in most cases they were not marked (< 25% reflectivity) and in 2 eyes the vitreous was nearly normal.

Coats' disease was diagnosed in 5 unilateral cases and only one child was younger than one year (Table 5). A normal eye-length was measured in 2 cases. Ultrasonography demonstrated an extensive retinal detachment in all cases. The reflectivity was always lower than in the retinoblastoma cases and it was maximally 50% at tissue sensitivity (2 cases 20%) (Figure 7). In one

Table 4. Clinical associated signs in 8 pseudogliòma cases

Pseudoglioma		
	N: 8 eyes	
Age:	< 6 months	12.5%
	< 1 year	25%
Inflammation:		100% synechie
Tension:	↓	38%
E.R.G.:	absent	50%
	nl	25%
L	nl	5/8
	↓	1/8
Cornea:	nl	50%
	↓	12.5%
L :	nl	5/8
	↓	1/8

Table 5. Clinical associated signs in Coat's disease

Coat's Disease
5 Unilateral
Age 1–15 years: 1/5 < 1 year
Cornea: ↑ 1/5
L: nl 2/2
Elevation: (7–18 μs) always > 7

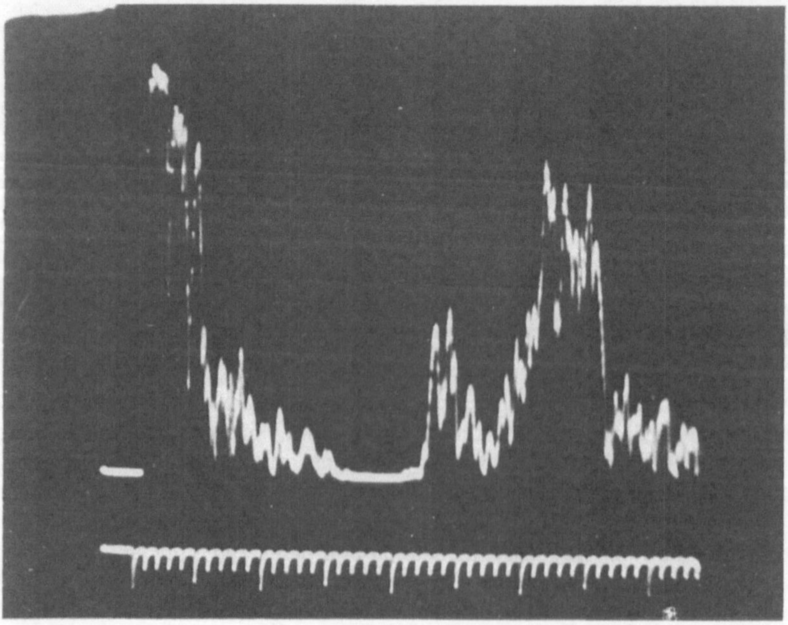

Fig. 7. A Scan of Coat's disease; medium to low-amplitude echoes in the posterior pole.

case (Manuela B) the differential diagnosis with retinoblastoma was not possible and this case was characterised by significant calcification. Coats' disease usually causes multiple echo spikes and if the reflectivity is high enough it can be confused with a tumour. Generally, however, the spikes are lower than in retinoblastoma.

Reese Dysplasia was diagnosed bilaterally in 2 children (ages 2 and 6 months). In all of these the anterior chamber was absent and posterior synechiae were present. Normal eye length measurements were obtained and ultrasound examinations demonstrated a retinal detachment with medium vitreous organisation. We found retinoblastoma responsible for 29 of the 122 leucocoria cases (24%) and it was present in 23% of 83 children with uni- or bilateral leucocoria (Table 6). With the help of A-scan ultrasonography we could diagnose retinoblastoma in 28 of the 29 histologically confirmed cases. In the whole leucocoria series of 122 cases we could not differentiate in 2 cases: one retinoblastoma case and one case of Coates' disease with significant calcification. It is, however, a fact that in many cases the anamnesis (retrolental fibroplasia), the associated clinical signs (microcornea in congenital malformations, posterior synechiae in inflammatory pseudoglioma) and the fundoscopic appearance of the lesion give sufficient information to orientate the diagnosis. We must remain aware of the fact that ultrasound alone cannot always differentiate between tumour and the pseudotumour group.

When we consider the associated clinical signs in our leucocoria series, we see that the *uni- or bilateral* presence of the leucocoria does not give helpful information because retinoblastoma was bilateral in 53% of our 19 affected children. P.H.P.V., Coats' disease and Pseudoglioma were always unilateral and R.L.F. was nearly always bilateral (89%) (Table 7). Concerning the *time-onset* of the disease, P.H.P.V. and Reese dysplasia always became manifest before the age of 2 years, while pseudoglioma and Coats' disease usually became manifest at a much greater age. Retinoblastoma manifested itself between the age of 3 months and 4 years (Table 8). Retinoblastoma cases usually had no history of ocular abnormalities at birth and they developed leucocoria or strabismus between 6 months and 2 years of age. *Eye-length* measurements remained nearly unchanged in retinoblastoma and in Coats' disease while some degree of microphthalmia was present in 62% of the R.L.F. cases, in 50% of the P.H.P.V. cases and in 39% of the congenital cataract cases (Table 9). As far as the *corneal diameter* is concerned, 50% of the Congenital cataract and Reese dysplasia, 33% of the P.H.P.V. and 26% of the R.L.F. cases had significant microcornea ($\leqslant$ 10 mm), while microcornea was never noticed in the retinoblastoma series (Table 10). *Electroretinography* was abnormal in a high percentage of P.H.P.V. (86%), R.L.F. (81%) and pseudoglioma (75%) cases but also present in 60% of the retinoblastoma cases. *Posterior synechiae* were typically present in all our pseudoglioma cases while in R.L.F. cases anterior synechiae were found in 27% and important changes of the anterior eye segment were frequently (44%) found.

In conclusion. A-scan ultrasound can differentiate many aetiologies of leucocoria and *typical* retinoblastomas with significant calcification can be diagnosed without error. However, we should not forget that A-scan

Table 6. Etiology of leucocoria in 122 eyes of 83 affected children

Leucocoria: 83 children	eyes	patients
Congenital cataract	33	21 = 25%
R.L.F.	34	19 = 23%
Retinoblastoma	29	19 = 23%
P.H.P.V.	9	9 = 11%
Pseudoglioma	8	8 = 10%
Coats' disease	5	5 = 6%
Reese dysplasia	4	2 = 2%
	122	83

Table 7. Unilateral or bilateral presence of the leucocoria in the 83 affected children

Leucocoria: 83 children	Unilateral	Bilateral
Congenital cataract	43%	57%
R.L.F.	11%	89%
Retinoblastoma	47%	53%
P.H.P.V.	100%	0%
Pseudoglioma	100%	0%
Coats'	100%	
Reese	0%	100%

Table 8. Age of the children at the moment of diagnosis

Age of Leucocoria: 83 children	< 6 months	< 1 year
Congenital cataract	57%	67%
R.L.F.	31%	47%
Retinoblastoma	16%	53%
P.H.P.V.	55%	100%
Pseudoglioma	12.5%	25%
Coats'	0%	20%
Reese	100%	100%

Table 9. Eye length changes in 122 leucocoria cases

Eye Length	↓↓	↓	nl	↑
Congenital cataract	18%	21%		15%
R.L.F.		62%		15%
Retinoblastoma		10%	80%	10%
P.H.P.V.		50%		12.5%
Pseudoglioma		12.5%		
Coats			100%	
Reese			100%	

Table 10. Corneal diameter in 122 leucoria cases

Corneal diameter: Leucocoria: 122 eyes			
	⩽ 9	⩽ 10	⩾ 12
Congenital cataract	24%	52%	
R.L.F.	3%	26%	20%
Retinoblastoma	normal		
P.H.P.V.	11%	33%	
Pseudoglioma		12.5%	
Coats'			20%
Reese		50%	

ultrasound alone is not sufficient in all cases and that careful consideration of the associated clinical signs and the use of other technical examinations (LDH plasma/aqueous ratio (Kabak and Romano, 1975): cytologic examinations (Shields and Augsburger, 1981): Fluorescein angiography: Scintillography (Yanake et al., 1978): Skull X-Rays and especially C.T. scan (Ellsworth, 1978, Goldberg and Danziger, 1977, Danziger and Price, 1979 and Brant et al., 1979) may give additional valuable information.

REFERENCES

Brant, Zawadzki, M. and Enzmann, D. R.: Orbital computed tomography calcific densities of the posterior pole. J. Comput. tomography, 3, 503–505, 1979.

Danziger, A. and Price, H.: CT Findings in Retinoblastoma. Amer. Journ. of radiology, 133, 783–785, 1979.

Ellsworth, R. M.: The Management of Retinoblastoma. Jap. J. Ophthal., 22, 389–395, 1978.

Gitter, K. A., Meyer, D., White, R., Ortolan, G. and Sarin, L.K.: Ultrasonic Aid in the Evaluation of Leukokoria. Amer. J. Ophthal. 65, 190–195, 1968.

Goldberg, L. and Danziger A.: Computed Tomographic Scanning in the Management of Retinoblastoma. Amer. J. Ophthal. 84, 380–382, 1977.

Kabak, J. and Romano, P. E.: Aqueous humorlactic dehydrogienase iso-enzymes in retinoblastoma. Br. J. Ophthal., 59, 268–269, 1975.

Ossoinig, K. C., Cennamo, G., Green, R. L. and Wyer, N. L.: Echographic results in the diagnosis of retinoblastoma. Doc. Ophthal. Proc. Series, Vol. 29, ed. J. M. Thyssen and A. M. Verbeeck, Dr. W. Junk Publishers, The Hague, 103–107, 1981.

Rochels, R. and Nover, A.: Echographische Differential diagnose der Leukokorie im Kindesalter. Ophthalmologica, Basel, 178, 215–219, 1979.

Shields, J. and Augsburger, J.: Current Approaches to the Diagnosis and Management of Retinoblastoma. Survey of Ophthal., 25, 347–371, 1981.

Tanaka, H., Minami, M. and Tsuchida, T.: Co-Bleomycin Scintigraphy for Diagnosis of Retinoblastoma. Jpn. J. Ophthal. 22, 412–419, 1978.

Author's address:
Ophthalmological Clinic
University of Ghent
Ghent
Belgium

CONTACT ULTRASONOGRAPHY IN THE EVALUATION OF DIABETIC TRACTION RETINAL DETACHMENT ASSOCIATED WITH VITREOUS HAEMORRHAGE

Y. L. FISHER
(New York, USA)

In ultrasonographic evaluation of the diabetic patient with dense vitreous haemorrhage, the recognition and localization of traction retinal detachment is critical in management since one major indication for immediate vitreous surgical intervention is detachment of the macula. Vitreo-retinal drawings created from contact combined A- and B-mode ultrasound scans are useful in the preoperative evaluation of diabetic patients with opaque media. In this study the overall accuracy in 79 cases assessed at surgery was found to be 93%. Errors resulted from the resolution limitations of the ultrasound equipment and from proliferative disease simulating detached macular retina.

Author's address:
Manhattan Eye, Ear and Throat Hospital
210 E. 64th Street
New York City
NY 10021
U.S.A.

Hillman, J.S./Le May, M.M. (eds.) Ophthalmic Ultrasonography

ISBN 978-94-009-7280-3

EVALUATION OF QUANTITATIVE ECHOGRAPHY FOR INTRAOCULAR MEMBRANE-LIKE LESIONS

A. SAWADA, Y. MASUYAMA, Y. BABA and Y. OYAMADA
(Miyazaki, Japan)

ABSTRACT

Quantitative echography using Kretztechnik 7200 MA was performed on 291 eyes with membrane-like lesions in the vitreous in the Department of Ophthalmology, Miyazaki Medical College Hospital. Differentiation between retinal detachment and proliferative changes with high reflectivity is difficult in some cases. A system of image storage is expected to give better resolution.

INTRODUCTION

Modern ultrasonic diagnosis is required not only to detect abnormality, but also to evaluate more precisely its nature. As one of responses to these demands, quantitative echography which can differentiate tissues from others on the basis of ultrasonic tissue characterization, has developed.

Since the introduction of vitreous surgery, differential diagnosis of membrane-like structures in the vitreous has been indispensable. Many criteria for membrane-like structures in A-scan and B-scan echography have been reported. In A-scan echography, reflectivity of tissues to the ultrasonic beam ranks above insertion, mobility, surface, thickness, extension and others. It is quantitative echography to evaluate the reflectivity of tissues more precisely.

Many works on quantitative echography have been published. Recently a series of works by Ossoinig and his collaborators have become a standard of A-scan quantitative echography. Quantitative echography, either intraocular or orbital, is divided into two parts. The one is for the inner reflectivity of space-occupying lesions and the other is for the surface reflectivity of point- or membrane-like lesions. It is the aim of the present study to evaluate quantitative echography for membrane-like lesions in the vitreous.

METHODS AND SUBJECTS

We use Kretztechnik 7200 MA as an A-scan instrument and Bronson-Turner Ophthalmic B-Scan as a B-scan instrument in the Department of Ophthalmology, Miyazaki Medical College Hospital.

Hillman, J.S./Le May, M.M. (eds.) Ophthalmic Ultrasonography

ISBN 978-94-009-7280-3

Table 1. Results of quantitative echography for membrane-like structures in the vitreous in Miyazaki Medical College

Diagnosis	Eyes	Δ dB in quantitative echography			
		⩽ 10	11–15	16–19	20 ⩽
Retinal Detachment	163	69	72	15	4
Vitreous Membrane Formation	78	0	2	11	65
Proliferative Diabetic Retinopathy	50	10	13	12	15
Total	291	79	90	38	84

Table 2. Retinal Detachment (RD) with Δ dB of 20 or more

Case	Δ dB	Diagnosis
1	20	RD secondary to uveitis
2	21	Longstanding RD with vitreous hemorrhage in aortic syndrome
3	22	RD secondary to uveitis
4	22	Longstanding RD with an intraocular iron foreign body left for years

Quantitative echography was performed with Kretztechnik 7200 MA as Ossoinig and others have described. The difference (Δ dB) in the dB setting between sensitivity of the tissue in question and that of the sclera was used for determination of reflectivity of the tissue to the ultrasonic beam. Ossoinig and others divided the values of Δ dB into three gradings, (1) Δ dB ⩽ 15 (detached retina), (2) 16 ⩽ Δ dB ⩽ 19 (borderline) and (3) 20 ⩽ Δ dB (membrane). For the detailed analysis, we have divided the values of Δ dB into four gradings, namely, (1) Δ dB ⩽ 10, (2) 11 ⩽ Δ dB ⩽ 15, (3) 16 ⩽ Δ dB ⩽ 19 and (4) 20 ⩽ Δ dB.

RESULTS

A-scan quantitative echography was performed in 163 eyes with retinal detachment, 78 eyes with vitreous membrane formation and 50 eyes with proliferative diabetic retinopathy. The results of A-scan quantitative echography in these 291 eyes are shown in Table 1.

Of 163 eyes with retinal detachment, 144 eyes (88.3%) showed a difference in reflectivity (Δ dB of less than 15, which was regarded as the detached retina. Fifteen eyes (9.2%) showed a difference of 16–19.

It is the matter to be noticed that the remaining four eyes (2.5%) showed a difference of 20 or more. Table 2 shows cases of retinal detachment with the value of Δ dB of 20 or more. The values in all cases were less than 22, which

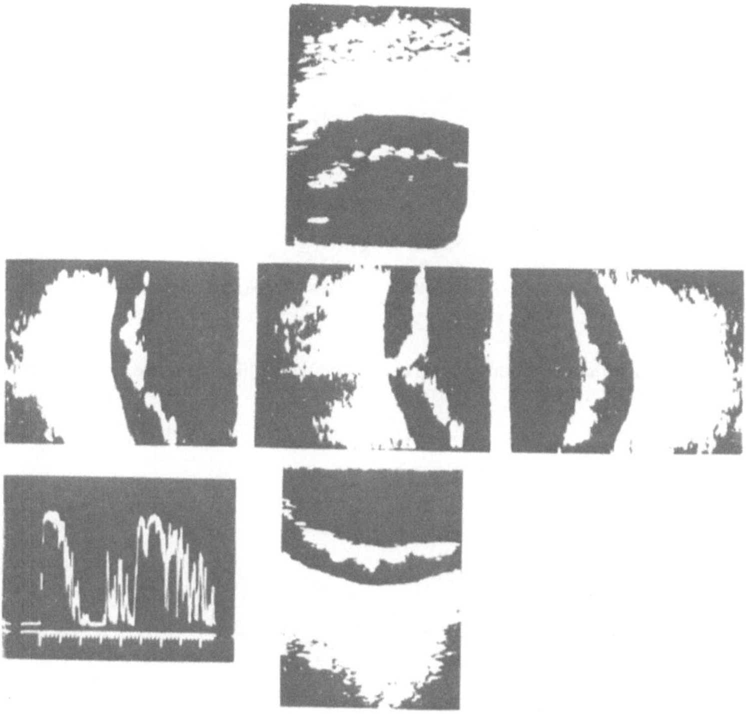

Fig. 1. Retinal detachment (MPP) secondary to uveitis after blunt trauma. In B-scan echograms a dense shrunken membraneous structure covered the whole fundus and was connected with the optic disc. In an A-scan echogram spikes from the folded membrane were medium to low in reflectivity.

were very slightly over the limit of detached retina in Ossoinig's criteria. Two cases were longstanding retinal detachment with vitreous hemorrhage in aortic arch syndrome and with intraocular iron foreign body retained for more than two years. The other two were retinal detachment secondary to uveitis. The third case was a 16-year-old boy. Retinal detachment followed by severe uveitis was found at the first consultation two months after blunt trauma. The ophthalmoscopic findings agreed with that of MPP. The ERG was extinguished. In B-scan echograms (Figure 1), a dense shrunken membraneous structure, massive in part, was stiffly connected to the fundus around the optic disc. In an A-scan echogram, spikes from the folded membrane were medium to low.

Echographic findings in MPP are controversial, because ultrasonic reflectivity in MPP is not definite. In another case with MPP, a bridge was formed in the temporal part of the right fundus, of which ΔdB was 3 (Figure 2). In the third case with MPP the reflectivity was quite weak ($\Delta dB = 19$) (Figure 3).

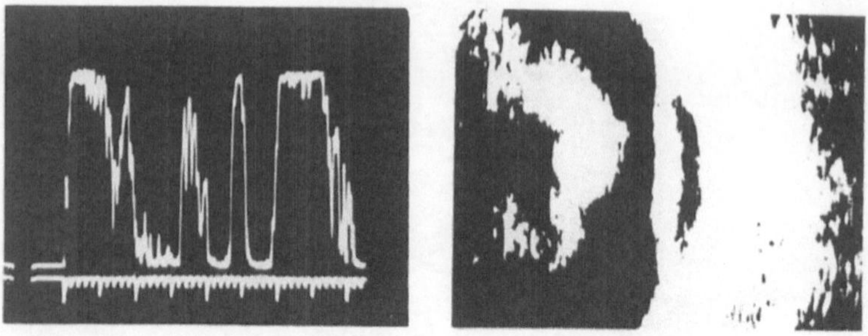

Fig. 2. A- and B-scan echograms in a case of MPP. A highly reflective bridge formation was displayed. Delta dB was 3.

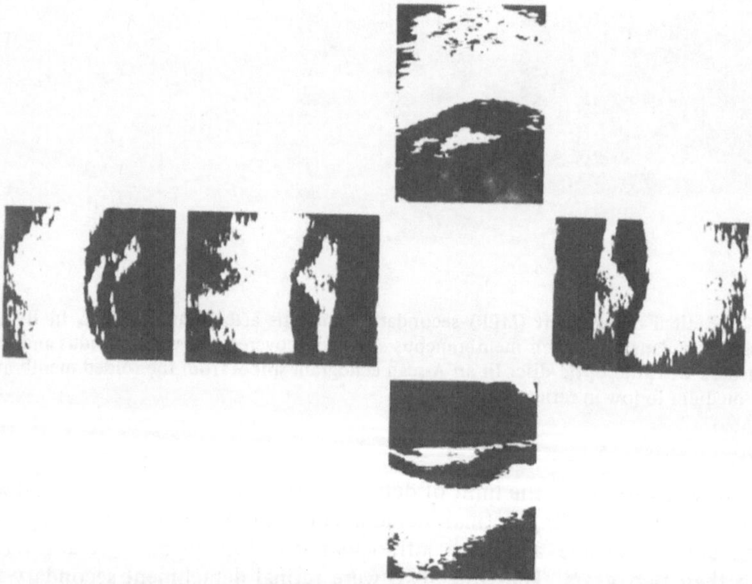

Fig. 3. B-scan echograms in a case of MPP, in which the reflectivity was so weak (Δ dB = 20).

Of 78 eyes with vitreous membrane formation, two eyes (2.6%) showed a difference in reflectivity of 12 and 14, which fell under the grading compatible with retinal detachment. Figure 4 is the echograms in a 76-year-old woman, in which Δ dB was 14. The characteristic feature common to these two cases was hemorrhage which occurred into the space between the detached vitreous and the retina. The posterior surface of detached vitreous, to which blood cells stuck fast, formed very strong source of echoes. In these cases the membraneous surface was split and hemorrhage spread diffusely in the course of time.

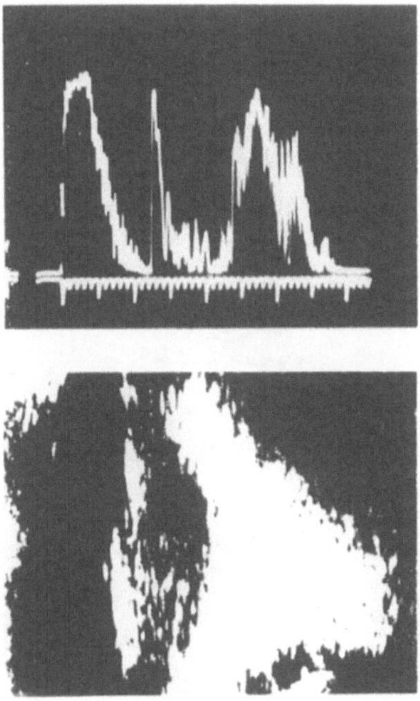

Fig. 4. A- and B-scan echograms in vitreous hemorrhage with vitreous detachment. A strong spike from the posterior surface of detached vitreous was noted.

Of 50 eyes with proliferative retinopathy, 23 eyes (46.0%) showed a difference of less than 15, which was regarded as retinal detachment. Twelve eyes (24.0%) were on the borderline and 15 eyes (30.0%) showed a difference of 20 or more. Fifty cases of proliferative diabetic retinopathy were almost equally distributed into four groups with different grading of reflectivity. Echograms with low reflectivity (Δ dB = 27) are shown in Figure 5. Echograms with high reflectivity (Δ dB = 10) are shown in Figure 6. In such cases of proliferative diabetic retinopathy with high reflectivity, no discrimination from retinal detachment could be found, provided it was based only on the reflectivity. Other findings should be taken into consideration.

When vitreous hemorrhage occurred in eyes with proliferative diabetic retinopathy, echographic findings become complicated. Figure 7 shows changes of reflectivity after vitreous hemorrhage between the detached vitreous and the retina.

Quantitative echography was used as an indicator, which showed changes in the internal quality of tissues. For example, Figure 8 shows changes of Δ dB in the treatment of subconjunctival injection of urokinase in the right eye of 55-year-old woman. At the initial consultation a tumor protruding from the fundus was found. In a short time findings of subretinal hemorrhage were manifested. Later on vitreous hemorrhage occurred. With the subconjunctival injection of urokinase the reflectivity of dense material in the vitreous decreased.

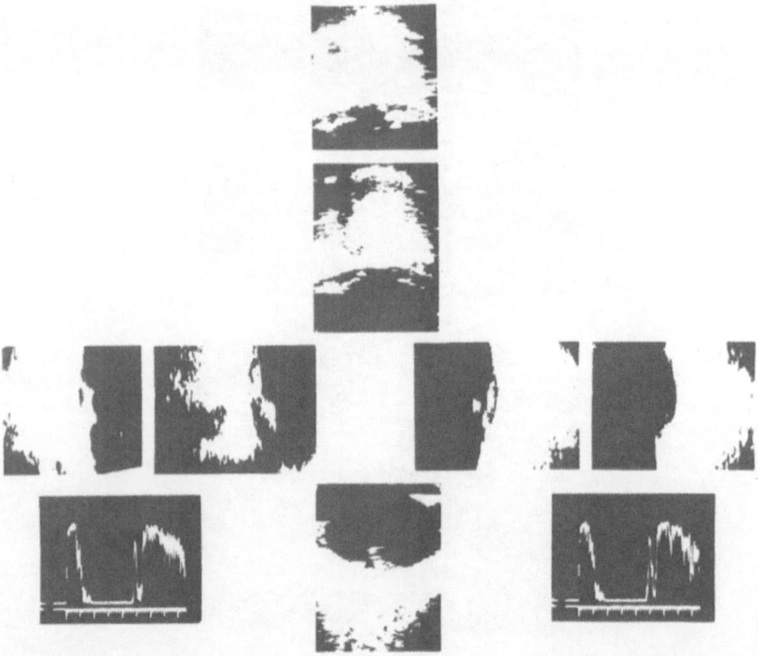

Fig. 5. A- and B-scan echograms in diabetic retinopathy, in which the reflectivity of membrane-like structures was very low (Δ dB = 27).

In some cases it was possible to follow up the values of Δ dB to decide the time of vitreous surgery. In a 66-year-old man with dense material in the vitreous was found. After the values of Δ dB increased from 17 to 26 and the vitreous membrane formation was confirmed, vitreous surgery was performed with satisfactory results.

On the other hand, it has been expected that quantitative echography can predict the development of retinal detachment in eyes with dense vitreous membrane or with proliferative diabetic retinopathy. In our experience, the prediction is possible in some cases. Figure 9 shows the echograms before and after the development of retinal detachment in a cases of proliferative diabetic retinopathy. The values of Δ dB changed from 18 to 13. In another case with dense vitreous hemorrhage the value of Δ dB changed from 17 to 10 with the development of retinal detachment.

DISCUSSION

The results of A-scan quantitative echography in 291 eyes with membrane-like structures in the vitreous were analyzed. In almost all cases the results coincided with Ossoinig's criteria except for a few points. Ultrasonic reflectivity varied in longstanding retinal detachment and in proliferative diabetic

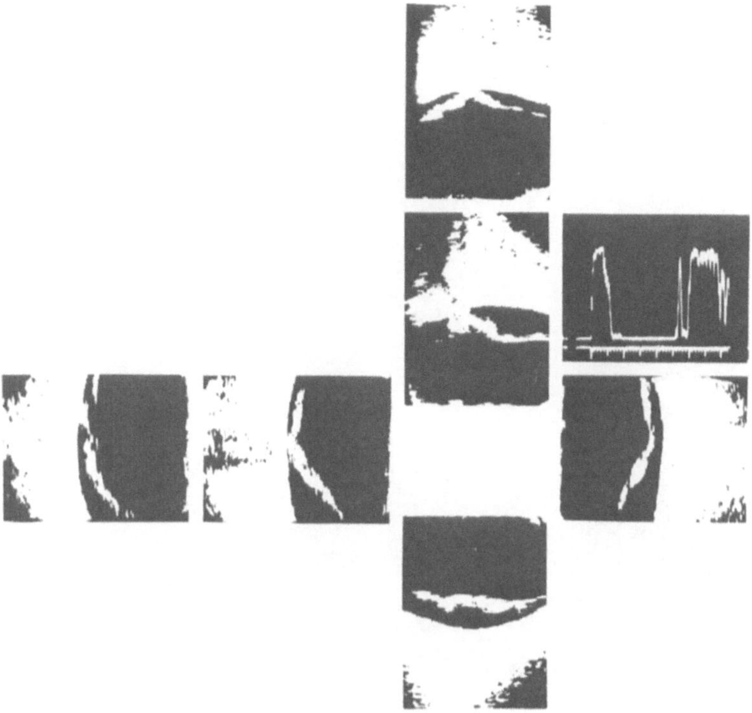

Fig. 6. A- and B-scan echograms in diabetic retinopathy, in which the reflectivity of membrane-like structures was so high (Δ dB = 10).

retinopathy. Although the relation between the duration and the acoustic characteristics of the detached retina is controversial (Hillman and Ridgway, 1975, Freyler and Egerer, 1977, Coleman et al., 1977, Takeuchi, 1981), proliferative changes in the tissues in question can modify the reflective character of the tissue to the ultrasonic beam. Also low reflectivity in some secondary retinal detachment was explained on histopathological findings that the detached retina in uveitis was swollen and cellular components in the detached retina were relatively decreased (Sawada et al., 1979).

High reflectivity in vitreous hemorrhage with vitreous detachment is also explainable from histopathological findings.

Another important thing in A-scan quantitative echography is precise control of ultrasonic beam direction. The present combination of A-scan with B-scan is still unsatisfactory in this respect. B-scan-guided (or isometrically guided) A-scan quantitative echography would be preferable. In a newly developed equipment, TRISCAN, the image in A-, B- and D-mode (isometric display) can be stopped and stored at any point at will. After that quantitative and vector analysis can be performed in detail. With equipment

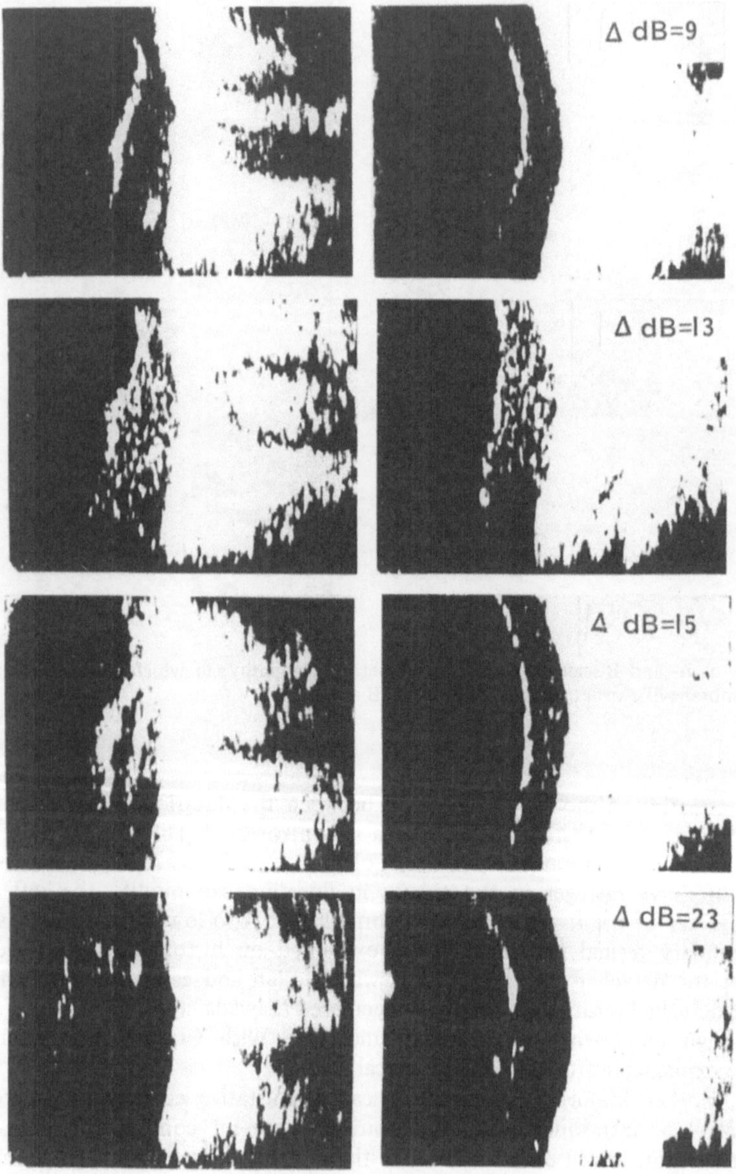

Fig. 7. Changes of Δ dB after vitreous hemorrhage between the detached vitreous and the retina in preceding diabetic retinopathy.

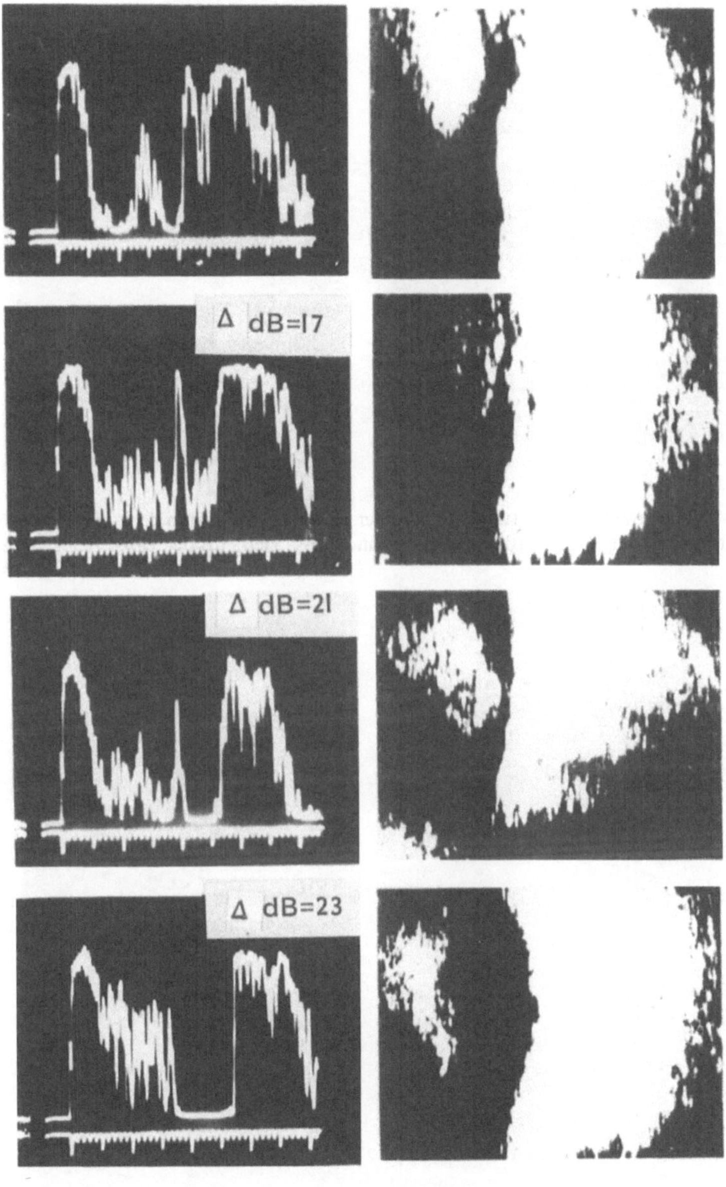

Fig. 8. Changes of Δ dB in the treatment of subconjunctival injection of urokinase in subretinal – vitreous hemorrhage.

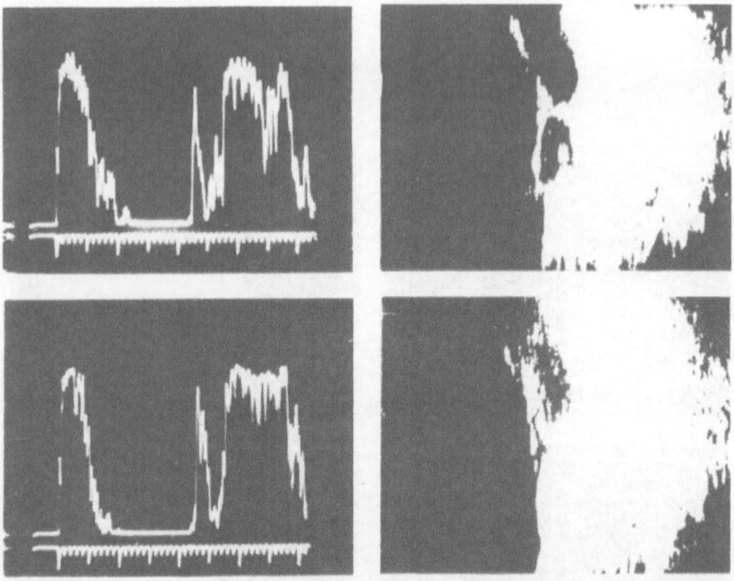

Fig. 9. Echograms before (upper) and after (lower) the development of retinal detachment in preceding proliferative diabetic retinopathy. Delta dB decreased from 18 to 13.

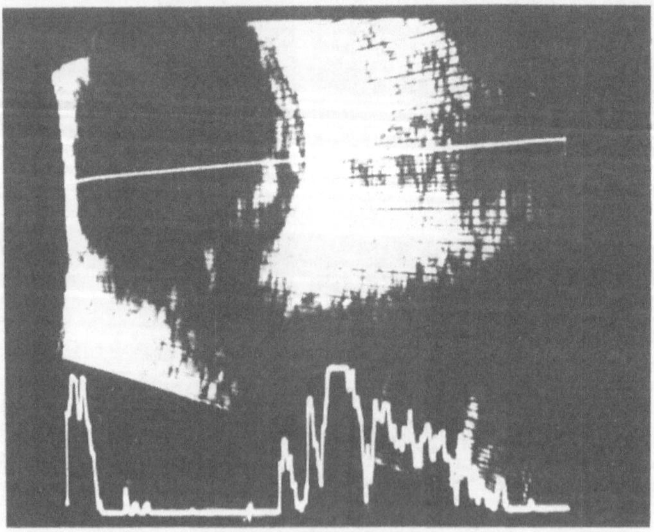

Fig. 10. Echograms in B-CV mode (combination of B and A) in a case of vitreous hemorrhage (TRISCAN).

of this kind, precise application of the ultrasonic beam is possible. Therefore, quantitative echography is expected to be sharper and more diagnostic. Figure 10 shows an echogram in B-CV mode (combination of B and A) in a case of vitreous hemorrhage. Delta dB was 23 in A-scan quantitiative echography using 40 dB logarithmic amplification. We have just started to use the equipment. The results will be reported on the next occasion.

CONCLUSION

The results of A-scan quantitative echography in 291 cases of membrane-like lesions in the vitreous were analyzed. Ultrasonic reflectivity was not constant in longstanding retinal detachment and in proliferative diabetic retinopathy. Correlation with histopathological findings should be studied. For precise control of ultrasonic beam direction, the facilities of stopping and storing of images were required. TRISCAN could meet the requirement.

REFERENCES

Coleman, D. J., Lizzi, F. L. and Jack, R. L.: Ultrasonography of the eye and orbit, p. 200, Lea & Febiger, Philadelphia, 1977.

Freyler, H. and Egerer, I.: Echography and histological studies in various eye conditions. Arch. Ophthalmol. 1977, 95: 1387–1394.

Hillman, J. S. and Ridgway, A. E. A.: Retinoschisis and retinal detachment, an ultrasonic comparison, Ultrasonography in ophthalmology (ed. by Francois, J. and Geos, F.) p. 63–67, S. Karger, Basel, 1975.

Ossoinig, K. C., Frazier, S. L., Watzke, R. C. and Diamond, J. G.: Combined A-scan and B-scan echography as a diagnostic aid for vitreoretinal surgery, New and controversial aspects of vitreoretinal surgery (ed. by McPherson, A.) p. 106–125, C. V. Mosby, St. Louis, 1977.

Sawada, A., Inahara, M., Masuyama, Y. and Baba, Y.: Significance of quantitative echography in membrane-like structures in the vitreous. Acta Soc. Ophthalmol. Jpn. 83: 1434–1444, 1979.

Sawada, A., Inahara, M. and Kogakura, H.: Experimental interpretation of vitreous echograms, XXIII Concilium Ophthalmologicum, Kyoto, 1978 (ed. by Shimizu, K. and Oosterhuis, A.) p. 1575–1577, Excerpta Medica, Amsterdam, 1979.

Sawada, A., Masuyama, Y. and Baba, Y.: Relation between histologic findings and echographic characteristics in experimental longstanding retinal detachment, Diagnostica Ultrasonica in Ophthalmologia (ed. Gernet, H.) p. 103–106, R. A. Rey, Münster, 1979.

Takeuchi, S.: Ultrasonic diagnosis of massive periretinal proliferation, Ultrasonography in Ophthalmology (ed. Thijssen, J. M. & Verbeek, A. M.) p. 13–20, Dr W. Junk, The Hague, 1981.

Authors' address:
Department of Ophthalmology,
Miyazaki Medical College
Kihara, Kiyotake, Miyazaki 889–16
Japan

ERRORS IN DIAGNOSTIC ULTRASOUND. A CRITICAL REVIEW OF 68 PATIENTS UNDERGOING DIAGNOSTIC ULTRASOUND BEFORE VITRECTOMY

R. MÜLLER-BREITENKAMP, H. G. TRIER, B. VÖLKER and U. MESTER
(Bonn, W. Germany)

Preopererative diagnostic ultrasound is increasingly important with respect to vitreal surgery. Because of opaque media, echography is often the only method to evaluate the indication and prognosis for the operation. It needs experience to be capable of interpreting the echogram, and a close co-operation between surgeon and echographist is necessary to improve the accuracy of interpretation by comparing the echographic diagnosis with the real condition retrospectively.

A pars plana vitrectomy was done on 120 patients. In 52 cases visual preoperative examination was possible, for the other 68 eyes the echographic examination only was diagnostically relevant. In Table 1 a survey of the basic diseases of all cases is given. The examination was carried out by means of A-mode equipment KRETZ 7200 MA, and by contact B-mode equipment SONOMETRICS Ocuscan 400.

The evaluation of the A- and B-mode examination was based on:

1. Topography,
2. Reflectivity,
3. Kinetic behaviour.

of the echo-giving intraocular structures.

The mobility of structures, or their rigidity, respectively, was evaluated, and the point of attachment of haemorrhages, and membranes topographically defined. For A-mode examination a 'region of interest' was chosen (Ossoinig et al., 1977, Kerman and Coleman, 1978).

For the sake of the patient, vitreous surgery was carried out in each case, even if no greater advantage was to be expected with regard to the echographic findings.

In 60 cases, the echographic diagnosis was confirmed by the vitrectomy, while in the residual 8 eyes, the echographic interpretation was only partly true, or erroneous.

Some of these misinterpreted cases shall be discussed, because they represent certain typical errors.

Case 1 (Figure 1): 37 year old patient; vitreal haemorrhage for 18 days after traumatic contusion of the eyeball on both sides. As a comparison, a characteristic echogram of choroidal detachment, and another one of retinal

Hillman, J.S./Le May, M.M. (eds.) Ophthalmic Ultrasonography
© 1983, Dr W. Junk Publishers, The Hague/Boston/Lancaster
ISBN 978-94-009-7280-3

Table 1. Vitrectomy cases: clinical conditions

1.	Diabetic retinopathy	45
2.	Ocular trauma	36
3.	Retinal detachment	21
4.	Ocular inflammation	4
5.	Vitreous hemorrhage of unknown genesis	14
		120
	Visual preoperative examination possible	52
	Diagnosis by ultrasound only	68

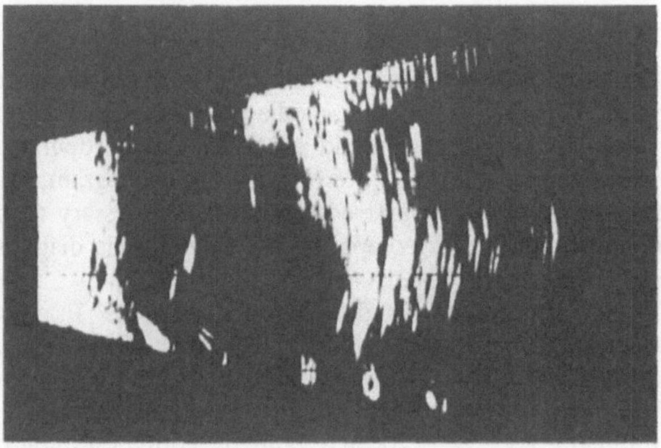

Fig. 1. Arterial vitreous bleeding. Convex membrane structures, obtuse-angled detached on the eye wall. US-diagnosis: Tentative choroidal detachment.

detachment is given (Figure 2 and 3). The comparison of these three echograms clearly shows that in certain cases it can be extremely difficult to distinguish between choroidal and retinal detachment, if the membrane configuration is echographically similar; in particular, if the membrane cannot be characterized by its dynamic behaviour.

With regard to the case mentioned the membrane, preoperatively interpreted to be a choroidal detachment, turned out on vitrectomy to be in fact a bullous retinal detachment.

Case 2 (Figure 4): 50 year old patient; vitreal haemorrhage of unclear origin, of 3 months duration.

In Figure 5 the similar echogram of a confirmed funnel-shaped retinal detachment with vitreal haemorrhage is demonstrated.

A comparable image is shown in Figure 6. This, however is a case of vitreal haemorrhage with vitreal detachment but without retinal detachment. In this case also, the preoperative interpretation was erroneous: there was no retinal detachment, only a dense vitreal haemorrhage.

With regard to the similar structures shown by B-mode display, the

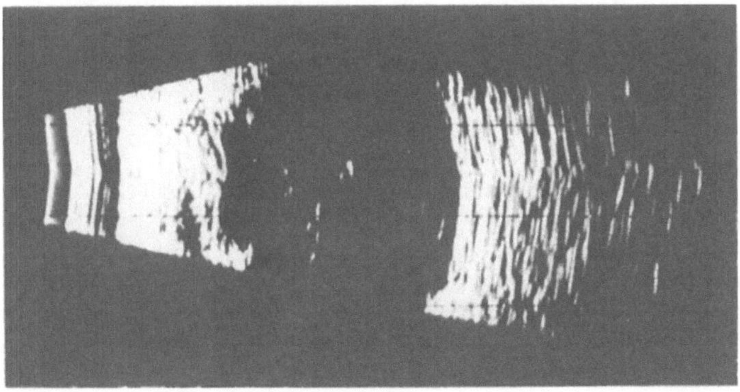

Fig. 2. Typical convex, obtuse-angled membrane structures in a confirmed choroidal detachment.

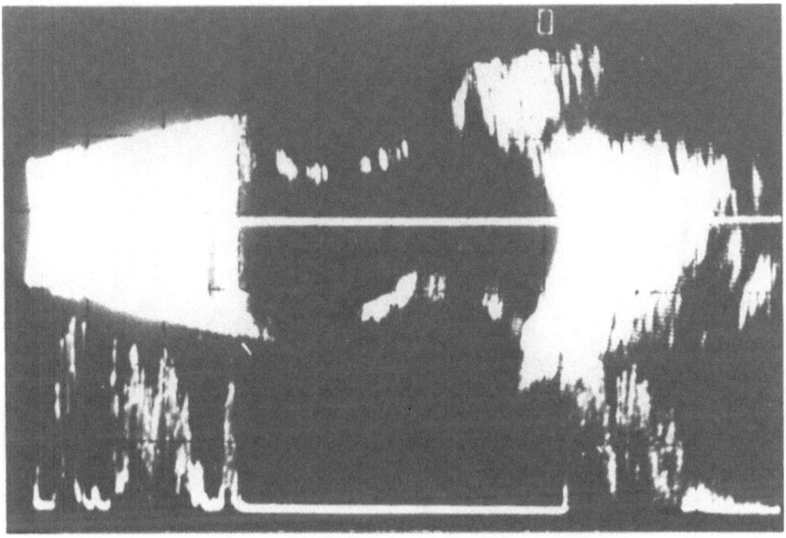

Fig. 3. Convex membrane structure in a confirmed retinal detachment.

difficulties of echographic differentiation in such cases are obvious. Here too, no further differentiation by A-mode techniques was obtainable.

Case 3 (Figure 7): 25 year old woman; diabetes mellitus, with dense vitreal haemorrhage.

In comparison Figure 8: In this case mainly the low reflectivity of the membrane in A-mode display was the cause of misinterpretation for 3 experienced echographists. Vitrectomy revealed that the retina, echographically described as being attached, was in fact detached in the shape of a severe MPP detachment.

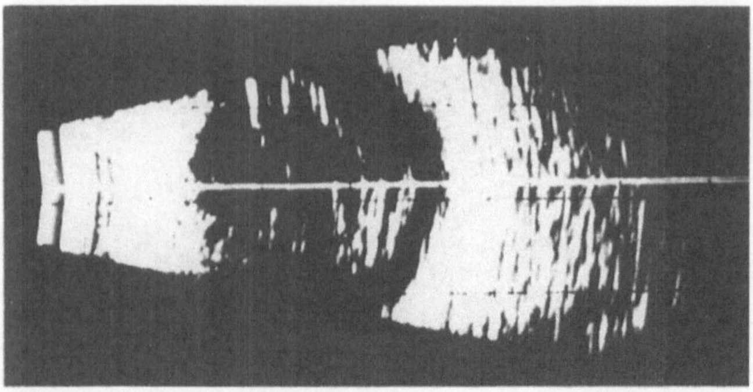

Fig. 4. Approximately cone-shaped echo-dense lesion in the central vitreous body with sharp borders to the echo-free space in front of the ocular wall; echographically attachment to the optic disc. US-diagnosis: Central vitreal haemorrhage with funnel-shaped retinal detachment.

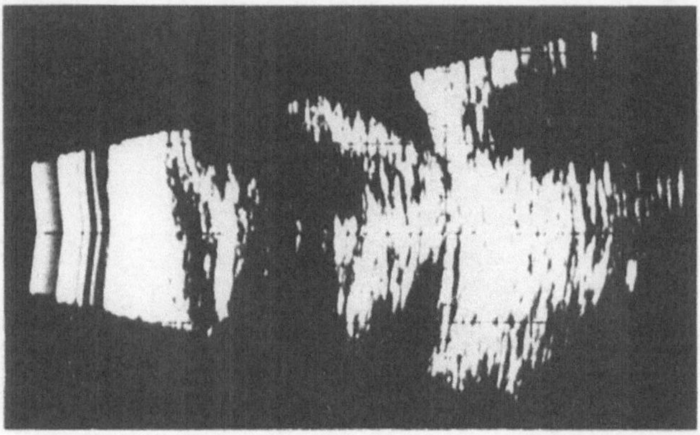

Fig. 5. Funnel-shaped membrane attached to the optic disc. US-Diagnosis: Diabetic vitreal haemorrhage and retinal detachment.

Similar comparisons were formerly reported by several authors (Jack et al., 1974, Bigar et al., 1977, Fuller et al., 1977, Ossoinig et al., 1977, Takeuchi et al., 1979, Jerneld et al., 1980, Findi 1981, Shimizu and Minoda, 1981, Mester et al., 1981). The results demonstrated that there is not always conformity to be expected. In 3–15% misinterpretation with respect to vitreoretinal lesions was found by Jack et al., 1974, Ossoinig et al., 1977, Bigar et al., 1977, Fuller et al., 1977, and Jerneld et al., 1980.

In our experience, better results in difficult cases are sometimes achievable by video-recording, thus enabling repeatable and thorough observation and comparison of the dynamic behaviour of intraocular membranes.

In many cases sound absorbing structures are present in front of the lesion examined. Then, quantitative A-scan evaluation of vitreal membranes reflectivity has to be carried out rather in comparison to the sclera (Ossoinig,

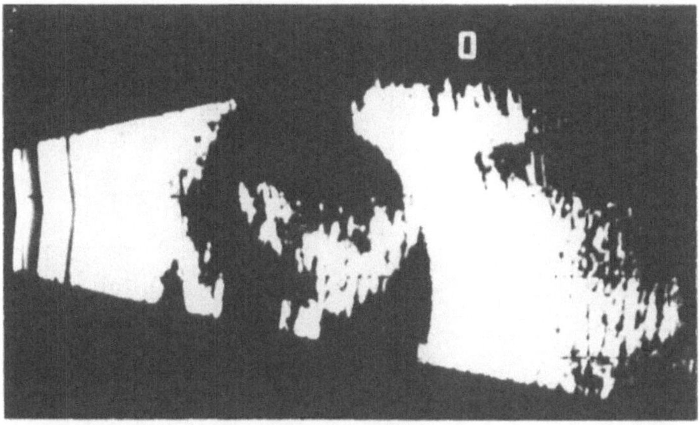

Fig. 6. Dense echo-giving structures in the posterior vitreal area with sharply defined margin and attachment to the optic disc. Confirmed diagnosis: organized vitreal haemorrhage with posterior vitreal detachment.

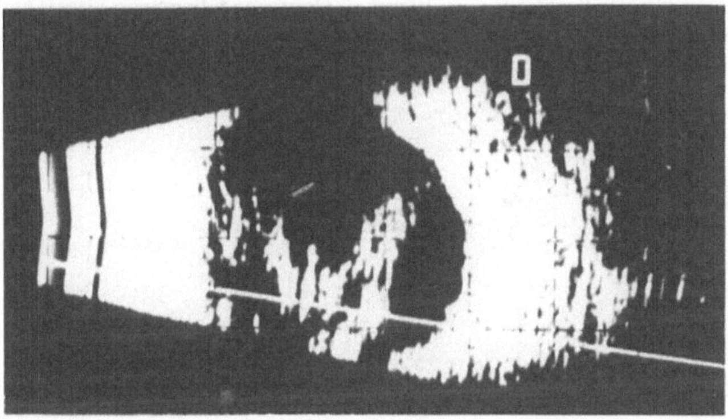

Fig. 7. Dense twisted membrane with faint attachment to the ocular wall. US-diagnosis: Vitreal haemorrhage, retinal detachment unlikely.

1979), than to a standard reflector. Nevertheless, the diagnosis may remain uncertain. From the cases discussed it may be deduced that an indirect approach to discover a retinal detachment would be very welcome. An indirect approach would mean that the retina, if assumed to be detached, should be missed in the echogram of the ocular wall. For this, a meticulous differentiation of the wall echoes of the eye ball would be necessary. Unfortunately, we were not yet able to obtain reliable results in this respect by means of the KRETZ 7200 MA- and Ocuscan 400-equipment.

The main problem is the simultaneous perpendicular adjustment of the sound beam to all backwall layers. Only, if this prerequisite were fulfilled, the lack of one interface, i.e. the retina echo, could accurately be observed. The same problem is known from A-scan localization of intramural foreign bodies.

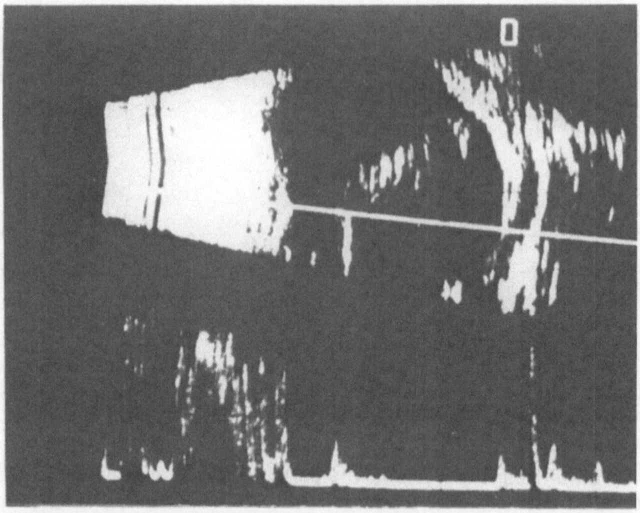

Fig. 8. **Similar vitreal alterations as in Figure 7. Confirmed diagnosis: vitreal haemorrhage in the anterior and central area, no retinal detachment.**

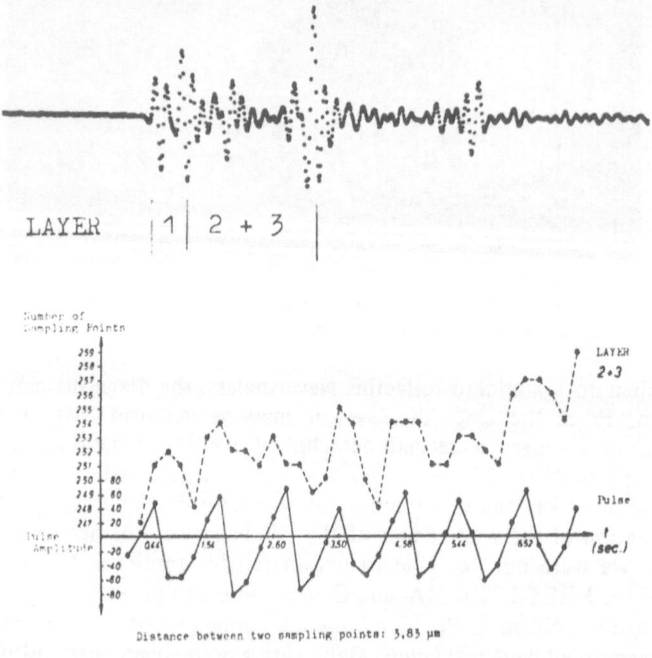

Fig. 9. **Choroidal pulsations. Top: 20 year old healthy volunteer's RF-signal of intact eyewall. Part 1 of the echotrace corresponds to retina, part 2 + 3 to the choroidal layer. Bottom: Pulsations of choroidal layer (upper curve), compared with finger pulse (bottom curve; S. Cords, Diss. Univ. Bonn, in prep.).**

It is known by experience that it often remains uncertain, whether the displayed echo corresponds to the anterior or posterior scleral surface.

The use of special RF-signals improved the resolution dramatically, but did not solve the problem of adjustment described above. Good adjustment provided, it is, however, possible to detect the retina reliably, though at present on an experimental basis only. In these cases, layer thickness and layer sequence are used as criteria.

For a broader application of the indirect approach in the diagnosis of retinal detachment the clear identification of the choroidal layer would be very useful. Experimental results have recently been obtained in our department, which demonstrated identification of the choroidal layer by its pulsations, recorded and evaluated by a computer-aided technique (Figure 9) (Trier et al., 1982).

To date, however, in diagnostic ultrasound evaluation of vitreal lesions there are some cases in which the pathology cannot be differentiated. Fortunately, this was the case in only 12% in our study.

ACKNOWLEDGEMENT

Figures 4 and 7 were taken from the paper by Mester et al. (in press).

REFERENCES

Bigar, F., Bosshard, Ch., Klöti, R. and Tschopp, H.: Combined A- and B-scan echography. Preoperative evaluation of vitrectomy patients. Proc. Xth Meet. Jules Gonin Club, Lausanne 1976, in: Turning Points in Retinal Surgery. Mod. Probl. Ophthal. 18, pp. 2–11 (Karger, Basel 1977).

Findi, M. L.: B-scan ultrasonography: the previtrectomy diabetic study. Ocutome/Fragmatome Newsletter 6, 2: 6–9 (1981).

Fuller, D. G., Laqua, H. and Machemer, R.: Triangle retinal detachment. Ultrasonic identification of massive periretinal proliferation in eyes with opaque media. Mod. Probl. Ophthal. 18: pp. 68–72 (Karger, Basel 1977).

Jack, R. L., Hutton, W. L. and Machemer, R.: Ultrasonography and vitrectomy. Amer. J. Ophthal. 78: 265–274 (1974).

Jerneld, B., Algvere, P., Singh, G.: An ultrasonographic study of diabetic vitreo-retinal disease with low visual acuity. Acta. Ophthal. 58: 193–201 (1980).

Kerman, B. M., Coleman, D. J.: B-scan ultrasonography of retinal detachments. Ann. Ophthal. 10: 903–911 (1978).

Mester, U., Völker, B., Müller-Breitenkamp, R. & Trier, H. G.: Echographie vor Vitrektomie: Kritische Auswertung nach 120 Operationen. S. Ber. 141. Vers. Verein Rhein.-Westf.. Augenärzte, Düsseldorf, Okt. 1981 (in press).

Ossoinig, K. C., Frazier, S. L., Watzke, R. C. and Diamond, J. G.: Combined A-scan and B-scan echography as a diagnostic aid for vitreoretinal surgery, in: New and Conversial Aspects of Vitreoretinal Surgery. A. McPherson, ed., pp. 106–125 (C. V. Mosby Co. St. Louis, 1977).

Ossoinig, K. C.: Standardized echography: basic principles, clinical applications, and results. Intern. Ophthal. Clin. 4: 127–211 (1979).

Shimizu, K. and Minoda, K.: Preoperative evaluation of vitreous surgery by combined study of ultrasonography and electroretinography. Jap. J. Ophthal. 25: 202–209 (1981).

Takeuchi, S., Kato, S. and Ota, Y.: The significance of ultrasonic diagnosis prior to vitreous surgery. Jap. J. Clin. Ophthal. 33: 967–973 (1979).
Trier, H. G., Decker, D., Lepper, R. D., Irion, K. M., Reuter, R., Kottow, M., Müller-Breitenkamp, R. and Otto, K. J.: Ocular tissue characterization by RF-signal analysis: Summary of the Bonn/Stuttgart in vivo study. Proc. SIDUO IX, Leeds (in press).

Authors' address:
Universitäts-Augenklinik
Sigmund-Freud Str. 25
D-5300 Bonn 1
Federal Republic of Germany

FIVE YEARS OF ULTRASONOGRAPHIC DIAGNOSIS IN COMBINED SURGERY THROUGH THE PARS PLANA

A. REIBALDI, M. DI PILATO and T. AVITABILE
(Bari, Italy)

The approach through the pars plana in vitreo-retinal surgery has widened the horizons of ocular surgery. This has been possible because of echographic examination by means of which we can know completely the vitreo-retinal situation in the finest detail.

This enables us to perform, apart from single operations like vitrectomy or lensectomy, combined operations such as lensectomy and retinal detachment, vitrectomy and removal of foreign bodies.

Our aim is the demonstration of the diagnostic reliability of echography in this particular type of pathology in the light of the report of cases examined at the University of Bari in the last 5 years.

CASE REPORT

It is made up of 121 cases of hospitalized and outpatients examined in our Clinic during the period between January 1977 and December 1981. We include in this report cases showing at least a double pathology of a surgical type operated in the Ophthalmologic Clinic of Bari. The echographic diagnosis was confirmed at surgery.

According to the pathogenesis we have divided the pathology into traumatic and non-traumatic. In the first case another subdivision has been made into contusion and perforating trauma. Among the contusion traumas we have diagnosed 15 cases where there was the coexistence of vitreous haemorrhage and retinal detachment. Among the perforating traumas, we have observed: 12 cataract with foreign body; 15 vitreous haemorrhage with retinal detachment; 31 vitreous haemorrhage with foreign body; 14 vitreous haemorrhage with retinal detachment and foreign body.

In cases of non-traumatic pathology we have observed 28 cases: 23 of these were diabetic with vitreous haemorrhage, retinal detachment and different stage of proliferans, while 5 non-diabetic showed vitreous haemorrhage with retinal detachment.

For the examination we used a Standardized Kretz 7200 A-Scan with a 8 MHz probe. All the cases considered had a follow-up of between 4 years and 6 months.

Hillman, J. S./Le May, M. M. (eds.) Ophthalmic Ultrasonography
©1983, Dr W. Junk Publishers, The Hague/Boston/Lancaster
ISBN 978-94-009-7280-3

RESULTS

In those subjects with traumatized eyes we had the following results:

- the 12 cases of cataract with foreign body were all diagnosed.
- of 6 cataracts with vitreous haemorrhage and retinal detachment only 5 were diagnosed.
- in 30 subjects with vitreous haemorrhage with retinal detachment we have had 2 negative results while in the 31 subjects with vitreous haemorrhage with foreign body only one was negative.
- with 14 cases of vitreous haemorrhage with retinal detachment and foreign body there were 12 positive results.

In those subjects with non-traumatized eyes with 23 cases of vitreous haemorrhage plus proliferans plus retinal detachment, we have been able to diagnose 21, while the 5 cases showing vitreous haemorrhage plus retinal detachment have all been diagnosed.

This data is summarized in the following tables:

Traumatized eyes (contusion and perforation)

	No cases	Postive	Negative	Reliability
Cataract + F.B.	12	12	–	100%
Cataract + vitreous haemorrhage + retinal detachment	6	5	1	83.33%
Vitreous haemorrhage + retinal detachment	30	28	2	93.33%
Vitreous haemorrhage + F.B.	31	30	1	96.77%
Vitreous haemorrhage + retinal detachment + F.B.	14	12	2	85.71%

Non-traumatized eyes

	No cases	Positive	Negative	Reliability
Vitreous haemorrhage + retinal detachment + diabetic proliferans	23	21	2	91.30%
Vitreous haemorrhage + retinal detachment	5	5	–	100%

From the data presented we can see that for traumatized eyes in 87 of the 93 cases examined (93.55%), and for non-traumatized eyes in 26 of the 28 cases (92.85%) the surgical operation confirmed our echographic diagnosis. Finally the overall reliability has been of 93.28%.

CONSIDERATIONS AND CONCLUSIONS

In the presence of such complex pathology as the coexistence of cataract and/or vitreous haemorrhage in different phases of organization and/or retinal detachment and/or foreign body it is extremely important with the help of echography to determine not only with extreme precision the various lesions present but also to consider other elements which can be indispensable for the success of the same operation.

Above all in presence of vitreous haemorrhage it is important to look for a posterior vitreous detachment apart from the other major pathology.

The presence of such pathology, in fact, will put us in a position to perform the vitrectomy faster even in absence of great membranes or vitreous tractions as the presence of a retinal break can always be possible, which, without the vitreous support can lead to a retinal detachment. In these cases it is necessary to associate a prophylactic encirclement with vitrectomy in order to contain the vitreous as far as possible.

Another extremely important point is the possibility of knowing how far the vitreous membranes are from retinal tissue. For this reason we feel it necessary for the vitreous surgeon to have as direct familiarity with echography as the ultrasonographist with the vitreous surgery.

The remarkable percentage of diagnostic reliability we have obtained in this particular type of pathology (93.28%) has significantly contributed to the reconstruction of these eyes.

We would like finally to summarize briefly the parameters supplied by echography in cases of combined intervention through the pars plana.

a. Time of execution of the same surgery

In cases of opaque media only by echography can we establish for example, the vitreous haemorrhage is going to organise or reduce, or in later observed cases if signals or pre-phthysis are appearing.

b. How to operate

Only knowing the exact vitreous-retinal situation and the final position of a foreign body is it possible to choose the instrument to introduce (vitrectomy, scissors) and where.

In conclusion, we wish to stress the importance of the associated use of A-Scan and B-Scan methods. According to our experience bi-dimensional echography gives a topographic diagnosis while standardized A-Scan gives a tissue diagnosis. In this respect we agree with Ossoinig that correct calibration of the equipment is really fundamental for this type of pathology. Finally, we cannot but confirm the extreme value of the ultrasonographic examination in this type of pathology even if we are sure it represents one of the hardest points to interpret.

SUMMARY

With the advent of the approach through the Pars Plana for the surgical management of various ocular lesions the role of ultrasonographic diagnosis in ophthalmology has recently enlarged.

In order to evaluate the usefulness, the reliability and the disadvantages of such a means of investigation in ocular pathology, with a view to performing combined surgery, such as lensectomy, with vitrectomy, with foreign body removal and retinal detachment or vitrectomy with retinal detachment and foreign body removal, the authors have studied the data derived from their five years' experience with such pathology.

The case material consists of 121 cases of hospitalized or outpatients examined at the Ultrasonography section of the Institue of Ophthalmology of Bari University.

Finally, in the light of the results obtained the role of ultrasonography in every type of combined surgery is stressed.

REFERENCES

Cardia L., Reibaldi A., Sborgia C., Santoro S.: Acquisizioni e limiti della vitrectomia via pars plana. 13° Con. S.O.M., Chieti, 29–30 giugno-1 luglio 1979

Coleman D. J.; Ultrasound in vitreous surgery. Trans. Am. Acad. Ophthal. Otolaryngol., 76:467–479, 1971

Coleman D. J., Franzen L. A.; Vitreous surgery-pre-operative evaluation and prognostic value of ultrasonic display of vitreous hemorrhage. Arch. Ophthal., 92:375–381, 1974

Coleman D. J., Jack R. L.: B-scan ultrasonography in the diagnosis and management of retinal detachment. Arch. Ophthal., 90:29–34, 1973

Coleman D. J., Lizzi F. L., Jack R. L.: Ultrasonography of the eye and orbit. Ed. Lea & Febiger – Philadelphia, 1977

Deutman A. F.: Echography and vitreous surgery. In proceedings 8th S.I.D.U.O. (Nijmegen 1980), Ed. by J. M. Thijssen and A. M. Verbeek – Dr. W. Junk Publishers – London 1981 Pp. 1–3

Gallenga P. E., Mazzeo V., Cennamo G., Reibaldi A.: Moderni aspetti semeiologici per la chirurgia del vitreo. XIII Conv. S.O.M. Chieti, 29–30 Giugno, 1 Luglio 1979.

Hassani S. N.: Real time ophthalmic ultrasonography. Ed. Springer – Verlag 1978

Ossoinig K. C., Frazier S. L., Watzke R. C. et al.: Combined A-scan and B-scan Echography as a Diagnostic Aid for vitreoretinal surgery. In A. McPherson (Ed.), Proceedings of the conference on New and Controversial Aspects of vitreoretinal surgery. (Houston, 1975). St. Louis: Mosby, 1977 Pp. 106–125

Reibaldi A., Capotorto B., Lorusso V. V.: Usefulness of echography in the vitrectomy. U.B.I.O.M.E.D. IV Visegrad (Hungary) 25–28 September 1979

Reibaldi A., Delle Noci N., Lorusso V. V.: La nostra esperienza sull'utilità dell'ecografia nella vitrectomia. 4° Cong. S. I.S.U.M. 9–10 Novembre 1979 Modena

Reibaldi A., Lorusso V.V., Giancipoli G.: Prophylaxis of retinal detachment in endovitreous hemorrhage experimentally driven.–In proceedings 8th S.I.D.U.O. (Nijmegen 1980) Ed. by J. M. Thijssen and A. M. Verbeek – Dr. W. Junk Publishers London 1981 Pp. 55–57

Shimizu K., Minoda K.: Preoperative evaluation of vitreous surgery by ultrasonography. In Proceedings 8th S. I.D.U.O. (Nijmegen 1980) Ed. by J. M. Thijssen and A. M. Verbeek – Dr. W. Junk Publishers London '81 Pp. 33–38

Verbeek A. M., Bayer A. L., Thijssen J. M.: Echographic diagnosis after intraocular silicone oil injection. In proceedings 8th S.I.D.U.O. (Nijmegen 1980) Ed. by J.M. Thijssen and A. M. Verbeek – Dr. Junk Publisher London 1981 Pp. 59–66

Authors' address:
Institute of Ophthalmology
University of Bari
Bari
Italy

PRE-VITRECTOMY ULTRASONIC EXAMINATION OF THE TRAUMATISED EYE

FRANCO PASSANI, LUIGI BARCA and GIORGIO VENTURI
(*Florence, Italy*)

INTRODUCTION

New intraocular microsurgical techniques have provided new opportunities for the treatment of the severe complications that can occur as a consequence of major ocular trauma. It has been shown that the surgical procedures are best performed before the internal structural changes which may develop soon after the traumatic event either penetrating or contusive (Coles and Haik).

Rapid B-scan evaluation represents the only available means of examination to accurately plan vitrectomy in an eye with opaque ocular media so that observation of the retina is precluded by conventional techniques. Various echographic aspects of structural change will be discussed.

LENS CHANGES

Echoes originating from within the lens are always of pathological nature.

The presence and the type of lens change that can be recognised with the B-scan are of great importance in cases where corneal opacity is present and combined procedures of corneal graft and extraction must be planned; for example the presence of calcium in a cataract, seen ultrasonically as high amplitude echoes producing strong attenuation of the sound beam (Fig. 1a) suggests removal would be best accomplished without using phacoemulsification and vitrectomy instruments.

On these occasions an immersion B-scan system is preferred as it delineates the anterior structures of the globe. Rupture of the posterior capsule with subsequent extrusion of lens material into the anterior vitreous body (Fig. 1b) can be easily recognised; thus indicating the need for early combined lens extraction and vitrectomy procedures in order to avoid possible vitritis and any possibility of a resultant sympathetic ophthalmitis.

A subluxation of the lens can be evaluated ultrasonically only with difficulty but complete dislocation can be recognised more easily. (Fig. 1c).

Hillman, J. S./Le May, M. M. (eds.) Ophthalmic Ultrasonography

ISBN 978-94-009-7280-3

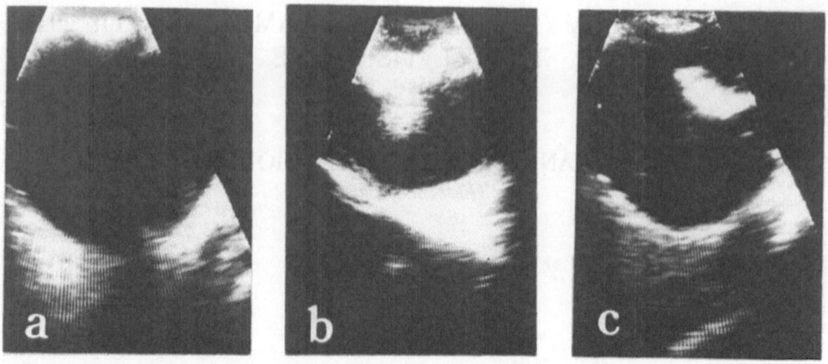

Fig. 1. Horizontal B-scan sections. (a) Calcified cataract producing strong attenuation of the sound beam. (b) Posterior lens rupture with lens material in anterior vitreous gel. (c) Dislocated cataractous lens.

VITREOUS CHANGES

Fibroplasia, vitreal incarceration and traction at the retinal surface can be nowadays eliminated by pars plana virectomy. The indications for this kind of surgical therapy must be rationalised and we cannot base judgements on clinical appearance alone but must use ultrasonic information as a means of assessing intraocular damage.

The presence of echoes arising from haemorrhage localised within the vitreous body immediately following trauma can indicate the location of the intraocular bleeding.

The presence of vitreal lacunae coexisting within vitreous haemorrhage can suggest the probable progression to a posterior vitreous detachment.

In cases where there is posterior vitreous detachment, the presence of haemorrhage may be confined to the vitreous gel alone, the retrohyaloid space alone or on occasions involve both compartments. (Fig. 2a) 'Real-time' examination of eyes in which there is posterior vitreous detachment is very important in the detection of vitreo-retinal adhesions which have to be severed at vitrectomy in an attempt to avoid traction retinal detachments around such adhesions. (Fig. 2b) Generally light haemorrhage with dispersion of blood cells in the vitreous body may not be detected ultrasonically. The presence of an anterior or posterior vitreous incarceration may be suggested by an asymmetrical contour of the gel and may occur at a site of penetration or at either the entry or the exit site of a foreign body. (Fig. 2a) Complicating a foreign body penetration one may see a track of haemorrhage traversing the vitreous along the pathway followed by the foreign body; this track may indicate the position of the foreign body.

Such tracks can be more easily seen in young patients who have a more compact vitreous gel and may lead to fibroblastic modification with subsequent retinal traction. The early detection of such modification is important to the vitreous surgeon. Vitrectomy in removing the vitreal scaffold avoids retinal traction and permitting the the visualisation of the retina allows

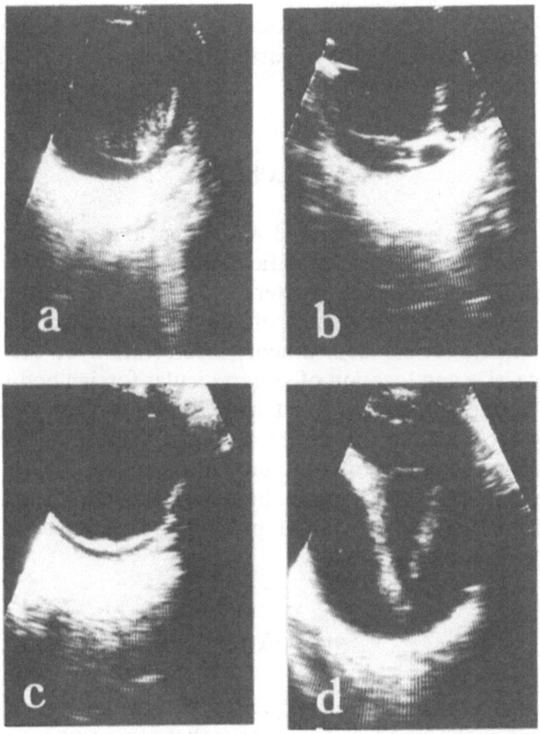

Fig. 2. Horizontal B-scan sections. (a) Detached vitreous gel incarcerated into posterior retina; intragel haemorrhage; orbital foreign body with 'ringing' artefact. (b) Detached vitreous gel inserting into localised traction retinal detachment. (c) Shallow posterior retinal detachment. (d) Total retinal detachment; detached retracted vitreous gel ('Triangle' sign of massive preretinal retraction).

combined transvitreal and transcleral surgery of retinal detachments, retinal holes and retinal breaks.

RETINAL CHANGES

Post traumatic retinal detachments have an ultrasonic appearance of high amplitude echoes anterior to those from the choroid and sclera. (Figs. 2c and 2d).

Often it is possible to detect sub-retinal haemorrhage complicating a penetrating injury; the ultrasonic image is characterised by high amplitude echoes filling the sub-retinal space.

The presence of retinal holes cannot be recognised on a B-scan but giant tears and giant dialyses can be identified.

Occasionally as a consequence of penetrating injury in the region of the pars plana a retinal detachment of the opposite pars plana may occur and be detected ultrasonically. This may extend to involve the entire ora serrata region and has been described by David McLeod and Marie Restori as a "purse-string" retinal detachment.

CONCLUSION

Rapid B-scan examination performed in either a contact or water-bath fashion can be used to recognise opacification or rupture of the lens with or without dispersion of cataractous material; the location and consistency of intravitreal haemorrhage; the presence of a complete or incomplete posterior vitreous detachment; retinal detachment; incarceration of the vitreous gel and the presence, size and location of an intraocular foreign body.

Ultrasound is undoubtedly of great help to the surgeon in planning the kind of surgery according to the extent of damage and in deciding the most convenient quadrant for entry of vitrectomy instruments.

Ultrasound may also be of value in the assessment of eyes in which haemorrhage complicates surgery and precludes direct observation of the anatomical surgical result.

SUMMARY

New intraocular microsurgical techniques have provided new opportunities for the treatment of the severe complications that can occur as a consequence of major ocular trauma. Rapid B-scan evaluation represents the only available means of examination to accurately plan vitrectomy in an eye with opaque ocular media so that observation of the retina is precluded by conventional techniques. Rapid B-scan examination performed in either a contact or water-bath fashion can be used to recognise opacification or rupture of the lens with or without dispersion of cataractous material; the location and consistency of intravitreal haemorrhage; the presence of a complete or incomplete posterior vitreous detachment; retinal detachment; incarceration of the vitreous gel and the presence, size and location of an intraocular foreign body.

REFERENCES

Coleman D. J.: The role of vitrectomy in traumatic vitreopathy. Amer. Acad. of Ophthal. and Otolar. 406–413, 1976.

Coleman D. J., Franzen L. A.: Vitreous surgery: Preoperative evaluation and prognostic value of ultrasonic display of vitreous haemorrhage. Arch. Ophthal. 92:375–381, 1974.

Haik G. M., Coles W.: Intraocular injuries: Their immediate surgical management. Philadelphia, Lea and Fabiger, 1972.

McLeod D., Restori M.: Real time B scanning of the vitreous. Trans. of the Ophthal. Soc. of the unit. King. 97:547–550, 1977.

McLeod D., Restori M. and Wright J. E.: Rapid B Scanning of the vitreous. British

Journal of Ophthal. 61: 437–445. 1977.
Mody K. V., Blach R. K., Leaver P. K. and McLeod D.: Closed vitrectomy after trauma. Trans. Ophthal. Soc. Unit. King. 55–58, 1978.

Authors' address:
Ia Cattedra di Clinica Oculistica
Universita' degli Studi di Firenze
Firenze
Italy

ULTRASONIC CHARACTERISTICS OF OCULAR TRAUMA, – ESPECIALLY DIAGNOSTIC APPLICATION OF OPHTHALMIC ULTRASONIC HIGH-SPEED ELECTRONIC SCANNING DISPLAY

SADANAO TANE and AKIRA KOMATSU
(*Kawasaki, Japan*)

Ultrasonic examinations were performed in 491 traumatic eyes in 352 patients by using a St. Marianna's ophthalmic high-resolution ultrasonic diagnostic equipment and the ophthalmic ultrasonic high-speed electronic scanning apparatus which we had recently developed. Useful results were obtained, confirming that the ultrasonic tomography is also useful for ocular trauma diagnosis. With this equipment, B-mode tomograms of the eyes are made by B-mode in water bath immersion method and mechanical compound scan. Useful diagnostic information could be obtained from the cases, whose diagnoses were occasionally difficult to confirm even by the conventional ophthalmic examinations or various X-ray examinations, by making tomograms of various phases of intraocular abnormalities (retinal detachment, vitreous hemorrhage or opacities, luxated lens, etc.) accompanied by optic media opacity, by diagnosing intraocular foreign bodies, and by making echograms of orbital trauma, etc. These results show an increase in accuracy in the diagnoses. Resolution in the B-mode tomography of eyes performed with the newly developed equipment was more improved than that performed with the conventional equipments.

Excellent reproducibility and quantification of the image is obtained through mechanical compound and electronic scanning by St. Marianna's ophthalmic ultrasonic diagnostic equipment and the ophthalmic ultrasonic high-speed electronic scanning apparatus developed by the author et al. The morphological diagnostic efficiency concerning traumatized eyes was thus markedly improved. Transducers types consisted of 5, 10, and 15 MHz PZT or a lithium niobate type.

Bronson-Turner and Ocuscan 400 contact B-scan equipments that makes simple rapid testing possible without the water immersion method has been employed in some patients. Ultrasonic examination was not performed in traumatized eyes with fresh perforations in order to avoid the risk of infection.

Here are the findings in several patients exhibiting typical and interesting echograms as presented during our clinical experiences.

AB-scan tomogram of a patient with complete luxation of the lens into vitreous body due to an intense ocular contusion is shown by Figure 1. The Zinn's zonule was shown to remain. The position of the luzated lens was indistinct by ophthalmoscopic examination on account of hypherma.

Hillman, J.S./Le May, M.M. (eds.) Ophthalmic Ultrasonography
©1983, Dr W. Junk Publishers, The Hague/Boston/Lancaster
ISBN 978-94-009-7280-3

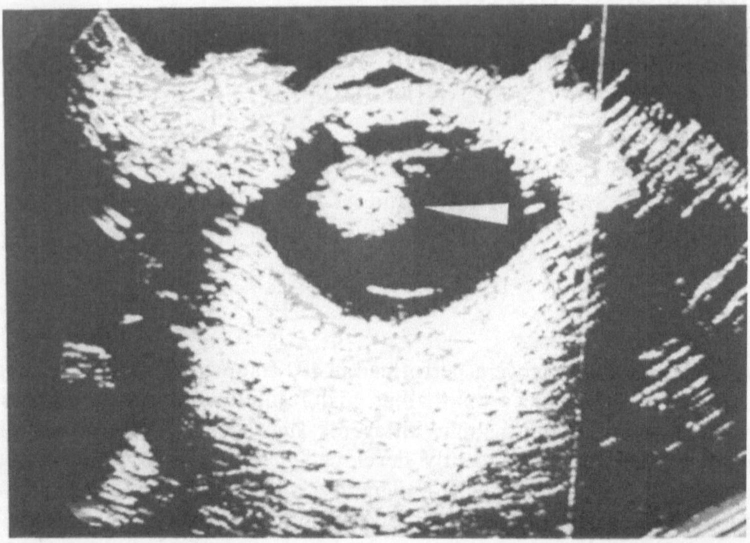

Fig. 1. **B-scan ultrasonogram of a complete luxation of the lens into vitreous body due to an intense ocular contusion.**

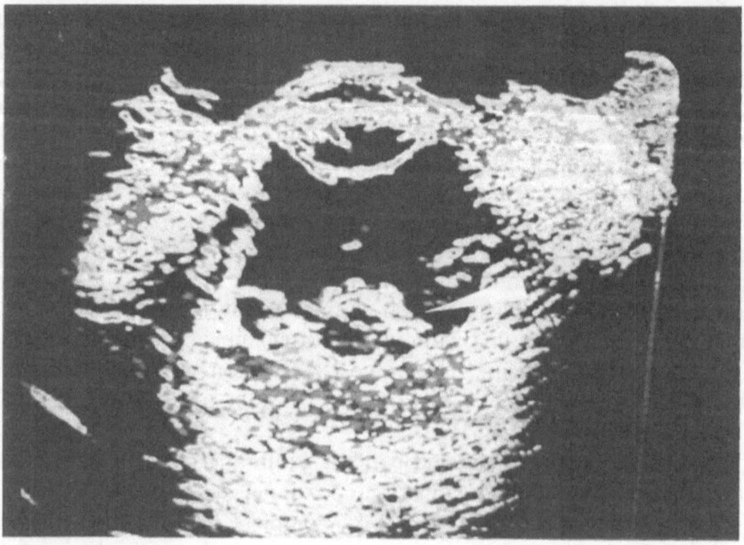

Fig. 2. **B-scan ultrasonogram of a vitreous hemorrhage localized near the posterior pole of the ocular fundus.**

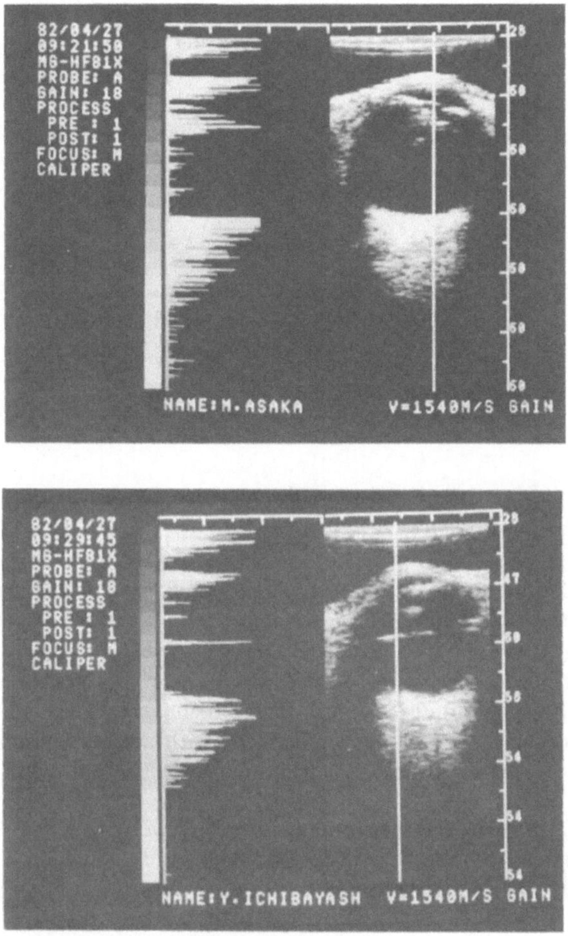

Fig. 3. A and B-scan ultrasonogram of the ophthalmic electronic high speed scanning display of the formation of a vitreous membrane after the absorption of long standing traumatic vitreous hemorrhage.

Figure 2 shows the vitreous hemorrhage localized near the posterior pole of the ocular fundus. This appears because of the ocular contusion.

In Figure 3 of the ophthalmic high-speed electronic scanning display, the formation of a vitreous membrane is shown to remain after the absorption of long standing vitreous hemorrhage. A vitrectomy was carried out in these patients with excellent results.

Figure 4 shows the B-scan ultrasonotomographic picture of an eye with traumatic retinal detachment. A membranous high amplitude echo was obtained from the detached retinal surface. It was possible to differentiate this from the vitreous membrane echo having a relatively low amplitude.

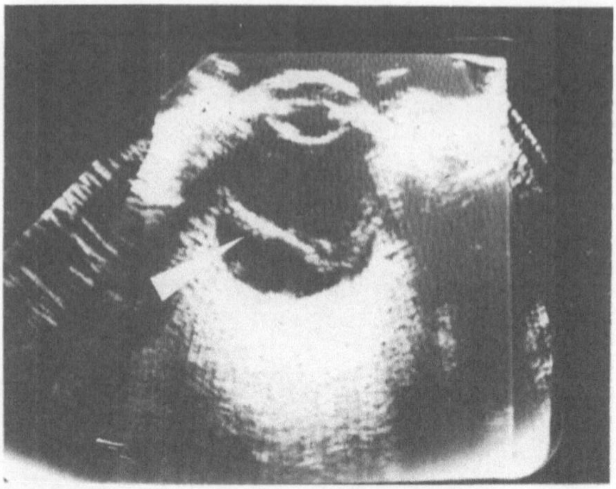

Fig. 4. B-scan ultrasonogram of a traumatic retinal detachment.

Figure 5 shows the findings of a traumatic total retinal detachment by means of the ophthalmic electronic high-speed scanning display. An elastic fluctuating movement of the retinal surface was noted by the dynamic observation diagnosis and real time observation under contact B-scan. This is useful in the differential diagnosis. Figure 6 shows a B-scan ultrasono-tomogram demonstrating a retinal detachment with a large amount of vitreous hemorrhage precluding the tesselation of the eye ground through the corpus vitreum.

Figure 7 shows the B-scan tomogram of an eye with a slug deposited into the iris surface. Multiple echoes were noted behind the foreign body echo. By using sensitivity tomography, the position of the foreign body was distinctly identified. The ultrasonic examination method is also useful in the diagnosis of wood and plastic pieces not visualized in the X-ray picture.

The clinical advantages of this examination method according to the echographic findings of traumatized eyes may be summarized in the following four items.

First, the intraocular and intraorbital findings may be demonstrated by the ultrasonic method even when ophthalmoscopic examination is impossible due to clouding of the transparent part of the eye. The various causes of clouding include intraocular hemorrhage, vitreous opacity and traumatic cataracts.

Second, this method is useful in the diagnosis and localization of foreign body within the eyeball and orbit. It is especially useful in X-ray transparent foreign bodies.

Third, this method is safe and allowed for several repeated examinations.

Fourth, the ophthalmic ultrasonic electronic high-speed scanning apparatus is far superior, specifically in resolution and gray scale assuring high reproducibility and safety excluding skill factors in diagnosing ocular traumas.

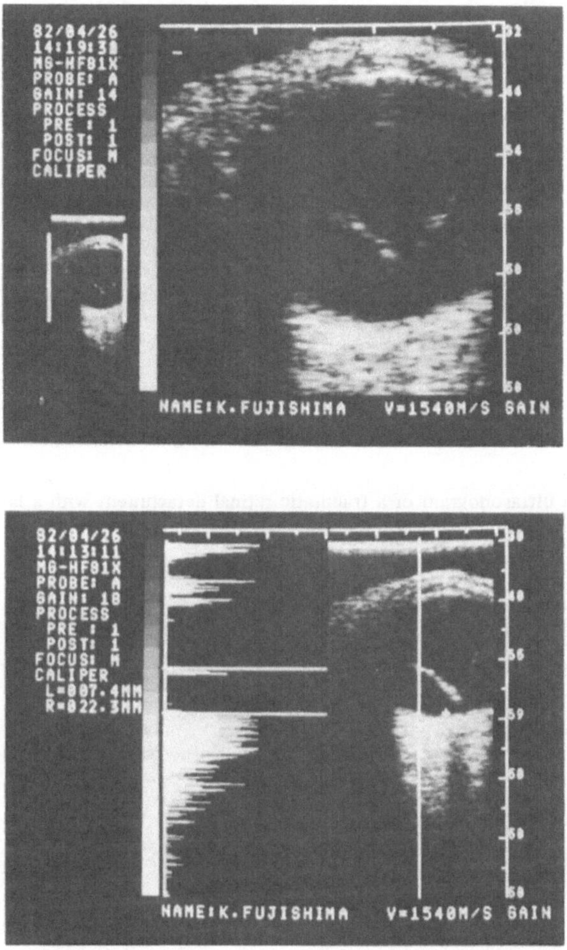

Fig. 5. B-scan ultrasonogram of a traumatic retinal detachment by means of the ophthalmic electronic high-speed scanning display.

CONCLUSION

The ultrasonic method, in combination with various methods of conventional ophthalmologic examinations was found to be quite useful in providing more accurate test information in the diagnosis of eye trauma. It is also a useful supplement in overcoming the drawbacks of other methods.

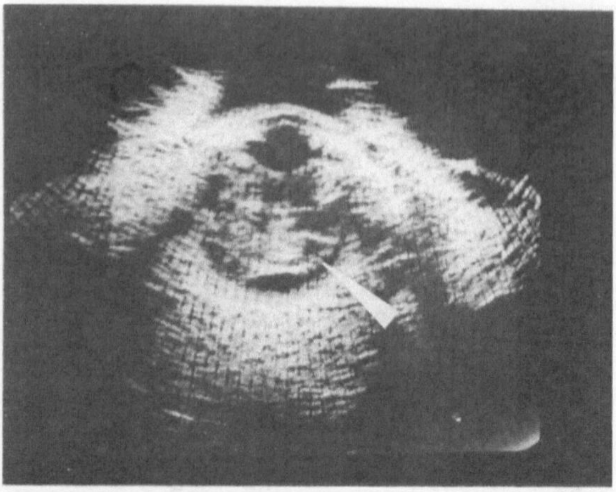

Fig. 6. A-scan ultrasonogram of a traumatic retinal detachment with a large amount of vitreous hemorrhage.

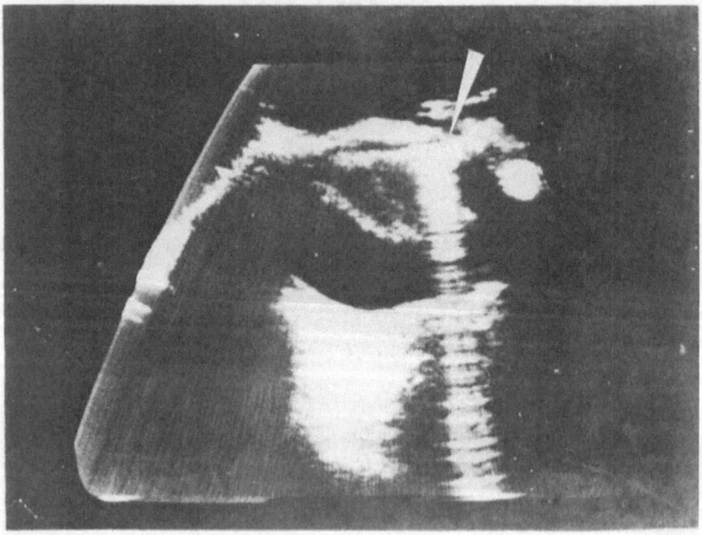

Fig. 7. B-scan ultrasonogram of a slug deposited into the iris.

Authors' address:
Department of Ophthalmology
St. Marianna University School of Medicine
2095 Sugao
Miyamae-ku
Kawasaki-shi
Kanagawa-ken 213
Japan

M-MODE ECHOGRAPHY PATTERN STUDY IN RETINAL DETACHMENT

A. BONAVOLONTA' and G. CENNAMO
(*Naples, Italy*)

ABSTRACT

At present, A- and B-scan echography enables differential diagnosis between vitreo-retinal diseases, secondary retinal detachment and neoplasia.

This is possible utilizing quantitative, topographical and kinetical echography with the standardized A-scan method, and, essentially topographical data with B-scan method. The evaluation of the role of M-mode echography in this pathology is the scope of this work.

At present, A and B-scan echography enables differential diagnosis between vitreo-retinal diseases such as secondary detachment and neoplasia. (Fig. 1, 2).

This is possible utilizing quantitative, topographical and kinetic echography with A-scan method (Ossoinig K. C. 1979), and, essentially topographical data with the B-scan method (Coleman D. J. 1977). The evaluation of the role of M-mode echography in this pathology with the intention of correct diagnosis and the choice of the most suitable surgical procedure, when required, is the scope of this work. The immersion technique was used in this

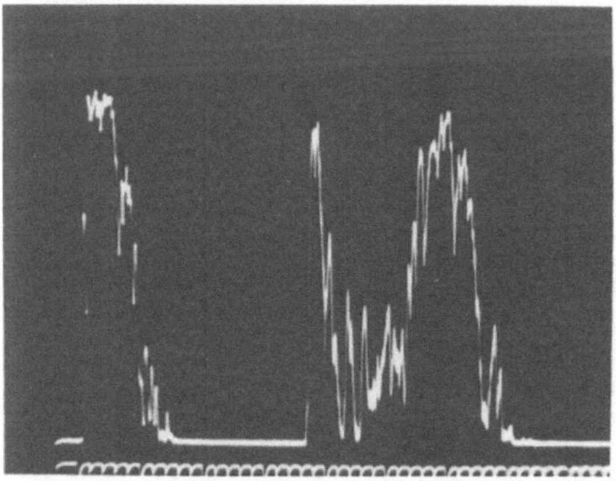

Fig. 1. Malignant melanoma of the choroid with standardized A-scan.

Hillman, J. S./Le May, M. M. (eds.) Ophthalmic Ultrasonography
© 1983, Dr W. Junk Publishers, The Hague/Boston/Lancaster
ISBN 978-94-009-7280-3

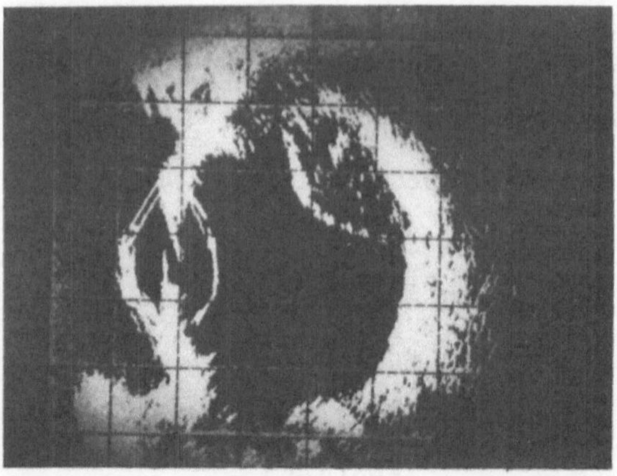

Fig. 2. Malignant melanoma of the choroid with immersion B-scan technique.

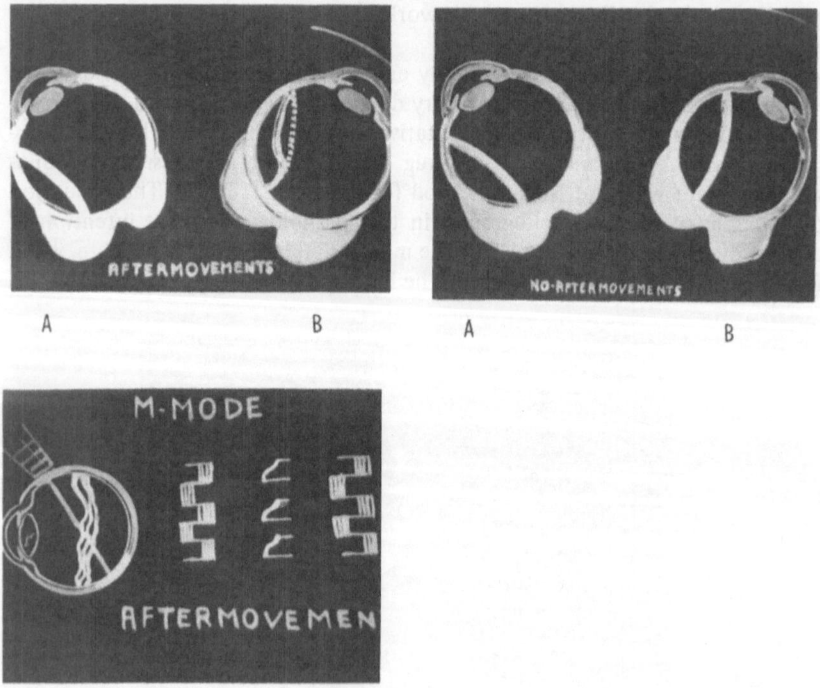

Fig. 3a, b, c. With M-mode echography it is possible to pinpoint the inertial motions within the global structure after each ocular movement.

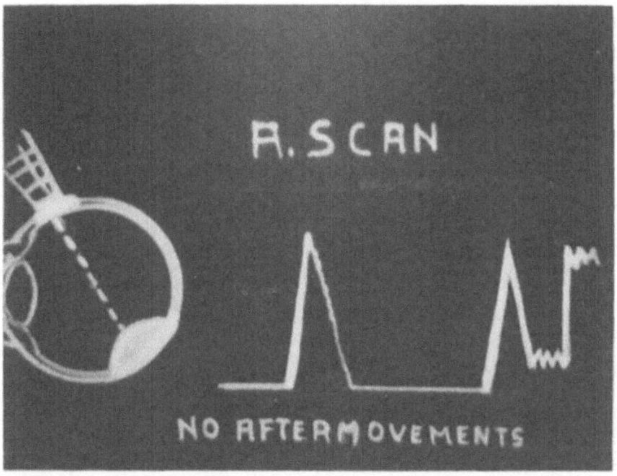

Fig. 4. The standardized A-scan echography shows absence of movement in case of a solid structure.

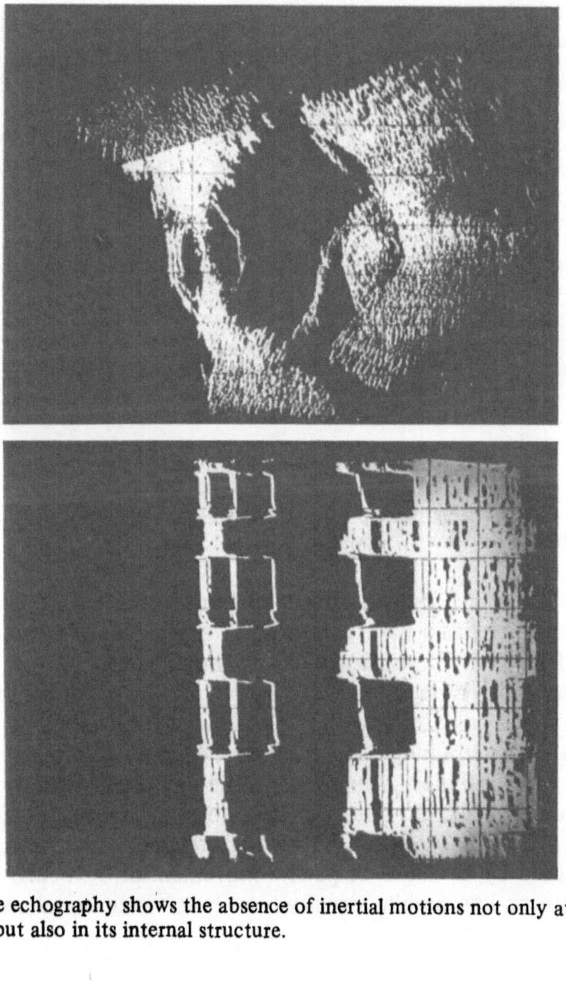

Fig. 5. M-mode echography shows the absence of inertial motions not only at the surface of the tumor, but also in its internal structure.

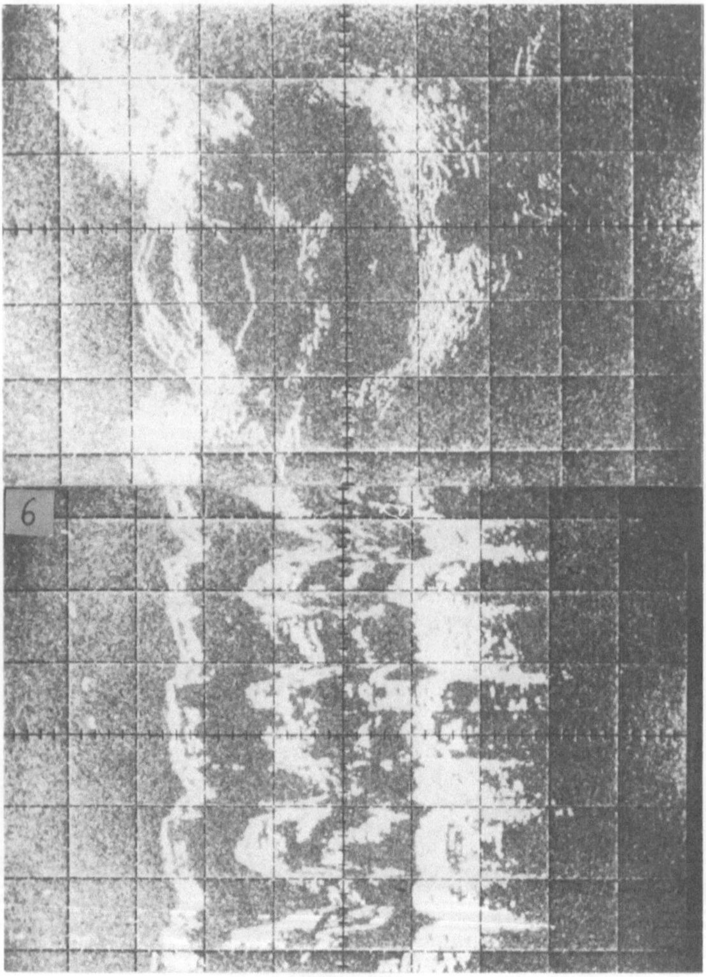

Fig. 6. In a case of vitreal pathology with absence of vitreo-retinal adhesion, M-mode shows considerable undulatory movements.

study with an Ophthalmoscan 200 apparatus with 15 MHz probe. The M-mode test was realized with a 10-second time span. This method enables the study of the active motilities of the ultrasonogram.

The active motility study was obtained by having the patient move his eye to a determined position and then immediately returning to the starting position while maintaining the probe in the same direction. Thus, it was possible to pinpoint inertial motions within the global structure after each ocular movement (Fig. 3a, b, c). In the A- or B-scan methods, the behaviour of the echographic image is proportionately related to the inertial movement which is caused by an active or passive movement of the ocular globe. In the case of more or less mobile structure, such as vitreoretinal pathology, the

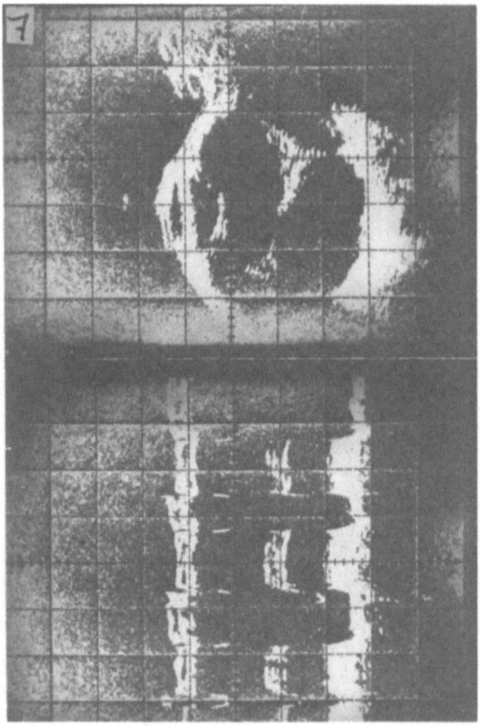

Fig. 7. A case of vitreo-retinal traction. The reduction in width and height of the tracing in M-mode representation is in relation to the gradation of the vitreal structure traction at the retinal level.

echographic image is gradated, while an absence of movement indicates a solid structure such as a neoplasm (Fig. 4) (Bonavolonta' A. 1980).

156 subjects were examined in this study: they were divided into three groups depending upon pathologies presented:

(1) 39 patients with choroid malignant melanoma.

(2) 59 patients with vitreous haemorrhage.

(3) 58 patients with an idiopathic retinal detachment.

The results obtained may be summarized as follows:

In the case of a solid neoplasm, no movement is discernible on the M-mode display not only at the point corresponding to the surface of the tumor, but also to that corresponding to its internal structure (Fig. 5).

A choroid detachment is indicated by small undulatory movements corresponding to the principal echo – similar to the vertical movements seen in A-scan. Furthermore, under these undulatory movements, a disordered pattern in the display is visible; this corresponds to diffuse haemorrhage, within the choroid detachment when it is present.

A vitreal pathology – haemorrhage or exudate – will result in undulatory movements that may diminish depending upon the presence of vitreoretinal adhesion points (Fig. 6). In such a case, the reduction in width and height of

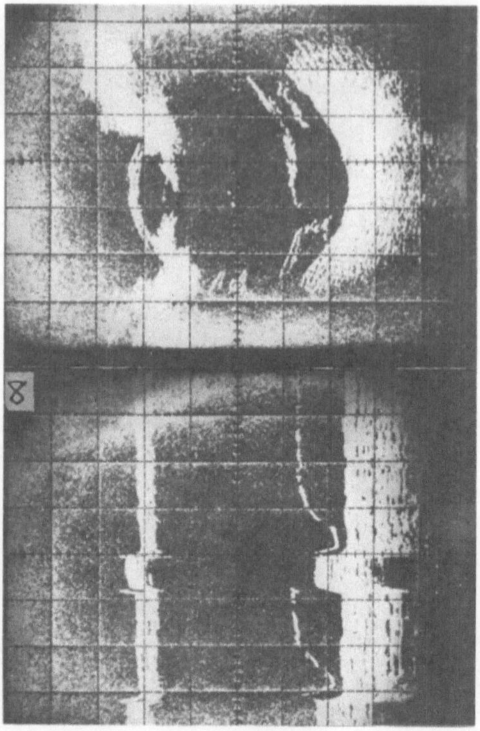

Fig. 8. An idiopathic retinal detachment with absence of vitreo-retinal tractions shows very wide undulations in M-mode echography.

the echo is in relation to the gradation of the vitreal structure traction at the retinal level (Fig. 7).

An idiopathic retinal detachment shows very wide undulations or waves which proportionately diminish in size in relation to the validity of the eventual vitreoretinal tractions (Fig. 8). Based upon the above, we conclude the following: M-mode can not be utilized as a substitute for standardized A- or B-scan echography; however, because it furnishes quantitative information, it may be used in a complementary role along with the more traditional methods.

In particular:

In the case of vitreous diseases: M-mode furnishes useful data regarding possible vitreal membranes and their relationship to the retinal surface.

M-mode provides a more exact evaluation of possible vitreo-retinal traction in cases of idiopathic retinal detachment. Above all, these data are of extreme importance in decisions regarding surgical options.

Diathermy with drainage of the eventual subretinal fluid is indicated only in those cases without valid vitreo-retinal traction, however, in moderately valid vitreo-retinal traction, cryotherapy or diathermy with scleral buckling procedure may be the more suitable procedure.

In cases of extremely valid vitreo-retinal traction, encircling procedure with scleral buckling associated with gas injections would be necessary.

REFERENCES

Bonavolonta' A., Cennamo G., Greco G. M.: Ruolo dell'esame ecografico nel trattamento e prognosi del distacco di retina. Aggiornamenti 1981 in Ecografia Internistica, Neurosonologia, Ecoftalmologia, Atti V Congresso Nazionale SISUM, Milano 1980.

Ossoinig K. C.: Standardized Echography: Basic Principles, Clinical Application, and Results. Reprinted from: International Ophthalmology Clinics. Ophthalmic Ultrasonography: Comparative Techniques, Winter. 1979, Vol. 19, No 4. (Published by Little, Brown and Company, Boston, Massachusetts.)

Coleman D. J., Lizzi F. L., Jack R. L.: Ultrasonography of the Eye and Orbit, Lea and Febiger, Philadelphia, 1977.

Authors' address:
Istituto di Clinica Oculistica
II Facolta' di Medicina e Chirurgia
Universita' degli Studi
80131 Naples
Italy

ULTRASONOGRAPHIC PATTERN OF THE EYEBALL OPERATED ON FOR RETINAL DETACHMENT

A. REIBALDI, M. DI PILATO and M. M. TRITTO
(Bari, Italy)

SUMMARY

The aim of this paper is to present the ultrasonographic patterns of eyes operated on for retinal detachment. In particular the differences between the various types of buckling, usually carried out in surgery of retinal detachment (scleral pocket, soft button, hard button of silicone, encirclement, vitreous supplementation) are pointed out, by means of ultrasound. Furthermore, some particular findings, such as the presence of endobulbar supramid thread, are reported.

INTRODUCTION

The aim of our work is to illustrate the echographic aspects of eyes which have been operated on for retinal detachment. This requirement has been dictated by the need to understand the anatomical condition of these eyes, the media of which are more susceptible to opaqueness and are therefore liable to be operated on. We studied 2172 eyeballs which had been operated on for retinal detachment in our hospital between January 1972 and December 1981. These eyes were divided into groups according to the different types of operation: (a) encirclement with a thread or silicone band; (b) scleral buckling; (c) encirclement and scleral buckling; (d) vitreous supplementation. Although evacuating centesis was used in 1193 cases, it is not generally recognized as accepted practice as it has not produced any change in echographic pattern. In order to examine the eyes which had been operated on we used a standardized Kretztechnik 7200 A-Scan with an 8 MHz probe and a Bronson-Turner B-Scan with a 10 MHz probe. We usually carried out two examinations, the first after one month, the second after six months from the date of the operation, only taking into account those eyeballs in which a perfect reattachment had been achieved.

ENCIRCLEMENT

Echographically speaking we can distinguish two different aspects: (a) the one obtained by an encircling thread which in our case was Mersilene or

Hillman, J. S./Le May, M. M. (eds.) Ophthalmic Ultrasonography

ISBN 978-94-009-7280-3

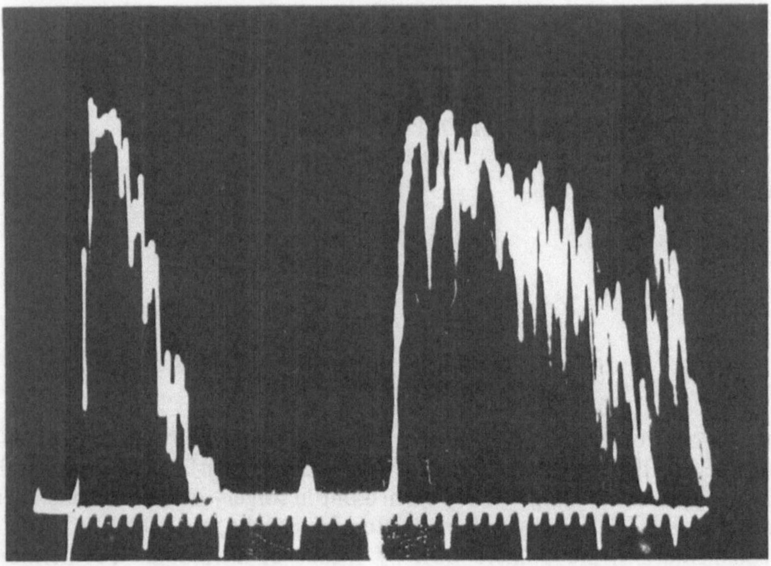

Fig. 1.

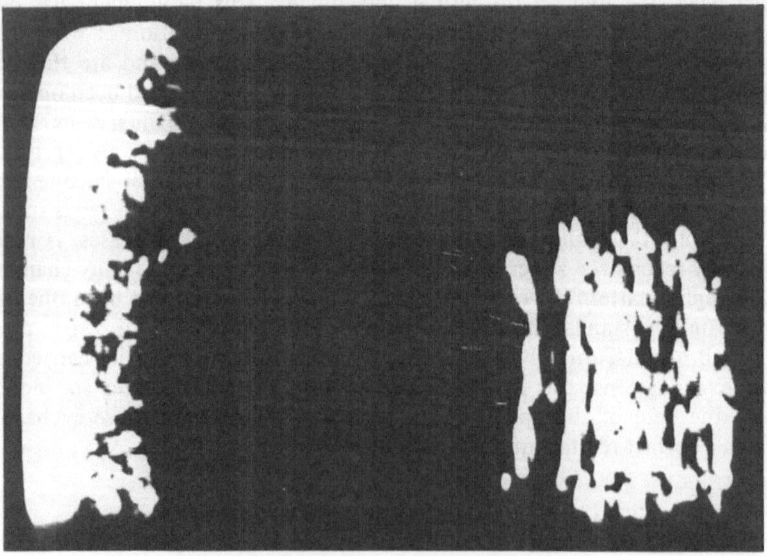

Fig. 1a.

Supramid (which are echographically indistinguishable from each other) – we abandoned this method in our clinical practice in 1974/5; (b) Encirclement with a silicone band.

In the first case the A-Scan pattern obtained with a probe perpendicular to the point of deeper indentation, presents the following characteristics: the length of vitreal silence seems to be shorter; the group of peaks which we will call 'posterior' and is made up of the retina, choroid and sclera is normal but followed by a short series of 1 or 2 peaks which are slightly lower. This is evidence of the reduction of the ultrasonic beam on crossing the thread. The B-Scan pattern with scanning parallel to the encirclement gives us an almost normal image of the eyeball if the reduction of the vitreal space caused by indentation is not taken into account; scanning perpendicular to the encirclement zone can on the other hand reveal a hyper-reflective point caused by the thread in the wall of the indentation zone: on lower sensitivity the pattern appears as a hyper-reflective retroscleral point; this manoeuvre helped us in many cases in pin-point the thread in the retino-choroidal thickness; when it had reached the sclera in a number of points, the B-scan result consisted of the image of the thread connecting two points of the indentation. On A-scan the result consisted of the presence of the highest endovitreal peak.

Encirclement with silicone band produces on A-Scan a pattern (Fig. 1) similar to that of encircling thread; the differences are: (a) a greater distance between the posterior complex and the closing peak of the encirclement; (b) a greater number of slightly lower peaks compared with those caused by the thread.

B-Scan with scanning parallel to the band likewise causes a (Fig. 1a) hyperdense area which is longer than that caused by the thread and also shows a line of shadow which runs behind and parallel to it. Scanning perpendicularly to the encirclement shows evidence of an indentation which is analogous to that obtained with the thread.

SCLERAL BUCKLING

In our clinical practice scleral buckling basically consisted in two techniques: the placing of a soft silicone sponge button attached to the sclera by a thread according to the position of the lesion; or the placing of a suitably shaped hard silicone button in the bed of an intrascleral pocket.

Episcleral buckling with a soft sponge button is the most easily recognised by its echographic characteristics: on A-Scan the peaks of the posterior complex may be followed by an opening peak at its maximum height, which is followed by a series of peaks that vary in number and are of average height. The opening peak may at other times be hidden by the posterior complex. The peaks are followed by a closing peak which may sometimes be double as a result of the effect of the ultrasonic beam on the thread which fixes the button in place. The following peaks often undergo a reduction in height. On B-scan the presence of the button denotes a typical 'C' shaped sclero-choroidal indentation, followed by a clean sonic shadow (Fig. 2).

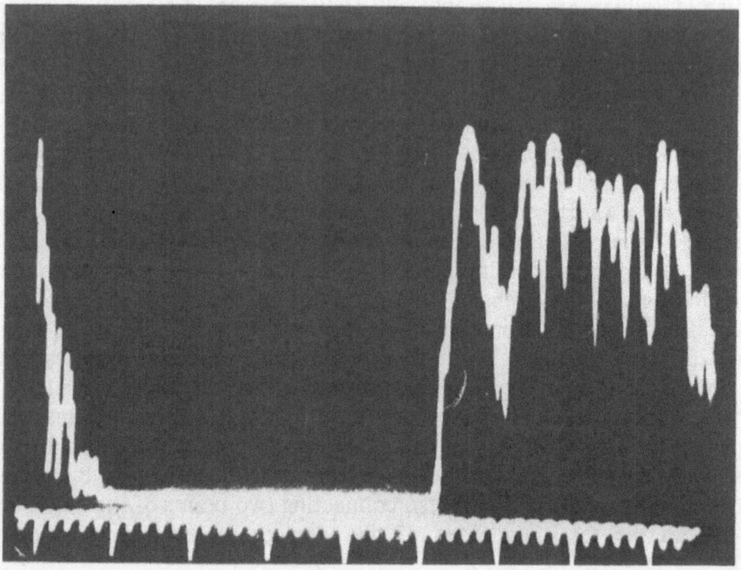

Fig. 2.

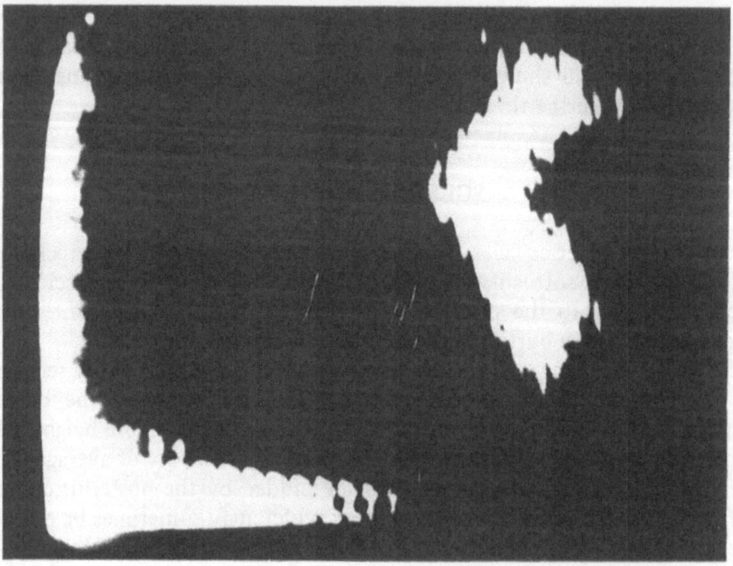

Fig. 2a.

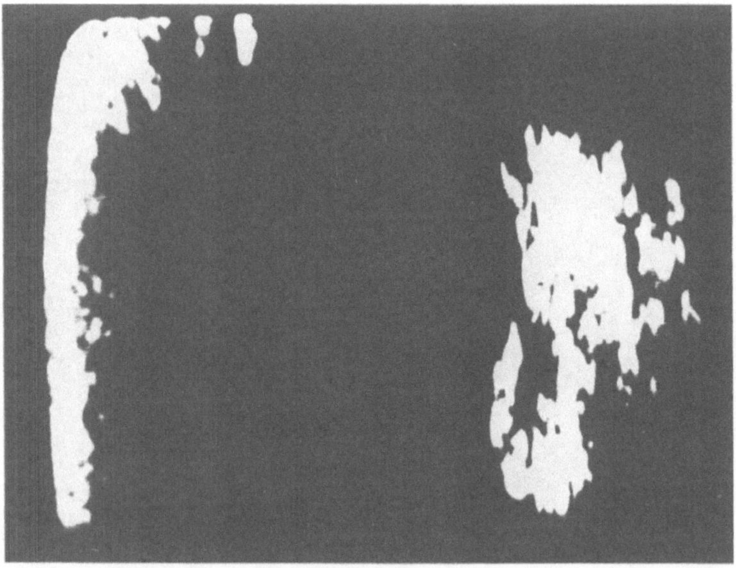

Fig. 3.

Intrascleral buckling on A-scan determines the appearance of a series of medium high peaks, which follow the posterior complex and which are followed by two peaks. These two peaks are sometimes clear, one showing the back of the intrascleral button, the other the flap of the sclera that closes the pocket. In some cases a virtual return to base line can take place after the first peak. This is evidence of a fairly clear interface between the scleral buckling and the scleral flap. On B-scan the result is typical: the indentation appears to be followed by a hyporeflective area which is the shadow of the scleral buckling between two tissue sensitive lines made up of the posterior complex at the front of the button, and at the back the scleral flap (Fig. 3).

SCLERAL BUCKLING AND ENCIRCLEMENT

In this case the operation consisted in the placing of a silicone band at a variable distance from the limbus and in the positioning of a hard fluted silicon button fixed under the encirclement according to the position of the lesion.

Echographically such an operation has the following aspects: on A-scan a number of medium high peaks followed by a closing peak of maximum height follows the posterior complex. The following peaks undergo a marked decrease in height (Fig. 4).

On B-scan the pattern is typical in the scanning which fall to the same level as the encirclement: a hyper-reflective area, attached to the posterior complex followed by an area of shadow of the same shape as the button running under

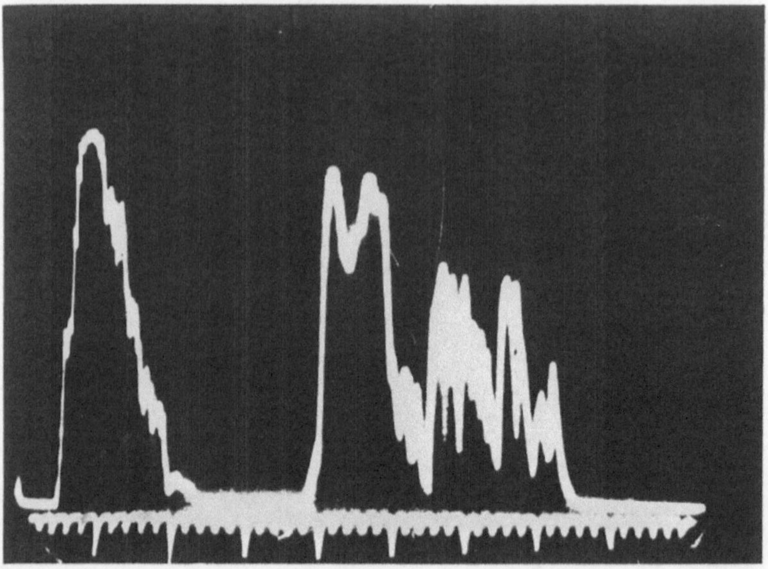

Fig. 4.

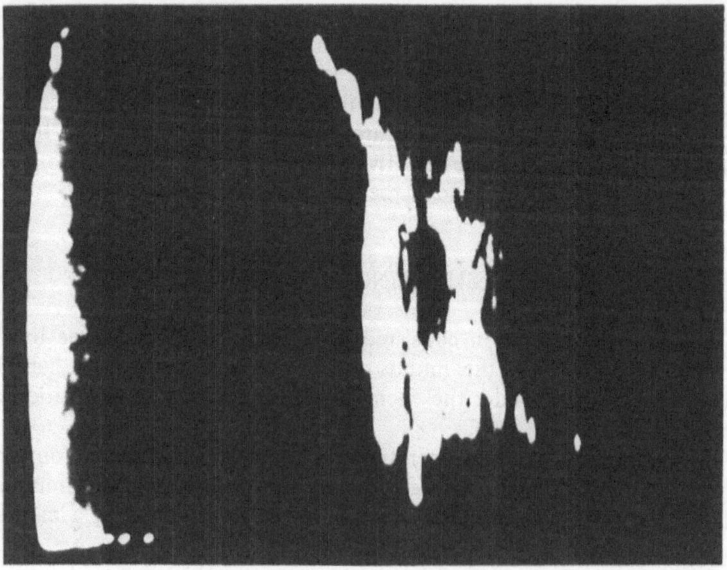

Fig. 4a.

the encirclement manifests itself. Furthermore the indentation caused by the button appears as a small endovitreous curve compared to the indentation caused by the encirclement (Fig. 4a).

VITREOUS SUPPLEMENTATION

In our experience vitreous supplementation associated in various ways with encirclement, encirclement and scleral buckling, scleral buckling, was obtained by the introduction of either a physiological solution, Healon, or silicone oil into the vitreous chamber.

The first two substances did not produce any change in pattern either on A or B-scan compared with the normal pattern.

Silicone oil on the other hand has the following characteristics: if the bubble is introduced correctly, that is singly, it behaves like an endovitreal foreign body, causing on A-scan a shortening of the pattern, which is why the posterior complex is not recorded either; if on the other hand the silicone appears as a number of small bubbles these produce interfaces, as result of which the pattern appears to be made up of a series of medium high peaks, sometimes even high peaks, which occupy the whole vitreous body: in this case it is with quantitative A-scan that we are able to distinguish (because of its different reflectivity) the pattern from serious organized haemorrhages or from massive vitreous retraction.

On B-scan, too, the pattern is affected by the homogeneity of the silicone: in the first case there is a large window comparable to that caused by a hardening of the tissue which masks the structures behind totally or in part. In the second case, however, (that is in the presence of interfaces) there is the image of a large foreign body, situated in front with numerous interfaces that suggest large blood clots in the vitreous, whereas behind we find that the posterior structures are incomplete.

CONCLUSION

In the light of the above results it is clear that in the eyeball operated on for retinal detachment new anatomical situations appear that are echographically quite different. In fact, according to the varying height and number of the peaks between the opening peak and the closing peak, it is possible in A-scan to distinguish an encircling thread from an encircling band, and to distinguish both from scleral buckling with a soft sponge button. The difference between encircling band and scleral buckling with encirclement is less typical; the latter produces a reduction in the echo to the end of the pattern.

If there are problems on A-scan in the differentiation of the various types of encirclement from scleral buckling pocket, then, on B-scan these problems can be overcome. On B-scan all the patterns described present typical aspects (the 'C' shape of the soft button, the shadow of the encircling band).

Diagnostic problems in B-scan could arise in differentiating the intrascleral pocket from scleral buckling and encirclement. We can distinguish these two aspects by the different distance of the button from the vitreo-retinal apparatus and in the second case by the encirclement.

In conclusion we maintain that the possibility of identifying echographically the type of operation on the eyeball is an advantage in the planning of future operations on those eyeballs whose media have become opaque.

REFERENCES

Flament J.: Aspect échographique des poches sclérales (note préliminaire). Bull. Soc. Ophthal. Fr. 1970, 70, 1, 165–168.

Larsen J. S., Syradalen P.: Ultrasonic study on changes in axial eye dimensions after encircling procedure in retinal detachment surgery. Acta Ophthal. (Kbh). 1979, no 3, 57, 337–343.

Poujol J., Toufic N.: Difficulte et valeur de l'examen echographique dans le decollement de retine opere. Cl. Ophthal. 1977, no 3, 181–198.

Reibaldi A., Di Pilato M., Balacco-Gabrieli C.: Valutazione nel tempo mediante ultrasuoni dell'entità dell'indentazione dei piombaggi sclerali. Studio sperimentale. Boll. Ocul. vol. 1981, 60, 9–10.

Sollner F., Ossoinig K., Wustemberg L.: Echografische befunde nach sklera eindellender operationen. S.I.D.U.O. IV, Paris May 1971. Diagnostica ultrasonica in Ophtalmologia. Centre National d'Ophtalmologie des Quinze-Vingts. Paris 1973, 199–204.

Toufic N.: Ultrasonographie et èlectroretinographie dans le décollement et rétine opéré. Jullet 1975, Monographie de 37 pages (ronéo) C.N.O. des Quinze-Vingts, Paris.

Wustenberg L., Ossoinig K., Sollner F.: Echographische untersuchung nach sklera eindellen den operationen. Klin. Mbl. Augen. 1972, 161, 1, 121.

Authors' address:
Institute of Ophthalmology
Bari University
Bari
Italy

DIFFERENTIAL DIAGNOSIS OF DISCIFORM LESIONS USING STANDARDIZED ECHOGRAPHY

SANDRA FRAZIER BYRNE
(*Miami, USA*)

Disciform fundus lesions may be readily diagnosed in both opaque and clear media with standardized echography. When opaque media harbors a disciform macular lesion, echography is essential in detection and differentiation, thus providing important prognostic information. In clear media, standardized echography serves as an independent method for differentiating disciform lesions from choroidal neoplasms.

In eyes with opaque media the posterior segment is initially screened with the standardized A-scan for lesion detection. Lesions are then localized, differentiated, and measured with the "special examination techniques" (1, 6, 10) using standardized echography (combined standardized A-scan and contact B-scan instrumentation), as described by Ossoinig. Each of these modalities is used to determine specific information which is assimilated to arrive at a final differential diagnosis.

TOPOGRAPHIC EVALUATION

B-scan is well suited for delineating topography of lesions (location, shape and extension) (1, 2, 6, 10, 11). Disciform lesions most commonly arise in the macula (senile macular degeneration), although they sometimes occur in eccentric locations. B-scan documentation of topography is achieved by obtaining photoechograms of perpendicular sections through maximally elevated portions of a given lesion. Such documentation is necessary to establish the lesion's superior-inferior and temporal-nasal extent (Fig. 1). Photoechograms relative to the optic disc are helpful since the disc serves as a convenient landmark for sequential examinations. Focal lesions are usually relatively smooth and dome-shaped while more diffuse fundus involvement results in significant surface irregularity.

QUANTITATIVE AND KINETIC EVALUATIONS

The "tissue sensitivity setting" (8, 9, 12) of the standardized A-scan is of paramount importance in assessing internal spike height (including structure, reflectivity and sound attenuation). Disciform lesions are typically

Hillman, J.S./Le May, M.M. (eds.) Ophthalmic Ultrasonography
©1983, Dr W. Junk Publishers, The Hague/Boston/Lancaster
ISBN 978-94-009-7280-3

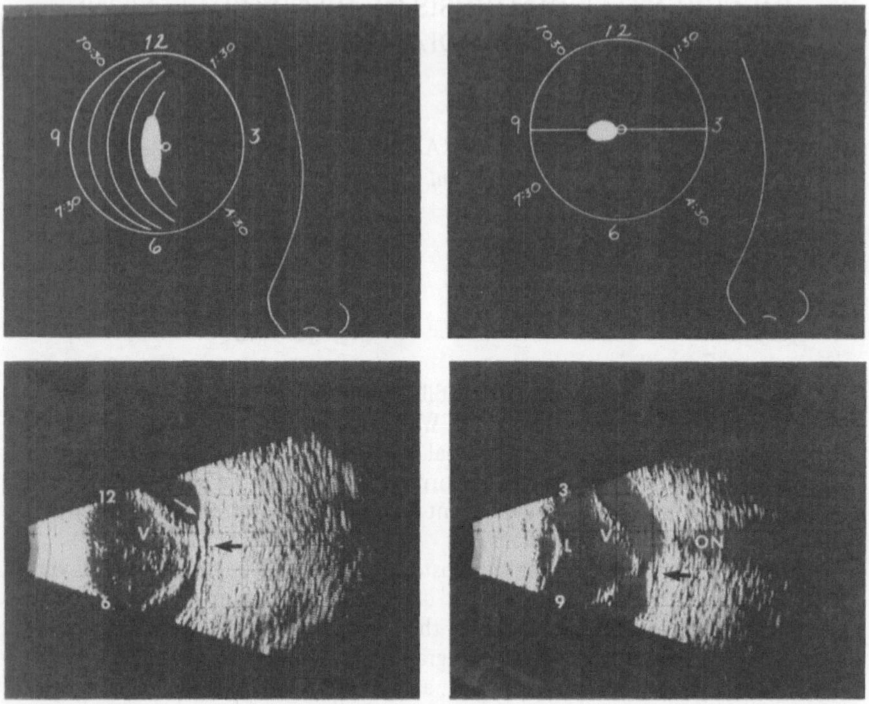

Fig. 1. **Schematic drawings and corresponding B-scan echograms through vitreous hemorrhage (with posterior vitreous detachment) and disciform lesion at the macula. Vertical section (left) shows superior-inferior extent of lesion in the posterior plane. Horizontal section (right) demonstrates horizontal axial section through lens, optic disc and macula. L = lens, V = vitreous hemorrhage, white arrow = surface of elevated sensory retina, black arrow = macula (thickening of subretinal layers).**

membraneous in structure due to the presence of subretinal neovascular membrane and/or extravasated blood beneath the sensory retina, pigment epithelium and choroid. When elevated, each of these fundus interfaces produces a distinct, high amplitude echo spike with the standardized A-scan (Fig. 2). A low B-scan sensitivity setting is often useful in documenting this finding, although differentiation from neoplasm with overlying retinal detachment is only possible by combining the topographic B-scan display with quantitative and kinetic criteria as obtained with the standardized A-scan (Fig. 3).

At tissue sensitivity, organized portions of disciform hemorrhages produce high internal reflectivity due to coagulated, stagnant blood (6, 7, 11). A-scan evaluation of organized lesions at 50 per cent spike height (the most sensitive portion of the S-shaped amplifier) indicates no lesion mobility (solid consistency). When significant fresh subretinal bleeding occurs, extensive, elevated and mobile hemorrhagic retinal detachments are frequently noted. Figure 4 demonstrates a disciform lesion with an overlying, elevated hem-

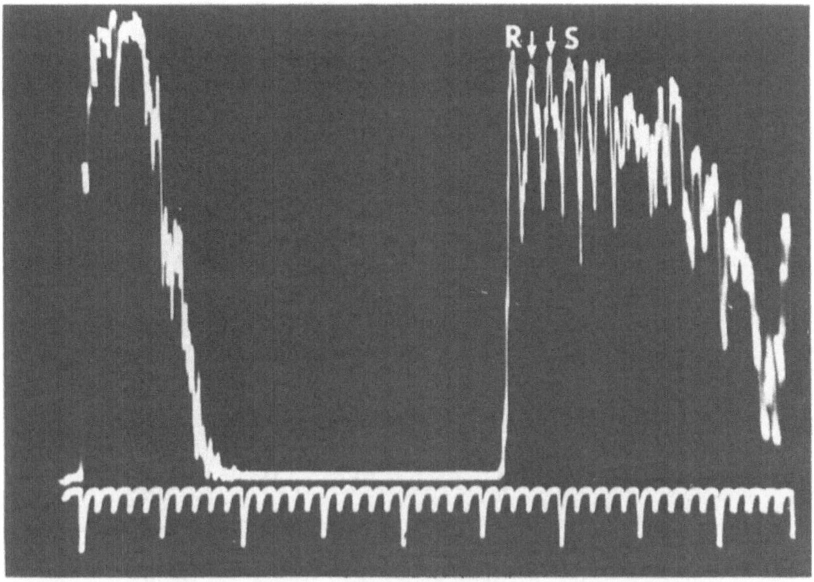

Fig. 2. A-scan at tissue sensitivity setting demonstrates typical membraneous structure of disciform lesion. R = retina, left arrow = surface of elevated pigment epithelium, right arrow = surface of elevated choroid, S = sclera. Each of these normal interfaces is elevated and accentuated due to extravasated blood.

orrhagic retinal detachment. Such fresh subretinal hemorrhage normally involves the posterior, temporal, and inferior retina, although total detachment sometimes develops. The extent of hemorrhagic retinal detachment is of great significance to the ophthalmologist in assessing future visual potential, and in evaluating whether or not vitrectomy is feasible for the recovery of peripheral vision.

Extensive disciform lesions are usually comprised of coagulated and fresh hemorrhage, thus creating irregular standardized A-scan echograms of variable internal reflectivity and mobility. If typical senile macular degeneration is present, an organized, highly reflective, solid portion is invariably noted in the macula (Fig. 5 and 6). Baseline measurements of maximal lesion elevation are taken with the standardized A-scan at initial examination by securing multiple A-scan photoechograms at low measuring sensitivity (Fig. 6). These measurements are invaluable for sequential examinations where decreased elevation strongly suggests the diagnosis of disciform lesion (Fig. 7).

Another frequent finding in organized portions of disciform lesions is the presence of calcium deposits – a critèrion which greatly aids the differential diagnosis. These extremely high reflective point-like sources (which acoustically behave like foreign bodies), produce significant sound attenuation. Large calcium deposits may be visualized with both B and A-scan, but small foci are only detectable with the more sensitive standardized A-scan using oblique sound beam incidence. With this oblique approach, the diagnostician

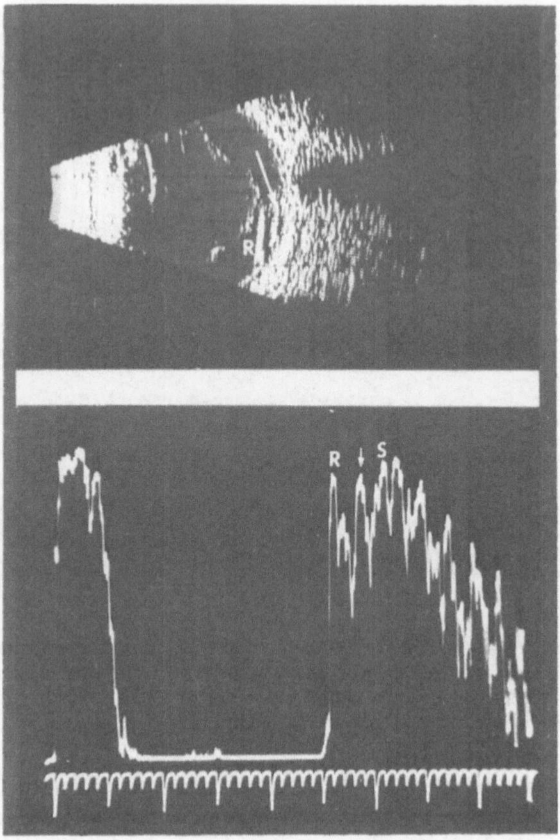

Fig. 3. Another disciform lesion in an eye with vitreous hemorrhage demonstrating elevation and accentuation of sensory retina and choroid. B-scan is at low sensitivity to better delineate membraneous structure. The tissue sensitivity setting of the standardized A-scan is essential in evaluating reflectivity of the subchoroidal space in suspected disciform lesions to rule out neoplasm. R = sensory retina, arrow = choroid, S = sclera.

(2) need only center the foreign body-like signal within the sound beam to obtain a 100 per cent tall spike. The lesion and underlying scleral signals produce low spikes during this maneuver due to tangential sound beam exposure (Fig. 8).

DIFFERENTIATION FROM NEOPLASMS

Malignant Melanoma

Malignant melanoma, when elevated by at least 2.0 mm. from the inner scleral surface, produces typical echographic patterns. These lesions are most

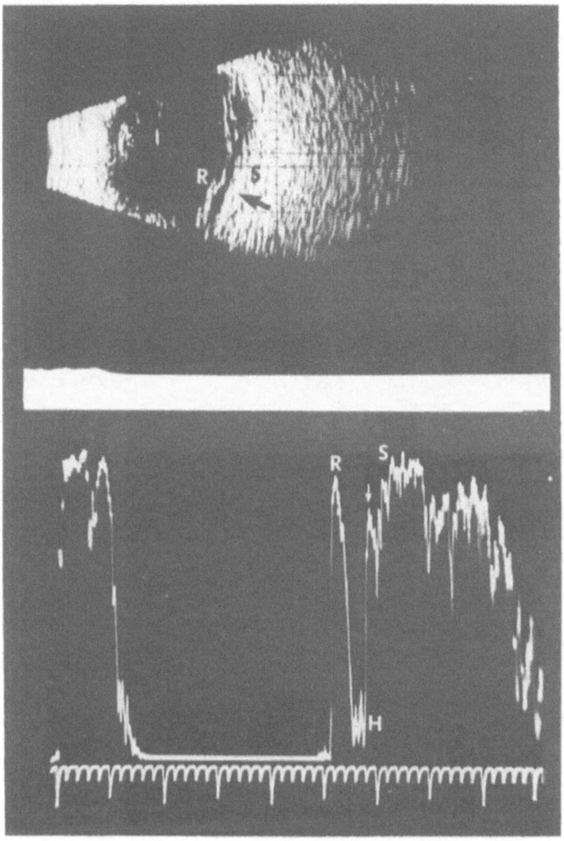

Fig. 4. Disciform lesion with extensive, elevated, fresh subretinal hemorrhage. The A-scan shows retinal detachment (R) followed by fresh subretinal blood (H). Arrow = more organized hemorrhage in posterior fundus layer, S = sclera. Typical aftermovement of the retinal spike was demonstrated during the dynamic kinetic evaluation.

commonly dome-shaped or mushrooming in appearance with B-scan. More importantly, with standardized A-scan they yield a regularly structured, low to medium reflective, solid echogram with significant internal vascularity (Fig. 9) (3, 4, 5, 6, 7, 10, 11). When elevated less than 2 mm. they may be irregularly structured or even highly reflective. In these cases, followup examination is necessary for further differentiation. Additionally, while clinical distinction between malignant melanoma and disciform lesion in clear media is not always clear-cut, echography makes a significant contribution in making this necessary differentiation.

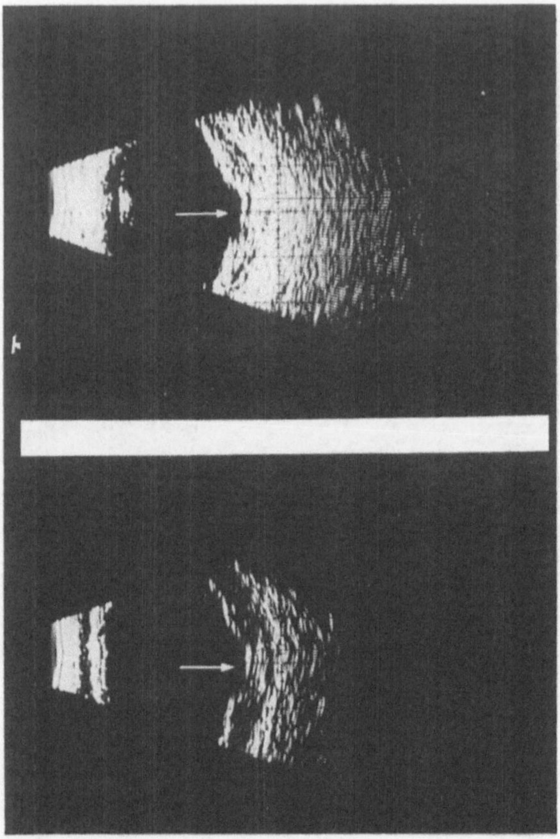

Fig. 5. B-scan at maximal sensitivity (top) and reduced sensitivity (bottom) of organized disciform lesion at the macula (arrow) with extensive collateral hemorrhagic retinal detachment.

METASTATIC TUMORS

Metastatic tumors may be localized or diffuse, and when significantly elevated often demonstrate a dumbbell shape on B-scanning. This central excavation is postulated to be caused by necrosis (13). With the standardized A-scan, internal structure is typically irregular (variable spike height) or regular with high reflectivity (constant, high spike height), consistency is solid and vascularity is rarely seen (Fig. 10) (3, 6, 7, 10).

Since differentiating metastatic from disciform lesions may be difficult (both may be highly reflective or irregularly structured), other factors must be considered. Metastatic lesions are rarely accompanied by vitreous

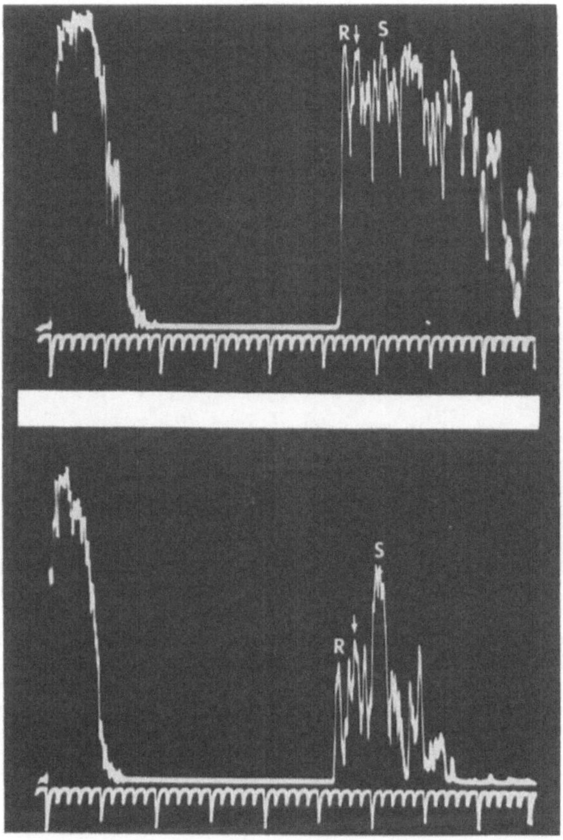

Fig. 6. A-scan of organized disciform lesion shown in Figure 5 at tissue sensitivity (top) and low, measuring sensitivity (bottom). R = sensory retina, arrow = choroid, S = sclera. High spikes beneath choroidal interface correspond to organized blood.

hemorrhage or associated hemorrhagic retinal detachment and internal calcification has not been documented. Followup examination often allows differentiation when the diagnosis cannot be established at initial examination. An additional helpful sign in diagnosing "senile macular degeneration" is the detection of macular thickening (greater than 1.5 mm.) in the fellow eye. In clear media, problems occasionally arise in clinically differentiating melanoma from disciform lesion, or melanoma from metastatic tumor as opposed to metastatic tumor from disciform lesion. Also, careful ophthalmoscopic examination frequently demonstrates drusen, thus supporting the echographic diagnosis.

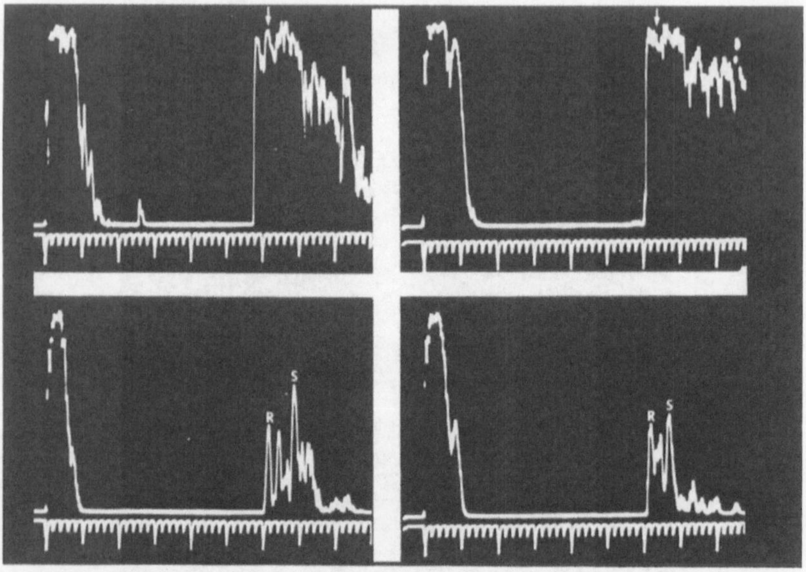

Fig. 7. **Left, disciform lesion at initial examination. Tissue sensitivity setting (top) shows high internal reflectivity (arrow). Lower echogram at measuring sensitivity displays maximal elevation. Right, same lesion at three month followup. Elevation of lesion has decreased, securing diagnosis. Arrows = internal lesion spikes, R = sensory retina, S = sclera.**

FOLLOWUP EXAMINATION

Sequential followup examinations are important in substantiating the diagnosis of disciform lesion by proving decrease rather than increase in lesion size (11). Any small, localized, solid, highly reflective or irregularly structured fundus lesion is initially classified as "disciform-like lesion". Neoplasms such as metastatic tumor and sometimes malignant melanoma, may exhibit these disciform-like characteristics when minimally elevated. With followup examination, neoplasms grow and change structurely, causing corresponding reflectivity alterations. Metastatic tumors become more elevated and often more irregular in internal structure, whereas melanomas frequently become more regular and less reflective even before enlarging (Fig. 11 and 12). Disciform lesions may initially present with some internal irregularity due to alternating areas of fresh and organized blood. At end stage, these lesions organize completely (highly reflective), and decrease in size (disciform scar). Followup examinations should be performed six weeks after the initial examination, and if there is no change, repeated in three months, six months, twelve months and annually thereafter.

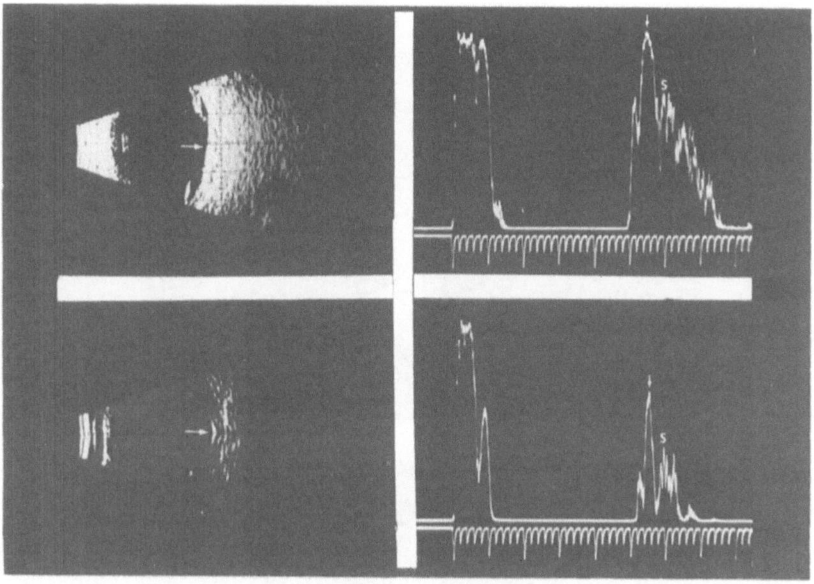

Fig. 8. A and B-scan montage of disciform scat containing large focus of calcium at high sensitivity (top) and reduced sensitivity (bottom). Arrow = calcium deposit, S = sclera. Note sound attenuation (shadowing) of sclera and orbital spikes. Echograms on bottom better illustrate sound attenuation by using low system sensitivity settings.

CONCLUSION

Standardized echography provides a highly reliable method of detecting, differentiating, and following disciform lesions of the fundus. This capability is of great importance in ruling out neoplasms, and in aiding the ophthalmologist with the assessment of future visual potential upon resolution of vitreous hemorrhage. Reliable diagnoses must, however, be based upon the use of standardized echography by an echographic diagnostician (2).

ACKNOWLEDGEMENTS

The author wishes to thank Trish Feally for typing this manuscript as well as Debbie Weinstein, Randy Hughes and Susan Eswine for the graphics.

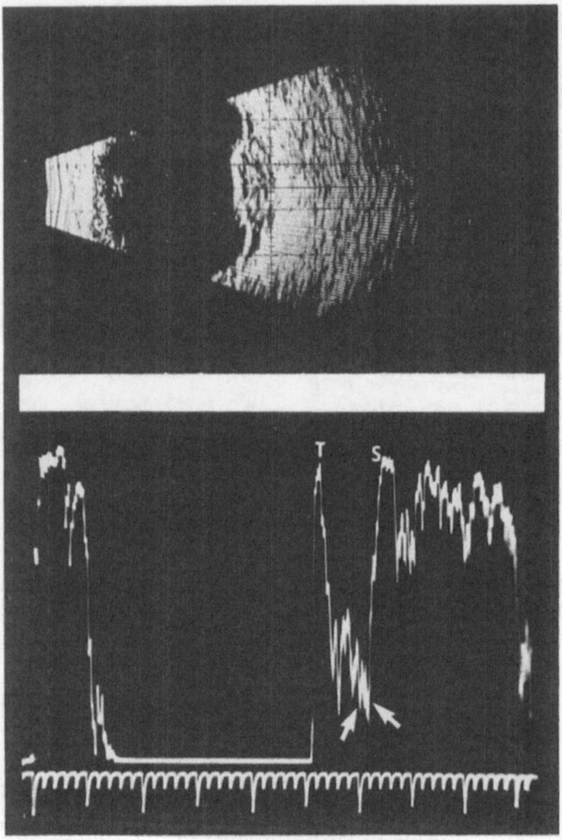

Fig. 9. B and A-scans of malignant melanoma. B-scan demonstrates lesion shape and location with concurrent serous retinal detachment. A-scan indicates typical regular arrangement of low spikes beneath the retinal/tumor surface (T) produced by dense, closely packed tumor cells. Arrows = blurred spikes indicating vascularity, S = sclera.

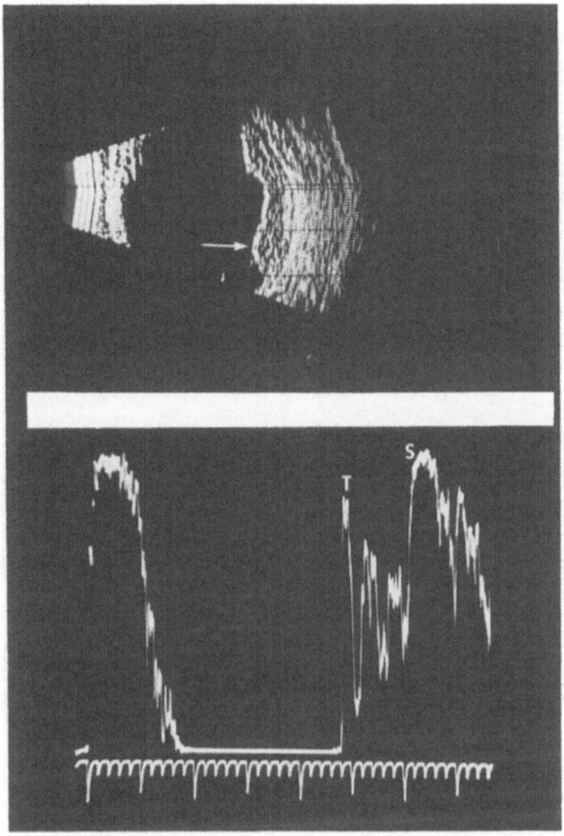

Fig. 10. B and A-scan montage of metastatic carcinoma. Note central excavation (dumbbell shape) on B-scan. A-scan section was taken from tumor portion of greatest elevation (arrow). T = retina/tumor interface, S = sclera. Note marked irregularity of internal tumor echogram corresponding to large and small tumor interfaces arranged in irregular distribution.

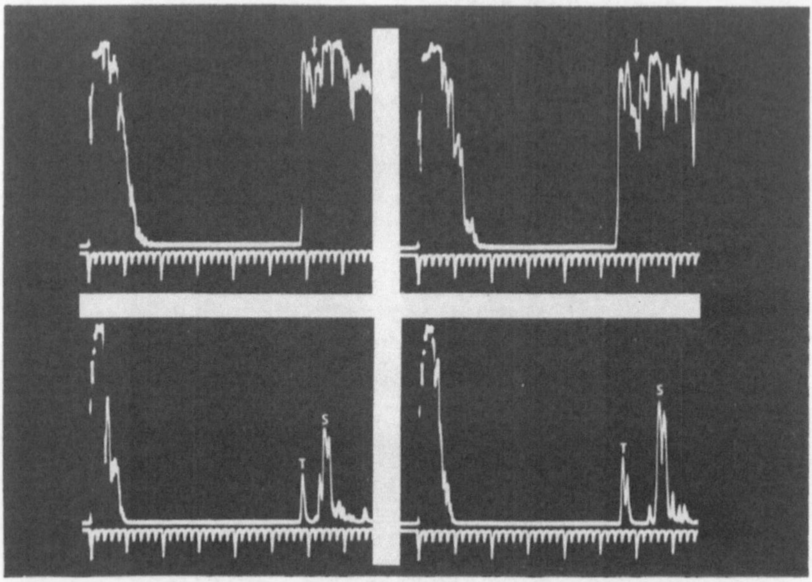

Fig. 11. Left, metastatic tumor at initial examination taken at the tissue sensitivity setting (top) and measuring sensitivity (bottom). Right, same tumor at three month followup. Internal structure (top) is slightly more irregular and elevation is increased. Arrows = internal lesion spikes, T = retina/tumor surface, S = sclera.

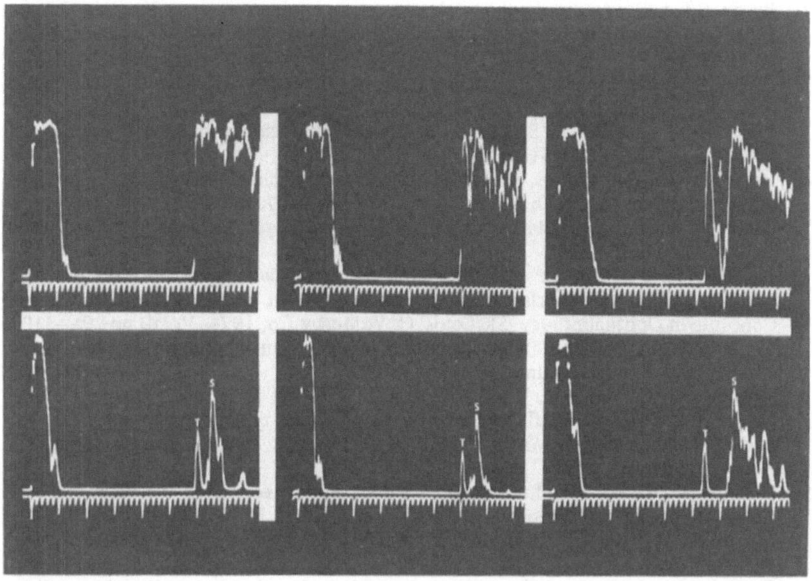

Fig. 12. Malignant melanoma at initial presentation (left), three months (center) and six months later (right). Upper echograms were taken at tissue sensitivity setting; lower sections show maximal elevation at measuring sensitivity. Arrows = internal lesion spikes, T = retina/tumor surface, S = sclera. Left, high internal reflectivity – disciform-like lesion. Center, medium internal reflectivity, no significant growth – suspicious for malignant melanoma. Right, low internal reflectivity, increased elevation – typical for malignant melanoma.

REFERENCES

1. Byrne, S.F.: Standardized echography: A-scan examination procedures, in Dallow, R. L. (ed): INT OPHTHAL CLIN, 19/4. Boston: Little Brown and Co, 1979, pp 267–281.
2. Byrne, S. F., Saclarides, E.: Standardized ophthalmic echography and the health care professional. JONT, 1/1, 1982, pp 19–27.
3. Fuller, D. G., Snyder, W. B., et al.: Ultrasonographic features of choroidal malignant melanomas. ARCH OPHTHALMOL, 97:1465–1472, 1979.
4. Hodes, B. L., Chormokos, E.: Standardized A-scan echographic diagnosis of choroidal melanoma. ARCH OPHTHALMOL, 95:593, 1977.
5. Ossoinig, K. C.: Quantitative echography – the basis of tissue differentiation. JCU, 2:33–46, 1974.
6. Ossoinig, K. C., Blodi, F. C.: Preoperative differential diagnosis of tumors with echography: III. Diagnosis of intraocular tumors, in Blodi, F. C. (ed): Current Concepts in Ophthalmology. St. Louis, C. V. Mosby Co, 1974, Vol 4, pp 296–313.
7. Ossoinig, K. C., Bigar, F., Kaefring, S. L.: Malignant melanoma of the choroid and ciliary body. Bibl Ophthalmol 83:141–154, 1975.
8. Ossoinig, K. C., Patel, J. H.: A-scan instrumentation for acoustic tissue differentiation: II. Clinical significance of various technical parameters of the 7200 MA unit of Kretztechnik, in White, D., Brown, R. E. (eds): Ultrasound in Medicine, 3B. New York: Plenum, 1977, pp 1949–1954.
9. Ossoinig, K. C., Patel, J. H.: A-scan instrumentation for acoustic tissue differentation: III. Testing and calibration of the 7200 MA unit of Kretztechnik, in White, D., Brown, R. E. (eds): Ultrasound in Medicine, 3B. New York: Plenum, 1977, pp 1955–1964.
10. Ossoinig, K. C.: Echography of the eye, orbit and periorbital region, Arger, P. H. (ed): Orbital Roentgenology, New York: Wiley, 1977, pp 224–269.
11. Ossoinig, K. C.: Standardized echography: Basic principles, clinical application and results, in Dallow, R. L. (ed): INT OPHTHAL CLIN, 19/4. Boston: Little Brown and Co, 1979, pp 127–210.
12. Till, P.: Solid tissue model for the standardization of the echo-ophthalmograph 7200 MA (Kretztechnik). Documenta Ophthalmol, 41(2):205, 1976.
13. Personal communication – Ossoinig.

Author's address:
Department of Echography
Bascom Palmer Eye Institute
P.O. Box 016880
Miami, FL 33101
USA

IN-VIVO MEASUREMENTS OF VITREOUS AND RETINAL ACCELERATION

ALAN L. SUSAL and JAMES T. WALKER
(Stanford, USA)

ABSTRACT

Ocular motion produces accelerative movement of the cortical vitreous and detached retinal segments. Such motion generates forces within the eye leading to retinal holes and tears and tractional retinal detachments. It is now possible to clinically measure in-vivo acceleration of ocular tissues using fast-frame, real-time ultrasound. The new equipment employs an electronically-scanned array to image in A- and B-modes at 60 frames per second and record these images on videotape. Studies of ocular tissue motion enables us to more fully understand the development of peripheral horseshoe retinal tears and posterior polar holes as well as degenerative changes within the vitreous body.

INTRODUCTION

The vitreous and detached retina have inertial movement to them which is independent of the motion of the global walls. This motion manifests as a velocity and acceleration, the acceleration leading to forces within the eye which can cause retinal tears, retinal traction and retinal detachments. Newly-developed ophthalmic ultrasonic imaging apparatus now enables us to evaluate the motion of the vitreous and detached retinal segments and to obtain clinical data regarding the accelerative changes these structures exhibit.

MATERIALS AND METHODS

Ultrasonic studies on the motion of the vitreous and detached retinal segments are possible primarily as the result of newly-developed linear array ultrasonic systems for use in ophthalmology. The linear array systems use a multiple transducer ultrasonic array of 35 elements which is electronically switched to quickly scan the eye region without any mechanical motion (Fig. 1). The electronic scanning is performed at 60 frames per second NTSC, U.S. standards (Walker J. T. et al. 1979) (or 50 frames per second European standards) and each frame is presented in perfect registry with preceding

Hillman, J. S./Le May, M. M. (eds.) Ophthalmic Ultrasonography

ISBN 978-94-009-7280-3

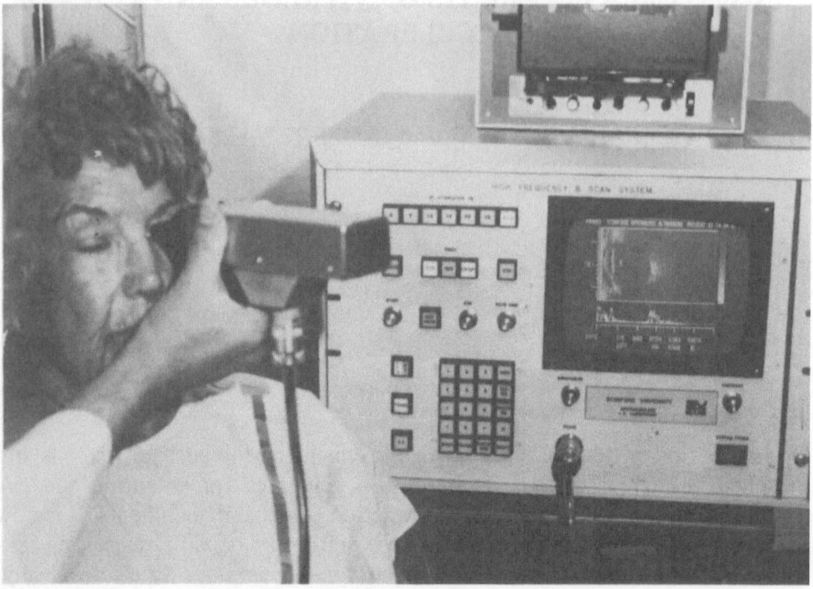

Fig. 1. Prototype linear-array, electronically-scanned ultrasonic system developed for ophthalmic real-time application. Contact scanning is being performed through the closed eyelids.

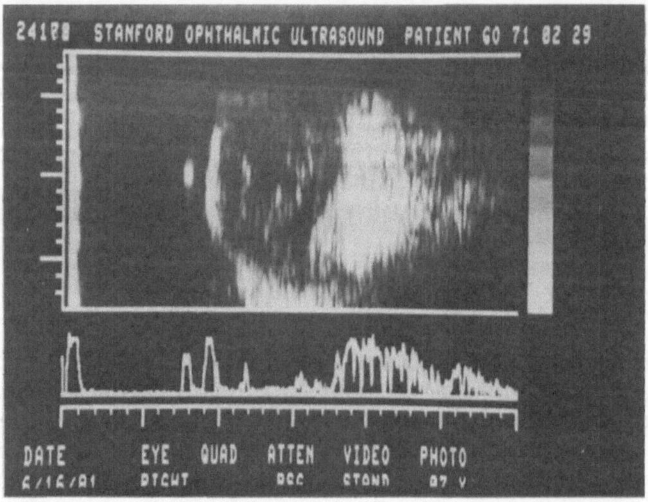

Fig. 2. Patient with asteroid hyalosis and elevated solid macular lesion. Note the multiple calcific deposite in the vitreous.

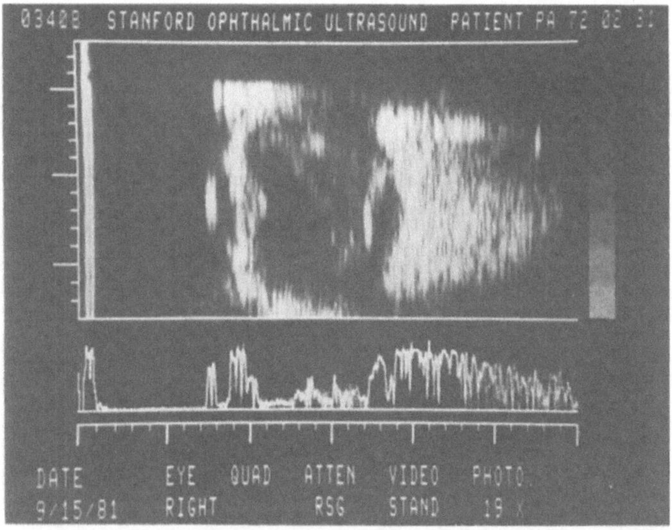

Fig. 3. Total retinal detachment with intravitreal haemorrhage. Patients with mobile retinal detachments demonstrate a whip-like retinal motility upon eye movements.

frames without any jittery motion induced by mechanically swept transducers. Since the transmitter and part of the receiver are also included in the hand-held probe containing the linear array, the sensitivity of the apparatus is considerably improved, enabling low-amplitude echoes in the vitreous to be imaged for the first time (Susal A. L. 1982).

The electronically-scanned images are presented on a standard television display with 64 levels of digitized gray scale giving a B-mode image of 580× 256 pixels. These images are recorded on standard television compatible videotape equipment (Susal A. L. et al. 1980).

Patients with asteroid hyalosis (Fig. 2) and mobile retinal detachments (Fig. 3) were chosen for this study. The discrete echoes from the calcific deposits in the hyalosis or specific retinal segments of detached retinas were imaged and recorded on videotape as the patients moved their eyes from side to side to induce motion. Each frame on the clinical videotape contains an ultrasonic image separated in time by 1/60th of a second from the next. Sequential ultrasonic images were thus obtained which documented the movement of the vitreous and detached retina and which were used to make distance measurements from a chosen portion of the global wall (Fig. 4). These distance measurements (separated from one another by 1/60th of a second) were then used to calculate velocity and acceleration.

RESULTS

Sequential photos of the movement of calcific deposits in asteroid hyalosis were used to calculate the cortical vitreous velocity and acceleration using the format given in Table 1. The cortical vitreous studied here had a moderate

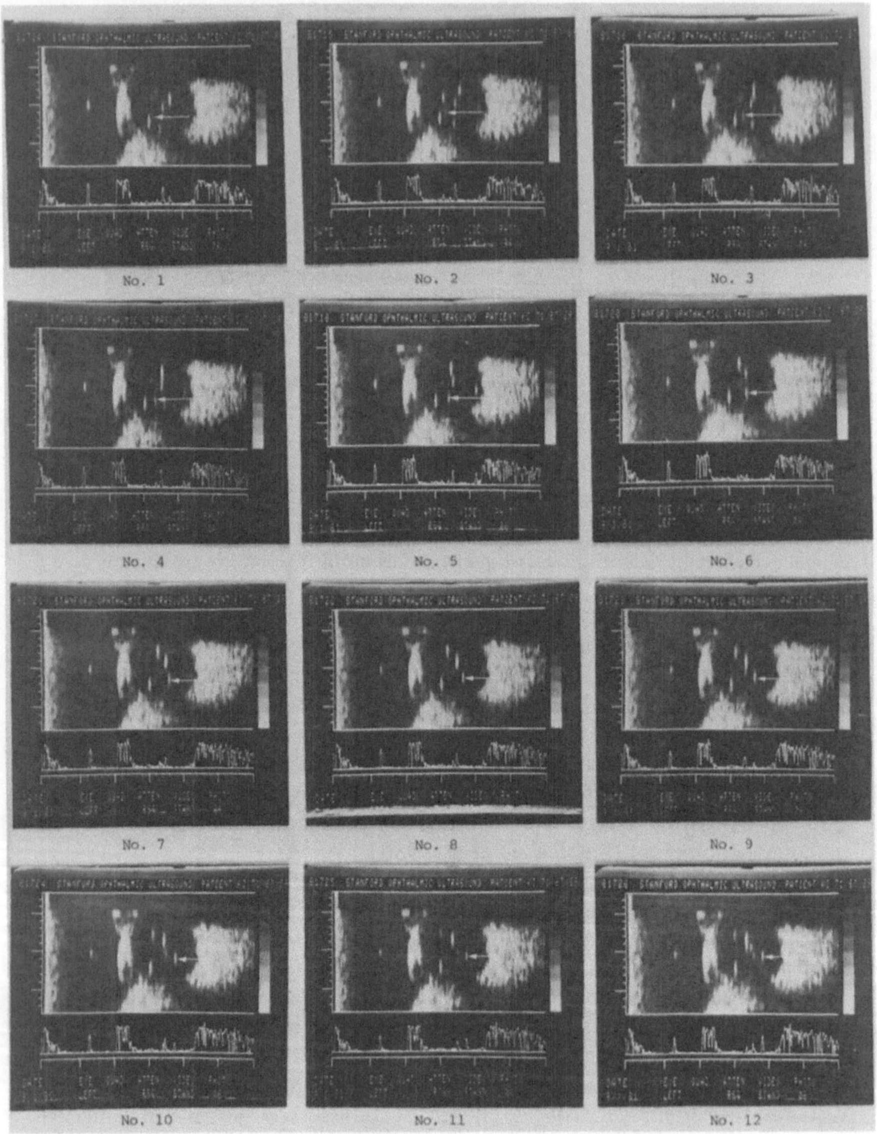

Fig. 4. Sequential videotaped ultrasonograms of a patient with asteroid hyalosis. Note the movement of the calcific deposit (arrow) from frame to frame. (Frame numbers in upper left-hand corner).

degree of vitreous degeneration (associated with the asteroid hyalosis) thus, exhibiting moderate accelerative movement. Cortical vitreous velocity and acceleration were calculated at 0.030 m. per second and 1.80 m. per second per second.

Table 1. Differences in the distance the target-point moves between subsequent ultrasonic images (separated by 1/60 sec.) is used to calculate the velocity and acceleration.

Videotaped (ultrasonic) images are 1/60 second apart

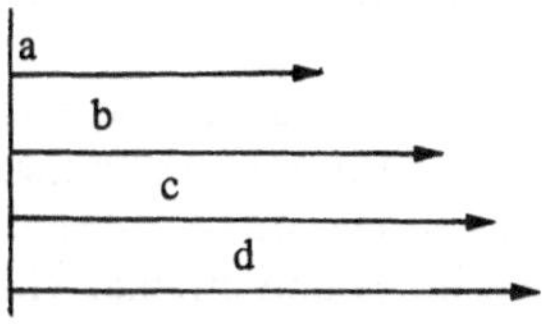

Distance (mm)	Distance Difference (mm)	2nd Distance Difference (mm)	Velocity (m/sec.)	Acceleration (m/sec.^{2})
a			$\frac{60\,(b-a)}{1000}$	
	b − a			
b		c + a − 2b	$\frac{60\,(c-b)}{1000}$	$\frac{(60)^2(c+a-2b)}{1000}$
	c − b			
c		d + b − 2c		$\frac{(60)^2(d+b-2c)}{1000}$
	d − c		$\frac{60\,(d-c)}{1000}$	
d				

Table 2. Results of representative vitreous and detached retinal movement calculations. A mobile retina with whip-like traveling waves can move faster than the cortical vitreous.

	Velocity	Acceleration
Cortical vitreous	0.030 m/sec.	1.80 m/sec.^{2}
Detached retina	0.090 m/sec.	7.92 m/sec.^{2}
(Acceleration of gravity = 9.80 m/sec.^{2})		

Acceleration from the detached retinal segments were measured and calculated to be 7.92 m. per second per second with retinal velocity 0.09 m. per second (Table 2).

DISCUSSION

The degree of vitreous degeneration, the breakdown from the gelatin-like hyaloid network of the young vitreous to the tumbling, swirling cortical vitreous movement pattern of the degenerated vitreous, mainly determines the motion measurements obtained here (McLeod D. and Restori M. 1977). Greater vitreous movement is seen in patients with moderate to severe vitreous degeneration.

With the cortical vitreous anchored at the vitreous base, the formed degenerated vitreous exhibits a swirling, rotating movement pattern which moves in a tangential fashion near the peripheral retina, but which moves in a rapid, linear manner posteriorly in eyes with partial or complete posterior vitreous detachments. The tangential motion of vitreous hinged at the vitreous base helps to explain the development of horseshoe retinal tears at the retinal periphery, where vitreoretinal adhesions induce shear forces which tear the retina. As the posterior vitreous hyaloid is progressively detaching, vitreo-retinal adhesions cause horseshoe tears with the operculum hinged closer to the vitreous base.

In partial posterior vitreous detachments, the posterior cortical vitreous moves in a rapid manner in a direction more perpendicular to the posterior pole. This causes linear tractional forces on the disk and posterior retina tending to create the round retinal holes and circular vitreous opacifications often seen with posterior pathology.

A fresh rhegmatogenous retinal detachment will demonstrate a tethered-rope movement pattern upon real-time sonography. The whip-like perturbations of traveling waves along the retinal membrane cause sudden, quick movements which give the detached retina a greater velocity and acceleration compared to the vitreous. These sudden retinal motions cause forces which are directly transmitted to adjacent retinal segments, promoting the rapid progression of rhegmatogenous retinal detachments.

Accelerative forces in the vitreous and the detached retina can be used to calculate absolute force measurements if a valid movement model is employed. This work is the basis of further studies.

CONCLUSIONS

Newer ultrasonic apparatus enables us to image the motion patterns of the cortical vitreous and the detached retina and to calculate velocity and acceleration values for that motion. Motion studies of the vitreous and retina aid in understanding the development and progression of retinal tears and retinal detachments. These observations also enable the physician to evaluate the degenerative movement of the cortical vitreous. Real-time ophthalmic ultrasound provides new observations on the eye which enables us to more fully evaluate vitreo-retinal pathology.

REFERENCES

McLeod, D. and Restori, M.: Real-time B-scanning of the vitreous. Trans. Ophthalmol. Soc. U.K. 97:547–550, 1977.

Susal, A. L., Walker, J. T. and Meindl, S. D.: Small organ dynamic imaging system. Jour. Clin. Ultrasound 8:421–426, 1980.

Susal, A. L.: Dynamic ultrasound examination of the eye. Submitted to Amer. Jour. of Ophthalmol., 1982.

Walker, J. T., Susal, A. L. and Meindl, J. D.: High resolution dynamic ultrasonic imaging. Proc. Photo-Optical Inst. Eng. 152:54–58, 1979.

Authors' addresses:
Alan L. Susal
Division of Ophthalmology
Stanford University Medical Center
Stanford, CA 94305
USA

James T. Walker
Applied Electronics Laboratory AEL-211
Stanford University
Stanford, CA 94305
USA

POSTERIOR SCLERITIS – THE ROLE OF ULTRASONOGRAPHY IN THE FOLLOW-UP OF THE DISEASE

R. F. GUTHOFF and GURINDER SINGH
(*Hamburg, W. Germany*)

SUMMARY

The course of the disease in 7 patients with a follow-up between 8 months and 6 years is presented. The initial clinical signs had been quite similar including acute hyperopia and choroidal folds. Ultrasonographically the well known enlargement of the posterior eye walls seemed to be due to a thickening of choroid, sclera and Tenon's capsule. In some cases the dural diameter of the optic nerve was found to be enlarged. During follow-up, in a few cases all symptoms disappeared within 1–2 weeks whereas in most of the patients the thickening of the choroidal tissue remained for years despite local and systemic steroid treatment.

Posterior scleritis, according to the literature (1, 2) is still an aetiologically undefined entity. Clinically it presents as acute hyperopia correctable by convex lenses. Ophthalmoscopically it shows mostly as horizontal folds of the posterior pole. Flourescein-angiography helps to define these folds as of choroidal origin (3, 4) without any damage to the retinal pigment epithelium layer. A few reports like by Cappaert, Purnell and Frank (1977) showed the correlation of posterior scleritis with Systemic Lupus Erythematosis and sinus disease. The role of steroids in its management still remains questionable (1, 2, 5).

The lack of histopathological studies, at least to our knowledge, to this moment can be only substituted by flourescein-angiography and ultrasonographical findings. We would like to present our experience with ultrasonographic follow-up of 7 patients to suggest the involvement of various tissues during the unpredictable course of this disease.

MATERIAL AND METHODS

10 eyes of 7 patients were examined clinically and by Ultrasound using Bronson-Turner B-scan and lately by Xenotec 303 (Ultrascan). The longest follow-up is for 6 years while the last patient included in this study presented with symptoms only 8 months ago. All the patients are still under observation. Flourescein-angiography and CT-scan had been performed additionally.

Hillman, J.S./Le May, M.M. (eds.) Ophthalmic Ultrasonography

ISBN 978-94-009-7280-3

RESULTS

All the seven patients were males, 3 of them presented with bilateral symptoms. (Table 1). The age varied from 14–49 years at the onset of the disease. The range of acquired hyperopia, which in all the cases led to the presenting symptom of blurred vision ranged from 1.5–3.5 diopters. Ophthalmoloscopic findings of folds on the posterior pole were associated with Ultrasonographic sign of Choroidal thickening in all 10 eyes, while Tenon's space enlargement could be demonstrated only in 6 patients. Unexpectedly, optic nerve thickening was additionally found in 4 patients as diagnosed by measuring the dural diameter and also shown by CT-scan. (11, 12).

Table 1. Clinical data of patients with posterior Scleritis during the follow-up

Sex	All males
No. of eyes	10 (3 patients with bilateral involvement)
Age at onset of disease	14–49 years
Follow-up	8 months–6 years
Range of acquired Hyperopia	1.5–3.5 Diopters
Choroidal thickening	10
Tenon's space involvement	6
Optic nerve thickening	
– ultrasonographically	4
– CT-scan	3
Persistence of choroidal thickening	6 (follow up 1–6 years)

During the follow-up, the posterior pole folds as well as ultrasonographically proven Choroidal thickening persisted in 6 of 10 eyes partly slowly regressing but still present up to the longest follow-up of 6 years.

DISCUSSION

The earlier reports dealing with the ultrasonographic signs of posterior scleritis by Cappaert, Purnell (1) and others (5) stress the flattening of the posterior pole as the most striking ultrasonographic finding. With increased resolving power of the equipment, differentiation of the ocular coats has been possible in B- and M-mode techniques used by Coleman 1969 (6, 7) Giglio et. al. 1967 (8) and Lepper 1981 (9). As demonstrated in Fig. 1 even with the commercially available instruments today the so called flattening of the posterior pole can be differentiated into several layers. Comparing identical ocular regions the lowering of amplification by 20 dB shows that while scleral curvature remained unchanged the the flattening was actually caused by a pre-scleral thickening only. According to the basic works of Coleman (6, 7) and the clinical findings of uneffected retinal and pigment epithelium structures this layer represents mainly a thickened choroid. In Fig. 2 the ultrasonographic follow-up of an unusually rapid regression in 14 year old boy is shown. The child was referred to the hospital with the provisional diagnosis of papillitis having vision reduced to 0.1. He was first seen by us on 4th Nov., 1981 and presented choroidal folds in both eyes. The

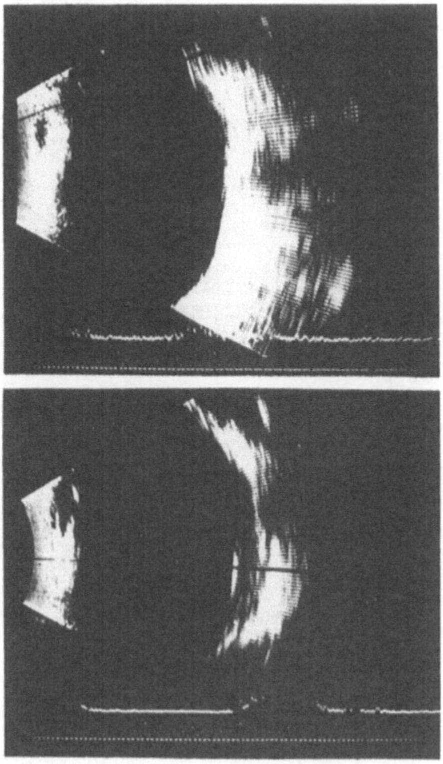

Fig. 1. B-Scan Ultrasonograms of the posterior pole in a acute stage of posterior scleritis. (a) with high amplification the flattening of the posterior pole appears to be the only pathological finding. (b) reducing the amplification by 20 dB the structures of the ocular coats are resolved into different layers.

vision improved from 0.1–0.8 just after correction of acute hyperopia by 2.5 diopters. The acute stage lasted only a few days and on the 11th Nov. the uncorrected vision increased to 1.0 despite the fact that a discrete swelling of the posterior pole was still demonstrable ultrasonographically. A few months later these findings also returned to normal with a vision of 1.2.

The more frequent chronic presentation of the disease preserves this choroidal thickening and acquired hyperopia. It was demonstrable even after a 6 years follow-up of a man aged 25 at the time of the initial symptoms.

As mentioned before, in 4 cases the dural diameter of the optic nerve was enlarged as can be appreciated in Fig. 3. In the right orbit the S-shaped optic nerve is seen within normal limits of width, compared to the left side where there is a definite thickening of the nerve. It is hard to comment on different reflecting surfaces seen on the B-scan sonogram – a separation of nerve surface and dural surface might be possible.

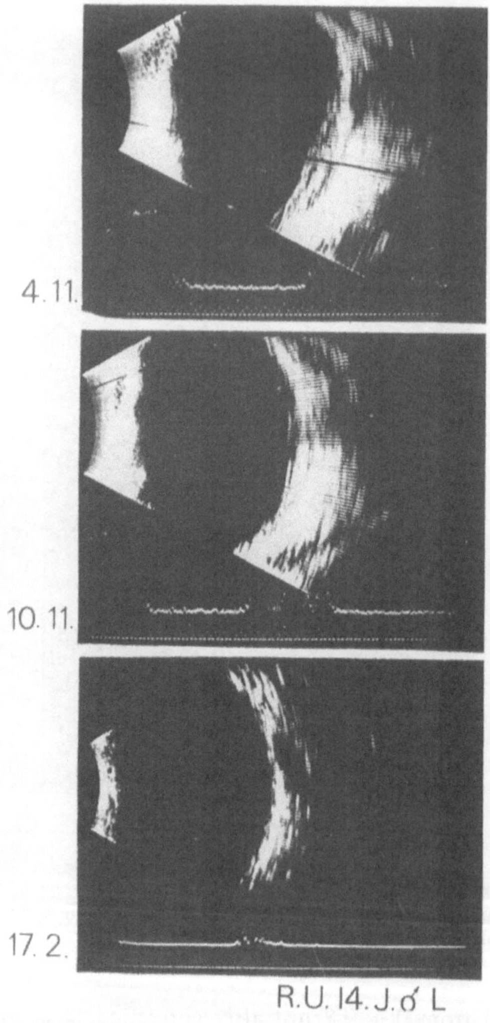

Fig. 2. **Rapid regression of posterior scleritis in a 14 year old boy. According to the shortening of axial length acute hyperopia of 2, 5 diopters returned to emmetropia within 14 days.**

What conclusions could be derived from these results?

(1) The fact that in all our chronic cases the ultrasonographically demonstrated choroidal thickening persisted and the acquired hyperopia remained constant leads us to the conclusion that only choroidal thickening and not scleral shrinkage as suggested earlier (Cappeart, Purnell (1), Norton (3)) occur in the course of the disease.

(2) The so called Posterior Scleritis involves Choroid and Tenon's space as described by other authors (1, 2, 10). Our additional findings of Optic Nerve thickening and the absence of scleral shrinkage makes us think that it is

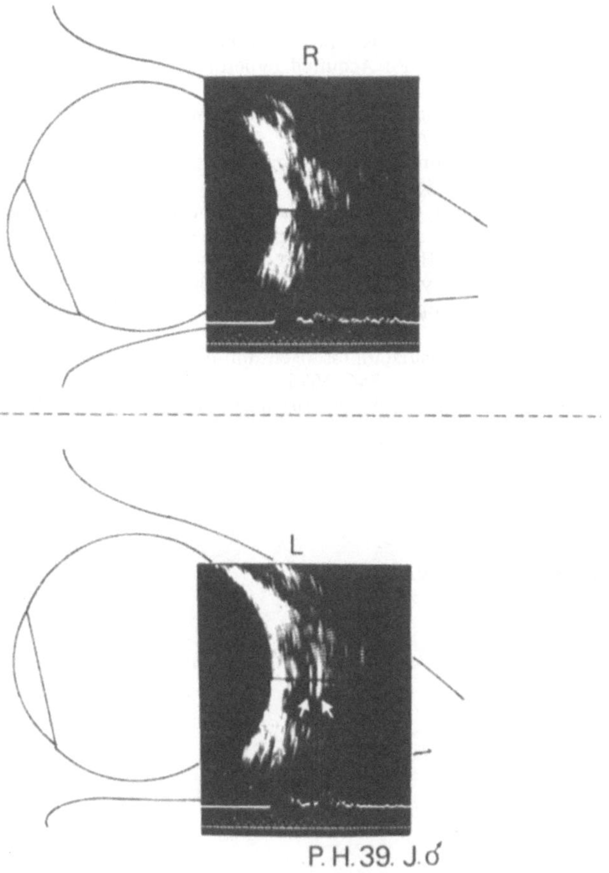

Fig. 3. Optic nerve thickening in unilateral posterior scleritis. Different reflections (arrows) may represent inner and outer dural surfaces.

a vasculitis of unknown etiology with increased permeability of the vasculature around the posterior pole, not localised mainly to the scleral tissue.

(3) The course of the disease seems to be benign and unpredictable. In the chronic cases correction of the acquired hyperopia is advocated and it reduces the patients complaints satisfactorally. Additional investigations like neurological and radiological studies could be limited to a certain extent.

REFERENCES

1. Cappaert, W. E., Purnell, E. W., Frank, K. E.: Use of B-scan Ultrasound in the diagnosis of benign choroidal folds. Am. J. Ophthal. 84, 375–379, 1977.
2. Verbeek, A. M.: Echographic findings in 34 patients with choroidal folds. Doc. Ophthal. Proc. Series, Vol 29, edited by J. M. Thijssen and A. M. Verbeek, 1981. Dr. W. Junk Publishers, The Hague, p. 367–374.
3. Norton, E. W. D.: A characteristic flourescein-angiographic pattern in choroidal folds. Proc. R. Soc. Med. 62:119, 1969.

4. Newell, F. W.: Choroidal folds. Am. J. Ophthal. 75, 930, 1973.
5. Kalina, R. E.,. Mills, R. P.: Acquired hyperopia with choroidal folds. Ophthalm. 87, 44–50, 1980.
6. Coleman, D. J., Weiniger, R.: Ultrasonic M-mode technique in Ophthalmology. Arch. Ophthalm. 82: 475–479, 1969.
7. Coleman, D. J.: Measurement of choroidal pulsation with M-scan ultrasound. Am. J. Ophthal. 71, 363–365, 1971.
8. Giglio, E. J., Ludlam, W. M.: High resolution ultrasonic equipment to measure intra-ocular distances. J. Am. Optometry 38, 367–371, 1967.
9. Lepper, R. D., Trier, H. G., Reuter, R.: Ultrasonic measurements at the posterior wall of Living human eyes. Ophthalmic Research 13, 1–11, 1981.
10. Cangemi, F. E., Trempe, C. L., Walsh, J. B.: Choroidal folds. Am. J. Ophthal. 86, 380–387, 1978.
11. Schroeder, W.: Schallaufzeitmessungen im distalen Sehnervenquerschnitt. Klin. Mbl. Augenheilk. 169, 743–746, 1976.
12. Guthoff, R. F., Schroeder, W.: Measurements of the optic nerve by Ultrasound and CT-Scan. Orbit in print.

Authors' address:
Universitäts-Augenklinik
Martinistrasse 52
Hamburg 20
Federal Republic of Germany

DIAGNOSTIC ULTRASOUND IN MASSIVE CHOROIDAL HAEMORRHAGE

L. KOLOZSVÁRI
(*Debrecen, Hungary*)

Choroidal detachment caused by circumscribed uveal haemorrhage can readily be diagnosed by means of ultrasound. Many authors (Bertényi 1977, Buschman 1966, Coleman 1977, Poujol 1981, etc.) have clarified the acoustic characteristics of this condition using A- and B-scan ultrasonograms.

Although much more rare massive choroidal haemorrhages do sometimes occur. Expulsive haemorrhages during or after surgery are known the best of all. Most of the German textbooks mention only this type of massive haemorrhage of the uvea. The extensive bleeding can have a fatal outcome for the eye, however, in some fortunate cases vision can be retained by suturing the wound in time and perhaps by scleral puncture.

Expulsive haemorrhages can also appear spontaneously and they occur following perforations resulting from the severely damaged tunica fibrosa.

Massive choroidal haemorrhage can be found also in the intact globe. This is called choroidal apoplexy according to Donders (Duke-Elder 1966). Due to the lack of fundus reflex, increased intraocular pressure, positive transillumination finding and painful eye, the possibility of an intraocular tumour comes to our mind. In case of damaged ocular wall as having been mentioned above, increased intraocular pressure can easily rupture the globe and produce a clinical picture similar to that of spontaneous expulsive bleeding.

In our clinic 6 massive uveal haemorrhages were diagnosed during the past 6 years (up to June 1982) by means of ultrasound. Three of them, 2 males and 1 female, suffered from choroidal apoplexy. The ages of the males ranged between 46–50 years, the female patient was 70 years old. The age of the three female patients with expulsive haemorrhage ranged between 66–70 years.

The oldest case was examined using a Picker Echoview IV. unit with a 7.5 MHz/5 mm slightly focused transducer. On the basis of the ultrasonogram the possibility of a solid lesion arose. Though blood could be observed behind the lens biomicroscopically, the painful eye with intraocular tension of about 60 mmHg and the positive transillumination finding supported the suspicion of tumour. Enucleation was carried out. Massive haemorrhage was proved histologically.

Recently ultrasonography has been carried out by means of the unit of the Firm Kretztechnik 7100 MA with a transducer 6 MHz/5 mm. The echography

Hillman, J. S./Le May, M. M. (eds.) Ophthalmic Ultrasonography

ISBN 978-94-009-7280-3

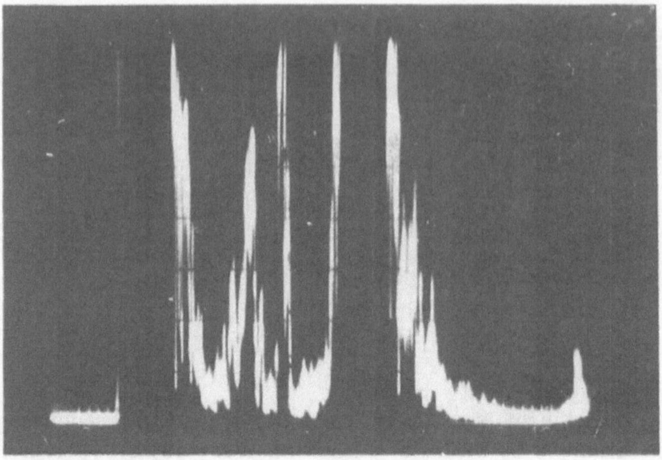

Fig. 1. Echogram of choroidal apoplexy.

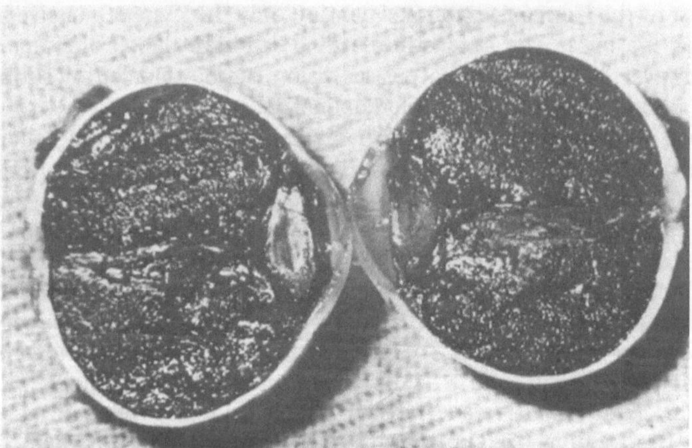

Fig. 2. Macroscopic picture of an eye following choroidal apoplexy.

of the eyeballs always began with maximum amplification (80 dB), in the case of quantitative echography the sclera was used as test object (Ossoinig 1971).

The next case showed symptoms similar to those of the former one. Echographically a structure could be discerned in a position corresponding to the axis of the globe. It was of great reflectivity with high, manifold echoes and with Δ dB values ranging between 10–12. Between the high spikes and the initial echoes, and between those and the posterior wall complex, respectively, a number of low, mobile echoes appeared (Fig. 1). However, they disappeared almost entirely on lowering the sensitivity of the apparatus 6–10 dB. Consequently, massive uveal haemorrhage was diagnosed. Because

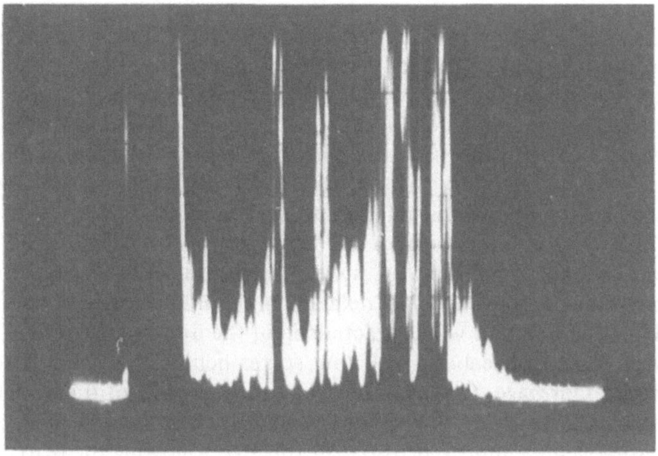

Fig. 3. Echogram of choroidal apoplexy.

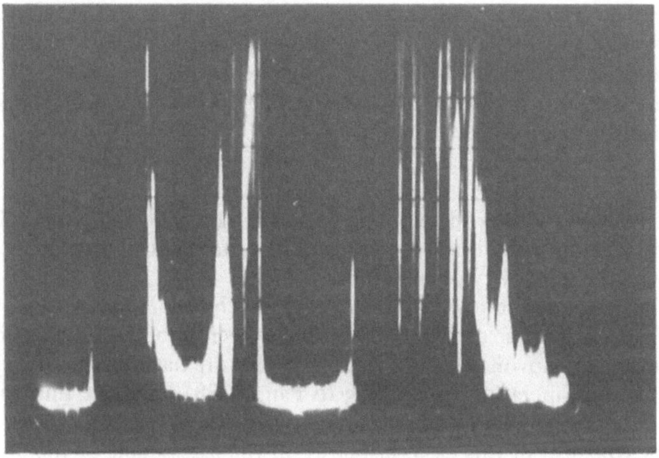

Fig. 4. Echogram of choroidal apoplexy 4 weeks later, (the same case).

of the unrelievable pain, the otherwise blind eye was enucleated. Macroscopically bleeding could be observed in the bisected globe between the sclera and the furled retina which was pushed to the center. The choroid could not be recognised in the blood clot (Fig. 2).

The third patient lost visual acuity in one eye 6 weeks prior to ultrasound examination. He was sent to our clinic with a diagnosis of absolute glaucoma. The echogram was similar to the former one (Fig. 3). Consequently, choroidal apoplexy was diagnosed. A month later the same ultrasonogram was found essentially, the intensity of the low spikes decreased becoming even lower between the high echoes and the posterior wall (Fig. 4).

In case 4 echography was carried out following expulsive haemorrhage. The echogram was similar to those mentioned previously. During a 5 months' follow up period reflectivity of the chorio-retinal bundle did not change, however, the echoes reflected by the neighbouring blood clot diminished perceptively. Here also the structure with high reflectivity seemed to shadow the posterior region up to the retina acoustically. The diseased eye was enucleated because of phthisis bulbi dolorosa.

The fifth patient underwent a moderate expulsive haemorrhage in the course of cataract operation. In spite of corneal scars 3 large touching elevations resulting from choroidal detachment could be observed ophthalmoscopically. The echogram was characteristic of the disease. The retina and the choroid reflected high echoes with low spikes behind them, the latter ones suggesting haemorrhage. On examining the touching parts of the detachments echographically, obviously the echogram became more complicated. After 2 months visual acuity improved to 0.4 in this eye following the reattachment of the choroid and the retina.

In the last case a severe expulsive haemorrhage treated with scleral puncture occured during star operation. The eye healed with a visual acuity of 0.25. The echogram was prepared 4 years following the severe complication. The vitreous cavity, filled with aqueous humour because of the extensive vitreous loss, was acoustically homogeneous.

Summarising, in the case of massive uveal haemorrhage choroidal apoplexy has to be suspected if the echogram shows:

(a) bundles of high reflectivity in a position corresponding to the axis of the globe,

(b) high echoes with Δ dB values agreeing with those of the retina (10–15),

(c) and surrounded with low, very mobile echoes which quickly disappear on lowering the sensitivity of the unit,

(d) a decrease of the low, mobile echoes which become even lower behind than in front of the high spikes after a follow up peroid of 3–4 weeks or more.

Diagnostically no difficulties arise from the dramatic event of expulsive bleeding during operation. According to Pau (1958) only one third of cases of this serious condition occur intraoperatively. However, echography has an important role also in this case, primarily in the assessment of the prognosis of the disease. In the case of an echogram characteristic of choroidal apoplexy, prognosis is unfavourable, as in case 4. Partial expulsive haemorrhage, consisting of some haemorrhagic elevations resulting from choroidal detachment, can recover with visual acuity some weeks or months later (cases 5 and 6). Echographic characteristics are well known also in this case.

In the case of early and late postoperative expulsive haemorrhage echography is a more useful method for the differential diagnosis (Bellone and Gallenga 1975).

REFERENCES

Bellone G., Sirianni G. and Murru L.: Tentativo di emorragia espulsiva blocato durante intervento di cataratta. Considerazioni sulla base dell'indagine ecografica. Minerva

Oftal. (Torino) 17:162 (1975).
Bertényi A.: Ultrasound diagnostics of the postoperative choroidal detachments. Szemészet 114:104 (1977).
Buschmann W.: Einführung in die ophthalmologische Ultraschalldiagnostik. Georg Thieme, Leipzig, 1966.
Coleman D. J., Lizzi F. L., Jack R. L.: Ultrasonography of eye and orbit. Lea and Febiger, Philadelphia, 1977.
Duke-Elder S.: Massive haemorrhages from the choroid. In: System of Ophthalmology. Vol. IV. pp. 27–34. London, Henry Kimpton, 1966.
Ossoinig K.: Grundlagen der klinischen Echo-Ophthalmologie. Verlag der Medizinischen Akademie, Wien, 1977.
Pau H.: Der Zeitfaktor bei der expulsiven Blutung. Klin. Mbl. Augenheilk. 132:865 (1958).
Poujol J.: A characteristic echographic sign of choroidal detachment – the reappearance of the angle of junction with the ocular wall. Documenta Ophthal. 29:265 (1981) ed. by J. M. Thijssen and A. M. Verbeek. Dr. W. Junk Publishers, The Hague.

Author's address:
University Eye Clinic
H 4012 Debrecen
Hungary

H-1085 Budapest
Hungary

B-SCAN ULTRASONOGRAMS OF CILIARY BODY DETACHMENT

YUKIO IIJIMA and KAORU ASANAGI
(*Chiba, Japan*)

ABSTRACT

In order to display ciliary body detachment, the authors developed the water bath immersion technique using the Sonometrics Ocuscan 400. Using this technique, ciliary body detachment in vivo in 19 eyes with rhegmatogenous retinal detachment was observed for the first time. As a result, it was detected that the former concept of ciliary body detachment did not correctly represent the shapes of this detachment in vivo.

INTRODUCTION

The morphology of ciliary body detachment in vivo has not yet been fully clarified. The authors observed pictures of ciliary body detachment in eyes with rhegmatogenous retinal detachment for the first time in vivo, using their own independently developed B-scan ultrasonographic diagnostic method. The following new findings regarding morphology of ciliary body detachment were obtained.

METHODS

The water-bath immersion technique with the patient in the supine position was adopted, using the Ocuscan 400, a diagnostic ultrasonic contact A-scan and B-scan system, manufactured by Sonometrics (ultrasonic frequency 10 MHz) (Fig. 1).

The unique points of this method are that the examiner can hold the scanning handpiece on making an examination, and that the oscillations of the scanner at the time of examination can be prevented by fixing the hand to the supporting stand.

When the ciliary body was examined, the authors paid particular attention to holding the lid open with the speculum; that the eye balls could be rotated to allow the ciliary body region to come immediately above; that the depth of water would be about 15 mm; and that the ultrasonic beams could be applied perpendicular to the ciliary body region. The ciliary body region was

Hillman, J.S./Le May, M.M. (eds.) Ophthalmic Ultrasonography

ISBN 978-94-009-7280-3

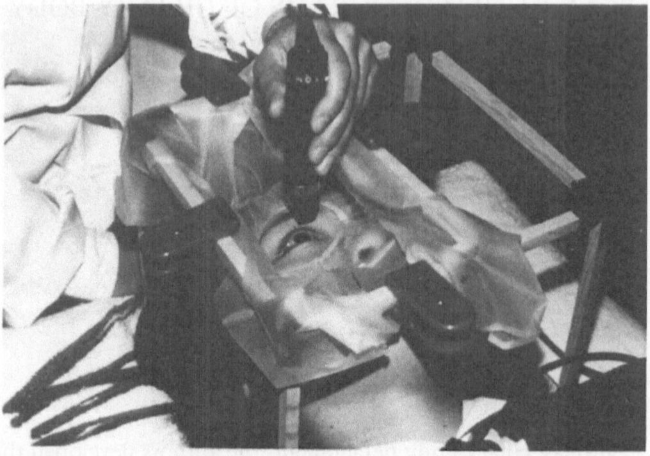

Fig. 1. **B-scan ultrasonographic method adopted by the authors.**

depicted in B-scan ultrasonograms of the sagittal section, and the pictures of two scans on the transducer were recorded by Polaroid camera.

The position of the ciliary body region

Figure 2 shows the B-scan ultrasonogram of an eye with rhegmatogenous retinal detachment being rotated to allow the ciliary body region to come immediately above. When the position of the ciliary body (CB) was decided, the region of adherence (arrow) of the detached retina (RD) to the eye wall was considered to be the posterior periphery of the CB, and the boundary (arrow) of the cornea (C) and the sclera on the B-scan ultrasonogram was considered to be the anterior periphery of the CB. The CB in Fig. 2 is normal. The indicated position is not an anatomical one, but a position for the sake of convenience of the study, and is regarded as a criterion for the decision as to the positions of other CB pictures.

SUBJECTS

The material used was 16 eyes in which choroidal detachment was noted ophthalmoscopically, and 4 eyes in which choroidal detachment was not observed; however, the existence of ciliary body detachment was suspected from accompanying ocular hypotony, among 115 eyes of patients with preoperative rhegmatogenous retinal detachment who had visited Chiba University Hospital over a one-year period from May 1, 1981 to April 30, 1982, and on whom the B-scan ultrasonic examination of their ciliary body regions had been performed.

However, the material included one eye on which this examination had already been performed once in the period when choroidal detachment was

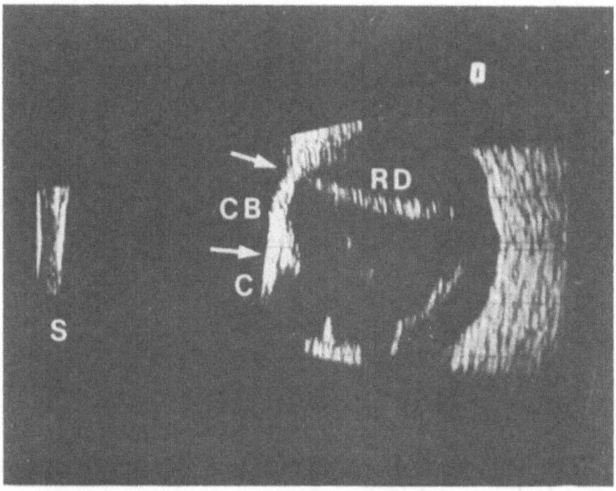

Fig. 2. B-scan ultrasonogram of the normal ciliary body region in an eye with rhegmatogenous retinal detachment. The position of ciliary body region is shown with two arrows and the sign of CB. S: the tip of the scanner, C: the cornea, RD: a detached retina, CB: the ciliary body region.

not noted, and once in the period when it was noted, and, in effect, the material amounted to 19 eyes of 19 patients (Table 1).

Table 1. The materials. Twenty-fold inspections of ciliary body regions of 19 eyes with B-scan ultrasonic waves were performed. The frequencies of ciliary body detachment in 4 regions of an eye classified by type are shown on the right side of the table.

materials				types of the B-scan ultrasonograms of the ciliary body detachment				
case number	name	age		a	b	c	d	e
case 1	Y.T.	59			1	3		
2	T.O.	67				2	2	
3	S.N.	66			1		2	1
4	R.F.	48			1	2		1
5	K.S.	46						4
6	T.K.	60		1	2			1
7	M.I.	51				4		
8	S.O.	61	Dec. 9, 1981	1	1	2		
			Dec. 26, 1981					4
9	M.T.	32		1		2	1	
10	S.S.	53					2	2
11	S.T.	70			2	2		
12	K.N.	44			1			3
13	T.S.	43						4
14	F.H.	56		2	1	1		
15	T.T.	72				1	2	1
16	J.N.	82				4		
17	K.D.	69				2		2
18	K.K.	40		1	1	2		
19	M.K.	66						4

In all these cases, B-scan pictures of ciliary body detachment, to be shown below, were observed. The observations and recordings of the pictures of ciliary body detachment were made at 4 regions, i.e. the upper side, lower side, temporal side, and nasal side, per one eye in all cases. Since the pictures of ciliary body detachment sometimes differed according to the site of recording, the present study made use of "echograms" of ciliary body regions from 80 sites and 80 polaroid pictures as data.

RESULTS

A fundamental shape of B-scan ultrasonograms of ciliary body detachment

B-scan pictures of ciliary body detachment were not uniform but multiform in shape. However, these multiform pictures were based upon a single basic form. The essentials of the basic form were that the wall of the eyeball of the ciliary body region was in principle separated into 2 layers, i.e. the inner layer and outer layer, and that the mode of separation was different between the anterior portion of the ciliary body region and posterior portion, the anterior portion being slit-like and in parallel, and the posterior portion, in a cuneiform expansion. In other words, the basic form consisted of the anterior portion in parallel and slit-shape, and the posterior portion in a cuneiform expansion, as shown in Fig. 3.

Although the anterior portion was described as separation in a slit shape, sometimes no separation was observed in it, whereas in the posterior portion, the cuneiform expansion was subdivided by several stages of separation, sometimes with no finding of separation, as with the anterior portion. In addition, the position of the boundary between the anterior portion and the posterior portion was not fixed, but variable in accordance with the state of disease. These variations in various combinations were added to the basic form, which seem to have manifested themselves as multiform B-scan ultrasonograms of ciliary body detachment.

Classification of B-scan ultrasonograms of ciliary body detachment

The multiform B-scan ultrasonograms of ciliary body detachment can be classified, on consideration of the above basic form, into 5 types as follows. This classification is convenient for grasping the whole picture. Comments are given below for each type; the frequency for each eye is shown in Table 1.

Type a

This is a type showing no separation in both anterior and posterior portions (Fig. 4).

This type differs from the normal picture (Fig. 2) of the ciliary body region in that the posterior half sector of the ciliary body region looks hypertrophied. This led the authors to believe that the type (a) shows very mild ciliary body detachment. It was noted in 6 (7.5%) of 80 ciliary body regions.

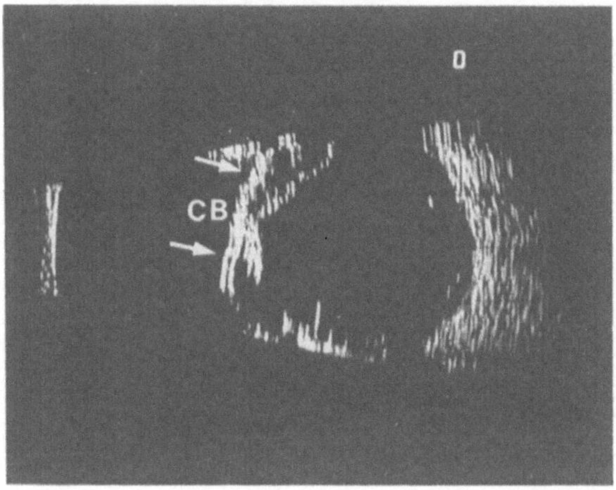

ciliary body region is separated in the form of a slit, while the posterior portion is separated in cuneiform expansion. This shows the basic form of ciliary body detachment, classified as Type e.

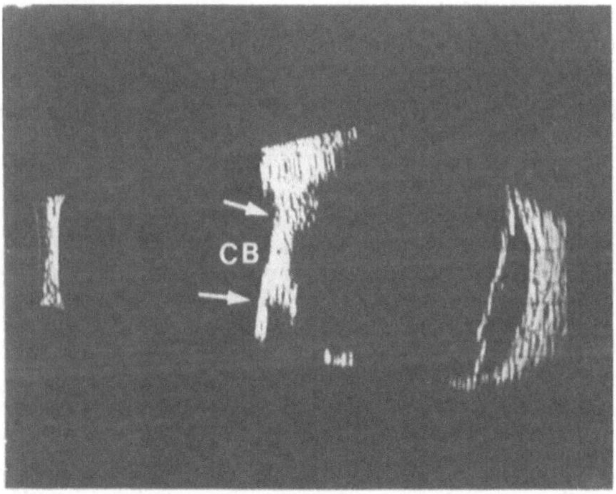

Fig. 4. B-scan ultrasonogram of ciliary body detachment. No separation is noted both in the anterior and posterior portions. This B-scan ultrasonogram differs from the normal one in that the posterior half looks hypertrophied. Classified as Type a.

Type b

No separation was noted in the anterior portion of the ciliary body region, but in the posterior portion a mild and parallel separation was observed (Fig. 5).

This type was observed in 11 (13.75%) of 80 ciliary body regions.

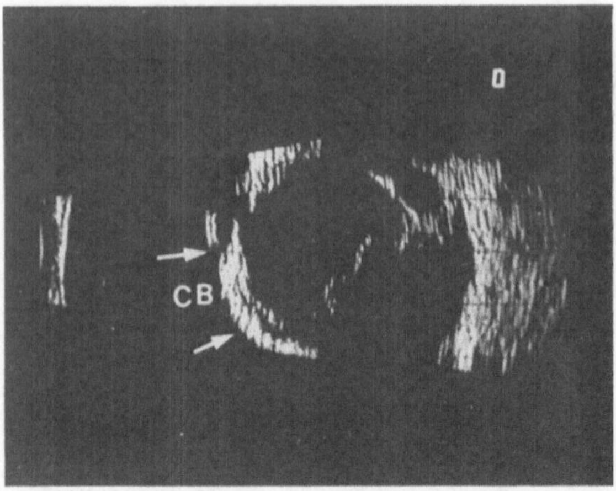

Fig. 5. B-scan ultrasonogram of ciliary body detachment. No separation is noted in the anterior portion, while separation in slight parallel is noted in the posterior portion. Type b.

Type c

In this type, separation of the anterior portion like a slit in parallel was observed, while the posterior portion was separated in parallel to a slight degree (Fig. 6)

This type was observed in 27 (33.75%) of 80 ciliary body regions.

Type d

In this type, no separation was noted in the anterior portion of the ciliary body region, whereas in the posterior portion, cuneiform separation in various degrees was seen (Fig. 7).

This type was observed in 9 (11.2%) of 80 ciliary body regions.

Type e

In this type, separation of the anterior portion like a slit in parallel was observed, while the posterior portion was separated in cuneiform expansion in various degrees (Fig. 3).

This type represented the basic form of the B-scan ultrasonogram of ciliary body detachment. It was noted in 27 (33.75%) of 80 ciliary body regions.

This type included a case showing the highest degree of separation (Fig. 8), which was noted in an eye showing bullous choroidal detachment in the highest degree. However, the basic form was retained in this case, even though the degree of separation was highest.

As has been explained so far, the existence of some types (Types a, b and d) in which no separation was noted in the anterior portion or in the whole

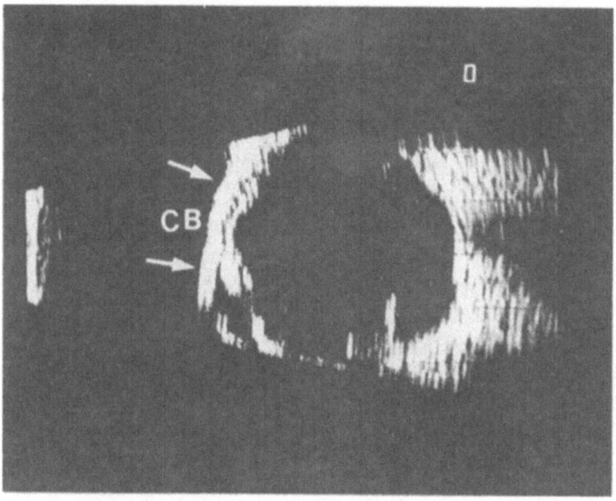

Fig. 6. B-scan ultrasonogram of ciliary body detachment. Separation is observed in a slit-shape in the anterior portion. In the posterior portion, separation is in slight parallel. Type c.

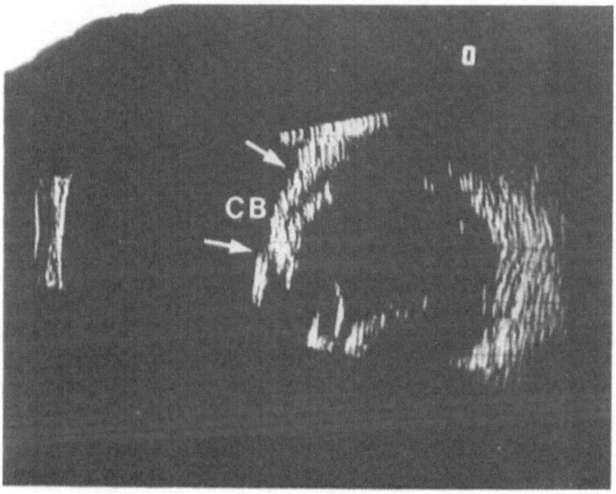

Fig. 7. B-scan ultrasonogram of ciliary body detachment. There is no separation in the anterior portion, but in the posterior portion cuneiform separation is observed. Type d.

ciliary body region was found. This is interpreted to mean that the degree of ciliary body detachment was too slight to depict separation with our B-scanning at 10 MHz.

DISCUSSION

Our observations were also found to apply to small cases of ocular contusion, uveitis and spontaneous cilio-choroidal detachment. This fact suggests that

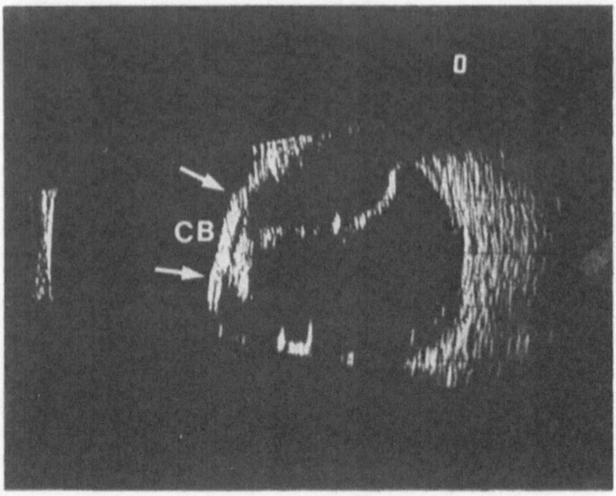

Fig. 8. B-scan ultrasonogram of ciliary body detachment showing the highest degree of separation among all cases investigated. Type e.

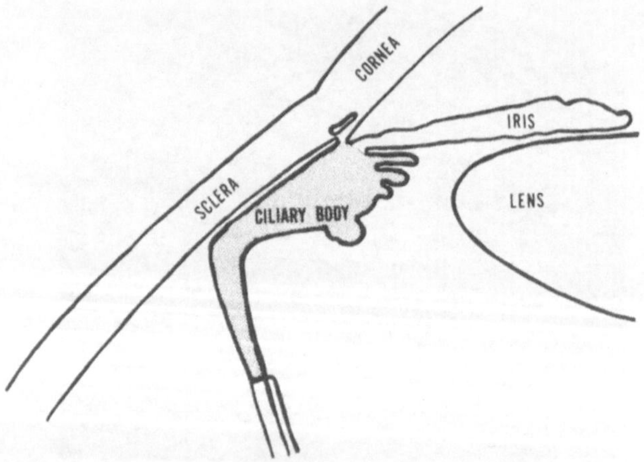

Fig. 9. Ciliary body detachment in vivo on the basis of our results.

the findings obtained in the present study are not limited to a particular single disease, but are common to other cases of ciliary body detachment having the same mechanism of onset, i.e. a transudation of fluid from the uveal vessels[1].

Figure 9 shows the morphology of ciliary body detachment in vivo on the basis of our results. The ciliary body is bent at the region along its longer axis, and the ciliary body is detached, in slight parallel, from the sclera in the sector anterior to the site of bending, while in the posterior sector it is detached in cuneiform expansion, with the site of bending as the axis.

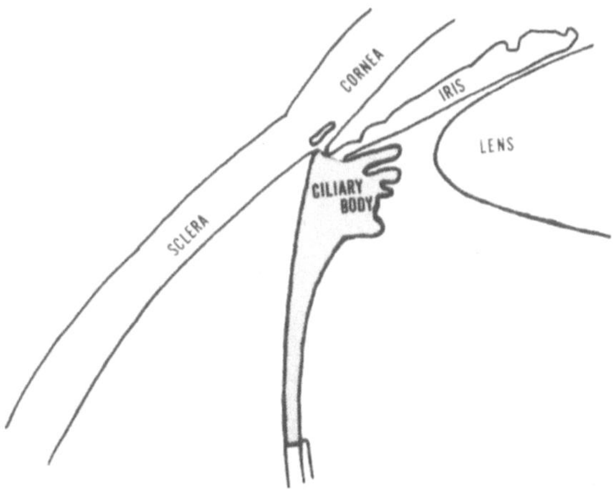

Fig. 10. The former concept of ciliary body detachment.

The concept of ciliary body detachment has previously been explained in the form of a monograph chart as per Duke-Elder[1]. According to the monograph chart, the ciliary body is simply detached in cuneiform expansion from the sclera, with the scleral spur as the axis (Fig. 10).

Our results are clearly not in agreement with this concept. The reason for the difference is that the conventional concept is not based on observation in a living organism, but on histopathologic findings.

The former concept of ciliary body detachment, in short, does not represent the morphology in vivo. This not only necessitates further observations of the shapes of ciliary body detachment in vivo with various other types of disease, but also suggests that more investigations into the concept of ciliochoroidal detachment and its various symptoms, including the changes in the anterior chamber depth and the state of refraction, as well as ocular hypotony, are required.

CONCLUSION

The authors observed pictures of ciliary body detachment in vivo in eyes with rhegmatogenous retinal detachment for the first time, using the B-scan ultrasonographic method, detecting that the conventional concept of ciliary body detachment does not correctly represent its shapes in vivo.

REFERENCE

1. Duke-Elder, S. and Perkins, E. S. Diseases of the uveal tract. pp. 939–960. Henry Kimpton, London, 1966.

Authors' address:
Department of Ophthalmology
School of Medicine
Chiba University
1-8-1, Inohana
Chiba 280
Japan

ULTRASONIC DIAGNOSIS OF INTRAOCULAR CYSTICERCUS

EDUARDO MORAGREGA
(*Coyoacán, Mexico*)

ABSTRACT

A, B and D scan echographic studies were performed on 17 patients who had previously been diagnosed ophthalmoscopically as having intraocular cysticercosis and on 8 patients who were diagnosed on the basis of these echographic studies. The 8 last patients had severe inflammation, retinal detachment and one probably a retinoblastoma. The echographic diagnosis were corroborated by surgery after anti-inflammatory-treatment. We believe that in our environment, intraocular cysticercosis should be ruled out when uveitis is present in an adult and when leukocoria is present. This is the first report of a 25 patient series with intraocular cysticercus studied and diagnosed with A and B-scan simultaneously.

HISTORY

1819 – A cysticercus was observed in the anterior chamber by Schott and Soemering.
1838 – The first subconjuntival cysticercus was observed by Baum.
1853 – The first cysticercus within the vitreous humor was reported by Coccius.
1870 – The first subretinal cysticercus was reported by Jaeger.
1888 – The first histopathologically confirmed case of intraocular cysticercus in Mexico was reported by Dr. Ricardo Vertiz.

GENERAL BACKGROUND

Cysticercosis of the eye, well known and defined is caused by ingesting the ova of Taenia Solium, which hatch in the human intestine and become haxacant embryos that evolve and migrate through the blood stream in a period of 60–70 days. These six-hooked tapeworm larvaes reach different areas of the eye and adnexa, depending on the arterial-stream taken (Sánchez Fontan*). Forty-two percent of all cases of cysticercosis are located in the eye and eyeball region according to Vosgien.

Hillman, J. S./Le May, M. M. (eds.) Ophthalmic Ultrasonography

ISBN 978-94-009-7280-3

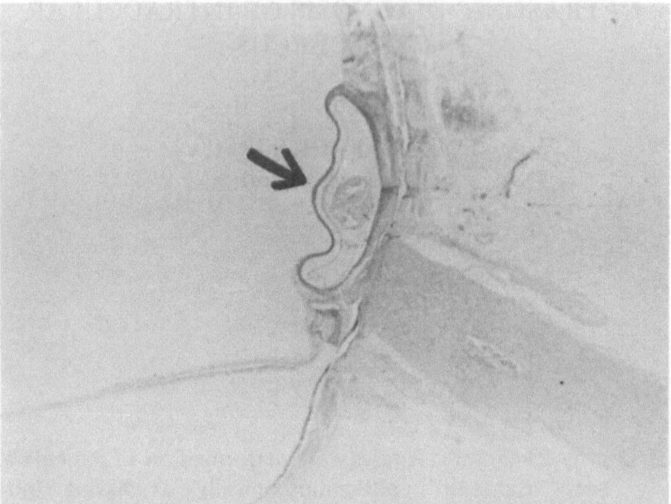

Fig. 1. Histologic section, showing a cysticercus behind the retina, (arrow) near optic nerve. The cyst is elongated because of the pressure of the retina. The scolex is seen in the center (Moragrega E., Gómez-Leal A.).

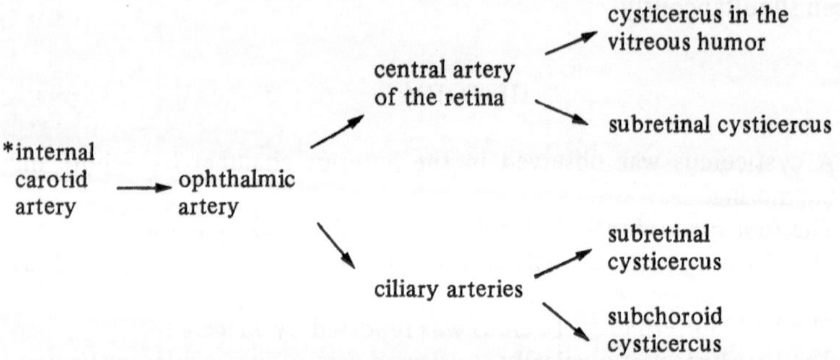

MATERIAL AND METHOD

The ultrasonic diagnostic equipment used, included a Kretz 7200 MA A-scanner, a Bronson/Turner B-scanner, and a Xenotec 404 ABDX-scanner. Twenty-five patients from the Hospital of the Association to Prevent Blindness in Mexico and private practice, were studied from June 1978 and June 1982, 17 patients have been previously diagnosed as having intraocular cysticercosis (by ophthalmoscopy), and 8 patients had severe inflammation and retinal detachment.

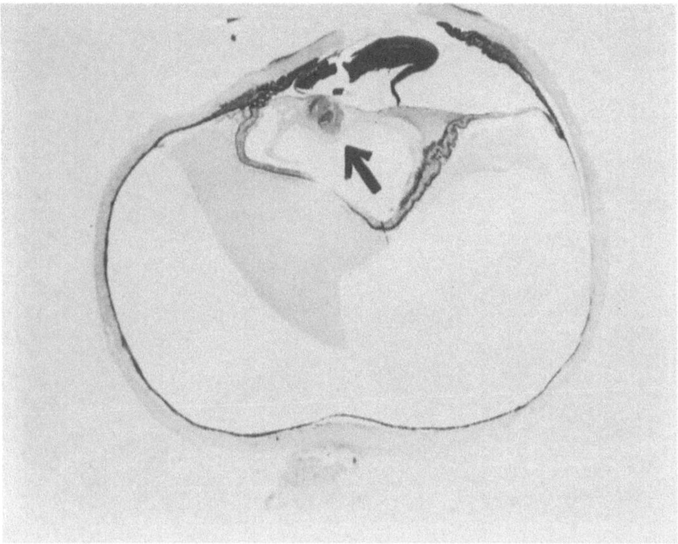

Fig. 2. Histologic section with a cysticercus in the vitreous with inflammatory changes around the parasite (arrow) (Moragrega E., Gómez-Leal A.).

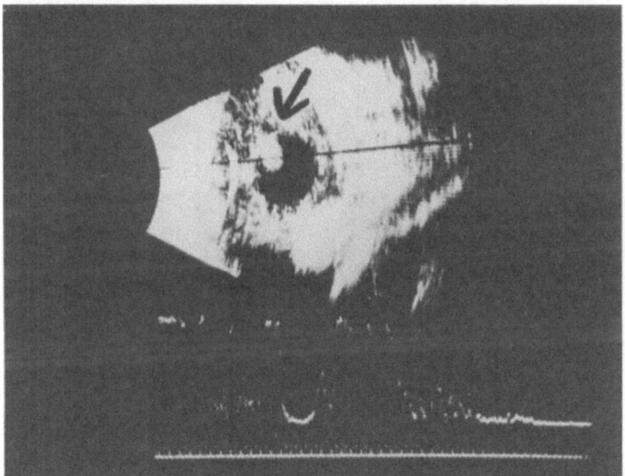

Fig. 3. Echogram of a vitreous cysticercus, the B-scan shows severe inflammation surrounding the cyst and the scolex within, (arrow) (Moragrega E., Gómez-Leal A.).

RESULTS

Examination of the cases in which the diagnosis was known beforehand made it possible to diagnose three other cases accurately and enable us to provide what we considered to be a typical image of cysticerci under the retina and free in vitreous.

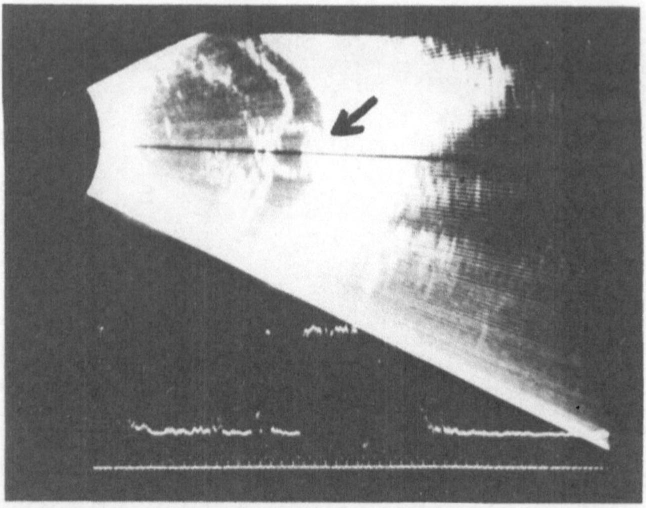

Fig. 4. Echogram of a subhyaloidal cysticercus, round image with greater eccentric density of the parasite head pointed by the arrow. (Moragrega E.).

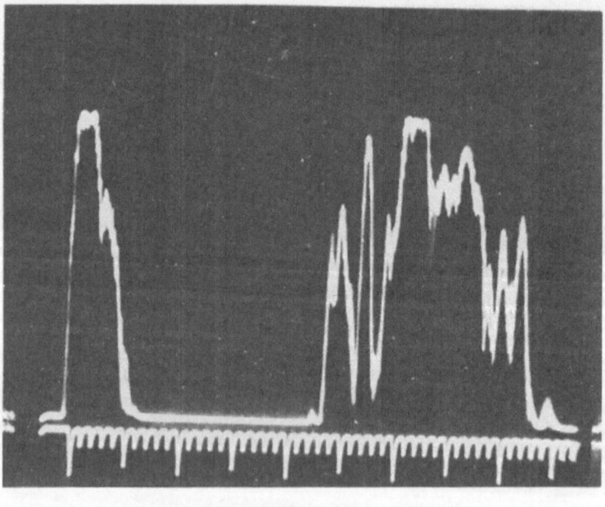

Fig. 5. A-scan with the echoes that delineate the cyst, and the high one in the center due to the scolex. (Moragrega E.).

SUBRETINAL CYSTICERCUS

The A-scan image shows a strong echo reflecting the raised or detached retina, an equally strong echo reflects the anterior part of the cyst and is followed by weak echoes unless the beam passes through the scolex (parasite's head) and

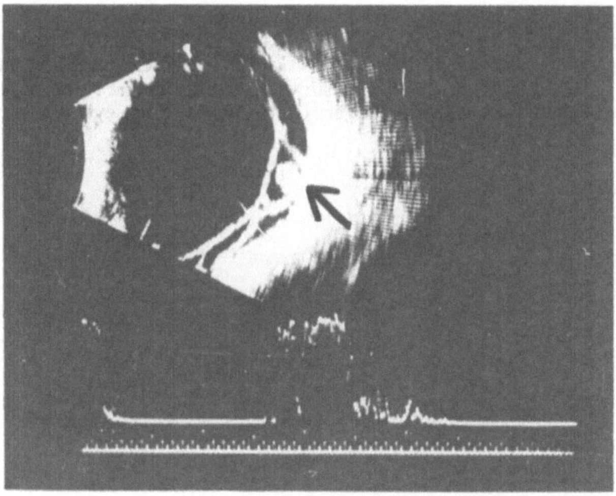

Fig. 6. In this echogram we can see a subretinal cysticercus. The arrow points to the cyst and the scolex is between the retina and choroid. (Moragrega E.).

produces a very strong echo, finally the echo reflecting the posterior part of the cyst and choroid.

The B-scan image is quite typical, the retina may be seen in the vitreous like a dense membrane behind which there is a complete image of a cyst with an eccentric density that reflects the scolex. Low density moving echoes may be observed within the cyst, particularly at 80 db.

FREE IN VITREOUS CYSTICERCUS

In this case the one dimensional A-scan image outlines the cyst with two strong echoes between which weak moving echoes are reflected, although there may be a strong reflection (100%) if the ultrasonic beam hits the scolex, that is always located eccentrically rather than in the center. The image described may be surrounded by low and medium reflecting echoes caused by inflammation and membranes.

The B-scan provides a complete image of the cyst in the vitreous chamber, the image is round and shows greater density in the eccentric area where the scolex is located. There are also moving echoes within the cyst.

It should be remembered that these studies are all of them real-time which means that the image of the oscilloscope represents what is taking place within the eye at that moment, including the typical amoebic movements of the cysticercus.

REFERENCES

1. Agundis, T. M.: Consideraciones clinicas acerca de la cisti-cercosis ocular. Arcu. Asoc. Evitar la Ceg. en Méx. 2a. epoca tomo XIII #60, 1971.

2. Santos, R.: Management of subretinal and vitreous cysticercosis. Role of photocoagulation and surgery. A. J. O. Vol. 86, Aug. 1979, psg. 1501–1504.
3. Solanes, N. P.: Tropical diseases, in Gordon's medical management of ocular diseases. Edited by Dunlap EA Hagerstown M. D. Harper and Row.
4. Rubem Pochasewsky and Alan Suger: Cysticercosis of the eye, ultrasonic findings. A. J. R. 133, 128–129,

Author's address:
Cirujano Oftalmologo
Vincente Garcia Torres 46
04030 Coyoacán
Mexico

HOW TO OBTAIN MAXIMUM MEASURING ACCURACIES WITH STANDARDIZED A-SCAN

KARL C. OSSOINIG
(Iowa, City, USA)

The standardized 7200 MA A-scan instrument of Kretztechnik can provide the most accurate ultrasonic measurements that are available. This is true for measurements of axial eye length and of any other normal or abnormal tissue thickness within the eye and orbit provided the correct procedures in calibrating the instrument, in displaying maximum signals at low "measuring sensitivity" and in taking the measurements from Polaroid pictures are followed. To obtain accurate clinical measurements, one other crucial requirement must be met: the distance to be measured must be properly identified first, i.e., an act of tissue identification must precede any measurement. Standardized A-scan is uniquely capable of providing such tissue identification. For this purpose, it is applied either at the very high standardized "tissue sensitivity" (e.g., for identifying the maximum diameter of a tumor or the maximum thickness of the optic nerve and the extraocular muscles) or at the low "measuring sensitivity", e.g., for identifying the thickness of the retinochoroid layer (through perpendicularity of the sound beam at both the inner retinal and inner scleral surfaces) or for identifying the axial eye length (through optimal alignment of the acoustic beam with the axis of the globe). Standardized A-scan then accurately measures the identified distance, preferably at the low measuring sensitivity. This paper will discuss (1) the optimal calibration of the electronic measuring scale of the 7200 MA, (2) the need for peak-to-peak measurements and (3) methods for taking the measurements from Polaroid pictures in a practical and accurate manner.

I. Calibration of the Electronic Measuring Scale in the 7200 MA:

There are almost 450 standardized A-scan instruments (7200 MA Kretztechnik) in use today and their number grows continually. These units potentially provide the most accurate results available at this time in axial eye-length measurements. However, the accuracies achieved depend on the appropriate calibration of the electronic measuring scale. Little is found on this extremely important part of acoustic measurements in the manual of the instrument. It is therefore both valuable and necessary to describe the procedure that produces the only accurate calibration of the electronic measuring scale in this instrument.

Figure 1 indicates the switches and dials used for the display of the electronic

Hillman, J. S./Le May, M. M. (eds.) Ophthalmic Ultrasonography

ISBN 978-94-009-7280-3

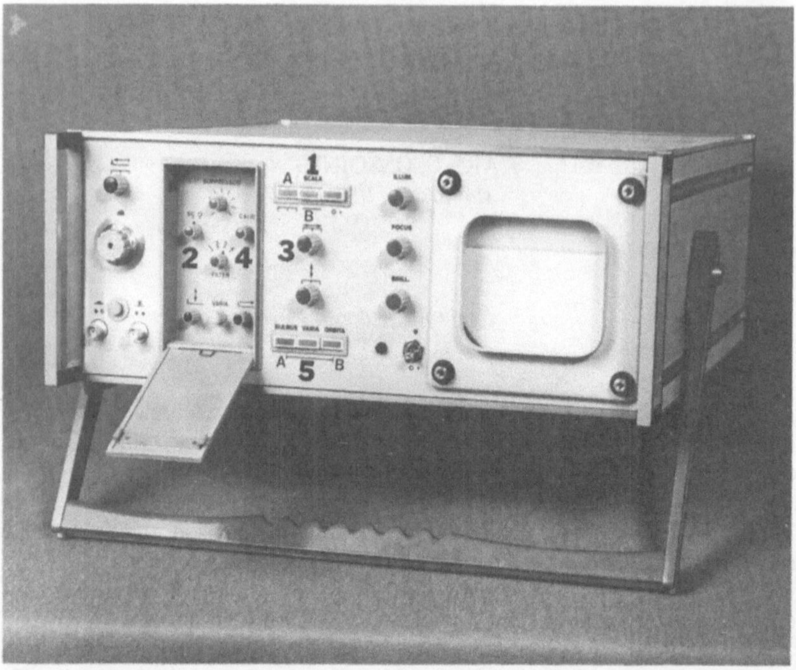

Fig. 1. **Push buttons and dials for the display and calibration of the electronic measuring scale in the standardized A-scan unit (7200 MA Kretztechnik).** ***1*** **push button to display the measuring line with (*A*) or without (*B*) measuring units;** ***2*** **on-off dial for display of quartz-clock time-base (changes measuring line to rectangular stepline);** ***3*** **Horizontal shift dial (does not change calibration);** ***4*** **calibration dial (changes duration of single measuring units);** ***5*** **push buttons for various horizontal expansions (*A* for intraocular examinations, *B* for orbital examinations).**

measuring scale and its calibration. *Figure 2* shows the display of the measuring line without (*left*) and with the electronic units (making it a measuring scale; *right*), and without (*top*) and with a step-like quartz time-base (a stepline with consecutive double steps consisting of positive and negative rectangular signals; *bottom*). The built-in quartz clock provides an extremely accurate display of time intervals that are independent of temperature and age of the instrument.

The plain horizontal measuring line is displayed on the screen when the push button shown as *1B* in *Figure 1* is used. Measuring units overlie this measuring line when the push button *1A* is pressed instead. By switching the quartz dial (*2* in *Figure 1*), one can superimpose the measuring line or scale over the quartz time-base. The interval between any point of the ascending left limb of one double step (*left arrow* in *Figure 2*) to the corresponding point of the ascending limb of the next following double step (*right arrow* in *Figure 2*) equals exactly 20 microseconds. It should be noted that half a double step, for instance the distance between corresponding parts of the ascending and descending limbs of one positive quartz signal, does not cor-

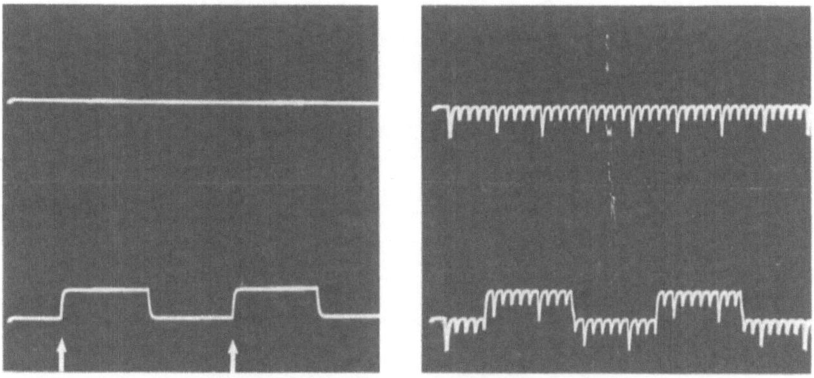

Fig. 2. Variations in the display of the measuring line. *Top left* plain horizontal measuring line; *top right* straight horizontal measuring line with overlying measuring units (*measuring scale*); *bottom left* plain measuring line combined with quartz time-base (rectangular stepline); *bottom right* quartz time-base with overlying measuring units; *arrows* point out the ascending (left) limbs of two consecutive double steps (quartz signals). One double step (positive and negative quartz signal) indicates precisely 20 microseconds (interval between the two arrows).

respond to exactly 10 microseconds and therefore should never be used for the calibration procedure.

By turning the horizontal shift dial (*3* in *Figure 1*), the measuring units are shifted horizontally over the underlying plain measuring line. By using the calibration dial (*4* in *Figure 1*), the time span of each measuring unit can be lengthened or shortened depending on the direction the dial is turned. Note that the duration of the measuring units, and thus the calibration of the scale, are note changed when just the horizontal shift dial is used.

Figure 3 shows one of the long measuring spikes (*arrows*), and illustrates what happens to this spike when it is shifted toward the left and across the ascending limb of a double step (by using the horizontal shift dial). First, the spike shifts toward the left and approaches the ascending limb riding along the upper portion of the stepline (first line in *Figure 3*). Then it descends along the ascending limb of the stepline, being superimposed on this limb to varying degrees. It appears as a very short spike underneath the limb (*large arrow* in second line of *Figure 3*), then growing longer but still being shorter than its full length (*large arrow* in the central line of *Figure 3*). Thereafter, it grows to full length and shifts away from the limb riding along the lower portion of the stepline (bottom line in *Figure 3*). It is only during the descent along an ascending limb of the stepline that the long spike can be clearly localized and accurately timed on the basis of its length that appears below this ascending limb. Once the long spike has reached its full length (fourth line in *Figure 3*), one cannot be sure if it is still under the limb or has already shifted slightly away from the limb.

Since a double step of the quartz line corresponds to exactly 20 microseconds, one measuring unit will be exactly one microsecond when 20 mea-

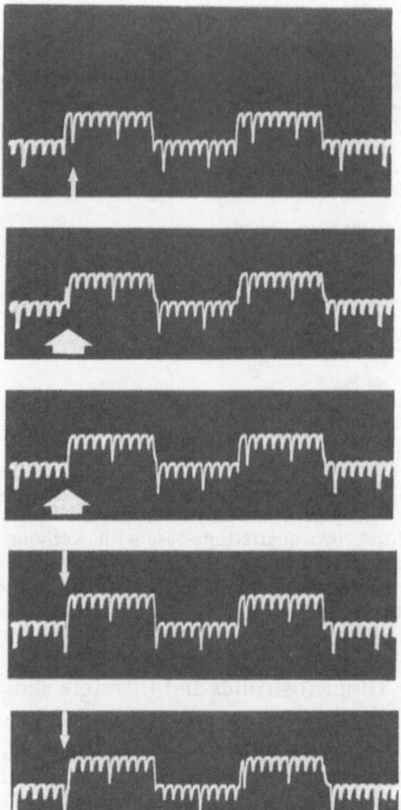

Fig. 3. **One of the long measuring spikes is shifted along the stepline of the quartz time-base from right to left crossing an ascending left limb of the double step, which is used for the calibration procedure. *Small arrows* point out the long measuring spike as it approaches (*top* line) and leaves (last two lines) the ascending limb; *large arrows* mark positions of the long measuring spike (in overlying the left ascending limb) which are useful for the calibration (*second* and *third* lines): in these positions, the long measuring spike may be used as a reference spike for the calibration procedure.**

suring units are shifted and stretched (or narrowed) so that they cover exactly one double step of the quartz base (*Figure 4, top*). To achieve this, a long measuring spike and the second following long spike (first and last spikes of a 20-unit block) are superimposed identically over two successive ascending limbs of the quartz stepline (*large arrows Figure 4, top*). Then these first and twenty-first spikes of the 20-unit block display exactly the same length (underneath the ascending limbs) indicating that they are in the same phase of alignment with the time-base, just 20 microseconds apart. As was explained before, it is only possible during their descent along ascending limbs of the stepline that two measuring spikes can be placed into identical phases relative

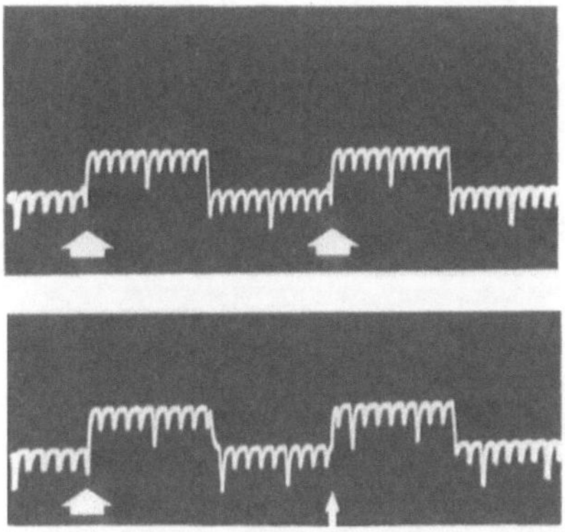

Fig. 4. Calibration of the measuring scale in microseconds (*top*) and in millimeters of tissue (*bottom*) utilizing one double step of the quartz time-base (Step 1 of calibration procedure). *Large arrows* mark clearly defined left and right reference points; *small arrow* indicates poorly defined mid-portion of a measuring unit used as right reference area when calibrating in millimeters.

to the time-base (see *top* line of *Figure 4* and *bottom* line of *Figure 5*). In *Figure 5*, which illustrates the first step of calibration (see below), large arrows then point at the only positions (in this figure) of the long spike which are useful for the calibration procedure. The other positions (*small arrows*) do not lend themselves to accurate definition of the long spike regarding the time-base, and none of these positions can be used for accurate calibration.

One may also calibrate the measuring units in millimeters of tissue (rather than in microseconds) by making a certain number of units (depending on the sound velocity in that tissue) cover each double step of the quartz line (e.g., 18.5 units in the case illustrated in the *bottom* pattern of *Figure 4*). As is obvious from this pattern, such calibration will never be really accurate since it is impossible to pinpoint the exact location of half a measuring unit. Therefore, the electronic measuring scale of 7200 MA should be calibrated in microseconds only. The measured intervals (microseconds) can easily be converted into distances (millimeters) by using conversion tables for the various tissue velocities.

In axial eye-length measurements, for instance, different sound velocities are involved in the lens and in the vitreous or aqueous humor. Were one to calibrate the electronic scale in millimeters, one would have to go through two different calibration procedures for one axial eye-length measurement or disregard the actual thickness of the lens (as is done in most eye-length measurements when using non-standardized A-scan units). Apart from being more accurate, it is, therefore, also more convenient to measure in microseconds and then convert the corresponding intervals into millimeters of aqueous humor, vitreous and lens, rather than to calibrate for each section and then measure it directly in millimeters.

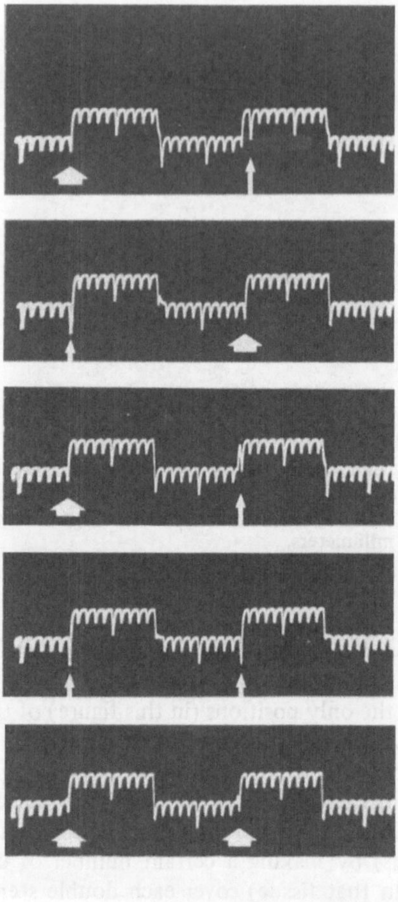

Fig. 5. Step 1 of the calibration procedure, which should be used first by beginners. A horizontal expansion as employed for intraocular examinations is used (push button *5A* in *Figure 1*). *Large arrows* mark positions of long measuring spikes that are appropriate for use as left or right reference points; *small arrows* mark the long measuring spikes (to be used as reference spikes) not yet placed into appropriate positions (first and third lines) or shifted beyond those appropriate positions (second and fourth lines). *Bottom* line indicates the calibration of the measuring scale achieved at the end of Step 1 (compare with *top* line in *Figure 4*).

CALIBRATION PROCEDURE:

For calibrating the electronic measuring scale or checking its accuracy prior to a measurement, one presses the push button for the display of the measuring scale (*1A* in *Figure 1*), switches dial *2* for the display of the quartz time-base, and then uses both the horizontal-shift (*3*) and the calibration (*4*) dials in an alternating fashion to show that calibration of the measuring scale is adequate or to achieve such calibration.

Step 1 (*Figure 5*): The aim of Step 1 is to produce the top pattern shown in *Figure 4*, where 20 measuring units are superimposed exactly on one double step. First, a single double step of the quartz time-base is displayed in the center of the screen by pushing the button for horizontal expansion used in intraocular examinations (*5A* in *Figure 1*). Next, any long spike near the left end of the measuring scale*) is used as a left reference spike for calibration, whereas the second (toward the right) long spike following this left reference point is used as the right reference point for calibration. The horizontal shift dial is turned to first align the left reference spike with the left ascending limb of the double step so that it is displayed as short as (or even better, shorter than) the neighboring short measuring spikes (*large arrow* in *top* line of *Figure 5*). Then the calibration dial is used to lengthen or shrink (in the situation as shown in *Figure 5*) the measuring scale so that the right reference spike (which marks the right end of the 20th measuring unit following the left reference spike) shifts into the same position on the ascending left limb of the next following double step (*large arrow* in *second* line of *Figure 5*) as the left reference spike is in regard to the ascending left limb of the previous double step (*large arrow* in *top* line of *Figure 5*). As can be seen from the second line in this figure, the alignment of the right reference spike with the calibration dial may cause the left reference spike to shift away from its appropriate previous position toward the left (*small arrow* in *second* line of *Figure 5*). This will not be the case if only a minimal tilt of the calibration dial is necessary to achieve calibration. But this will happen regularly when the measuring scale is quite a bit off calibration.

The next procedure is to readjust that left reference spike to the correct position using the horizontal shift dial (not the calibration dial!). When doing this, as shown in the third line of *Figure 5* (*large arrow*), the right reference spike shifts back out of its appropriate position (*small arrow* in *third* line). This is corrected by again using the calibration dial and shrinking the measuring scale and results in the situation shown in the *fourth* line in *Figure 5*: both reference spikes (*small arrows*) are poorly aligned. Through the use of the calibration dial, the left spike has shifted out of its correct position, while the right spike was shifted on purpose beyond the correct position to shorten the calibration procedure (by over-adjusting calibration to avoid a repetition of the previous situation). By simply shifting the whole measuring scale toward the right using the horizontal shift dial (not the calibration dial), both reference spikes are moved into correct positions as indicated by the *large arrows* in the *bottom* line of *Figure 5*, marking the end of Step 1 of the calibration procedure.

Step 1 of the calibration procedure was, in summary, executed by alternately using the horizontal-shift dial (to appropriately position the left reference spike) and the calibration dial (to correctly position the right reference spike). The fact that both reference spikes (being superimposed on

*The very first long spike on the left end of the measuring scale should not be used for calibration because the first measuring unit tends to be shorter than all the others.

two consecutive left limbs of the quartz time-base) show the same length, which should be slightly shorter than the neighboring short spikes (see *bottom* line of *Figure 5*), and the fact that, consequently, 20 measuring units cover one full double step, indicate that one measuring unit amounts to one microsecond.

Step 2 (*Figure 6*): The aim of Step 2 is to obtain even greater accuracy in calibration by using several consecutive double steps of the quartz time-base (and not just one double step as in Step 1), and by superimposing a corresponding number of measuring units on them. By pressing the push button for the horizontal screen expansion as used in orbital examinations (*5B* in *Figure 1*), the measuring scale is shrunk to half its previous horizontal expansion and displays twice as many double steps on the screen of the instrument. The top pattern in *Figure 6* illustrates the resulting increase in the sensitivity of the display regarding calibration: the left reference spike (*large arrow* in *top* line of *Figure 6*) and the second following long spike (previous right reference spike; see *bottom* line of *Figure 5*) still are in place, since pushing the Orbita button does not affect calibration nor shift the measuring scale in regard to the quartz time-base. When, however, scrutinizing the 60th spike following the left reference spike to the right (*small arrow* in *top* line of *Figure 6*), which is used as the new right reference spike, one can see that it is slightly off calibration (longer than the left reference spike). It requires only a brief maneuver using the calibration dial to correct this situation, resulting in the pattern shown in the *bottom* line of *Figure 6* where the two *large arrows* point out that both the left and the right reference spikes are positioned appropriately in this expanded version of the calibration procedure (as compared to Step 1).

Step 3 (*Figure 7*): The aim of Step 3 is to obtain the maximum accuracy of calibration by utilizing the entire electronic scale for the calibration

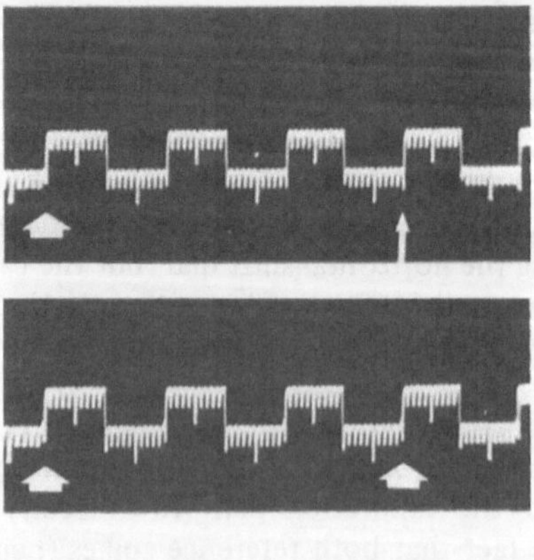

Fig. 6. Step 2 of the calibration procedure. The horizontal screen expansion is set as for orbital examinations (push button *5B* in *Figure 1*). *Top* inadequate calibration (in spite of all efforts taken in Step 1 of the calibration procedure) is evident when the push button for orbital examination is pressed; *bottom* final stage of Step 2 of calibration procedure. *Large arrows* reference spikes in appropriate positions; *small arrow* reference spike off appropriate position.

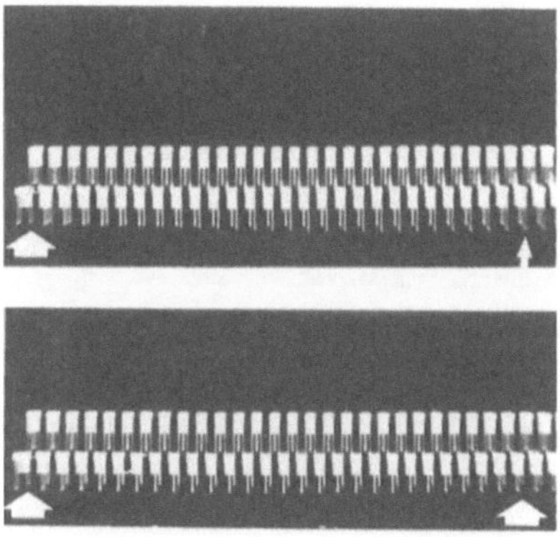

Fig. 7. Step 3 of the calibration procedure. Horizontal expansion is minimized so that the entire electronic measuring scale is shown on the screen of the instrument (achieved by releasing all three push buttons that control the horizontal screen expansion; see *5* in *Figure 1*). *Top* inadequate calibration (in spite of efforts taken in Step 2 of the calibration procedure) is evident when all push buttons for horizontal expansion are released. *Bottom* full, most accurate calibration achieved at the end of Step 3. *Large arrows* reference spikes in appropriate positions; *small arrow* reference spike off appropriate position.

procedure. Such a display is obtained by releasing all three push buttons that control the horizontal screen expansion (*5* in *Figure 1*). This maximizes the sensitivity of the display indicating accurate calibration. As the *top* line in *Figure 7* indicates, the 120th spike following the left reference spike (*large arrow*) already shows a slight deviation from the correct length (position along the ascending limb), in spite of the efforts taken in Step 2 of the calibration procedure. When looking at the new right reference spike (*small arrow* in *top* line of *Figure 7*), which marks the 28th double step toward the right, this deviation is very clear. It requires another adjustment of the calibration dial to correct the situation and achieve full calibration, as shown in the *bottom* line of *Figure 7*, where both the left and new right reference spikes (and each consecutive 20th spike [potential reference spike] in between) show exactly the same length as indicated by the *large arrows*. At the end of Step 3, the best possible calibration of the measuring scale is achieved. A potential error that may still be involved in this calibration will then be much less than one per mill of the distances to be measured with the standardized A-scan instrument, and will therefore be totally inconsequential regarding the results of the acoustic measurements.

Figure 8 illustrates a simple checking procedure performed at the end of the calibration of the measuring scale. By turning the horizontal shift dial minimally toward the right and left, all the long spikes that are aligned with ascending limbs, and thus show the same length as the left and right reference spikes (*large arrows* in the *central* pattern of *Figure 8*), will move simultaneously either up or down (shorten or lengthen) as shown in the *top* and *bottom* patterns of *Figure 8*. The calibration is perfect only when these vertical shifts occur simultaneously and not in a wave pattern. When this

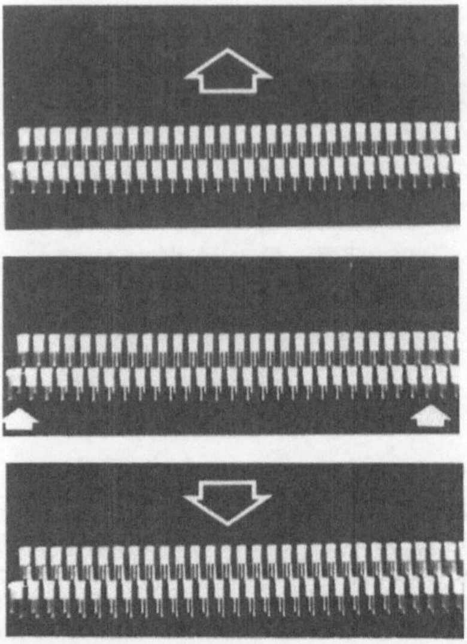

Fig. 8. Illustration of simple procedure to check whether the calibration of the measuring scale is complete (as indicated in *Figure 7*). By using the horizontal-shift dial (not the calibration dial!), the two reference spikes (*large arrows* in *central* pattern) and, together with them, every second large spike in between are displayed at about half their full length. They are then made to shift simultaneously upwards (shorten in length) and downwards (lengthen) together with every second long spike in between by turning the horizontal-shift dial minimally in either direction. Only the simultaneous up and down shifts, and the equal length, of all these reference spikes indicate full, most accurate calibration. If calibration is still slightly off, the long spikes will shift in a wave-like pattern rather than simultaneously.

highest level of calibration is achieved, measurements are not affected at all by inaccuracies that would have been caused by errors in the calibration of the electronic measuring scale.

To the beginner, the calibration procedure for the 7200 MA as described above may seem to be complicated and time-consuming. Actually, for the beginner it is. With some practice, however, an echographer learns to quickly check calibration and adjust it if necessary. The trained echographer will usually use Step 3 to check calibration and to correct minor deviations, and will resort to Step 2 only when the measuring scale is way off calibration. The trained echographer does not need to go back to Step 1 at all. It will take him only 5 to 10 seconds to check calibration (prior to a measurement), between 10 and 20 seconds to correct minor deviations in calibration, and 20 to 30 seconds to apply both Steps 2 and 3 when calibration is off considerably. Such checking or calibrating the measuring scale is a routine procedure applied whenever pictures for documentation are taken; it is as routine as setting the decibel dial for tissue sensitivity at the beginning of each examination. Regular checking of the measuring scale is necessary since calibration of the scale in the 7200 MA is very sensitive and promptly reacts to changes in temperature of the instrument (more in some units than in others). The addition of a fan housing (a recent advance in the design of the instrumentation) provides continuous cooling of the 7200 MA and has greatly improved the situation in terms of stabilizing the temperature within the unit. Nevertheless, a check of the calibration should be made before each measuring procedure, and should be repeated during the procedure every five minutes or so (if the measurement takes that long). By such an approach, one can fully realize the great potential of the 7200 MA for highly accurate measurements and insure that inaccurate calibration of the measuring scale does not affect the results of ultrasonic biometry.

II. Peak-to-Peak Measurements:

In order to obtain the most accurate measurements under clinical conditions, one must use a narrow beam and short ultrasonic pulses. This is achieved by

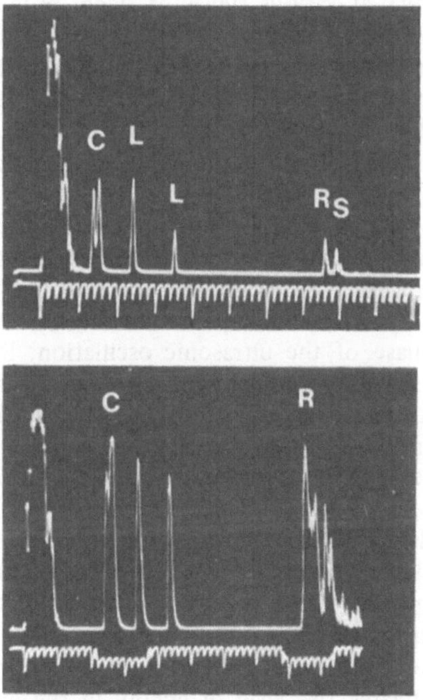

Fig. 9. Top echogram: axial echogram of eye obtained with immersion method using standardized A-scan. The spikes from the cornea (*C*; the two peaks represent the anterior and posterior corneal surfaces), the anterior and the posterior lens surfaces (*L*), and the inner retinal (*R*) as well as inner scleral (*S*) surfaces are displayed at low (measuring sensitivity) but maximum height (indicating alignment of the acoustic beam with the axis of the eye).

Bottom echogram: this echogram was obtained using the DOC unit (Digital Ocular Computer) in combination with the standardized A-scan instrument relying on electronic gates (steps in the measuring scale) for automatic measurement and calculation of distances in millimeters.

simply decreasing system sensitivity to a minimum level, just sufficient to clearly display the maximum echo signals from the pertinent interfaces whose distances are to be measured. At this low measuring sensitivity, it is easy to use the peaks of the maximized echo spikes for the measurement (*top* echogram in *Figure 9*). Such peak-to-peak measurements are often the only way to measure tissues at all, e.g., the thickness of thin layers such as the cornea or the retinochoroid layer, the maximum elevation of an intraocular tumor or the diameter of an orbital lesion. In many of these instances, one cannot even display the left bases of both surface spikes and must therefore use the peaks (or at least portions of the spike limbs next to the peaks) to take the measurements at all.

Peak-to-peak measurements are preferable over base-to-base measurements for yet another important reason. As *Figure 10* illustrates, peak-to-peak measurements are both more reliable and more accurate. This figure presents schematic drawings of an emitted ultrasonic pulse (*far left*) and of echo signals evoked by the pulse. The echo signals are shown at decreasing intensities (*top* to *bottom*), at various stages of signal processing (*left* to *right*), and in their final form as displayed on the screen of the cathode ray tube (*far right*). This signal processing (as depicted in *Figure 10*) includes full-wave rectification and high-frequency filtering. The original radio-frequency echo signals undergo high-frequency filtering to the point that the final rectified video signals show the high frequency only as small nodes along their ascending (left) limbs.

These drawings are, of course, simplified and disregard facts such as amplification and attenuation in both the tissues and the instrument, but they clarify and emphasize the point that the peaks of echo signals are the only consistent and stable reference points on the echo signals, always representing the same phase of the ultrasonic oscillation. By contrast, the left bases of the echo signals may represent different phases of oscillation at different signal intensities. The left base of an echo signal may correspond to the first, second, third, etc., phases of oscillation, depending on the reflectivity of the interface, the type of amplifier used and the degree of amplification applied. The *top line* in *Figure 10* depicts the (theoretical) situation when the echo intensity equals the intensity of the emitted pulse. In this case, the left base of the echo signal corresponds to the ascending portion of the first phase of oscillation; the peak of the echo signal corresponds to the positive peak of the fourth oscillation of the pulse. In the second line, the echo intensity is weaker, but the left base is still produced by the first phase of oscillation. The dotted line indicates the level of energy in the emitted pulse that is utilized for the display of the echo signal. In the third line, the echo intensity has become so little that the left base of this echo spike corresponds to the upper positive portion of the third phase of oscillation. In the bottom line, a very weak echo signal is displayed. Its left base is formed by the ascending portion of the fourth oscillation. By contrast, the peaks of all the echo spikes represent the same phase of oscillation always (regardless of signal intensities), i.e., the positive peak of the fourth oscillation in the case illustrated in *Figure 10*.

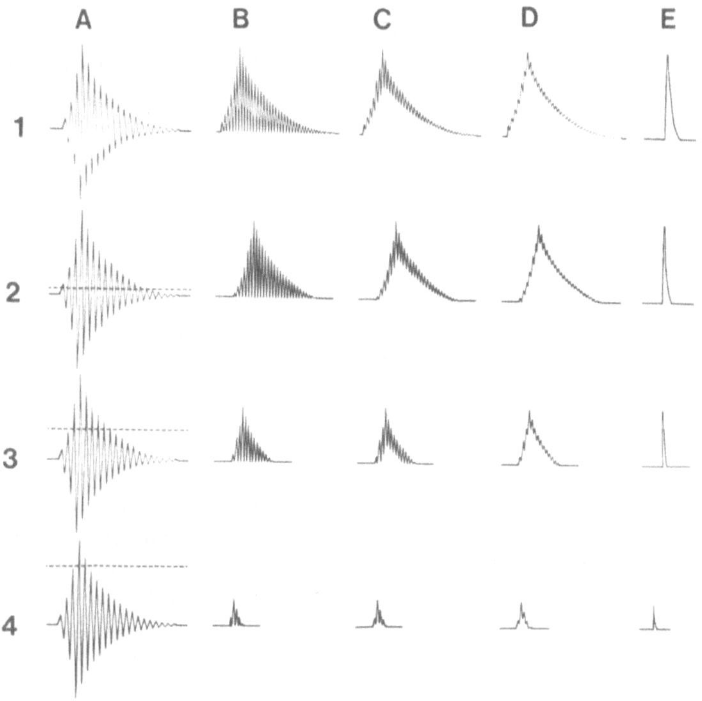

Fig. 10. Schematic drawings illustrating the fact that the peaks of echo spikes always correspond to the same phase of oscillation, whereas the left bases or other points along ascending left limbs of the spikes do not. *A* emitted ultrasonic pulse; *B–E* echo pulse at different stages of signal processing and in its final displayed form (echo spike, *E*). *1* all energy is reflected; the echo pulse contains as many positive amplitudes as the emitted pulse has both positive and negative amplitudes (full-wave rectification). By increasing high-frequency filtering, these oscillations are minimized and show up as tiny nodes along the left ascending limb on the final echo spike only (*E*). Note that the left base of the echo spike corresponds to the first positive amplitude of the emitted ultrasonic pulse (first phase of oscillation). The peak of the echo spike represents the peak of the fourth positive amplitude (fourth phase of oscillation). *2* echo pulse is weaker than emitted pulse; dotted horizontal line indicates what energy level participates in the build-up of the echo pulse. The left base of the echo spike corresponds to the first positive oscillation of the emitted pulse, while the peak of the echo spike traces back to the positive peak of the fourth phase of oscillation. *3* much less of the energy of the emitted pulse is contained in the returning echo pulse this time. The left base of this weaker echo spike corresponds to the third positive amplitude of the emitted ultrasonic pulse (third phase of oscillation). Note that the peak of the spike still represents the peak of the fourth positive amplitude of the emitted ultrasonic pulse (fourth phase of oscillation). *4* this very weak echo signal contains only the peak energy of the emitted ultrasonic pulse. Its left base is formed by the positive amplitude of the fourth phase of oscillation. The peak still corresponds to the same phase as in the other signals.

If one measures the interval between two echo signals whose left bases correspond to the same phase of oscillation, the measured interval will correctly represent the distance (provided the appropriate sound velocity is applied to the calculation). If one, however, were to measure the interval between a stronger and a weaker echo signal by using the left bases of the spikes, one would introduce an error corresponding to half a phase or up to several phases of oscillation which, translated into distances in tissues, would correspond to one half to several wave lengths and thus to errors from $\simeq$0.05 mm up to $\simeq$1.0 mm depending on the make of the amplifier (full-wave or half-wave rectification), the ultrasonic frequencies used and, most important, the differences in intensity of the two reference signals. This would result in a longer or shorter (incorrect) distance measured, depending on whether the stronger echo signal is first or second in the display. A similar, though possibly less severe, situation applies to ultrasonic measurements that use points along the ascending (left) limbs of the reference spikes, as is the case, for instance, in DOC automatic measurements illustrated in *Figure 9* (*bottom* echogram). Note that the system sensitivity had to be raised compared to the *top* echogram in *Figure 9* in order to assure that spike height surpassed the threshold for electronic measurements. This necessity decreases the accuracy of measurment by both decreasing the sensitivity of the system for aligning the acoustic beam with the axis of the eye and by lengthening the ultrasonic pulses and widening the ultrasonic beam as compared to the plain immersion technique and the measuring procedures described in the next section. This decrease in potential accuracy is in addition to the disadvantage of not including the position and thickness of the lens as an individual variable in axial eye-length measurements.

In unusually long distances, e.g., when measuring the axial eye length in highly myopic eyes, a small phase shift between the emitted pulse and the returning echo signal may occur (due to absorption of ultrasonic energy that reults in a shift in the frequency spectrum), i.e., the maximum amplitude of the oscillation (peak of spike) may shift from one to the next (half) phase of oscillation. When using peak-to-peak measurements, this occasional error is still minimal compared to the several times larger errors occurring when the left bases or the ascending limbs of the echo spikes are used as reference points for the measurement (e.g., in automatic electronic measurement by electronic gates).

Therefore, the only reliable and really accurate procedure for measuring distances with ultrasound is to use the peaks as reference points. This is not a new finding. Jansson, in his original work on axial eye-length measurement in the early 1960s, used both minimal system sensitivity and peak-to-peak measurements. We are only following his guidelines in this regard. The error in base-to-base measurements may be quite different in different A-scan instruments. It clearly is significant for the standardized A-scan 7200 MA instrument (which, incidentally, is the only currently available instrument that has been investigated in this regard). Only peak-to-peak measurements of maximal but weak echo signals as obtained at measuring sensitivity provide accurate results.

III. Measurement from Polaroid Pictures:

The frequent, small involuntary eye movements of a patient during the measuring procedure, and the resulting instabilities in the display of optimal echograms, do not allow measurements to be taken directly from the screen of the cathode-ray tube. Digital scan converters and their "frozen" displays will eliminate this problem. Meanwhile, Polaroid pictures are taken to "freeze" the axial eye-length echograms. At least three pictures of good quality (recognizable from the appearance of the echo spikes), obtained in three different approaches (to avoid repeating the same possible error in alignment), are measured and the average value of the axial eye-length measurements is calculated.

For the measurement of the echograms on the Polaroid pictures, two basically different approaches are possible. In one, the measurements are taken by hand using calipers, and either a sheet of scratch paper or a rectangular ruler is used to aid in the vertical projections of the higher peaks to the level of the lower peaks (*Figures 11* and *12*). During these measurements, care must be taken that the projection of the higher peaks is made in a direction truly perpendicular to the baseline, and that the mark designating the projected position of the higher peak is made at the same distance from the initial spike that the center of that peak is. The points of the calipers are placed exactly below the center of the peak of the lower spike and at the center of the projected mark of the higher spike to obtain a distance measurement parallel to the baseline of the echogram. Then the calipers are placed over the electronic measuring scale below the measured distance, avoiding the longer measuring spikes, and the corresponding value in microseconds is determined. Using the magnification on a Polaroid photo, distances may be estimated in increments as small as 0.1 microsecond. This limit determines the level of accuracy of the entire measurement; all other factors such as errors in alignment of the acoustic beam with the axis of the eye, the angle kappa (angle between the optical and visual axes of the eye), deviations from the theoretical sound velocities in the acqueous, vitreous and lens, etc., are smaller than the reading errors when measuring pictures (provided the appropriate examination technique and peak-to-peak measurements are performed). Therefore, the best available accuracy of axial eye-length measurements can be assumed to be ± 0.1 mm.

These measurements by hand require meticulous procedures such as the projection of the higher peaks downward to the level of the lower peaks, and the alignment of the calipers with the various measuring points in directions that are strictly parallel to the baseline. This measuring technique is also time-consuming. The skilled echographer will need several minutes to obtain the result of the measurement after the examination of the patient, particularly since repeated measurements of three high-quality pictures are required. Therefore, a computer-aided measuring procedure as shown in *Figures 13–15* is preferable (though not necessarily more accurate). Instead of the calipers, the examiner uses a cursor with a digitizing tablet ("Bit Pad One" by Summagraphics). It is not necessary to project any peaks downward to another

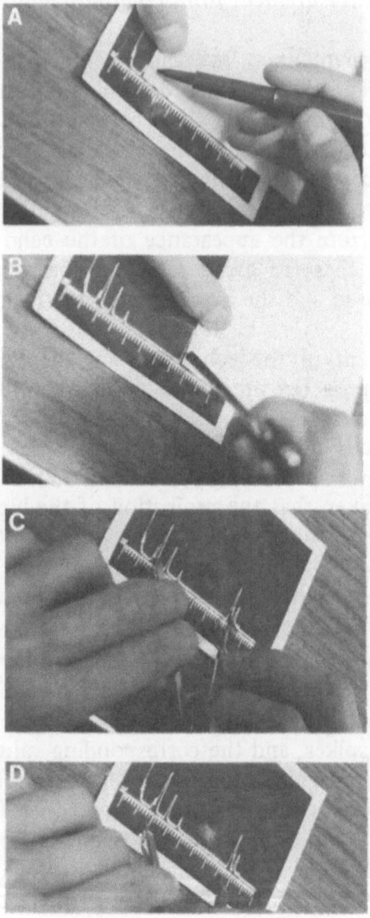

Fig. 11. Illustration of simple, but reliable and accurate measuring technique using the rectangular edge of a sheet of scratch paper and calipers (example of measuring distance cornea/retina). *A* the peak of the lower (left peak of corneal spike) of two echo spikes (whose distance is to be measured) is marked on the sheet of paper. *B* the peak of the higher of the two spikes (retinal signal) is projected down to the same height as the lower spike using the mark on the sheet of paper; a mark is made with a point of the calipers. Note that, for this projection, the lower margin of the paper is aligned carefully in a parallel fashion with the baseline or the measuring scale in the echogram picture (to produce a truly perpendicular projection of the higher peak). *C* the points of the calipers are adjusted with the peak of the left lower spike and the mark representing the higher peak (projected to the lower level). *D* the distance is compared with the electronic measuring scale and read in microseconds (down to 0.1 microsecond accuracy).

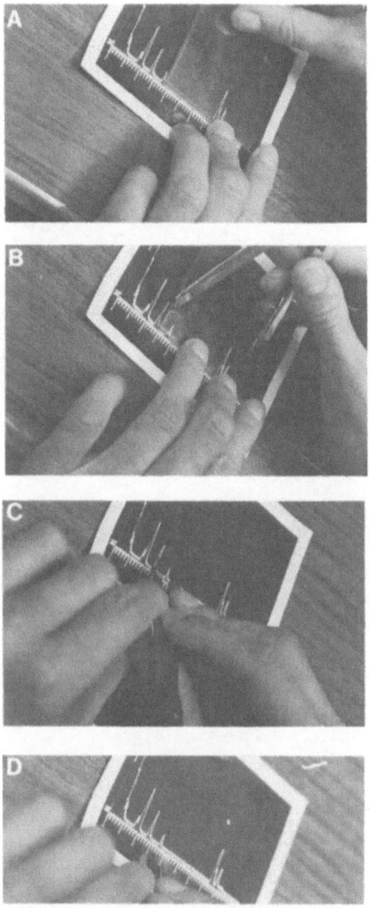

Fig. 12. Simple measuring procedure using calipers and a rectangular ruler (example of measuring lens thickness). *A* the height of the lower (posterior lens signal) of two spikes whose distance is to be determined is measured from the baseline. *B* the peak of the higher spike (anterior lens signal) is projected down to the same height as the peak of the lower spike with the help of the rectangular ruler; a mark is made with a point of the calipers at this projected height. Note that the ruler is aligned carefully with the baseline or the measuring line in order to allow for truly perpendicular downward projection of the higher peak. *C* the distance between the two spikes is now measured at the level of the peak of the lower spike with the aid of the calipers. *D* the calipers are now placed over the electronic measuring scale calibrated in microseconds to determine that distance in microseconds (down to 0.1 microsecond accuracy). Note that the measuring units underneath the distance that is measured in the echogram are used for the comparison to prevent possible distortions of the screen display from influencing the outcome of the measurement.

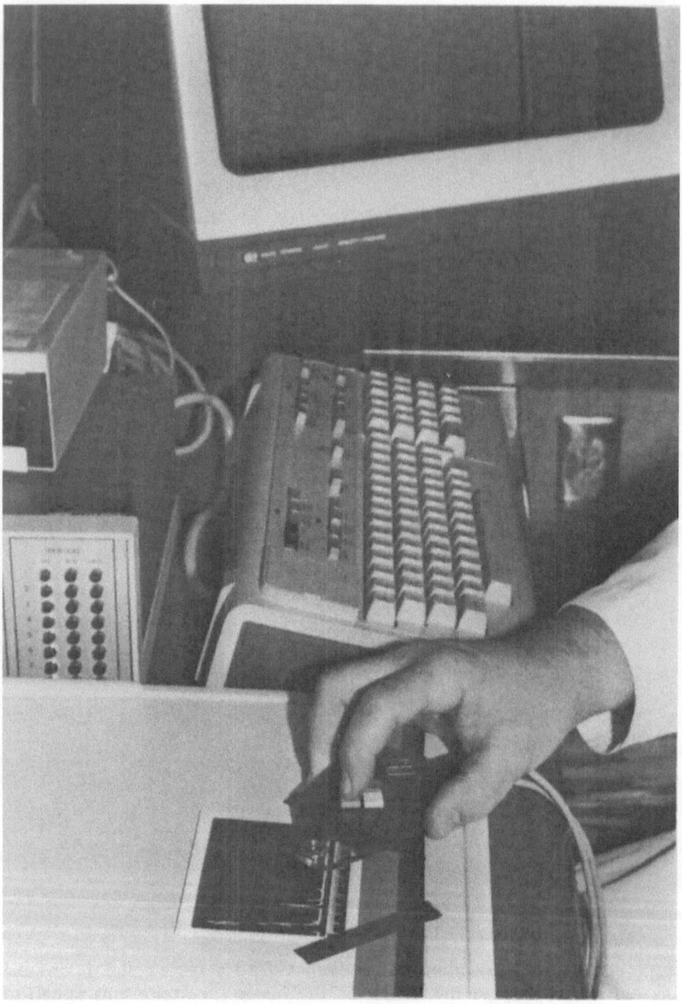

Fig. 13. **Computer terminal (*top*), digitizing tablet (*bottom*) and hand-held 4-button cursor for electronic measurement (for computer-aided measurement of axial eye length and computation of measurements in millimeters).**

level. The only necessity is to meticulously align the cursor with each of the peaks that are involved in the measurement (e.g., 5 point measurement for measuring the axial eye length as indicated in *Figure 15 top*). However, care must be taken to keep the Polaroid picture in place and aligned so that the baseline of the echogram is precisely parallel to the edge of the digitizing tablet and remains so throughout the measurement procedure. This is easily achieved by taping the picture on the surface of the tablet (as shown in

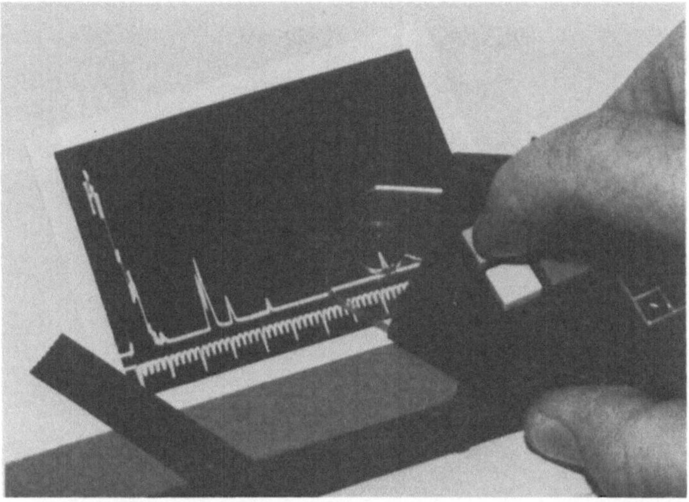

Fig. 14. For axial eye-length measurement, a "5-point" measurement is taken using the digitizing tablet: the 4-button cursor is placed successively over the two peaks of the corneal spike, the anterior and posterior lens spikes and the retinal spike. Then the cursor is placed over two spikes on the measuring scale which are 40 units (microseconds) apart. It is important to use the measuring units below the distance to be measured. In this picture, the cursor is placed just below the peak of the retina spike (end of 5-point measurement).

Figures 13 and *14*). However, the cathode-ray tube in the instrument must be aligned with the support frame for the Polaroid camera so that the baseline on the picture is exactly parallel to the edge of the picture. Once these requirements are satisfied, the measuring procedure is quick and requires only a few seconds (including the automatic calculation of the various distances along the axis of the eye in millimeters; ***Figure 15 bottom***).* In fact, the measuring procedure is so swift that it can easily be repeated several times in order to obtain a more accurate mean value for the result. When using the immersion mehod described with the standardized A-scan, taking three high-quality photographs of the axial eye length and measuring with the digitizing tablet, highly accurate millimeter values of the axial eye length and of its various components (such as anterior chamber depth and lens thickness) can be obtained for one patient within several minutes (including examination, measurement and calculation).

REFERENCES

1. Jansson, F.: Measurement of Intraocular Distances by Ultrasound. Acta Ophthalmol. (Copenh.), 74 (Suppl.):1–51, 1963.

*The program for axial eye-length measurement (by P. Montague) can be obtained from the Department of Ophthalmology of The University of Iowa.

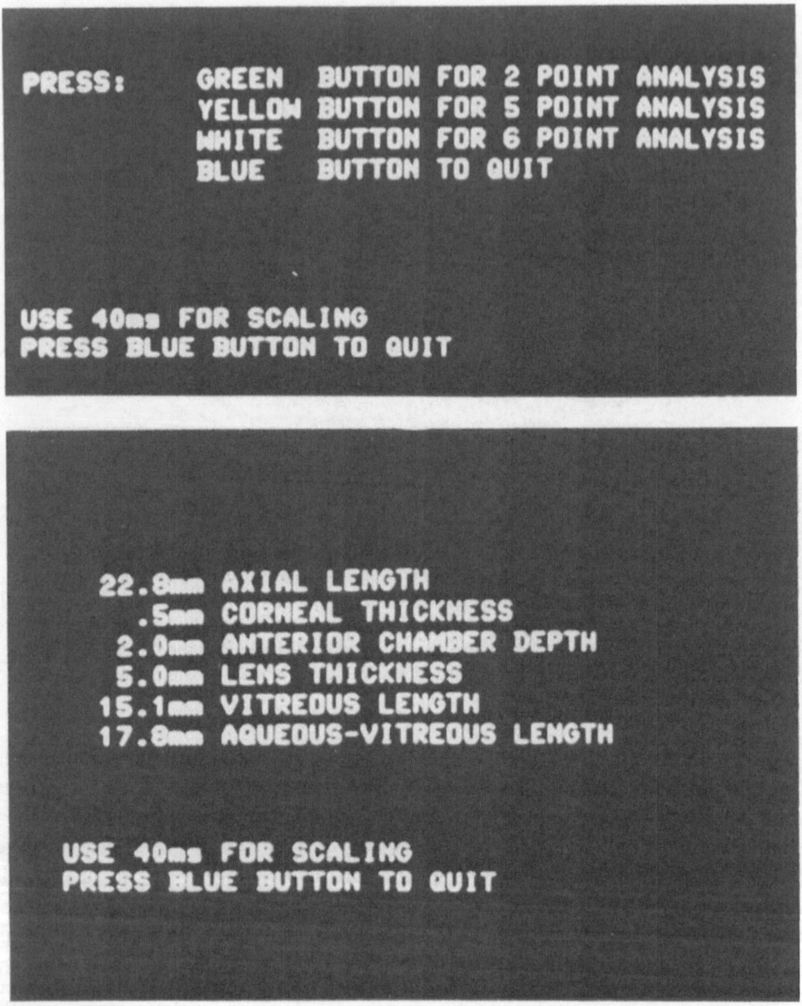

Fig. 15. Display on the terminal screen with the "menu" for measuring procedure (*top*) and the results of the measurement which are displayed immediately after the final measuring point (right measuring spike; see *Figure 14*) is electronically entered into the computer (*bottom*).

2. Ossoinig K. C.: Standardized Echography: Basic Principles, Clinical Applications and Results. In: Ophthalmic Ultrasonography: Comparative Techniques (Dallow R. L., ed.). Int. Ophthalmol. Clin., 19/4:127–210. Little, Brown and Co., Boston, 1979.

Author's address:
Dept. of Ophthalmology
University of Iowa
Iowa City, IA 55242
USA

BIOMETRY IN CALCULATING INTRAOCULAR LENS POWER

W. HAUFF
(Vienna, Austria)

SUMMARY

In 82 cataract patients the power of the pseudophakos to be implanted was determined. Axial length and anterior chamber depth were measured by ultrasound. The results of keratometry and the echographic data were used for lens power calculation. For accurate prediction the estimated postoperative anterior chamber depth is of importance. The advantages of measuring the axial length with an immersion technique are discussed. Using R. D. Binkhorst's formula in a series of 32 Binkhorst iris-clip lenses a mean error of + 0.16 D and a standard deviation of ± 0.81 D were obtained. In a group of 50 Kelman Quadraflex anterior chamber lenses the mean error was + 0.17 D and the standard deviation ± 0.66 D. An error of prediction greater than ± 2.0 D could not be observed.

INTRODUCTION

An 18 dioptre intraocular lens tends to restore the refraction before the development of cataract. Given the basic refraction the surgeon has to add 1.25 D for each dioptre of hyperopia; for each dioptre of myopia 1.25 D have to be subtracted (Binkhorst 1976). An increase in the refractive index of the crystalline lens accompanying the development of cataract can change the refraction to the myopic side. To trace the basic refraction one must obtain a record of previous refractions. In most patients basic refraction is doubtful or unknown.

The refractive power of the normal crystalline lens ranges from 15.5 D to 23.9 D and the corneal refractive power varies from 39.0 D to 47.6 D. R. D. Binkhorst (1981) measured axial length of living eyes varying from 21.50 mm to 26.97 mm.

When estimating the IOL power, errors of several dioptres may occur due to the variation of the power of the normal crystalline lens and the unknown relationship between refractive lens and corneal power and the axial length. Errors of 3 dioptres are frequent, ametropia of 9 dioptres has been reported (Hillman 1982).

Hillman, J.S./Le May, M.M. (eds.) Opthalmic Ultrasonography

ISBN 978-94-009-7280-3.

Preoperative lens power calculation using data of keratometry, postoperative anterior chamber depth and axial length measurement has gained in popularity. Three of the most popular formulas are those of Binkhorst and Loones, Colenbrander, and Fyodorov, Galin and Linksz. These formulas are simply related and after some algebraic manipulations have a similar form. Which formula is used makes little practical difference.

The results of IOL power calculation depend in part on the accuracy of ultrasonic axial length measurements and clinical A-scan units have an accuracy of 0.1 mm (Ossoinig 1979).

METHODS

We obtained keratometry measurements with the use of a keratometer (Zeiss) and measured the axial length with an A-scan instrument (7200 MA Kretz) using a 10 MHz sound probe described by Till (1978) to localize intraocular foreign bodies. The patients were examined in a supine position using an immersion technique with scleral shells as advocated by Ossoinig. For each measurement we took three Polaroid photographs from the screen on which the measuring scale was calibrated in microseconds (Fig. 1). The echo peaks of anterior and posterior corneal surface, of both lens surfaces and of the vitreoretinal interface were marked by vertical lines on the measuring-scale (Fig. 2). Anterior chamber depth, lens thickness and the distance to the vitreoretinal spike were taken directly from the scale in microseconds. Using appropriate sound velocities for different ocular tissues, microseconds were converted to millimetres and the addition of these three values gave the total axial length.

The intraocular lens power was predicted by a programmable pocket calculator TI 59 (Texas Instruments) by means of Binkhorst's formula.

SUBJECTS

We included in this study only eyes with 20/40 or better postoperative visual acuity and a stabilised refraction. 32 patients received a Binkhorst iris-clip lens and in 50 eyes a Kelman Quadraflex anterior chamber lens was implanted. The calculation of IOL power aimed at 1 D myopia but in 11 eyes the iseikonic lens was implanted.

The power of iris-clip lenses varied from 16.5 D to 24.0 D (Fig. 3), and the distribution of Kelman Quadraflex anterior chamber lenses ranged from 12.0 D to 22.5 D (Fig. 4). For each eye the absolute dioptric power difference between actual and predicted refractive error was recorded comparing the residual spherical equivalent with preoperative calculated refraction.

RESULTS

In the group of Binkhorst iris-clip lenses mean error ($\bar{x}$) was + 0.16 D with a standard deviation (SD) of ± 0.81 D (Fig. 5). 71.9% of the predictions were

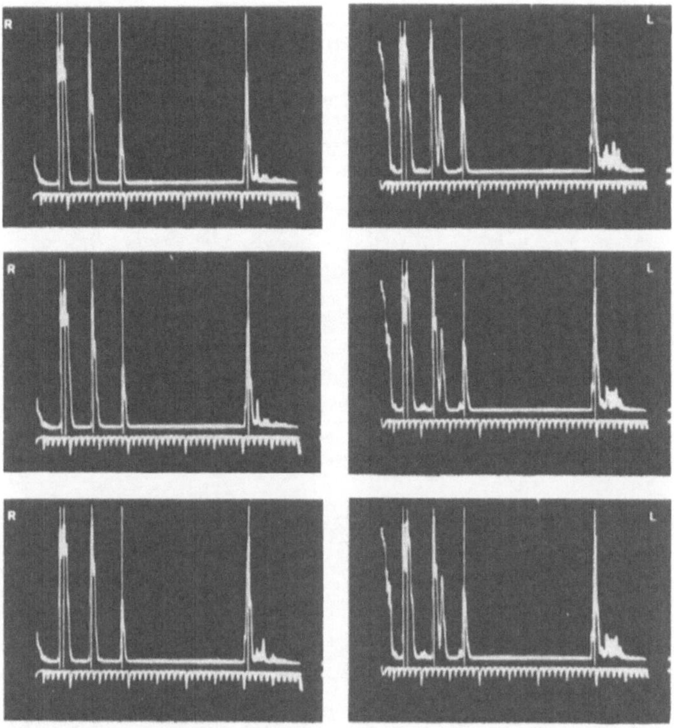

Fig. 1. For each measurement three Polaroid photographs were taken from the screen (measuring – scale calibrated in microseconds).

within the ± 0.5 D range and 87.5% within the ± 1.0 D range compared with the preoperative calculated refraction.

In anterior chamber lenses the error of prediction was less than or equal to ± 0.5 D in 70%, in 90% of these eyes we predicted within the ± 1.0 D range (Fig. 6). The mean error tended towards hypermetropia also ($\bar{x}$) = + 0.17 D, SD = ± 0.66 D).

DISCUSSION

The combination of biometry with 7200 MA Kretz unit and the calculation of IOL power by the use of Binkhorst's formula was reported by Hillman (1982). 50 eyes received an iris-clip lens and 70% of the predictions were within the ± 1.0 D range. Hoffer (1981) using his own variation of Colenbrander's formula described an error of ± 1.0 D in 70% and in a second study in 71%. Clevenger (1980) predicted IOL power of anterior chamber lenses and the error was less than or equal to ± 1.0 D in 75% of the cases. The comparable results of this study are 87.5% in iris-clip lenses and 90.0% in the group of anterior chamber lenses.

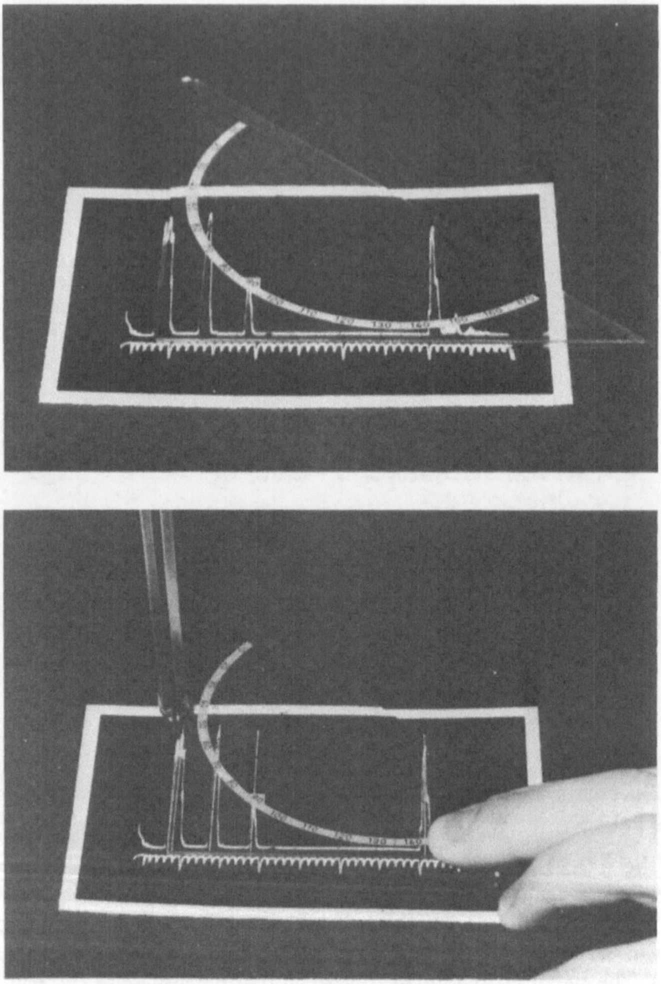

Fig. 2. Echo peaks of anterior and posterior corneal surface, of both surfaces of the lens and the vitreoretinal interface are marked by vertical lines; distances are taken from the measuring – scale in microseconds.

The maximal error of predicted refraction reported by Hillman ranged from + 3.0 D to − 4.0 D. Hoffer described errors of + 2.5 D and − 4.5 D. In our study of 82 calculated intraocular lenses an error of prediction greater than ± 2.0 D could not be observed.

The accuracy of intraocular lens power calculation depends on the estimation of the postoperative anterior chamber depth. For prepupillary lenses Cornelius D. Binkhorst (1974) proposed to use a standard measurement of 3.5 mm. Hoffer reported, that the accuracy of prediction using this standard value was lowered.

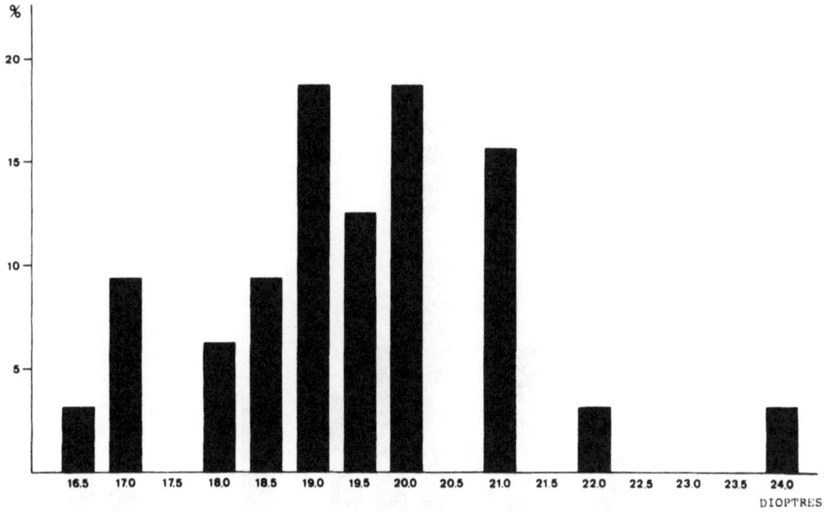

Fig. 3. Binkhorst iris-clip lenses: The distribution of IOL powers (dioptres in aqueous) (N = 32).

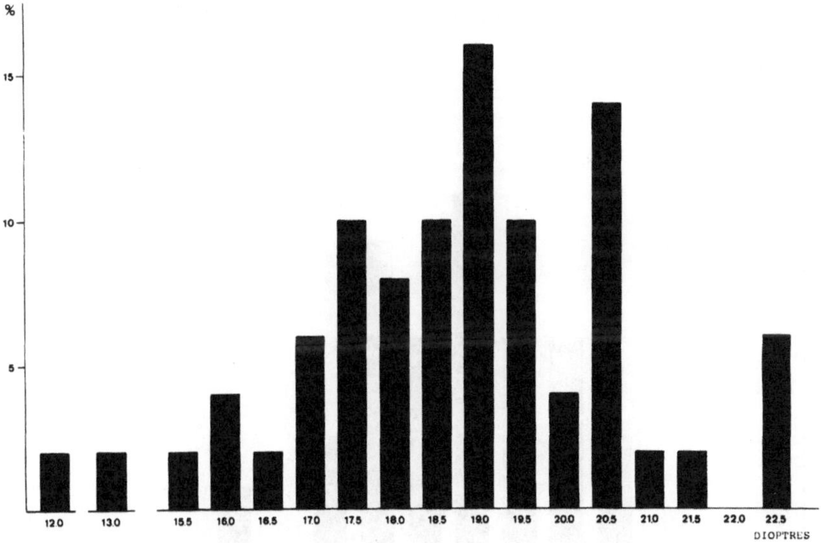

Fig. 4. Kelman Quadraflex anterior chamber lenses: The distribution of IOL powers (dioptres in aqueous) (N = 50).

In this series of iris-clip lenses we measured the distance from the vertex to the cornea to the anterior surface of the lens preoperatively by ultrasound. If the preoperative measurement ranged from 3.0 mm to 3.5 mm, we calculated the IOL power with a value of 3.3 mm. If this distance was shorter than

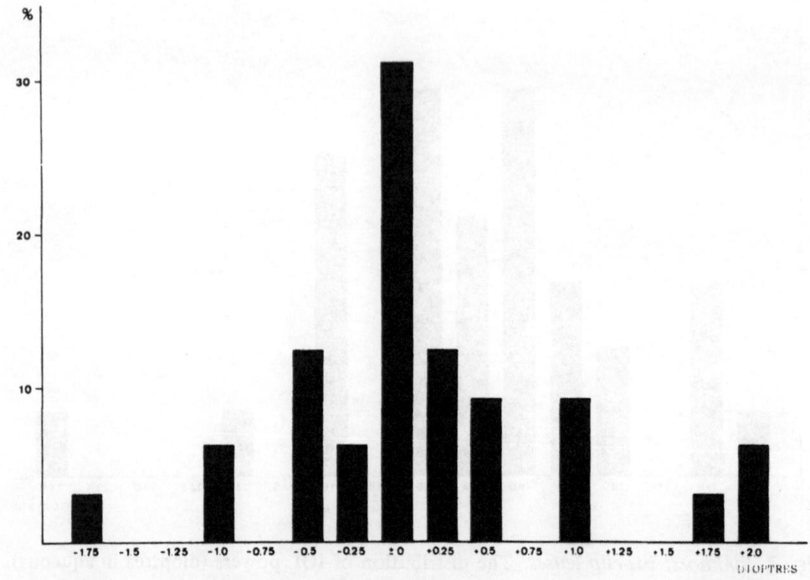

*Fig. 5. **Binkhorst iris-clip lenses:*** The differences in dioptres between the calculated predictions of postoperative refraction and the actual postoperative refractions (spherical equivalent): mean error $\bar{x} = + 0.16$ D, standard deviation SD = ± 0.81 D.

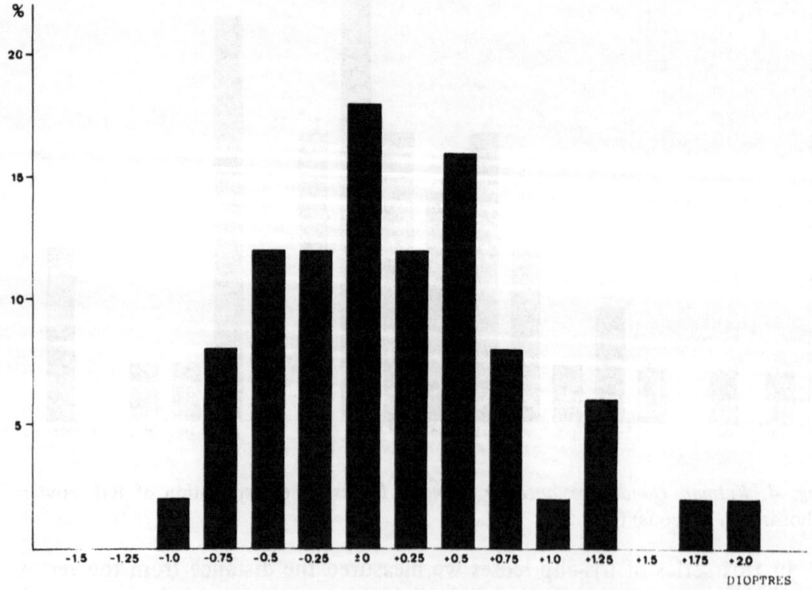

*Fig. 6. **Kelman Quadraflex anterior chamber lenses:*** The differences in dioptres between the calculated predictions of postoperative refraction and the actual postoperative refractions (spherical equivalent): mean error $\bar{x} = + 0.17$ D, standard deviation SD = ± 0.66 D.

3.0 mm, we used 3.1 mm; the only reason for following Binkhorst's proposal was a preoperative measurement greater than 3.5 mm. For calculation of Kelman Quadraflex anterior chamber lenses we used a standard measurement of 3.3 mm.

In all of the 82 calculations no retinal factor was added to the axial length measurement. An accurate axial length measurement is possible with the use of the 7200 MA Kretz unit. The exact procedure to examine the patient in a supine position using an immersion technique with scleral shells is important. To obtain maximal echo peaks of the anterior and posterior surface of cornea and lens and the vitreoretinal interface simultaneously we aimed the sound beam along the visual axis by hand. It is much more difficult to obtain cooperation from a patient while applanating the cornea. With the Sonometrics DBR unit it is almost impossible not to indent the cornea during applanation. Indentation leads to a shorter axial length measurement, thus giving too strong an intraocular lens power. The ultrasound probe never touches the eye with the use of an immersion method described by Ossoinig. Using a hypothetical common sound velocity of 1550 metres/second in ocular tissues and adding a retinal factor lowers the accuracy of axial length measurement and the prediction of intraocular lens power.

The aimed postoperative result is emmetropia or a low myopia (Huber 1981). Patients with an intraocular lens and a simple myopic astigmatism as a residual ametropia are independent of spectacles for most of the time. They need their glasses only for driving or prolonged reading. Calculation of intraocular lens power using a programmable pocket calculator is simple. Exact axial length measurements need time and care. The quality of postoperative vision depends on the accuracy of IOL power calculation resulting from an accurate axial length measurement.

REFERENCES

Binkhorst, C. D.: Power of the prepupillary pseudophakos. Brit. J. Ophthal. 56: 332 (1972).

Binkhorst, C. D.: Dioptrienzahl künstlicher Augenlinsen. Klin. Mbl. Augenheilk. 162: 354 (1973).

Binkhorst, R. D.: The optical design of intraocular lens implants. Ophthalmic. Surg. 6: 17 (1975).

Binkhorst, R. D.: Pitfalls in the determination of intraocular lens power without ultrasound. Ophthalmic. Surg. 7 (3): 69 (1976).

Binkhorst, R. D.: The accuracy of ultrasonic measurement of the axial length of the eye. Ophthalmic. Surg. 12: 363 (1981).

Clevenger, C. E.: Clinical prediction versus ultrasound measurement of IOL power. Amer. Intraocular Implant Soc. J.4: 222 (1978).

Colenbrander, M. C.: Calculation of the power of an iris clip lens for distant vision. Brit. J. Ophthal. 57: 735 (1973).

Fyodorov, S. N., Galin, M. A., Linksz, A.: Calculation of the optical power of intraocular lenses. Invest. Ophthal. 14: 625 (1975).

Hillman, J. S.: Intraocular lens power calculation for emmetropia: a clinical study. Brit. J. Ophthal. 66: 53 (1982).

Hoffer, K. J.: Accuracy of ultrasound intraocular lens calculation. Arch. Ophthalmol. 99: 1819 (1981).

Huber, C.: Myopic astigmatism a substitute for accommodation in pseudophakia. Docum. Ophthalmol. 52: 123 (1981).

Ossoinig, K. C.: Standardized echography: Basic principles. Int. Ophthalmol. Clin. 19: 127 (1979).

Till, P.: Spezialschallkopf zur Fremdkörperdiagnostik. Klin. Mbl. Augenheilk. 172: 252 (1978).

Author's address:
II. Universitäts – Augenklinik
Alserstrasse 4
A – 1090 Wien
Austria

MANUAL VERSUS ELECTRONIC MEASURMENT OF THE AXIAL LENGTH

H. JOHN F. SHAMMAS
(Los Angeles, USA)

During the past few years multiple ultrasound units have been specifically designed for axial length measurements; such a measurement is performed electronically within the unit and the result is displayed on the screen. Two years ago we adapted a Digital Ocular Computer (DOC) to our Kretz 7200 MA standardized A-scan; the DOC allows conversion of the ultrasound travel time into millimeters with an immediate readout (1).

The purpose of this prospective study is to compare electronic to manual measurements in 100 consecutive cases and evaluate the influence of each on intraocular lens (IOL) power calculations.

MATERIALS AND METHODS

One hundred eyes scheduled for extracapsular cataract extraction with an insertion of a posterior chamber lens had the axial length measured with the Kretz 7200 MA ultrasound unit using an immersion technique as advocated by Ossoinig (2). The patient is placed in a supine position. After instilling a drop of local anesthetic in the eye a scleral cup is applied keeping the upper and lower lids apart. The cup is filled with 1% methylcellulose and the ultrasound probe is immersed into the solution keeping it 5 to 10 mm away from the cornea.

The A scan probe is aligned with the visual axis of the eye. Four echospikes are then displayed on the oscilloscope representing from left to right, the cornea, anterior lens surface, posterior lens surface and retina (Fig. 1). The system sensitivity is decreased by 10 to 20 decibels and polaroid pictures are taken.

The axial length was first measured electronically using the digital ocular computer (D.O.C.) adapted to the Kretz 7200 MA. Two 'gates' are displayed on the oscilloscope screen: a 'corneal gate' in the region of the corneal spike and a 'retinal gate' in the region of the retinal spike. These two echospikes are maximized and placed within the appropriate gates. The measurement is taken between the leading edges of these two echo spikes (Fig. 1).

The axial length was then measured manually from the polaroid pictures between the peak of the echospike representing the anterior surface of the

Hillman, J.S./Le May, M.M. (eds.) Opthalmic Ultrasonography

ISBN 978-94-009-7280-3.

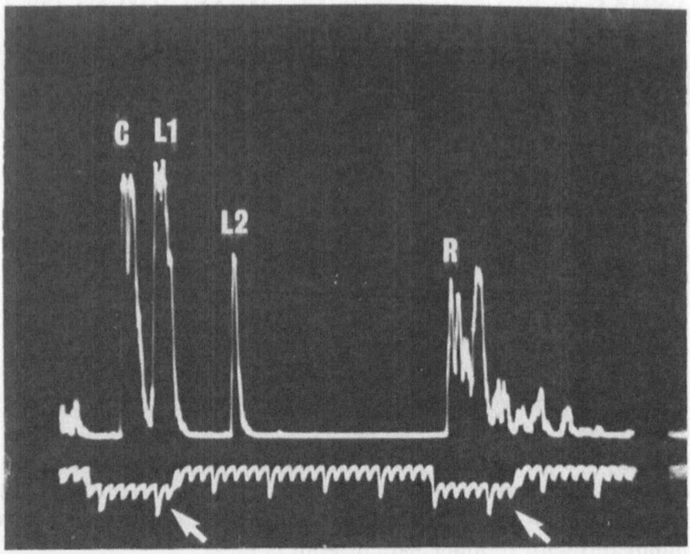

Fig. 1. Axial length is measured from the anterior surface of the cornea ('C') to the anterior surface of the retina ('R'). 'L_1 and L_2' represent the anterior and posterior surfaces of the lens respectively. Note the presence of gates (arrows) in the scale for electronic measurement of the axial length.

cornea and the peak of the echospike respresenting the anterior surface of the retina. The reading is taken in microseconds (t) from the unit's electronic scale; 't' is the travel time and represents the time it takes the ultrasound beam to reach the tissue and return to the probe. Since it represents twice the actual measurement, it is divided by two then converted to mm using an average velocity of 1548 m/s.

$$AL = \frac{t}{2} \times \frac{1548}{1000}$$

where AL is the axial length in mm.

We used the fudged formula (3) for IOL power calculations.

$$P = \frac{1336}{L - 0.1\,(L - 23) - C - 0.05} - \frac{1}{\dfrac{1.0125}{K} - \dfrac{C + 0.05}{1336}}$$

where

P = The power of the I.O.L for emmetropia in diopters
L = The axial length in millimeters
K = The average keratometer readings in diopters
C = The distance between the anterior vertex of the cornea and the I.O.L. in millimeters (estimated anterior chamber depth).

The formula was programmed on a Hewlett Packard 97 calculator using a modification of Drew's program (4). The dioptric power of the cornea K is substituted by K/1.0125 and the axial length L is substituted by $L - 0.1\,(L - 23)$. The postoperative anterior chamber depth was evaluated at 4.1 mm. The keratometer powers were measured using a Bausch & Lomb keratometer; also there was no postoperative change in the average keratometer redings over 1 diopter in any of the cases.

RESULTS

The axial length ranged from 21.76 to 26.43 mm when measured electronically with an average value of 23.48 mm ± 1.12 mm and from 22.00 to 26.50 mm when measured manually with an average value of 23.51 mm ± 1.13 mm. The difference between the two average values is not statistically significant ($p > 0.05$).

The electronic measurement of the axial length was longer than the manual measurement in 45 cases and ranged from + 0.01 to + 0.19 mm; it was shorter in 49 cases and ranged from − 0.01 to − 0.26 mm. The two measurements were identical in 6 cases. The average difference between the electronic and manual measurements was − 0.03 mm ± 0.01 mm. The difference between the two measurements was within ± 0.1 mm in 65 cases and within ± 0.2 mm in 93 cases.

The fudged formula for I.O.L. power calculations was used in all 100 cases. We predicted within ± 1.0 diopters in 95 eyes when the axial length measurement was performed electronically and in 93 eyes when the measurement was performed manually. The difference between the two is not statistically significant ($p > 05$). The errors ranged between − 1.90 D and + 0.95 D with the electronic measurement and between − 2.10 D and + 1.20 D with the manual measurement.

DISCUSSION

An accurate measurement of the axial length is the most important factor affecting I.O.L. power calculations. A 1 mm error affects the post-operative refraction by approximately 2.5 diopters. A manual measurement of the axial length can be time-consuming especially if properly performed; the system sensitivity is decreased until the echospikes representing the cornea, anterior surface of the lens, posterior surface of the lens and retina are extremely short. This technique ensures that all signals are at the same phase of oscillation. If the axial length is measured at a higher system sensitivity, the signals representing the cornea and the retina are not necessarily at the same phase of oscillation and an error in measurement of up to one wavelength (0.2 mm) can occur. In our study the axial length was measured at approximately tissue sensitivity − 15 dB. This setting is necessary for the electronic measurement; the DOC measures the axial length between the leading edges of the corneal and retinal echospikes at approximately 50% the height of the inital spike.

When an axial length is measured for IOL power calculations the reproducibility of the measurement becomes an important factor. Such a reproducibility has been tested in 155 consecutive cases (1). In each case multiple polaroid pictures of the ultrasound pattern were taken. The best two pictures were kept for axial length measurement and an average value used for the calculations. When manually measured, the difference between the axial length measurements in each case ranged from no change to 0.2 mm with an average value of 0.05 mm. When electronically measured the difference between the two measurements ranged from no change to 0.05 mm with an average value of 0.01 mm.

The fudged formula that we are using is a modified Colenbrander's formula (5). The first modification involved the corneal index of refraction; it is changed from 1.333 to 4/3 as suggested by Binkhorst (6). The corneal power such as read on the Bausch and Lomb Keratometer is decreased by a factor of 1.0125; the results would then be similar to those obtained with Binkhorst's formula. The second modification is the incorporation of a fudged factor linked to the axial length. This fudge factor is established by reviewing the 500 cases of axial length measurements and I.O.L. power calculations in which this factor is needed for higher accuracy (3). The axial length is increased by 0.1 mm for each 1 mm shorter than 23 mm and decreased it by 0.1 mm for each 1 mm longer than 23 mm. This fudge factor can be easily introduced into any theoretical formula by changing the axial length (L) to $L - 0.1 (L - 23)$.

CONCLUSIONS

The electronic measurement of the axial length is accurate and comparable to the manual measurement. Furthermore, an immersion technique for axial length measurement with an electronic readout yields highly reproducible results.

The fudged formula is a modification of Colenbrander's formula. It yields a 0.70 D stronger power lens for a 23.0 mm average length eye which is similar to results obtained with Binkhorst's formula. It also fudges the axial length by − 0.1 mm for each 1 mm longer than 23 mm and by + 0.1 mm for each 1 mm shorter than 23 mm. In our series the axial length was measured using an immersion technique and our fudged formula yielded an accuracy of 95% (predictions with ± 1 D).

REFERENCES

1. Shammas, H. J. F.: Axial length measurement and its relation to intraocular lens power calculations. American Intraocular Implant Society Journal: 8: 346, 1982.
2. Ossoinig, K.: Standardized echography: Basic principles. Int. Ophthalmol. Clin. 19: 127, 1979.
3. Shammas, H. J. F.: The fudged formula for intraocular lens power calculations. American I.O.I.S. Journal: 8: 350, 1982.
4. Drews, R. D.: Calculation of intraocular power. A program for the Hewlitt Packard 97 calculator. A.I.O.I.S. Journal 3: 209, 1977.

5. Colenbrander, M. D.: Calculation of the power of an iris-clip lens for distance version. Br. J. Ophthalmology 57: 735, 1973.
6. Binkhorst, R. D.: The optical design of intraocular lens implants. Ophthalmic Surgery 6: 17, 1975.

Author's address:
3510 Century Blvd.
Lynwood, CA 90262
USA

COMPUTERIZED BIOMETRY AND LENS CALCULATION

J. M. THIJSSEN, W. A. VERHOEF, F. PASMAN-SCHEPS and A. M. VERBEEK
(Nijmegen, The Netherlands)

INTRODUCTION

In a recent paper (Thijssen and Deutman 1981) we summarized the pre- and postoperative data from the calculation of the power of implant lenses by using echographic measurements. A systematic deviation was observed between the predicted emmetropizing lens power and the postoperatively deduced value (from the refractive error). Two causes were indicated: the assumption of a 0.5 mm thick retina should be corrected and 0.2 mm might be a more realistic value (Binkhorst). The second cause was assumed to be the inaccuracy of the ultrasonic biometry. This is because the high attenuation in cataract lenses reduces the posterior wall echocomplex. We, therefore, decided to make available a system that employs the RF echowaveform of a broadband transducer and to connect this system to a digital computer. The computer program stores a series of echograms and then evaluates the echopeaks accurately and, finally, automatically produces the iseikonizing and emmetropizing lens powers after proper averaging of the accumulated data. The procedure will be outlined in this paper and the first results discussed.

TECHNIQUE

The echographic system consists of a broadband transmitter/receiver (Panametrics 5052 PR) which is connected to the receiver input of a clinical A-mode device (Kretztechnik 7200 MA) as shown in Figure 1. The tranducer yields a high resolution and is focused at 25 mm (Panametrics). The biometry can be performed while using the display of the A-scan device and the broadband RF echogram is transmitted to a transient recorder (Biomation 8100). This recorder is interfaced to a digital computer (DEC PDP 11/34) which controls it by software means. So after a command by the ophthalmologist a series of 7 RF echograms is digitized (100 MHz ADC) and stored in the computer memory within 0.5 seconds. The stored data are transferred to a magnetic disk and may be displayed for visual inspection.

Hillman, J.S./Le May, M.M. (eds.) Ophthalmic Ultrasonography
© 1983, Dr W. Junk Publishers, The Hague/Boston/Lancaster
ISBN 978-94-009-7280-3.

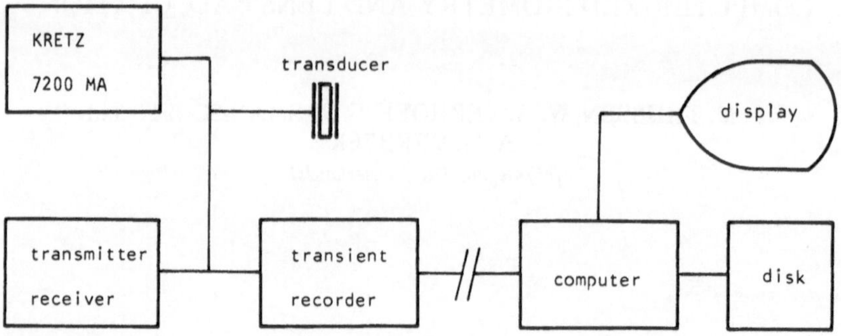

Fig. 1. Block diagram of equipment used for biometry.

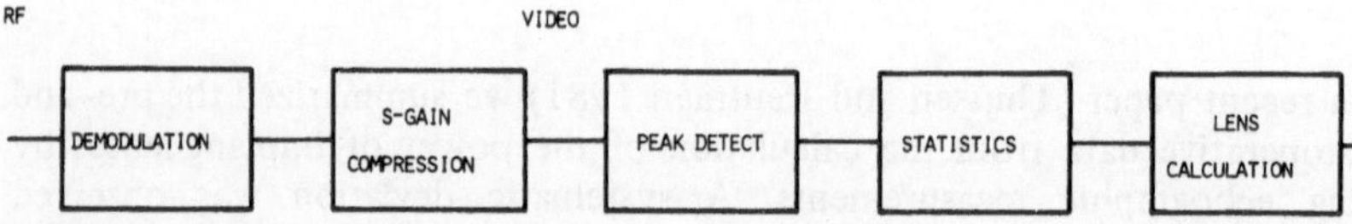

Fig. 2. Block diagram of computer programs employed to evaluate the echograms.

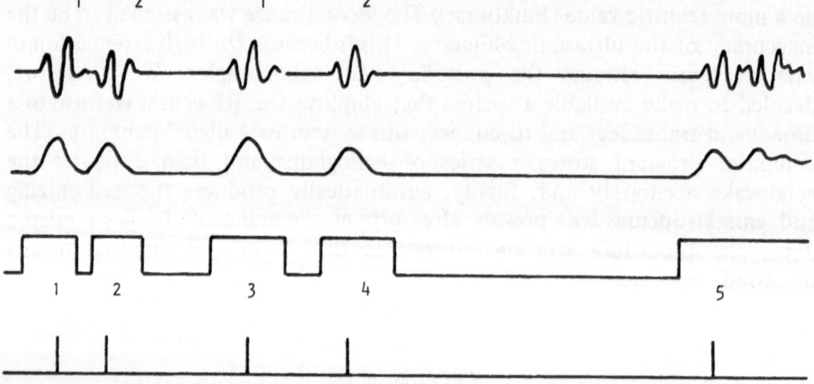

Fig. 3. Scheme of processing steps. First trace: RF echogram; Second trace: demodulated echogram; Third trace: time window in which peak has to be detected; Fourth trace: times of detected peaks.

DATA ANALYSIS

The overall scheme of the computer programs is shown in Figure 2. The various steps involved will be discussed now. After storage of 7 RF echograms the first step is to demodulate these signals one by one (cf. Figure 3 second trace) by means of an analytical signal method (cf. Whalen, 1971). The

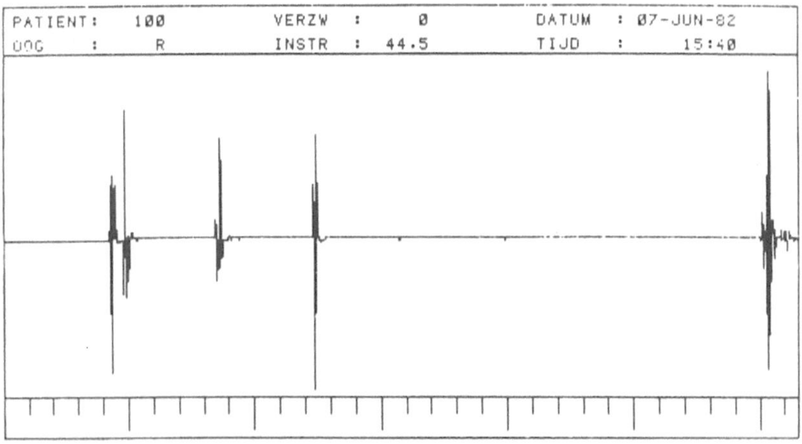

Fig. 4. Example of RF echogram from healthy eye (waterbath).

demodulated signal is then compressed by a sigmoid characteristic which is also present in the clinical echoapparatus. The latter processing step is not absolutely necessary but it has the advantage that it yields an A-mode picture quite similar to the usual ones. The demodulated signal is optimally suited for the estimation of peak maxima. The third trace in Figure 3 illustrates the strategy followed in this peak detection algorithm. The program detects the first maximum and then sets a window around it to be able to find the absolute maximum in that region. After detection of the anterior cornea echo a second window is set relative to the first maximum and the posterior cornea echo is detected. The third and fourth windows are used to estimate the anterior and posterior lens echoes and the fifth one encloses the retinapeak. In order to prevent disturbance by reduplication artifacts and noise a threshold level is involved. Like shown in Figure 3, bottom trace, the peak values of the video signal are thus estimated. An example is shown in Figures 4 and 5. The excellent axial resolution of the broadband system employed can be decided from the clear separation of the anterior from the posterior corneal peaks.

RESULTS

The first test of the whole set up concerned a series of estimations of the dimensions of 10 eyes with a total of independent measurements of 25. The accuracy of the computerized estimations amounts to 0.03 mm if the spread of the 7 echograms per measurement is considered (Fig. 6). When the various estimations on a single eye are compared the reproduceability of the measurements of all the dimensions appears to be of the order of 0.05 mm. The main cause of errors in the axial length is the absence of the retinal echo from the echogram, which may occur when the direction of the sound beam is off-axis.

The computerized estimates have been compared with the results

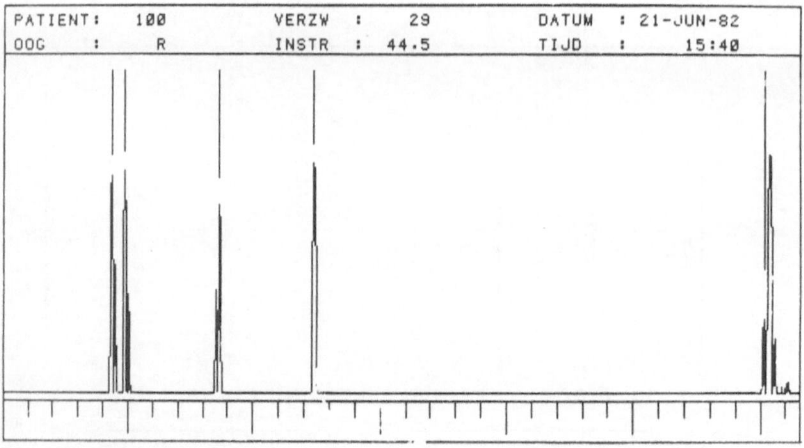

Fig. 5. Example of demodulated (video) echogram from Fig. 3.

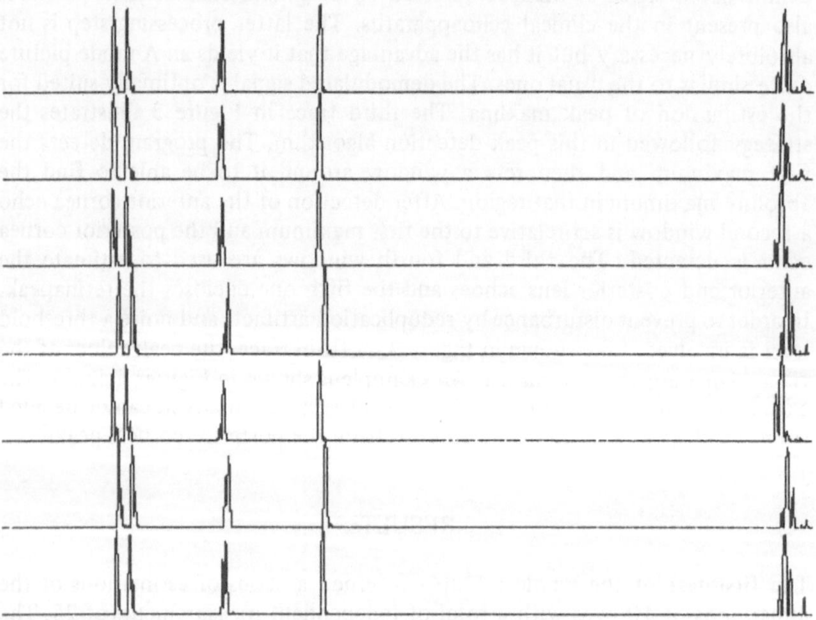

Fig. 6. Demodulated waveforms obtained in a single measurement.

obtained from the Polaroid photographs. It appeared essential to measure the calibration square wave of the Kretz apparatus from the same photograph because a warming-up effect caused an increase of the size of the oscilloscope display by a 1 to 1.5%. The reproduceability of the axial length measurements from the photographs was 0.15 mm. The difference of these data with the axial lengths obtained from the RF echograms by computer was on the average not significant, probably because healthy eyes of young subjects were involved.

DISCUSSION

The method used to estimate the peaks in the computerized echograms is similar to the strategy built in the electronic device of Van Marle (cf. Van Marle & Gommers, 1981). The difference is that in the presented method the windows within which a peak is to be detected are flexibly shifted depending on the time the last peak was estimated. Van Marle and Gommers indicated a reproducability between subsequent measurements of the order of 0.2 mm (with extreme values up to 0.4 mm). The same observation was made by the present authors. The main cause for this variability is the absence of the retinal peak in some echograms. Even within a series of seven echograms of a single measurement it occasionally happens that the retina is missing. The best way to avoid this problem is to change the sensitivity of the equipment until the retinal echo reaches approximately 50% height of the A-mode screen so that it can be clearly separated from the scleral echopeaks. The reproduceability of the axial length measurements from the photographs was 0.15 mm. The difference of these data with the axial lengths obtained from the RF echograms by computer was on the average not significant; probably because healthy eyes of young subjects were involved.

REFERENCES

Binkhorst, R. D.: Intraocular lens power calculation. Int. Ophthal. Clin. 19:83–94 (1979).

Van Marle, G. W. R. B. and Gommers, P. A. M.: Digitalized echo oculometry. In: 'Ultrasonography in Ophthalmology'. Eds. J. M. Thijssen and A. M. Verbeek. Doc. Ophthal. Proc. Series 29. Junk, The Hague 1981. Pp. 521–526.

Thijssen, J. M. and Deutman, A. F.: Predictive value of calculated dioptric power of prepupillary implane lenses. In: 'Ultrasonography in Ophthalmology'. Eds. J. M. Thijssen and A. M. Verbeek. Doc. Ophthal. Proc. Series 29. Junk, The Hague 1981. Pp. 239–244.

Whalen, A. D.: 'Detection of signals in noise'. Acad. Press, New York, 1971.

Author's address:
Biophysics Laboratory of the Institute of Ophthalmology
University of Nijmegen
6500 HB Nijmegen
The Netherlands

COMPUTERIZED OCULAR BIOMETRY: A NEWLY DEVELOPED COMPACT SYSTEM

R.-D. LEPPER and H. G. TRIER
(Bonn, W. Germany)

Since 1979, the Bonn group for ophthalmic ultrasound has used computerized systems for biometry of the eye, which were developed by the authors. Reports on the clinical results are given in the next paper by Lepper and Trier (1982). Since then, the ocular distances of about 5,000 patients have been measured to determine adequate implant lenses. Starting with only a few patients, the number has now increased to nearly 20 per day. This was feasible only with highly specialised equipment. In the first years, from 1979–81, a system consisting of a PDP 11 (Digital Equipment Corp.) with attached commercial and laboratory periphery was used (Lepper and Trier, 1981). On the basis of experience thus obtained, a new compact ultrasonic biometry-device was constructed. The new system, called BMS-811-Echo-comp, is composed of an ultrasonic A-mode equipment, transit time evaluating electronics, and a homecomputer Commodore CBM 4032, which is described elsewhere. Therefore, details are only given for two former components, which are installed together in a 19" compartment. The block diagram of the system is given in Figure 1.

The ultrasonic subunit transmits a unipolar pulse of manually adjustable amplitude. The transmitter voltage is limited to maximally 75 V. Different from other transmitters the pulse shape is chosen according to Figure 2. The trailing steep edge of the pulse corresponds to the transmission bang. The time interval following that bang until the next rise of the transmitter voltage is the receiving time for echoes. During the receiving time the transmitter offers an output impedance of 50 Ohm. This technique leads to several advantageous results. First, overloading of the receiver section is minimized, as there is no transmitter voltage tail running into the receiving time. Second, the transducer cable is terminated in its own impedance, thus avoiding any ringing effects.

The echoes are processed by a noiseless amplifier, and a balanced demodulator. The receiver consists of six moderately amplifying stages with broadband transistors. The total RF-amplification comes up to approximately 65 dB. Even in case of excessive lens opacification, back wall signals of sufficient amplitude are obtainable. The frequency response of the receiver is set in such a manner that frequencies below 5 MHz and above 30 MHz are rejected. The demodulator must be of balanced type to get rid of phase

Hillman, J.S./Le May, M.M. (eds.) Ophthalmic Ultrasonography

ISBN 978-94-009-7280-3.

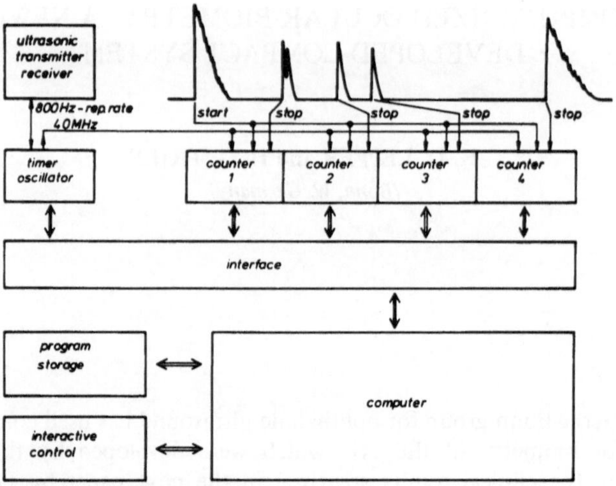

Fig. 1. Block diagram of the BMS 811-Echocomp.

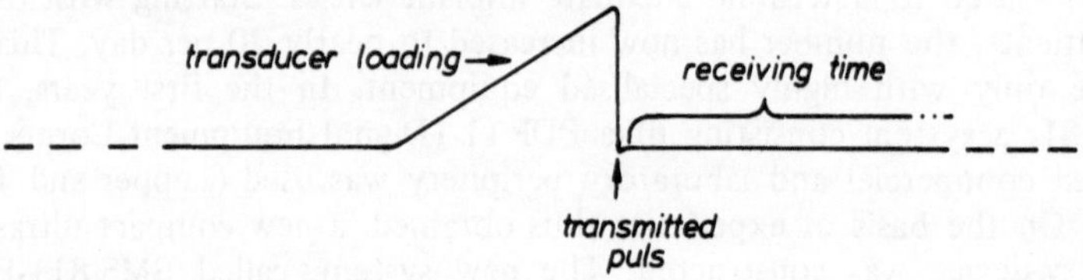

Fig. 2. Electrical output of the transmitter. The amplitude of the sawtooth can be changed manually in logarithmic scales.

ambiguities in the sound field. Figure 3 gives details. After demodulation the signal is fed into two stages: unfiltered into a Schmitt trigger unit, and low-pass filtered into the display unit. Thus, visual interpretation is improved without loss of resolution in the trigger unit.

The ultrasound subunit is designed for patients' maximum safety: the dosage is as low as possible, depending on the needs. Even in cases of catastrophic failure, the maximum current is limited to a few mA, the average current to far below 1 mA, and the maximum transmitter voltage to 75 V, as mentioned above.

The system is equipped with four digital counters for measuring the ultrasonic transit time from the transmitter pulse to corneal surfaces, anterior and posterior lens surface, and posterior ocular wall. Four gates and, correspondingly four trigger events are, therefore, necessary. On the screen the A-mode display, the position of the four gates, and the trigger points are depicted in two separate beams (Fig. 4). The resolution of the transit time evaluating unit should exceed that of the ultrasonic frequencies used. For this reason, 40 MHz counting frequency were chosen. Furthermore, the system should be controllable by the computer, gate-position included. In consequence, the transit time evaluating unit consists of four electronic counter boards, one timer board, and one interface board. These boards are bus-connected. Connection to the computer is made via a bus extension cable.

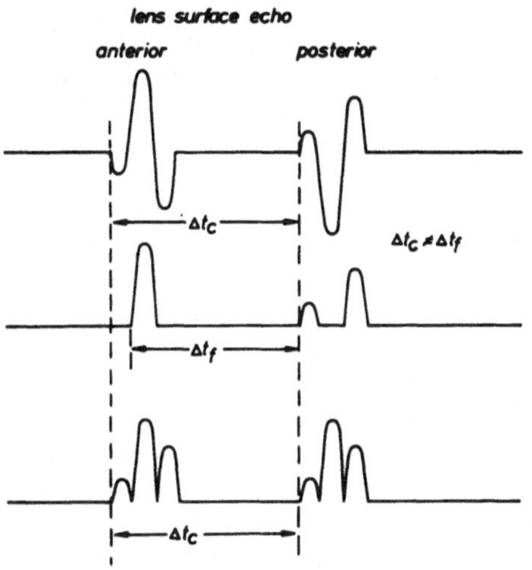

Fig. 3. Effects of phase steps of the echoes. A one way rectification leads to false measurements (Δt_f). Only the double way rectifier (balanced demodulator) gives the correct time interval Δt_c.

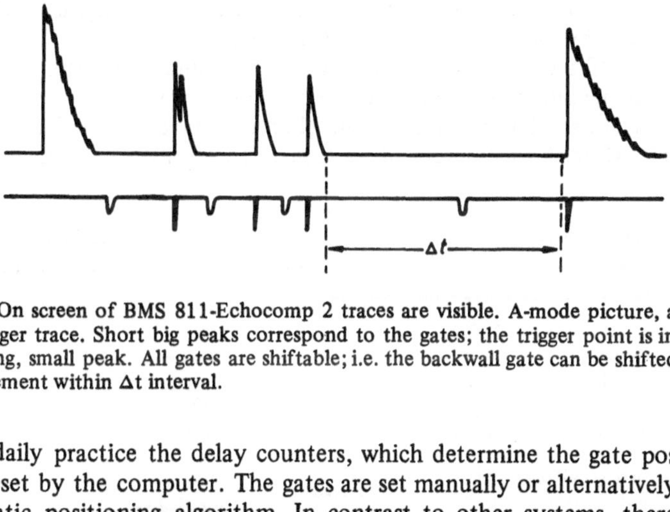

Fig. 4. On screen of BMS 811-Echocomp 2 traces are visible. A-mode picture, and gate and trigger trace. Short big peaks correspond to the gates; the trigger point is indicated by a long, small peak. All gates are shiftable; i.e. the backwall gate can be shifted during measurement within Δt interval.

In daily practice the delay counters, which determine the gate positions, are preset by the computer. The gates are set manually or alternatively by an automatic positioning algorithm. In contrast to other systems, there is no start and stop gate in the BMS 811-Echocomp. The BMS-gate has the function of enabling asynchronous trigger signals to stop a counter, i.e.: any next echo of sufficient height after the gate is registered regardless of the mutual distance of echo and gate. In consequence, the gates simply have to be adjusted ahead of the echoes to be measured with no interfering echo in between.

Manually the gates are positioned via computer key board. The positioning algorithm shifts all gates in parallel, so that the first gate approximates the following echo. If there is no echo, all gates are shifted towards the transmitting pulse. If the mutual distance of eye and transducer changes, the gates are moving adequately. Thus, the system offers echo tracing capability.

Trigger signals from the ultrasound subunit allow stopping of the counter, if their pertaining delay counters run out. Thus, assignment of each counter to its specific echo is assured. After a fixed time interval the content of the counters are read in by the computer, the system is then started anew. This process occurs in real time, every ultrasonic event is, therefore, registered at a rate of 800 measurements/sec. Whilst running, the timer clock is perpetually checked against the computer clock to monitor any timer malfunction. This process is done as a background job of which the user is not aware, except in cases of noticeable deviations, when the action to be taken is left to the user's discretion.

For each axial length determination 32 single measurements in 4/100 sec are evaluated. These data blocks are judged according to predetermined criteria. Only measurements that fulfill all these criteria are accepted as 'ok'. The others are marked according to the type of error. In general 4 types of error are diagnosed. The first type of error marks a false 'following up' of interfaces in the eye. For example: if the anterior lens surface is missed in one of the 32 measurements, this is indicated by an 'F'-type error. If one of the gates in one of the 32 measurements approaches its corresponding interface by less than one microsecond the system indicates a 'G'-type error. A very useful criterion is the variation of the 32 measured eye lengths. If the eye length 'jitters' by more than 0.3 mm within the data block, a 'J'-type of error is indicated. If there is no backwall echo to be found, the system indicates this too. Six measurements complete one measurement set.

The patient's relevant optical and clinical data are also fed into the computer. After the measurement of (usually) both eyes is completed, the

Datum 12.07.82 OP LINKS

Name Vorn. Ernst geb 22.05.05

Bemerkungen: Berechnung fuer VK-Linse

	RECHTS		LINKS
Brille	2.5 dptr		
HHradius	8.25 mm		7.95 mm
Vorderk.	2.47 mm		2.55 mm
Linse	5.54 mm		5.33 mm
Glask.	15.11 mm		15.63 mm
Augenl.	23.12 mm		23.51 mm
<HHS(br/iol)/avk>	14	-1.2	3.5
		Iseikonie	
IOL			19.24 dptr
Brille			-2.42 dptr
Bildgr.		103.34 %	
		Emmetropie	
IOL			16.69 dptr
Bildgr.			107.1 %
Dioptr.Anis.		3.64 %	
		Empfehlung	
IOL			18 dptr
Brille			-1.25 dptr
Bildgr.			105.16 %
Aniseik.			1.76 %

Fig. 5. Example for measurement protocol.

emmetropic, the iseikonic, and a 'best choice' lens can easily be determined. The best choice lens is selected under the responsibility of the user. He may select the dioptric power of an IOL or of the spectacles, alternatively. In both cases the consequences, i.e. dioptric power of the other optical element, image size, and dioptric aniseikonia are calculated and presented. The selection of suitable ultrasonic measurements, and the determination of the best choice are carried out interactively at the screen. Finally, the result is printed on paper as a complete measurement protocol on request (Fig. 5).

Needless to say, the total system response changes according to the status of the eyes involved, be they phakic, aphakic, or amblyopic.

ACKNOWLEDGEMENT

The authors are especially indebted to Mr. W. Klein for his invaluable help in building the system.

REFERENCES

Lepper, R.-D. and Trier, H. G.: A new device for ocular biometry. Docum. Ophthal. Proc. Series 29, ed. J. M. Thijssen & A. M. Verbeek (Dr. W. Junk Publ., The Hague, 1981).

Lepper, R.-D. and Trier, H. G.: Refraction after intraocular lens implantation: Results with a computerized system for ultrasonic biometry and for implant lens power calculation. Docum. Ophthal. Proc. Series vol. 38, ed. J. S. Hillman & M. M. Le May (Dr. W. Junk Publ., The Hague, 1983), pp. 243–248.

Author's address:
Universitäts Augenklinik
Abbestrasse 2
D-5300 Bonn-Venusberg
Federal Republic of Germany

REFRACTION AFTER INTRAOCULAR LENS IMPLANTATION: RESULTS WITH A COMPUTERIZED SYSTEM FOR ULTRASONIC BIOMETRY AND FOR IMPLANT LENS POWER CALCULATION

R.-D. LEPPER and H. G. TRIER
(Bonn, W. Germany)

Since 1979, about 5,000 Patients, or 10,000 eyes, respectively, were examined by ultrasonic biometry in the Bonn University Eye Clinic. As each eye has to be measured several times, the total number of measurements has amounted to tens of thousands. It is obvious that it would not be possible to cope with this number without a computerized biometric system.

Such a system, called BMS 811 Echocomp, has been developed by the authors, and was described in the preceding paper (Lepper and Trier, 1982).

A number of schemes for determining suitable intraocular implant lenses were developed, which were based either on empirical formulas, i.e. regression formulas, or on theoretical optical derivatives. Our calculations are based on modifications of formulas that were published by Gernet et al., in 1978.

Having rendered possible the echographic measurement of the ocular axial distances on a high technical level, the question arose as to what extent this determination proved clinically relevant. The post-operative visual acuity – with and without spectacles – indicates the success of a lens implantation. The accuracy of the lens power determination by means of echographic measurements can be proved by one parameter only, namely the difference between the predetermined and the post-operatively accepted optical power of the patients spectacles.

A systematic analysis of provable measurement errors was carried out. Only those patients who came at least one month later for lens implantation in the second eye could be followed up.

Measurement of the corneal curvature was done by means of a Zeiss ophthalmometer. As is generally known, 0.1 mm deviation in curvature equals approximately 0.5 dptr refractive error. Figure 1 demonstrates the pre- and postoperative average corneal curvatures of 344 patients. The broken line marks the unchanged state. Most of the measurements show minor changes from pre- to post-operative values. However, a certain trend towards flattening to an average postoperative corneal curvature is observable. This was also confirmed by a regression analysis. Figure 1 clearly indicates that the assumption of a fixed value for the corneal curvature is by no means adequate for IOL-determination.

By implanting an IOL the anterior chamber depth is altered. As any shift of an optical element influences the refractive status, this is also of importance

Hillman, J.S./Le May, M.M. (eds.) Ophthalmic Ultrasonography

ISBN 978-94-009-7280-3.

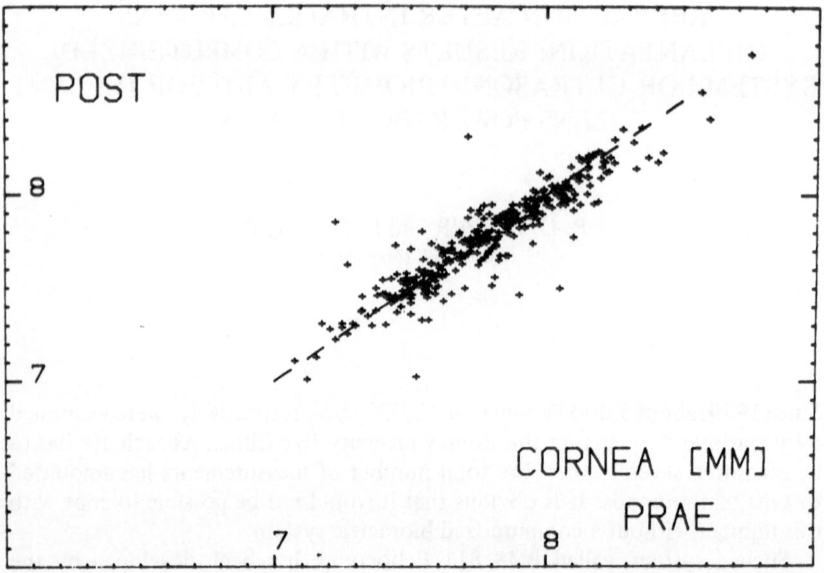

Fig. 1. Pre- and postoperative corneal curvature (344 eyes). The broken line indicates 'no change'.

for the IOL-determination. As a rule of thumb, 0.1 mm change in anterior chamber depth results in 0.1–0.2 dptr refractive error.

Figure 2 shows the preoperatively measured anterior chamber depth of 344 eyes. The considerable variations between less than 2, and more than 5 mm is due to the differences in eye length, and more or less pronounced swelling of the lens.

Figure 3 demonstrates the anterior chamber depth after implantation of a posterior chamber lens. Comparing these two figures one can easily notice an increase of anterior chamber depth, caused by the implantation.

The individual increase of the anterior chamber depth is depicted in Figure 4. On average, roughly 0.4 mm change was found. The first approximation for estimating the postoperative chamber depth preoperatively is to add a constant of 0.4 mm to the preoperative value for calculation. However, larger deviations from the real postoperative value were found in individual cases.

To obtain a more accurate estimate of the anterior chamber (a.c.) depth, the eye length ought also to be taken into account. A regression analysis, including both the a.c. depth and the eye length resulted in regression coefficients of 0.32 and 0.098, respectively. The regression constants were dropped. The difference between post-operatively measured chamber depth, and preoperatively calculated pseudovalue is depicted in Figure 5. The slope is steeper and the curve more compact. This figure shows clearly that bilinear correlation of both factors improves the prediction of postoperative anterior chamber depth. The 'true' bilinear regression does not give better results.

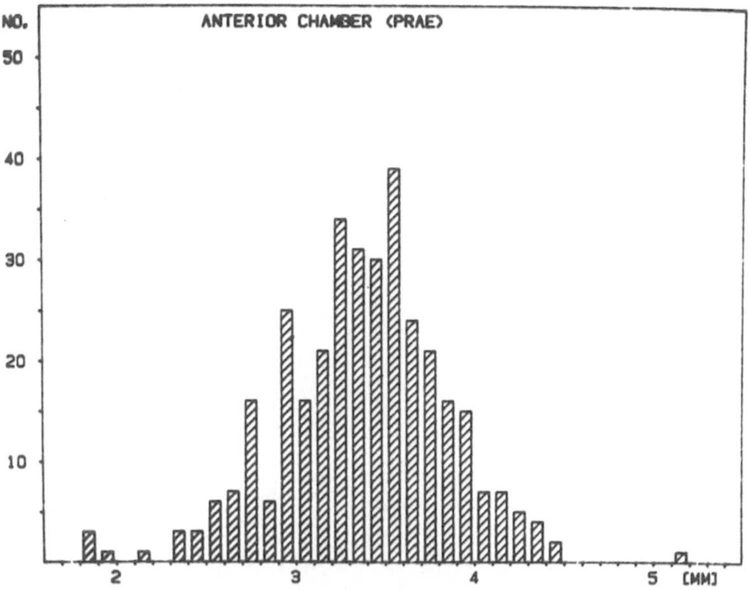

Fig. 2. Anterior chamber depth before lens surgery (344 cases).

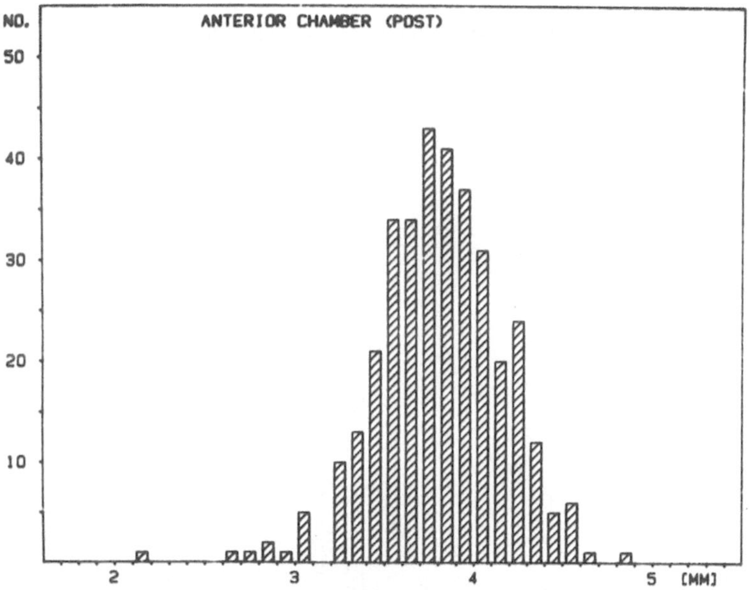

Fig. 3. Anterior chamber depth after implantation of posterior chamber IOL.

From the point of view of the patient who has to undergo this operation, the problem summarized in Figure 6 is the most important. Here, the distribution of postoperative refractive errors is demonstrated. 304 unbiased cases are included. Only patients who received an implant lens with a dioptric

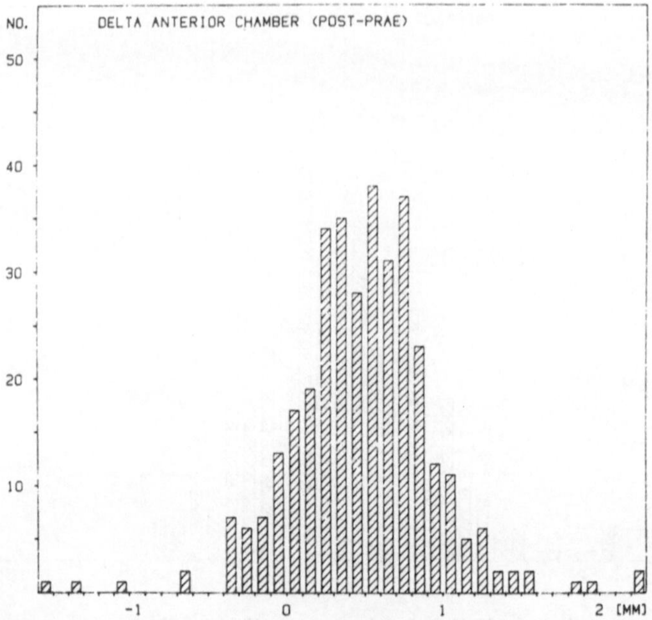

Fig. 4. Increase of anterior chamber depth due to lens implantation.

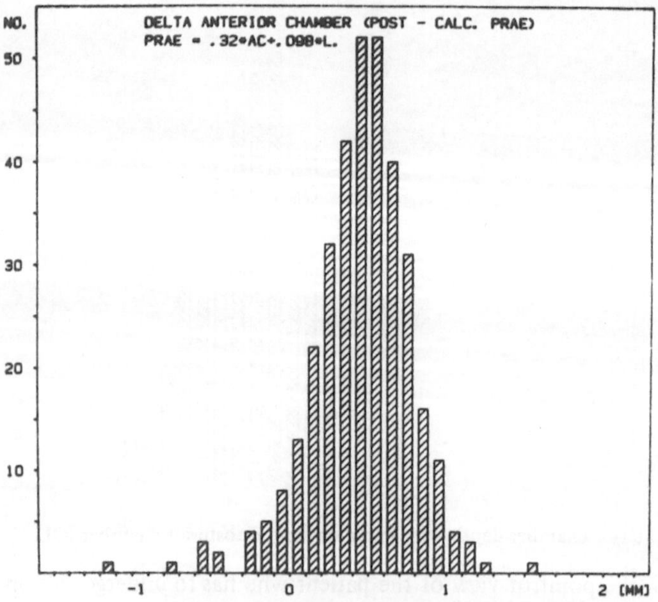

Fig. 5. Increase of anterior chamber depth from a predicted value to the measured postoperative value. The prediction is based on preoperative measurements of anterior chamber depth, and eye length, and the two corresponding linear regression functions.

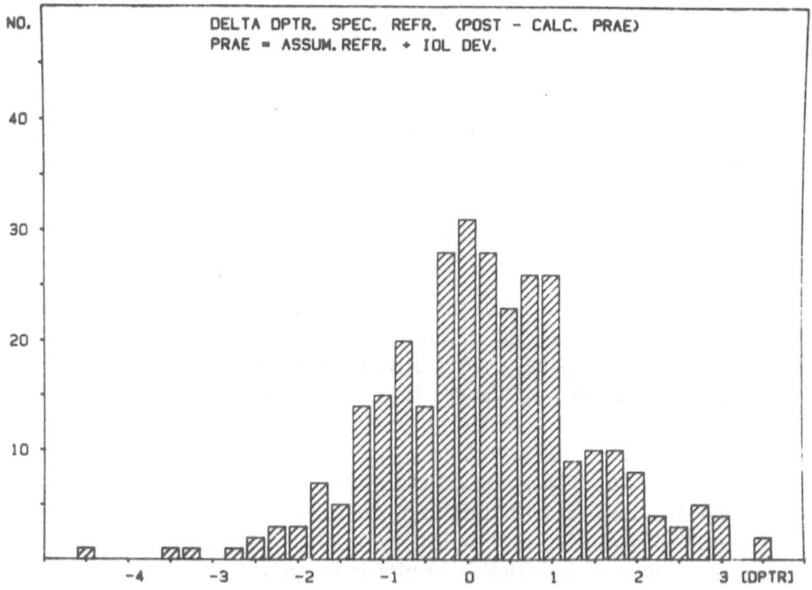

Fig. 6. Total refractive error after lens implantation. Shown is the difference between the actual dioptric power of the patient's eye glasses after implantation and the predicted value. (304 unbiased cases).

power that differed for more than 1 dptr from the proposed lens were excluded. In 1.3% (4 eyes) only, greater refraction errors than +/− 3 dptr were observed. In one of these 4 cases the visual acuity was 0.1 (6/60) only; in another the corneal curvature changed from 7.5 to 7.0 mm. The other two cases are not yet fully explained and need further observation. The group with refractive errors of more than +/− 2 dptr included 8.9% of all cases.

To get a deeper insight into the sources of refractive error the next data analysis included the known operational changes in corneal curvature. For the sake of simplicity the corrections were done on a first approximation basis only; i.e. the total refractive status was changed by 5 dptr per mm alteration of corneal curvature. The distribution of errors appeared more compact, but the tails were not minimized significantly. A similar result is achieved when the chamber depth variation is also included.

The reason for these distribution tails is at least twofold: one factor is the influence of macular degeneration, which results in a very bad visual acuity, or the Irvine Gass Syndrome, respectively. The other (mathematical) factor is based on the fact that the first order approximation is valid only in a limited range of the parameters involved.

Table 1 gives the regression analysis of 344 cases. Estimations of the postoperative corneal curvatures resulted in a correlation coefficient of 92% between pre- and postoperative corneal curvature. The regression factor, less than 1, confirmed the flattening effect of the operation on the corneal curvature.

Table 1. Regression analysis on 344 cases.

```
POSTOP CORNEAL CURV. = 0.897 + 0.883 * PRAEOP. C.C        [ CORR.COEF. 92 % ]

POSTOP ANTERIOR CMB. = 2.734 + 0.32  * PRAEOP  A.C        [ CORR.COEF. 43 % ]

POSTOP ANTERIOR CMB. = 1.472 + 0.098 * PRAEOP EYELENGTH [ CORR.COEF. 39 % ]

POSTOP ANTERIOR CMB. = 1.434 + 0.068 * PRAEOP EYELENGTH
                             + 0.223 * PRAEOP A.C.        [ CORR.COEF. 49 % ]

POSTOP ANTERIOR CMB. = 3.8   (CONSTANTLY)        =>       [ CORR.COEF.  0 % ]
```

The next four equations deal with the prediction of postoperative anterior chamber depth. If correlated unilinearly, the highest coefficient (43%) is obtained by calculating the postoperative chamber depth from the preoperative. If the preoperative eye length is taken into account, the coefficient is only 39%. The bilinear calculation, which considers a.c. and eye length, gave the best result, a correlation coefficient of 49% being achieved. Frequently, a constant postoperative chamber depth (3.8 mm) is postulated for calculation. However, the correlation coefficient is then 0%.

By means of statistics only an average quality may be described, but the individual number of insufficient results is scarcely found in the statistical description. If the number of insufficient results could be reduced at the expense of slightly decreased average accuracy, this would be clinically valuable. Further analyses in this direction are in progress. Generally, however, a satisfactory implantation result is achievable with the methods currently available.

ACKNOWLEDGEMENT

We are especially indebted to Prof. Dardenne and his team who performed the lens implantations.

REFERENCES

Gernet, H., Ostholt, H. and Werner, H.: Intraokulare Optik in Klinik und Praxis. (Rothacker, München 1978).

Lepper, R.-D. and Trier, H. G.: Computerized ocular biometry: A newly developed compact system. In: Hillman J. S. and Le May M. M. (eds.), Docum. Opthal. Proc. Series vol. 38. The Hague: Dr. W. Junk Publishers, 1983, pp. 237–241.

Author's address:
Universitäts Augenklinik
Abbestrasse 2
D-5300 Bonn-Venusberg
Federal Republic of Germany

CORRECTION OF ULTRASONIC DISTANCE MEASUREMENTS FOR THE CALCULATION OF THE REFRACTIVE POWER OF INTRAOCULAR LENSES

B. PRAHS
(Würzburg, W. Germany)

INTRODUCTION

Today's IOL patient does not only want an improved quality of vision over the aphakic correction, he wants the best possible optical correction in his individual case. Regarding the permanent discomfort a disadvantageous refraction may induce the little more expense of an IOL calculation is justified. The precision of IOL calculation mostly depends on the accuracy of axial length determination with ultrasound (Binkhorst 1978). Different studies (Binkhorst 1978, Hoffer 1981) on the accuracy of IOL power calculation based on keratometry and ultrasonic measurements have shown that a prediction of the postoperative refraction of about ± 1 D is possible. This accuracy was achieved with different equipment and different calculation formulas.

The theoretically derived calculation formulas are sometimes corrected with some factor on the grounds that the posterior surface of the cornea is more curved than the anterior surface (Colenbrander 1973), that there is a surgically induced flattening of the cornea (Binkhorst 1975) or that the visual cell layer does not correspond to the vitreoretinal peak of the A-scan (Colenbrander 1973, Oguchi, van Balen 1974, Binkhorst 1975).

With these factors a correction of about 2 D is possible. Another systematic aberration of about the same amount is induced by the ultrasound equipment and the way the ultrasonic measurement is done as will be shown.

METHOD AND MATERIAL

The axial length of these same cataract eye with nuclear sclerosis and capsular opacities was measured with 4 different echographs:

1. Kretz 7200 MA with 8 MHz transducer	
2. Ocuscan 400 (Sonometrics)	(a) with 10 MHz transducer
	(b) with 5 MHz transducer
3. Digital Biometric Ruler (DBR) (Sonometrics)	with 10 MHz transducer
4. Compu Scan Biometric Ruler (Storz)	with 10 MHz transducer

Hillman, J.S./Le May, M.M. (eds.) Ophthalmic Ultrasonography

ISBN 978-94-009-7280-3.

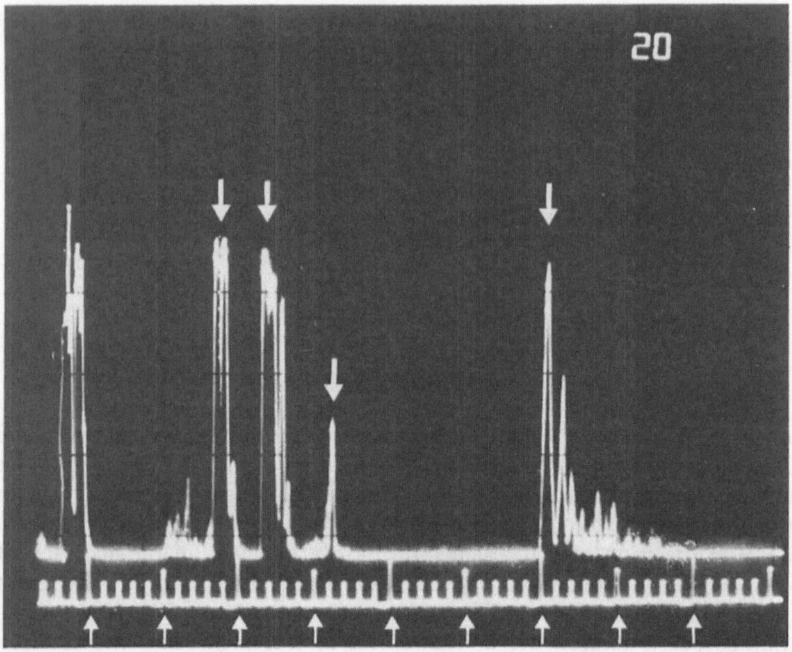

Fig. 1. A-scan (Ocuscan 400). The reading points on the echogram and the calibration scale are marked. Each reading point is calibrated by an interpolation between the two nearest calibration points of the scale.

The measurement was done after pupil dilation using an immersion device – a scleral cup filled with 5% methylcellulose. The ultrasound beam was aligned along the optical axis as shown by high echo peaks from the cornea, both lens surfaces and the vitreoretinal interface. For measurement 36 photographs were taken from the screen of the echograph with a motor camera (2 shots/sec.)

The echograms from the Kretz 7200 MA and Ocuscan 400 which fitted best the criterion of axial alignment were taken for photo evaluation. They were projected on a digitizer board (total enlargment: 17 ×).

The points of measurement of the echogram and those of the calibration scale were digitized (Fig. 1). The evaluation was performed by a computer interpolating between the two nearest calibration points (calibration steps: 10 μsec Kretz, 5 mm Ocuscan) and assuming a speed for ultrasound of 1641 m/sec for the lens and 1531 m/sec for the rest of the ocular tissues. To estimate the effect of random reading errors the same well defined distance was measured 20 times.

There is some uncertainty about the reading point in an enlarged echogram as the lines and peaks have a certain extension. To estimate this effect one echogram was evaluated 20 times and the mean error was compared to the one derived from the error propagation law with the mean reading error of a distance measurement inserted. Horizontal distortions on the screen of the echographs were determined by measuring the same calibration step (Kretz: 10 μsec, Ocuscan: 10 mm) on the right and left side of the screen.

Both Biometric Rulers worked with an assumed common speed of 1550 m/sec for ultrasound in ocular tissues. The same 10 MHz transducer was used for both Biometric Rulers. The echograms and results of the axial length measurement were displayed simultaneously on the screen of the echograph and were photographed with a motor camera. Those measurements which fitted the criterion of axial alignment and had a correct gate position were taken for evaluation.

RESULTS

The mean error of a distance measurement on the digitizer board was ± 0.22 mm (standard deviation). This was determined by measuring the same distance 20 times. Regarding the 17-fold enlargement this corresponds to a reading accuracy of ± 0.013 mm in the ocular tissues.

Horizontal distortions on the screen of the Kretz 7200 MA are obvious. The difference of a 10 μsec step on the calibration scale measured on the right and left side of the screen was 4.35%.

Due to this distortion the steps of the quartz calibration scale were not rectangular but showed slight slopes and round edges. Systematic errors can be expected by the uncertainty about the calibration reading point.

Photo Evaluation of Kretz 7200 MA Echograms

The same 26 echograms were evaluated 4 times. One time reading the calibration points at the top edges of the quartz scale and the other time at the bottom edges. To demonstrate the differences between peak to peak measurements and readings at the baseline each of these measurements was done with each of the 2 calibrations (Figs. 2 and 3). The evaluation was done by the same person.

Photo Evaluation of Ocuscan 400 Echograms

Horizontal distortions on the Tectronix screen of the Ocuscan 400 were not detectable with the accuracy of our reading method. Two set of 17 echograms each taken with a 10 MHz and 5 MHz transducer were evaluated with baseline and peak to peak measurements (Figs. 4 and 5).

Digital Biometric Ruler Measurements (an average of 12 measurements)

Ocuscan DBR: axial length = 21.88 ± 0.133 mm
Compu Scan: axial length = 21.82 ± 0.128 mm

calibration points	axial length (mean)	standard deviation
top edges of the scale	21.63 mm	± 0.086 mm
bottom edges of the scale	22.08 mm	± 0.115 mm

7200b1

Fig. 2. Photo evaluation of the Kretz 7200 MA echograms with 8 MHz transducer – baseline measurements.

calibration points	axial length (mean)	standard deviation
top edges of the scale	22.14 mm	± 0.076 mm
bottom edges of the scale	22.47 mm	± 0.085 mm

7200pp

Fig. 3. Photo evaluation of the Kretz 7200 MA echograms with 8 MHz transducer – peak to peak measurements.

DISCUSSION

The theoretical limitation to accuracy of biometry by ultrasound is a quarter of a wavelength and this is 0.04 mm for a 10 MHz transducer. To come close to this accuracy the reading errors and the aberrations due to distortions of the screen have to be kept small. This can be achieved by a sufficient enlargement of the screen photograph and the proposed reading procedure. The improvement of accuracy by enlargement is limited as the thickness of the echogram lines is increased also and this increases the uncertainty about the reading point. Evaluating the same echogram 20 times the reading error was ± 0.057 mm. According to the error propagation law a mean error of

transducer probe	axial length (mean)	standard deviation
10 MHz	21.81 mm	± 0.056 mm
5 MHz	21.73 mm	± 0.111 mm

Fig. 4. Photo evaluation of Ocuscan echograms baseline measurements.

transducer probe	axial length (mean)	standard deviation
10 MHz	22.20 mm	± 0.082 mm
5 MHz	21.80 mm	± 0.123 mm

Fig. 5. Photo evaluation of Ocuscan echograms peak to peak measurements.

± 0.054 mm follows for an axial length measurement with our reading accuracy.

This indicates that in our measurements with a 17-fold enlargement the lines of the echogram can still be regarded as thin. The proposed evaluation method divides the calibration scale in 9 calibration intervals (Fig. 1). The horizontal distortion is thereby reduced to 1/9.

Systematic aberrations between peak to peak measurements and baseline measurements could be expected. The first are gain dependent, the latter not. A maximal difference in axial length measurements of 0.84 mm was found. This corresponds to a difference of 2.6 D in IOL calculation. The gain dependence of baseline measurements explains only a part of the differences in the means of the axial length measurements. A difference of 0.4 mm with peak to peak measurements with the same echograph and different transducers (5 and 10 MHz) occurred. The difference is not due to random errors as shown by the t-test ($t_{17, 0.05} = 6.97 > 2.037$). Side lobe effects (Lepper, Trier 1980) and interference effects combined with stronger absorption of higher frequencies in the ocular tissues may have contributed to this difference. The standard deviations of all measurements with the same transducer did not differ significantly (F-test). The uncertainty about the reading point on the Kretz 7200 MA calibration scale has no effect on the reproducibility. The reason may be that the same person evaluated the echograms, obviously assuming the same point of the round edges of the quartz scale as calibration point. Different evaluaters may have obtained different results.

The alignment of the transducer probe along the optical axis is easier with an echograph with linear amplifier characteristic than with a logarithmic or 'S-curved' one.

Differences in high amplitudes are better displayed. No significant differences, however, between axial length measurements with 'S-curved' and linear amplifier characteristic could be detected in our data.

The results of both Biometric Rulers obtained with the same transducer probe are almost identical. This may be by chance. The standard deviations of the Biometric Rulers are bigger than those of photo-evaluated measurements. The reason may be that there is a difference in time between the shot of the photo and the measurement.

CONCLUSION

The theoretically derived calculation formulas for IOLs have empirical aspects as corrections are added in general. Starting with IOL calculation or changing the equipment there is an uncertainty about the necessary correction. A plane calibration block would solve only part of the problems, as in general a different gain adjustment is needed for the measurement on the calibration block and the ocular tissues. A change of the gain, however, changes the result of baseline measurements. Side lobe effects on tilted surfaces and frequency selective absorption effects cannot be taken into account.

As long as there is no well defined ultrasonic eye model available a practical solution would be to calibrate one echograph with another echograph on the same human eye(s).

Measurements should be related as close as possible to the calibration scale in order to avoid errors due to horizontal distortions of the screeen. The nearness of baseline measurement points to the calibration scale in an advantage of this method. A photo evaluation on polaroid photos is not sufficient as the mean error with an enlargement of only 2.5 x is already 0.13 mm (S.D.).

To avoid random errors multiple measurements should be evaluated. In photo evaluation, a computer supported device is of great help.

REFERENCES

1. Binkhorst, R. D.: The optical design of intraocular lens implants. Ophthalmic Surg. 6(3):17, 1976.
2. Binkhorst, R. D.: Biometric A-scan ultrasonography and intraocular lens power calculation, in Emery J. M. (ed.). 'Current Concepts in Cataract Surgery'. St. Louis, C. V. Mosby Co., 1978.

3. Colenbrander, M. D.: Calculation of the power of an iris clip lens for distance vision. Br. J. Ophthalmol 57:735, 1973.
4. Hoffer, K. J.: Intraocular lens calculation: The Problem of the short eye. Ophthalmic Surg. 12:269, 1981.
5. Oguchi, Y. and van Baelen, A. T. M.: Ultrasonic study of the refraction of patients with pseudophakos, in Ultrasound in Medicine and Biology. London, Pergamon Press, 1974.
6. Lepper, R. D. and Trier, H. G.: A new device for ocular biometry. Docum. Opthal. Proc. Series, Vol. 29, 1981.

Author's address:
Universitäts-Augenklinik
Josef-Schneider Strasse 11
D-8700 Würzburg
Federal Republic of Germany

ULTRASOUND VELOCITY IN DIFFERENT TYPES OF LENS OPACITIES

A. LOFFREDO, A. DE LELLIS and G. CENNAMO
(*Naples, Italy*)

ABSTRACT

Intraocular lens implantation gives a practical value to ocular biometry. The preoperative calculation of refraction is based on the ultrasound velocity in different fluids and tissues of the eye. While the ultrasound velocity may be considered constant in the aqueous humour and vitreous it may be different in various types of cataract. The results showed a significant difference in the ultrasound velocity in the opaque lens that may influence the ocular length calculation.

Ocular biometry has assumed recently a more practical value due to an increase in the use of intraocular lenses (IOL). The post-operative refraction may be calculated by means of the ocular biometry; its accuracy depends upon the axial length ultrasound measurement.

The ultrasound velocity in different ocular tissues plays an important role in the axial length determination.

Ultrasound velocity in the aqueous humour and in the vitreous can be assumed constant and equal to 1532 m/sec. The velocity changes in the lens because of various types of cataract.

Studies by Oguchi and Van Balen stated that the anterior chamber depth after intraocular lens implantation is related to the lens thickness. But this latter parameter depends in part upon the ultrasound velocity in various types of cataract.

A more accurate study of the correlation between the anterior chamber depth and the lens thickness may lead to a more accurate knowledge of the postoperative position of an I.O.L.

To ascertain by ultrasound biometry the lens thickness, it is necessary to know the ultrasound velocity in the opaque lens.

This latter parameter was determined by Jansson and Kock by Yamahoto et al., and by Coleman E.J. et al. The average ultrasound velocity in opaque lens is 1640.5 m/sec., according to Jansson and 1629 m/sec., according to Coleman. Pallikaris (1981) studied the ultrasound velocity in 37 opaque lenses, classified on the basis of their slit lamp appearance. The results of this research gave the opaque lens values of ultrasound velocity ranging from

Hillman, J.S./Le May, M.M. (eds.) Ophthalmic Ultrasonography

ISBN 978-94-009-7280-3.

1588 to 1692 m/sec., with an average of 1641.35 m/sec., and a standard deviation equal to ± 28 m/sec.

To evaluate the data in the literature reporting the ultrasound velocity in the lens for axial length and lens thickness calculation we determined this velocity in various types of cataract.

MATERIALS AND METHODS

For this research a Kretz 7200 MA apparatus with 8 MHz probe was utilized. The lenses were introduced into a small container of width less than 8 mm. (Fig. 1). The width of this container can be modified by means of a screw in relation to the volume of the lens. The lens surfaces were in direct contact with the transducer on one side and the reflecting wall of the end of the screw on the other side (Fig. 2.) In our opinion, this method prevents possible errors of measurement due to the interposition of a water solution between the lens and transducer. In fact in this latter condition the incorrect incidence on the lens of the ultrasonic beam may lead to the artefacts due to a wrong refraction.

Measurements were carried out at a constant temperature of 34°C ± 1°C; this is the temperature of the lens in physiological conditions.

Twenty nine lenses with different types of cataractous opacities were examined and classified as follows:

(1) Nuclear
(2) Cortical
(3) Intumescent
(4) Subcapsular (anterior or posterior).

As a reference group transparent lenses obtained from eyes enucleated for malignant melanoma of the choroid were examined.

The measurements were carried out immediately after the intracapsular extraction of the lens by means of cryoprobe. The ultrasound velocity for each lens was calculated using the biometric scale calibrated in microseconds according to Ossoinig. Soon after each measurement on the lens the biometric measurement was repeated using distilled water. In this way it was possible to calculate the ultrasound velocity in the lens knowing the ultrasound velocity in the distilled water at 35°C and for this reason the width of the container.

RESULTS

Our results showed a particular reduction in the ultrasound velocity for cataract opacities that is greatest for the intumescent cataract. On the contrary an increase of the ultrasound velocity was observed in the cataract with nuclear sclerosis.

The greatest difference in the average ultrasound velocity in comparison with that in the transparent lenses was of 45 m/sec., corresponding to a variation of 0.25 Dioptre.

The different ultrasound velocity in various types of cataract may be

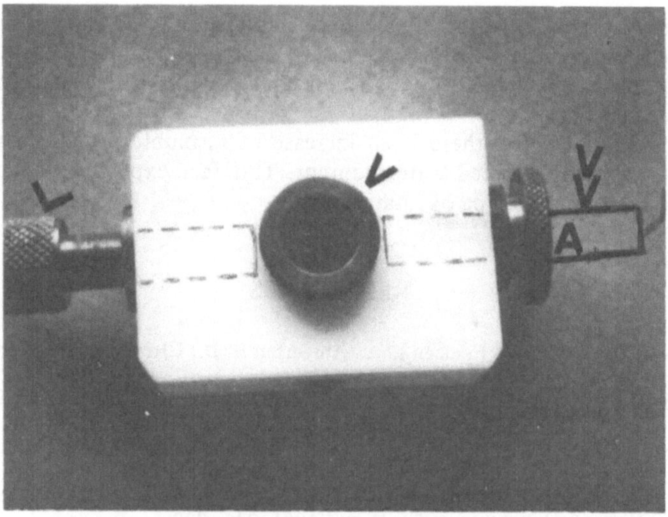

Fig. 1. Little container (L) width less than 8 mm. The width of this container can be modified by means of a screw (V) in relation to the volume of the lens. (A) Side in which is put the A-scan probe. (V̌) A scan probe.

A B C D

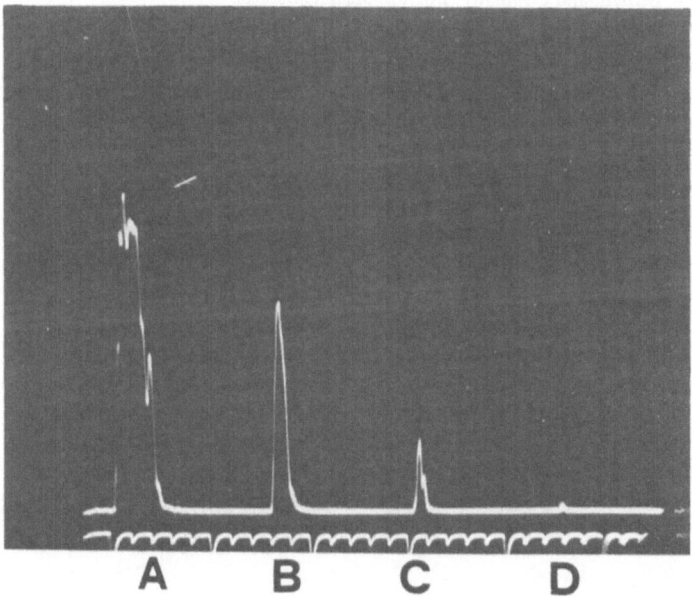

Fig. 2. Echogram from lens. In this case the lens surfaces were in direct contact with the transducer on one side (A) and with the reflecting wall of the end of the screw (B) on the other side. (C–D) Multiple signals. Thickness of the lens was taken from -B- and -C- for more precision.

explained by the different biochemical composition and water content of opacified lenses. In fact it is well known that in cortical and intumescent cataract there is a reduction in the protein content in the later stages on intumescence.

In nuclear opacities there is an increase of insoluble proteins associated with a normal or reduced water content. This fact explains a higher ultrasound velocity in this type of cataract.

REFERENCES

Coleman J. D., Lizzi L. F., Franzen L. A., Abramson H. D.: Ultrasonography in Ophthalmology. Bibl. Ophthalmol. 1975. 83:246.

Coleman J. D., Lizzi F. L., Jack R. L.: Ultrasound velocity of tissues. In Ultrasonography of the eye and orbit. Lea and Febiger. Philadelphia 1977. p 124.

Graymore Clive N.: Biochemistry of the Eye. Academic Press London New York. 1970.

Hillman Jeffrey S., de Dombal F. T.: Sources of error in the calculation of intraocular lens power. Docum. Ophthal. Proc. Series, Vol. 29, ed by J. M. Thijssen and A. M. Verbeek, Dr. Junk Publishers, The Hague. 1981. 225–232.

Okamoto H.: An idea for measurement of the axial length of the eye with Laser as visual target. Docum. Ophthal. Proc. Series, Vol. 29, ed. by J. M. Thijssen and A. M. Verbeek, Dr. W. Junk Publishers, The Hague. 1981. 205–210.

Ossoinig K. C.: Standardized Echography: Basic Principles, Clinical Applications, and Results. Reprinted from International Ophthalmology Clinics. Ophthalmic Ultrasonography: Comparative Techniques. Winter. 1979, Vol. 19, No. 4. Published by Little, Brown, and Company, Boston, Massachussetts.

Pallikaris I., Gruber H.: Determination of sound velocity in different forms of cataracts. Docum. Ophthal. Proc. Series, Vol. 29, ed. by J. M. Thijssen and A. M. Verbeek Dr. W. Junk Publishers, The Hague. 1981. 165–169.

Thijssen J. M.: The emmetropic and the iseikonic implant lens: Computer calculation of the refractive power and its accuracy. Ophthalmologica 1975. 171:467.

Author's address:
Istituto di Clinica Oculistica
II Facolta' di Medicina e Chirurgia
Universita' degli Studi
80131 Naples
Italy

ULTRASONIC BIOMETRY IN CONGENITAL GLAUCOMA. A CLINICAL STUDY

MASSIN, M. AND PELLAT, B.
(Paris, France)

INTRODUCTION

It is a platitude to say that many mistakes can be made during the measurement of the pressure of eyes with congenital glaucoma. The indentation tonometer is generally wrong because its foot is not adapted to the very disturbed corneal curvature and because the scleral rigidity is not known. The aplanation system which can be used when the patient is in the supine position is flimsy and very often does not work. The values are not always the same when the tonometer is placed on different parts of the enlarged cornea. Most of the anaesthetic drugs lower the intra-ocular pressure significantly (11 to 48% after BRINI) and one has to add 4 or 5 mm. Hg to the value found for correction.

Ultrasonic biometry is a much more reliable method for the diagnosis of congenital glaucoma when it is made in accordance with a few simple rules.

MATERIAL AND METHODS

We observed 60 children with congenital glaucoma from birth to the age of 6 years over a period of 3 years. All the examinations were performed under general anaesthesia in the operating theatre. At the same time the corneal diameter and the ocular pressure were measured and the fundus was examined. Very often an operation, goniotomy or trabeculectomy, followed immediately. For that reason we made all our measurements by placing the ultrasonic probe against the cornea, the non-contact method with interposition of water being impossible. None the less very good accuracy could be obtained under some conditions:

– the anterior slope of the echoes must be rectilinear.

– the probe must be placed without methylcellulose or any other liquid.

– no pressure must be exerted upon the cornea: special training is necessary for the operator.

– at least 3 photographs must be taken for each measurement, read with a magnifier and the average of the 3 calculated.

Our apparatus was a portable one which we described 10 years ago and was made by Roche Bioelectronic.

Hillman, J.S./Le May, M.M. (eds.) Ophthalmic Ultrasonography

ISBN 978-94-009-7280-3.

We tested the accuracy of our measurements by repeating them 35 times on the same eye and taking photographs each time. After calculation of the error we found that the accuracy with our 7 MHz probe was between 0.15 and 0.20 mm.

RESULTS

We found that ultrasound biometry of eyes with congenital glaucoma was very useful from several points of view: diagnosis, supervision of the evolution of the disease and of the efficiency of treatment and prognosis.

Diagnosis. It appeared rather easy to recognise congenital glaucoma by comparing the total axial length of the eye with that of a normal eye. Our reference was the curve established by Poujol in 1976 which gives the normal value and deviation for each age. Most of the glaucomas were at its superior part or above it, particularly during the first year of life. The only possible confusion is with congenital myopia but there is no megalocornea and the anterior segment is normal.

The second biometric sign of congenital glaucoma is the lengthening of the anterior segment (thickness of the cornea + depth of the anterior chamber). In our patients aged from 5 weeks to 1 year and not yet operated upon, the average lengths were:

– anterior segment:	4.21 mm
– lens:	3.56 mm
– vitreous:	13.77 mm
– total length:	21.67 mm

These should be compared with values for the normal neonate from the results of several authors:

– anterior segment:	2.57 mm (variation from 2.3 to 3)
– lens:	3.60 mm
– vitreous:	10.80 mm
– total length:	17.40 mm (variation from 16 to 19)

In this way it becomes possible to distinguish congenital glaucoma from two other diseases with an appearance of buphthalmia: the anterior megalophthalmia and the megalocornea.

In megalophthalmia the anterior segment is enlarged (4, 3 and 5 mm in two of our patients) but the lens is normal and so is the vitreous.

In megalocornea the corneal diameter is increased but the ultrasonic measurements remain normal.

It is of course important to check the measurements again after some months to be quite sure, but we can say that the 2 main echographic symptoms of congenital glaucoma are *the lengthening of the anterior segment* and *the increasing of the total length.*

Ultrasound in the evolution of glaucoma. Efficiency of the treatment. Figure 1 presents diagrammatically the mean lengths of all our glaucoma eyes between birth and the age of 10 years. We found that the growth of the eye, quick at the beginning of life, returned gradually to the normal curve

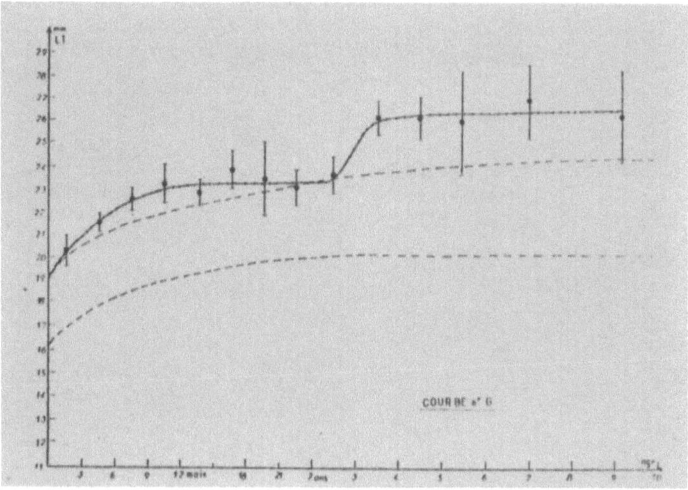

Fig. 1. Growth curve of buphthalmic eyes from birth to the age of 10 (Total length).

and reached it at the age of 2. It should be mentioned that all our patients had been operated on before the age of 1 year. There was a sudden growth of the eye at 3 years and it is only at 4 years that it stabilises. We cannot explain this phenomenon completely but it seems to be due to a recurrence of the ocular hypertonia in some of our cases.

By considering separately the growth of the posterior segment of the eye, that is to say the vitreous, we found it was strictly parallel to that of the total length (Fig. 2). So the anterior part of the glaucomatous eye (anterior segment + lens) remains unchanged during the 5 or 6 first years of life and *the vitreous grows alone.*

Our findings are confirmed by comparison with some already published surveys. Sampaolesi (1981) has reported that for 22 patients between 2 months and 2 years of age the anterior segment was 4.21 mm and the lens 3.50 mm, that is to say he found exactly the same values as we did for children under 1 year. However, he found a longer vitreous: 14.70 mm instead of 13.77 mm and a greater total length. His patients were a little older.

Gernet and Hollwich (1967) have reported 81 cases with a mean age of 3.5 years and found an anterior segment of 3.94 mm, a lens of 3.86 mm (total of both = 7.80 mm) and a posterior segment of 16.54 mm. In 83 eyes between 5 weeks and 6 years, we found an anterior segment of 4.37 mm, a lens of 3.57 mm (total of both = 7.94 mm) and a posterior segment of 14.4 mm. Again the anterior part is the same and the vitreous along is longer. Gernet and Hollwich's patients were a little older too and perhaps they have been less fortunate . . . but we can conclude that *the increase of length of the glaucomatous eye is due to its posterior part alone.*

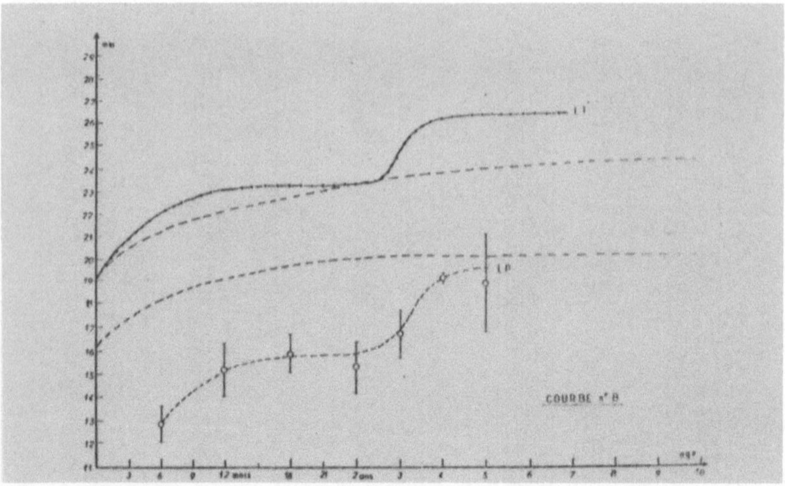

Fig. 2. **Growth curve of the posterior segment (LP) of buphthalmic eyes plotted against the total length growth curve.**

Sampaolesi (1981) found a *thickness of lens* lower than normal, as we did (3.50 mm). This is a new notion since the lens of Gernet and Hollwich was normal (3.86 mm). It is possible, as Sampaolesi says that this thinning of the lens is an emmetropizing factor.

In summary we have made a diagram of the growth of each part of the glaucomatous eye in terms of the total length (Fig. 3). We have also compared the growth of operated eyes with that of unoperated ones during the first year of life and the difference is significant (Fig. 4).

Prognosis. We have collected all our glaucomas operated upon during their first year of life and we have plotted them on Poujol's normal growth curve. After integration of the curves we could separate 4 zones (Figs. 5 and 6). In the lower zone, No. 1, white, all the eyes are normal. In the second one, hatched, the eyes may be normal or glaucomatous. The diagnosis is made by measuring the anterior segment which is definitely increased in case of glaucome. If there is still doubt a new measurement will be made some time later and the other signs of glaucome searched for. The third zone, the dotted one, contains only glaucomas, but when their total length is under 23 mm, the results of the surgery is generally good and the growth curve returns to the normal. On the contrary, in the upper zone, no. 4, the prognosis is bad. The total length remains above the normal curve, parallel to it but never returns to the normal. Several operations are usually necessary.

CONCLUSIONS

Ultrasonic biometry is a much more reliable method than the measurement of the ocular pressure to examine an eye with congenital glaucoma. It allows the

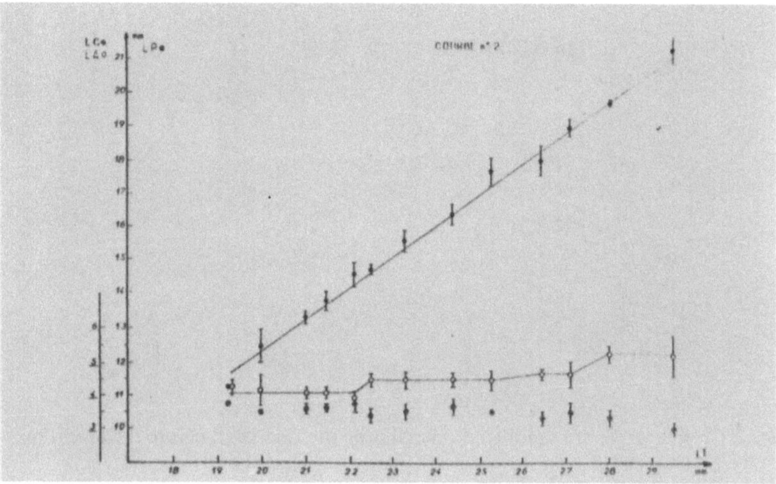

Fig. 3. Growth curve of the posterior segment •, of the anterior segment ○, and of the lens ⊙, plotted against the total length (LT).

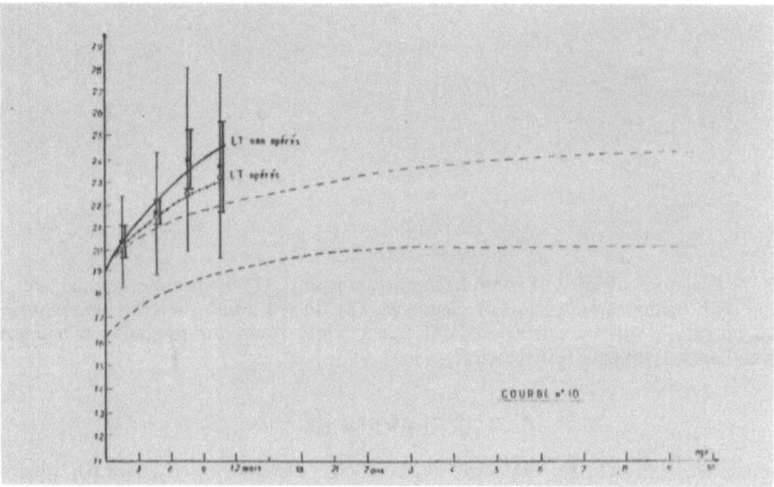

Fig. 4. Growth curve (total length) of operated and unoperated eyes.

diagnosis, showing the two main signs: *increasing of the total length, increasing of the anterior segment.* It demonstrates that the growth of the glaucomatous eye is made by the posterior segment only. It shows whether the operation has been successful and warns when a recurrence occurs. Finally we have drawn a graph which may help the prognosis.

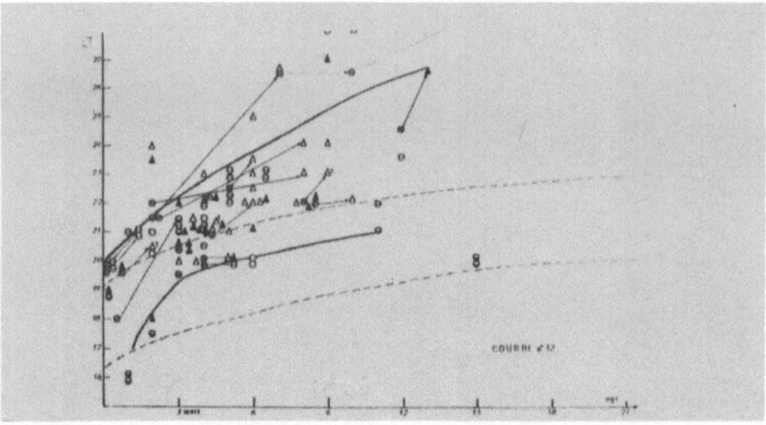

Fig. 5. Growth curve of buphthalmic eyes during the first year, before the operation.

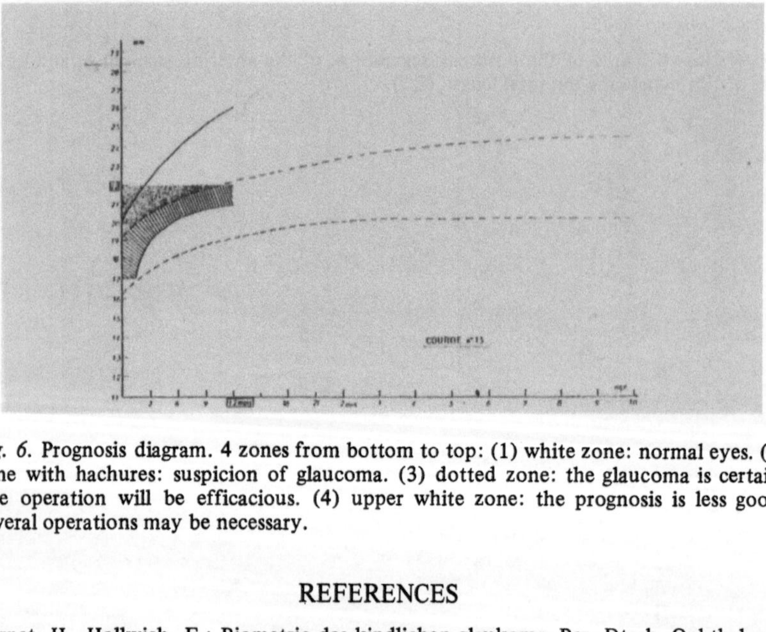

Fig. 6. Prognosis diagram. 4 zones from bottom to top: (1) white zone: normal eyes. (2) zone with hachures: suspicion of glaucoma. (3) dotted zone: the glaucoma is certain. The operation will be efficacious. (4) upper white zone: the prognosis is less good. Several operations may be necessary.

REFERENCES

Gernet, H., Hollwich, F.: Biometric des kindlichen glaukoms. Ber. Dtsch. Ophthal. ges Heidelberg, 1967, 68, 31–36.

Poujol, J.: Clinical biometry in child pathology. In: Proc. 1st meeting of WFUMB. White and Coll. Plenum press, New York 1977.

Sampaolesi, R.: Ocular echometry in the diagnosis of congenital glaucoma. In 'Ultrasonography in ophthalmology'. Documenta ophthalmologica. Proceedings of Series 29. Eds. J. M. Thijssen and A. M. Verbeek Junk, The Hague, 1981, pp. 177–189.

Author's address:
Hôpital National des Quinze-Vingts
28 Rue de Charenton
75571 Paris Cedex 12
France

ULTRASONIC BIOMETRY IN CONGENITAL GLAUCOMA

K. BLUTH
(Berlin, GDR)

INTRODUCTION

Congenital glaucoma still produces severe visual loss despite intensive surgical, medical, optical and amblyopia therapy. The axial length measurement by ultrasound is recognized as a valuable help for diagnosis and follow-up of congenital glaucoma.

Whereas some valuable cross-sectional studies on axial length have been carried out (Luyckx and Delmarcelle 1968, Gernet 1969, Hollwich and Gernet 1971, Ustimenko 1972, Sampaolesi 1981), very little information is available on longitudinal data of axial length in congenital glaucoma (Buschmann and Bluth 1974, Machekhin and Krivopaluva 1979). Information about normal growth of the human eye (Sorsby et al., 1961, Larsen 1971) is the basis for comparison with the growth rate of eyes with congenital glaucoma.

The aim of this presentation is to give some longitudinal data about changes of axial length and its components in congenital glaucoma.

MATERIAL AND METHODS

The longitudinal 10-year-study was made on 62 children with congenital glaucoma: 53 with bilateral and 9 with unilateral glaucoma (115 eyes). Their ages ranged from 0.2 to 14 years with a mean age of 3.89 ± 2.85 years. 107 eyes had primary glaucoma, 8 eyes had secondary glaucoma because of Lowe-syndrome, Rieger-syndrome, chromosomal anomalies (21, 12) v. Waardenburg-syndrome, aniridia. Inheritance could be proved in 3 cases. The incidence of prematures was 9.6%. The axial length measurements were performed on an average four times a year up to the age of 6 years and then once a year. The time of follow-up was between half a year and ten years. 67 children with normal eyes and normal refraction formed the second group (Table 1). 5 eyes were excluded because of anetropia (129 eyes; Table 2).

The children were investigated under general anesthesia, these examinations included intraocular pressure and corneal diameter measurements, ophthalmoscopy and echometry.

Hillman, J.S./Le May, M.M. (eds.) Ophthalmic Ultrasonography

ISBN 978-94-009-7280-3.

Table 1. Longitudinal study in glaucomatous and normal eyes

	Number of children	Female	Male
Glaucoma	62	24	38
Normal	67	32	35

Table 2. Average age in glaucomatous and normal eyes

	Number of eyes	Age (Mean ± SD)
Glaucoma	115	3.89 ± 2.85
Normal	129	3.23 ± 3.13

Ultrasonography is performed with the Kretztechnik unit (Models 7100 and 7200) and a 10 MHz transducer with a waterfilled plexiglass cylinder. Calculations of the eye distances were based on the different sound velocities in aqueous, vitreous (1532 m/sec) and lens (1641 m/sec), reported by Jansson 1963. No correction for retinal thickness was made.

RESULTS AND DISCUSSION

Correlation between axial length and age.

Linear growth curve of normal and glaucomatous eyes in relation to age was plotted according to the least square method.

(1) Figure 1 gives the linear growth curve for the normal eyes (n = 129) and the glaucomatous eyes (n = 115). Compared to the normal growth of the emmetropic eyes, the axial length of glaucomatous eyes is grossly enlarged ($y = 21.13 \pm 0.49\,x$, $r = 0.4$). The glaucomatous eyes can be divided into two groups with different growth rates: Group A (86 eyes) with a moderate growth rate and not so enlarged axial length and group B (29 eyes) with a more increased growth rate. The average increase of axial length was higher than 1.0–1.5 mm per year. Figure 2 shows the growth rate of normal eyes and group A of glaucoma. Table 3 shows growth rates of normal eyes. It demonstrates a rapid growth from birth to 18 month, moderate growth between 2 and 5 years and slow juvenile growth between 5 and 15 years.

(2) The vitreous length of glaucomatous eyes correlates in the increased length and increased growth rate with the axial length (Fig. 3).

(3) The anterior chamber depth increases in glaucomatous eyes more than in normal eyes (Fig. 4). In normal eyes the main increase is 0.05 mm per year between 2 and 6 years and between 6 and 13 years 0.02 mm per year.

(4) Lens thickness in normal and glaucomatous eyes is within normal limits. We found a significant reduction of lens thickness in glaucomatous eyes. ($y = 3.84 - 0.02\,x$, $r = 0.9$). Lens thickness in normal eyes was unchanged (Fig. 5). Francois and Goes (1970), also Gernet (1970) found an unchanged lens thickness in normal eyes from birth to 20 years. Delmarcelle (1969) described a decreasing of lens thickness from birth to 10 years, caused

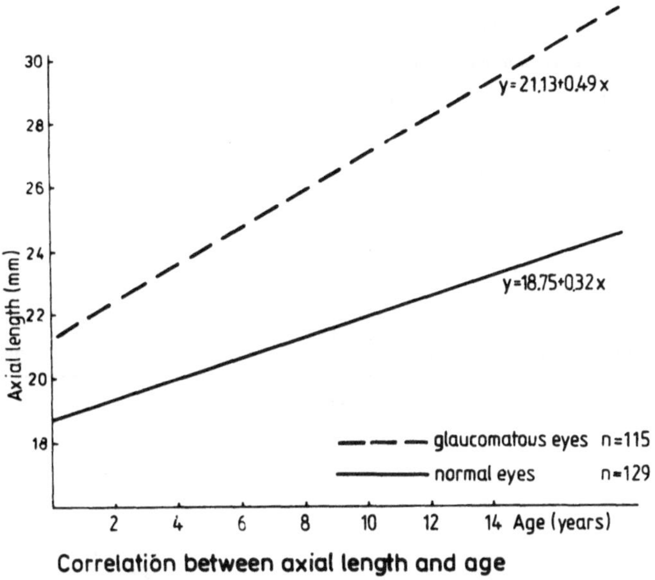

Fig. 1. Different growth curves in normal and glaucomatous eyes.

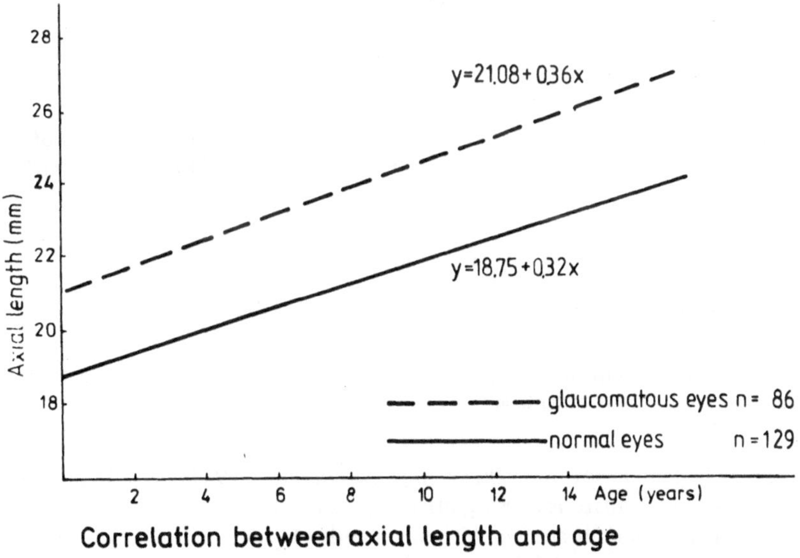

Fig. 2. Growth curve of normal eyes compared to glaucomatous eyes with controlled intraocular pressure.

Table 3. Growth of axial length, normal eyes

Average increase of axial length (mm)		
Derived from literature via mean sizes in different age groups		
Age period	Per month	Per year
Premature babies, 6–8 months old	2.5	
One year old		3.2–3.5
Two years old		0.9–1.0
Three years old		0.5
Four years old		0.3
Five to 15 years old		0.1 (0.2)
Average axial length in mature newborn babies		17.2 mm
Average axial length in emmetropic adults		23.4 mm

For References, see Buschmann and Bluth (1974).

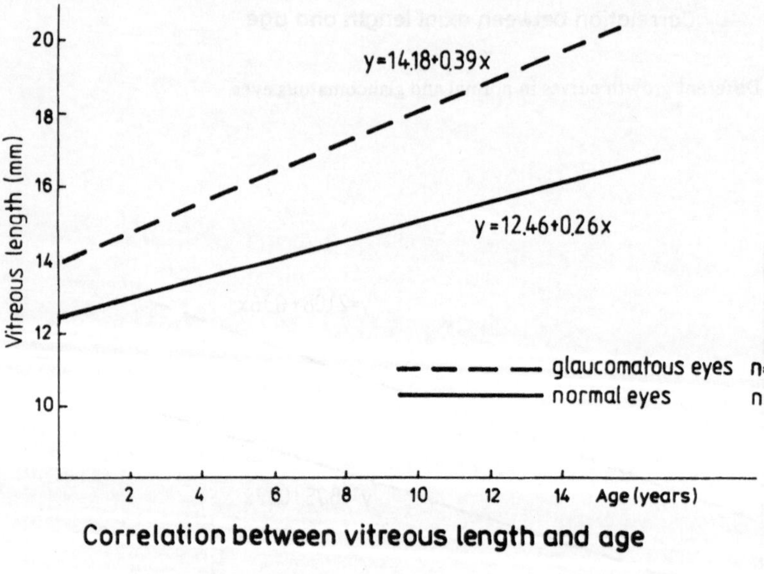

Fig. 3. Changes of vitreous length in normal and glaucomatous eyes with controlled intraocular pressure in relation to age.

by the enlargement of the ciliary ring. Sampaolesi (1981) found the lens thickness of glaucomatous eyes significantly reduced.

(5) The axial length and the vitreous length of glaucomatous eyes show a large distribution ($r = < 0.5$). Nevertheless the arithmetic mean and the standard deviation for axial length and its components were calculated for the estimated number of eyes (Table 4).

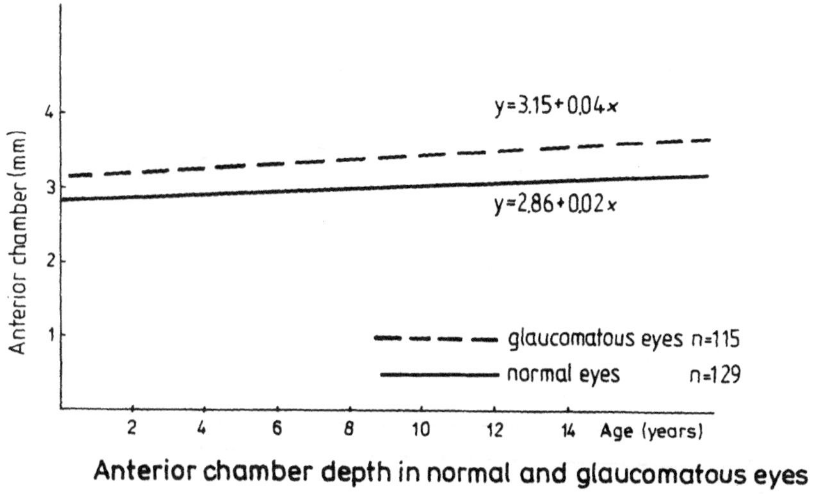

Fig. 4. Changes of anterior chamber depth in normal and glaucomatous eyes in relation to age. Changes in glaucomatous eyes are significant (r = 0.85).

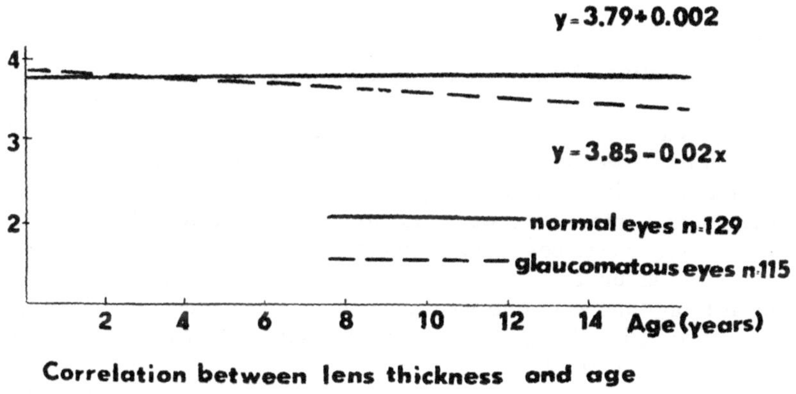

Fig. 5. Lens thickness in normal and glaucomatous eyes in relation to age (changes in glaucomatous eyes are significant).

Table 4. Average of axial length and its components in glaucomatous and normal eyes (Average age in Table 2)

	Normal	Glaucoma
Anterior chamber depth	3.02 ± 0.29	3.68 ± 0.43
Lens thickness	3.69 ± 0.34	3.79 ± 0.44
Vitreous length	13.88 ± 1.87	15.99 ± 3.14
Axial length	20.85 ± 1.98	23.67 ± 3.62

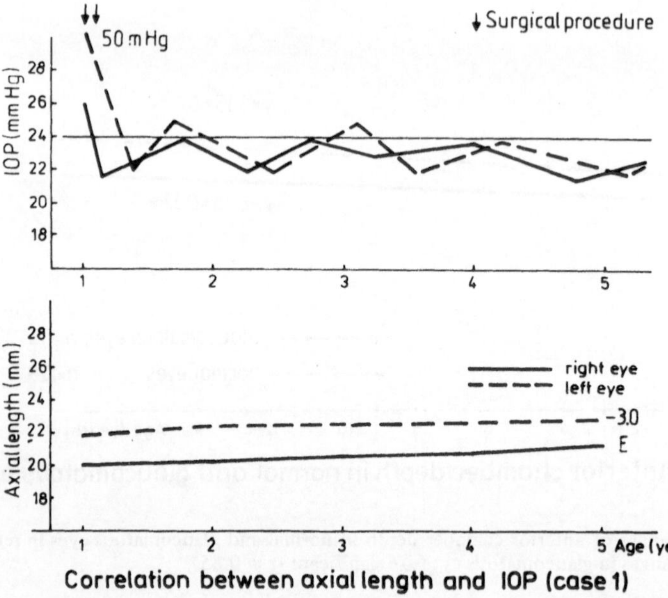

Fig. 6. **Bilateral congenital glaucoma with controlled intraocular pressure, normal growth rates, but different axial length in both eyes.**

Correlation between axial length and intraocular pressure

Ocular hypertension leads to biometric changes that are more important if hypertension has been early and prolonged. Increase over normal axial length growth rate shows insufficient therapy.

After surgical procedures we found in some cases a reduction of axial length, probably due to postoperative hypotension.

(6) In the group of glaucomatous eyes with moderate growth rate the intraocular pressure was controlled after surgical procedure, the abnormal increase of axial length was finished and the average growth rate similar to normal eyes (Fig. 6, case 1).

(7) In the group of glaucomatous eyes with increased growth pattern we found intraocular pressure peaks up to 40 mm Hg and more (Fig. 7, case 2). These eyes continued to have uncontrolled hypertension after surgery despite additional medication and show in this example axial length up to 36 mm and more.

(8) But also a high level of intraocular hypertension (24 mm Hg and more) leads to increased growth of the eye (Fig. 8, case 3).

Correlation between axial length and visual acuity

(9) The consequence of the large dimension of the eyes is myopia, which is partly compensated by an increase of the corneal curvature and the reduced

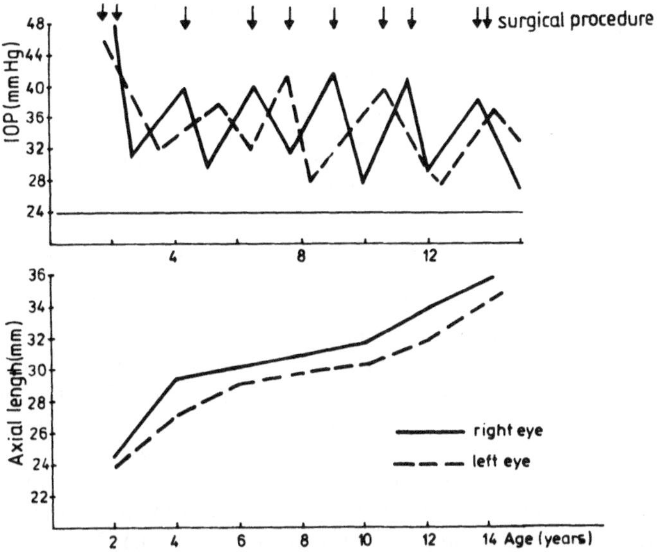

Corretation between axial length and IOP (case 2)

Fig. 7. Bilateral congenital glaucoma with high growth rates caused by uncontrolled intraocular pressure despite agressive therapy.

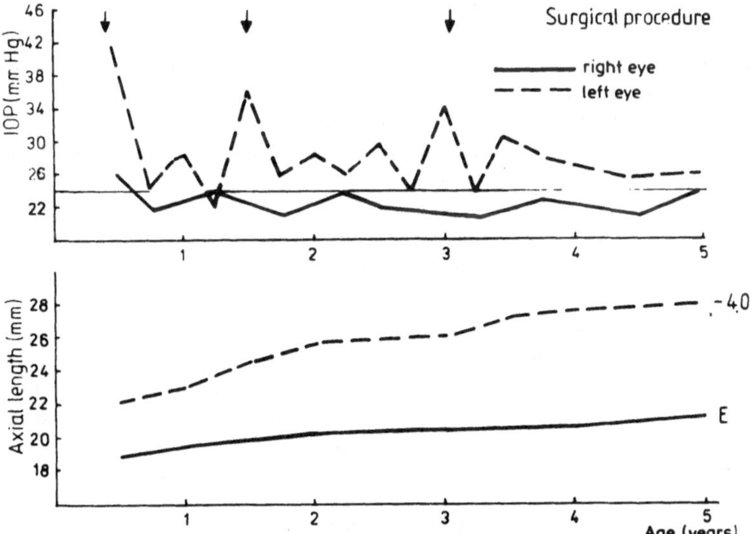

Correlation between axial length and IOP (case 3)

Fig. 8. Intraocular hypertension above 24 mm Hg lead to higher growth rate, myopia and amblyopia in this case.

Table 5. Correlation between axial length and visual acuity in glaucomatous eyes. Number of eyes 115 = 100%

	Axial length	Number of eyes	
Myopia	increased	24	21.5%
Amblyopia	increased	10	8.6%
Optic nerve damage	more increased > 27 mm	20	17.3%

dioptric power of the lens. We found myopia in 21.5% (24 eyes), of glaucomatous eyes.

(10) Amblyopia is found in 8.6% (10 eyes), so far as could be examined. The average age at diagnosis of congenital glaucoma was 4.2 months. The importance of an early input should be stressed because of amblyopia. Von Noorden (1970) demonstrated the necessity of early visual stimulation for development of normal vision in monkeys.

(11) Visual prognosis was not only determined by amblyopia, but also by optic nerve damage in more enlarged eyes. We found serious optic nerve damage in 20 eyes (17.3%) with axial length above 27 mm. This observation has confirmed our findings in 1974 (Buschmann and Bluth) (Table 5).

CONCLUSIONS AND SUMMARY

Eye growth of children with congenital glaucoma is analysed using longitudinal data of ultrasonic biometry. The longitudinal 10-year study was made on 62 children with congenital glaucoma and compared with 67 children with normal eyes.

We recognised two glaucoma groups depending upon the growth rate, one with moderate growth rate and controlled intraocular pressure and the other with an increased growth rate, uncontrolled intraocular hypertension and corresponding visual acuity despite aggressive therapy.

Eye growth curves show the exact correlation between the axial length and the duration of ocular hypertension.

Ultrasonic biometry facilitates the differentiation from congenital glaucoma, anterior chamber megophthalmia, megalocornea and axial myopia. Corneal diameter and axial length are quite well correlated in congenital glaucoma.

In the follow-up of congenital glaucoma axial length measurement is a fundamental factor in judging the necessity and efficiency of therapy. The measurement of ocular pressure gives only a short-term information on the situation, whereas axial length measurement reflects the average pressure in the control pėriod.

REFERENCES

Buschmann, W. und Bluth, K.: Regelmacige echographische Messungen der Achsenlange zur Kontrolle der Druckregulierung bei Hydrophthalmie. Klin. Mbl. Augenheilk., 165, 878–886, (1974).

Delmarcelle, Y., Luyxhx, J. and Weekers, R.: Etude biométrique antérieur de l'oeil dans le glaucoma àngle fermé. Bull. Soc. Belge Ophtal. 153, 638 (1969).
Gernet, H.: Résultats oculometriques àpropos du glaucoma infantile. Bull. et Mém. Soc. franc. Ophtal. (92), 41 (1969).
Gernet, H. and Hollwich, F.: Oculometrie des kindlichen Glaukoms. Ber. dtsch. Opthalm. Ges. (69), 341 (1969).
Gernet, H.: Valeur de base on oculométrie clinique. Bull. et Mém. Soc. franc. Ophtal. 83, 379 (1970).
Jansson, F.: Measurement of introcular distances by ultrasound. Acta. Ophthal. Kbh., Suppl. (74), 1 (1963).
Larsen, J.S.: The saggital growth of the eye. Acta Ophthal., Kbh. 49, 427, 441, 873 (1971).
Luyckx, J. and Delmarcelle, Y.: Recherches biometriques sur des youx présentant une mincrocornés ou une megalocornée. Bull. Soc. belge Ophtal., 149, 433 (1968).
Machekhin, V. A. and Krivopaluva: The possibilities of ultrasonic biometry in assessing the extent of stabilisation of glaucoma. Vestn. Oftal., 96, 17, (1979).
Von Noorden, G. K., Dowling, J. E. and Ferguson, D. C.: Experimental amblyopia in monkeys. I. Behavioural studies of stimulus deprivation amblyopia. Arch. Ophthalmol. 84, 206 (1970).
Sampaolesi, R.: Ocular echometry in the diagnosis of congenital glaucoma. Docum. Ophthal. Proc. Series, Vol. 29, 177 (1981).
Sorsby, A., Benjamin, B. and Sheridan, M.: Refraction and its components during growth of the eye from age of three. Medical Research Council SRS 301, London, H.M.S.O. (1961).
Ustimenko, L. L.: Zehnjährige Erfahrungen im Studium des diagnostischen Wertes der Ultraschallbiometrie in der Ophthalmologie. Oftal. J. (Moskau) 27, 488 (1972).

Author's address:
Department of Ophthalmology
Humboldt University
1040 Berlin
German Democratic Republic

ULTRASONIC BIOMETRY OF THE SAGITTAL GROWTH OF EYES IN CHILDREN

SADANAO TANE AND JUNKO KOHNO
(Kawasaki, Japan)

It is necessary to ascertain the growth curves of the refractive components of the eyes of children in elucidating the etiology of refractive anomalies and in studying myopia of prematurity, buphthalmos or eyes with abnormal axial length accompanied by macrocornea or microcornea.

In present study, we measured changes of refractive components of the eyes of many infants and children in proportion to their growth at one-year intervals by ultrasonic biometry and studied the growth curves of the axial length related to the findings of the eyes as well as general findings. In addition, we compared the results with the values previously reported and obtained the interesting findings.

As subjects, we selected infants and boys and girls up to the age of 20 because our purpose was to study the growth curves of the axial length. The refractive anomalies of their eyes were within ± 2 diopters. We excluded eyes with severe refractive anomalies and we selected healthy subjects with no abnormalities in the anterior segment of the eye, optic media or fundus. None of the subjects had a history of prematurity. We studied 465 eyes in 239 boys and 499 eyes in 259 girls, a total of 964 eyes.

In this study, we employed the high-power ophthalmic ultrasonic equipment developed at St. Marianna University School of Medicine and a digital electronic counter for measuring the axial length. We incorporated a microcomputer built into the digital counter, using the sound velocity in aqueous fluid, the lens and the vitreous body, 1532 m/sec, 1641 m/sec and 1532 m/sec, respectively, for the measurement and calculation, which was reported by Jansson in 1963. In other words, the anterior chamber depth, anteroposterior diameter of the lens, axial length of the vitreous body and total axial length of the eye were digitally displayed and recorded by simultaneous print-out. We requested the subjects to watch closely an optical target at a distance of 3 m and tried to exclude the influence of accommodation as much as possible. Errors were maintained within 0.1 mm to ensure the precision of this measurement. In addition, we employed a 3 and or 5 mm ϕ focused-type PZT transducer with 10 MHz and/or 15 MHz. The subjects were fitted with a cylindrical eye speculum after topical anesthesia with benoxyl and filling this speculum with physiological saline solution and we measured by the water-bath method. Measurement was undertaken in the non-mydriatic state.

Figure 1 and 2 shows the average and standard deviations of the

Hillman, J.S./Le May, M.M. (eds.) Ophthalmic Ultrasonography
© 1983, Dr W. Junk Publishers, The Hague/Boston/Lancaster
ISBN 978-94-009-7280-3.

Ages

男子眼軸長の平均値と標準偏差

Total ocular axial length

年令 / 眼軸長 (mm)	MONTHS 0-1	1-3	3-6	6-12	YEARS 1	2	3	4	5	6	7	8	9	10	11	12	13	14	15	16	17	18	19	20
16.50 - 16.99																								
17.00 - 17.49	3																							
17.50 - 17.99	5	2																						
18.00 - 18.49	6	2																						
18.50 - 18.99	4	7																						
19.00 - 19.49		9	2																					
19.50 - 19.99		3	2																					
20.00 - 20.49		1	1																					
20.50 - 20.99		1	9	6		1																		
21.00 - 21.49			1	6	4	8		2																
21.50 - 21.99				2	8	6	3	5	1		1		1											
22.00 - 22.49				2	6	3		3	2		5		2											
22.50 - 22.99						6	5	4	5	7	8	7	9	1										
23.00 - 23.49							1	1	2	7	30	9	19	12		3				4				1
23.50 - 23.99											26	4	23	3	4	2			3		2			
24.00 - 24.49										1	6		28	11	5	4		1	3					1
24.50 - 24.99										1	2		5	9	6	13		9						
25.00 - 25.49														1	1	4	3	3						
25.50 - 25.99															2	1								
26.00 - 26.49														1			1							
n	18	25	15	16	18	24	9	15	10	16	78	20	87	38	18	27	4	13	6	4	2			2
M	18.01	19.02	20.15	21.20	21.76	21.82	22.46	22.03	22.65	23.16	23.35	23.10	23.65	24.00	24.43	24.51	25.53	24.74	24.52	23.25	23.75			23.80
SD	0.49	0.70	0.82	0.52	0.35	0.61	0.55	0.64	0.45	0.50	0.53	0.40	0.60	0.74	0.56	0.66		0.24						
SE	0.116	0.141	0.206	0.129	0.083	0.125	0.184	0.164	0.143	0.125	0.060	0.090	0.065	0.121	0.131	0.130		0.066						
MAX	18.9	20.5	21.1	22.2	22.3	22.8	23.0	23.0	23.2	24.5	24.5	23.8	24.6	26.0	25.5	25.5		25.2						
MIN	17.3	17.8	19.2	20.5	21.1	20.9	21.7	21.0	21.8	22.5	21.8	22.5	21.9	22.8	23.6	23.1		24.4						
RANGE	1.6	2.7	1.9	1.7	1.2	1.9	1.3	2.0	1.4	2.0	2.7	1.3	2.7	3.2	1.9	2.4		0.6						

Fig. 1. The averages and standard deviations of the total ocular axial length of the normal male eyes on the aging.

Ages

女子眼軸長の平均値と標準偏差

年令 / 眼軸長 (mm)	0-1 (MONTHS)	1-3	3-6	6-12	1 (YEARS)	2	3	4	5	6	7	8	9	10	11	12	13	14	15	16	17	18	19	20
16.50 - 16.99	5																							
17.00 - 17.49	10																							
17.50 - 17.99	3	1																						
18.00 - 18.49	1		4																					
18.50 - 18.99	2		2																					
19.00 - 19.49			1	3	1																			
19.50 - 19.99			5					2																
20.00 - 20.49				1	3																			
20.50 - 20.99					7	3	1	2					3											
21.00 - 21.49					4	9	9	1	7	2			1											
21.50 - 21.99					3	6	2	4	3		3				4	1								
22.00 - 22.49					5	2	5	6	2	6	14		4	1	1	3			4					
22.50 - 22.99					2		7	4	2	7	41	8	15	19	2	3	2							
23.00 - 23.49							5		1	2	16	11	18	5	15	3	3							
23.50 - 23.99											7	14	13	15	11	8			4					
24.00 - 24.49											1		13	15	4	5		6	2					
24.50 - 24.99											1			3		5								
25.00 - 25.49													1		5									
25.50 - 25.99														1	1									1
26.00 - 26.49																								
n	21	1	12	4	25	20	29	19	15	17	83	33	68	59	43	28	5	6	10					1
M	17.32	17.55	18.98	19.38	21.25	21.25	22.13	21.73	21.77	22.39	22.81	23.25	23.17	23.55	23.49	23.62	22.88	24.07	23.20					25.75
SD	0.56		0.63		0.88	0.35	0.80	0.93	0.69	0.53	0.53	0.31	0.84	0.69	0.92	0.91			0.97					
SE	0.123		0.182		0.176	0.078	0.148	0.214	0.180	0.130	0.059	0.055	0.102	0.090	0.140	0.171			0.308					
MAX	18.7		19.7		22.9	22.0	23.4	22.8	23.0	23.3	24.8	23.8	25.0	25.0	25.5	24.9			24.2					
MIN	16.6		18.2		19.2	20.8	21.0	19.7	21.1	21.2	21.7	22.6	20.8	22.4	21.6				23.0					
RANGE	2.1		1.5		3.7	1.2	2.4	3.1	1.9	2.1	3.1	1.2	4.2	2.6	3.9	3.0			2.2					

ocular axial length

Total

Fig. 2. The average and standard deviations of the total ocular axial length of the normal female eyes on the aging.

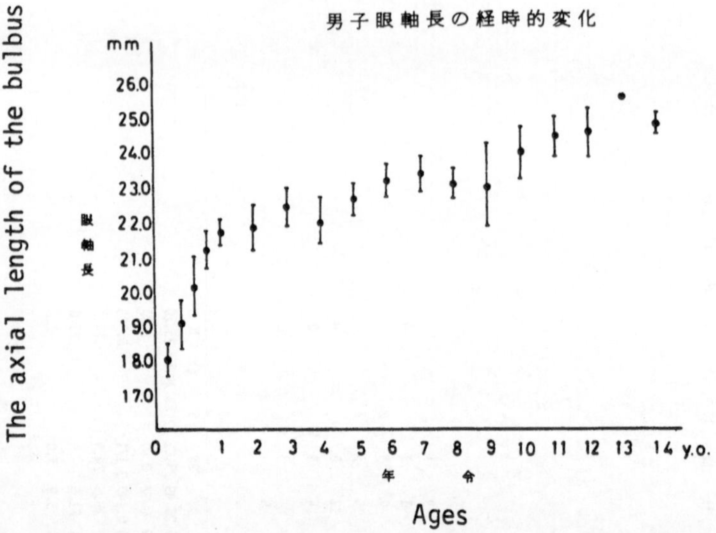

Fig. 3. The growth curve of the total axial length of the bulbus in boys in the aging.

total axial length of the eye in each age group. The Figure 1 shows those of the boys and the Figure 2 those of the girls. Figure 3 and 4 also shows annual changes obtained by the average and standard deviations. As shown here, we can consider three developmental periods up to one year in which rapid growth is observed, the period from one to seven in which mild growth is observed and the period from seven to 15 in which even milder growth is

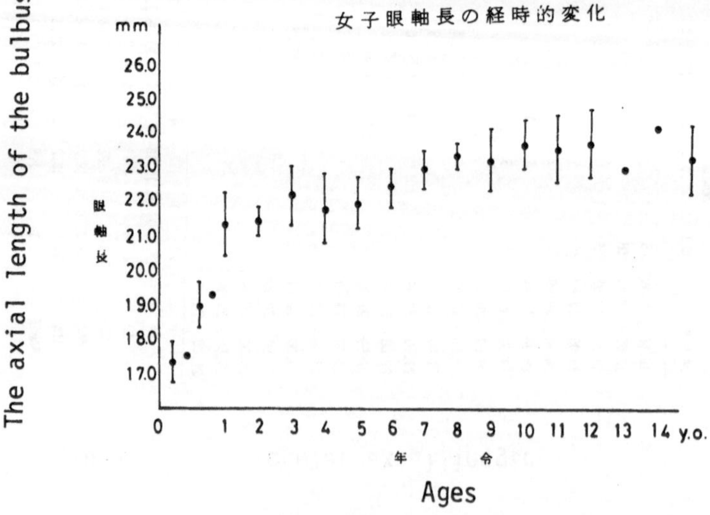

Fig. 4. The growth curve of the total axial length of the bulbus in girls in the aging.

Ages

男子前房深度の平均値と標準偏差

Anterior chamber depth

年令 / 前房深度 (mm)	MONTHS 0-1	1-3	3-6	6-12	YEARS 1	2	3	4	5	6	7	8	9	10	11	12	13	14	15	16	17	18	19	20
2.20 - 2.29		2																						
2.30 - 2.39		5	1																					
2.40 - 2.49		5																						
2.50 - 2.59		2		1																				
2.60 - 2.69	1	2		2																				
2.70 - 2.79	4	4	2																					
2.80 - 2.89	3	1	2						1															
2.90 - 2.99	2	1				1			1												2			
3.00 - 3.09	5			2					1															
3.10 - 3.19	1	2	9	6	1	1		1	2		4		2											
3.20 - 3.29	1	1	1	2		2		3	1		2	1	5											
3.30 - 3.39				2	1	4		3		1	2	7	3											1
3.40 - 3.49				1	5	5		3	1	1	7	3	10	1	5									
3.50 - 3.59					4	5	7		3	2	6	3	20	5	1	2								
3.60 - 3.69						5		1		4	15	4	8	4	1	6	3	2						1
3.70 - 3.79					5	1	1	1		2	17	2	12	10	1	5	1	1						
3.80 - 3.89					1		1			1	11		12	11	2	9		2						
3.90 - 3.99					1			1		2	6		7	3	2	3		3		1				
4.00 - 4.09								1		1	3		8	1	4	2		4	1	2				
4.10 - 4.19											2								4	1				
4.20 - 4.29								1			2			2	2			1						
4.30 - 4.39										2	1			1					1					
n	18	25	15	16	18	24	9	15	10	16	78	20	87	38	18	27	4	13	6	4	2			2
M	2.88	2.56	2.93	3.04	3.53	3.41	3.56	3.48	3.20	3.73	3.66	3.44	3.61	3.75	3.76	3.75	3.63	3.88	4.12	4.05	2.95			3.45
SD	0.17	0.29	0.28	0.26	0.20	0.19	0.11	0.33	0.26	0.29	0.26	0.15	0.23	0.20	0.29	0.13		0.17						
SE	0.039	0.057	0.071	0.065	0.047	0.038	0.038	0.085	0.083	0.072	0.029	0.034	0.025	0.032	0.068	0.025		0.046						
MAX	3.2	3.2	3.3	3.4	3.9	3.7	3.8	4.2	3.5	4.3	4.4	3.7	4.0	4.3	4.2	4.0		4.2						
MIN	2.6	2.2	2.3	2.5	3.1	2.9	3.5	3.1	2.8	3.3	3.1	3.2	3.1	3.4	3.4	3.5		3.6						
RANGE	0.6	1.0	1.0	0.9	0.8	0.8	0.3	1.1	0.7	1.0	1.3	0.5	0.9	0.9	0.8	0.5		0.6						

Fig. 5. The averages and standard deviations of the anterior chamber depth of the normal male eyes on the aging.

Ages

女子前房深度の平均値と標準偏差

Anterior chamber depth

年令 / 前房深度 (mm)	MONTHS 0-1	1-3	3-6	6-12	YEARS 1	2	3	4	5	6	7	8	9	10	11	12	13	14	15	16	17	18	19	20
2.20 - 2.29																								
2.30 - 2.39			1																					
2.40 - 2.49		1	2																					
2.50 - 2.59	1																							
2.60 - 2.69	5		4				2	1																
2.70 - 2.79	6		2				2																	
2.80 - 2.89	7		3		2	5	4																	
2.90 - 2.99				3	5	1	1	1	2															
3.00 - 3.09	2			1	2	6		1	4		2	1				1								
3.10 - 3.19					4	1	2	1	3	2	4	1	1	1		2								
3.20 - 3.29					7		6	1	2	1	11	4	3	7		2			1					
3.30 - 3.39					1	1	1		1		9	2	4	9	1	1			1					
3.40 - 3.49					1	2	4	3	1	6	11	9	9	7	4	3			1					
3.50 - 2.59					2	1	2	5	2	4	21	4	18	12	5	4	2		1					
3.60 - 3.69						2	2	1		1	13	6	7	6	8	2	1		1					
3.70 - 3.79					1			2			7	5	12	10	7	6	1		2					
3.80 - 3.89							2	2		1	1	1	4	3	3		1		2					
3.90 - 3.99						1	1	1		1	2		6	2	6	1			1					
4.00 - 4.09											1		3	2	2	1								1
4.10 - 4.19										1			1		3									
4.20 - 4.29											1				3	2		4						
4.30 - 4.39															1	3		2						
n	21	1	12	4	25	20	29	19	15	17	83	33	68	59	43	28	5	6	10					1
M	2.73	2.45	2.61	2.93	3.13	3.14	3.20	3.42	3.15	3.48	3.45	3.45	3.59	3.51	3.65	3.63	3.62	4.23	3.59					4.05
SD	0.13		0 17		0.23	0.33	0.36	0.33	0.20	0.26	0.22	0.19	0.22	0.22	0.26	0.39			0.23					
SE	0.028		0.048		0.046	0.073	0.068	0.077	0.052	0.063	0.024	0.034	0.026	0.028	0.040	0.073			0.074					
MAX	3.0		2.8		3.7	3.9	3.9	3.9	3.5	4.1	4.2	3.8	4.1	4.0	4.3	4.3			3.9					
MIN	2.5		2.3		2.8	2.8	2.6	2.6	2.9	3.1	3.0	3.0	3.1	3.1	3.3	3.0			3.2					
RANGE	0.5		0.5		0.9	1.1	1.3	1.3	0.6	1.0	1.2	0.8	1.0	0.9	1.0	1.4			0.7					

Fig. 6, The averages and standard deviations of the anterior chamber depth of the normal female eyes on the aging.

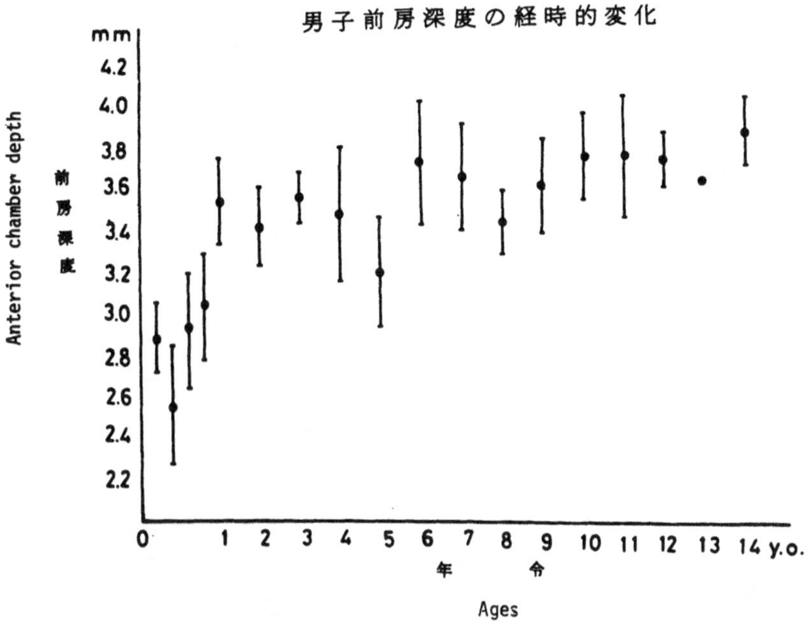

Fig. 7. The growth curve of the anterior chamber depth of the normal male eyes on the aging.

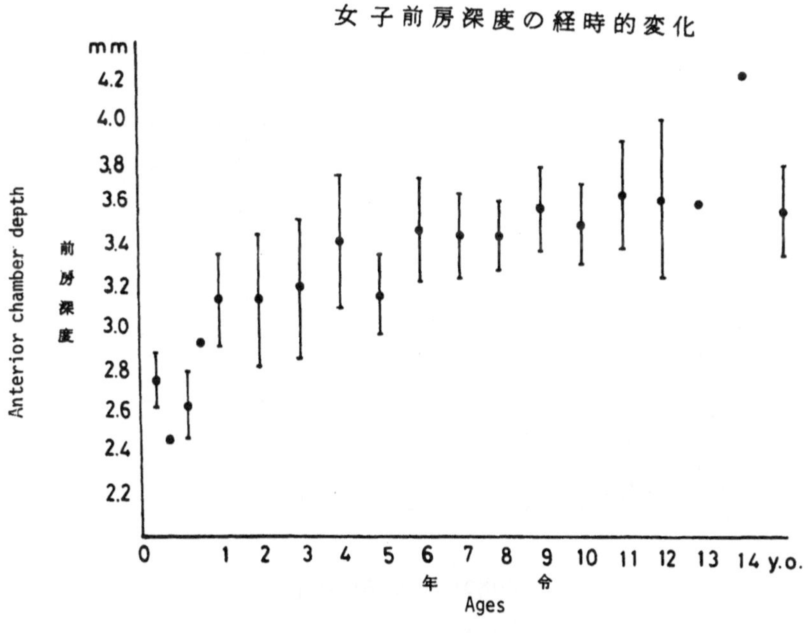

Fig. 8. The growth curve of the anterior chamber depth of the normal female eyes on the aging.

Ages

The lens thickness

男子水晶体厚の平均値と標準偏差

年令 / 水晶体厚 (mm)	MONTHS 0-1	1-3	3-6	6-12	YEARS 1	2	3	4	5	6	7	8	9	10	11	12	13	14	15	16	17	18	19	20
3.10 - 3.19											1		1		1			1						
3.20 - 3.29									1		2	1	2	1	1			1						
3.30 - 3.39	1	1							1		2	1	7	1		4		1	1					
3.40 - 3.49	1					1		1		3	5	1	12	3	1	7		3	2	1				
3.50 - 3.59	1	1		1	1			2	1	1	5		17	5	4	8	2	4	2					
3.60 - 3.69	5	1				1		4		3	4		9	4	2	4	1	1	1	1				
3.70 - 3.79	1				1	3	5	4	3	2	7	3	11	6	1	1	1			1				
3.80 - 3.89	1	2	1	1	3	3			2		7	1	12	7	5	2		1						
3.90 - 3.99	2		2	2	4	4	1	1		3	8	3	5	5	1									
4.00 - 4.09	3		4	2	3	6	3	1	2	1	10	3	3	4	2						2			1
4.10 - 4.19	1	6	3	1	3	4				2	12	1	3	2						1				
4.20 - 4.29		3	3	1		1					4	5	3			1		1						1
4.30 - 4.39	1	7	2	4				1		1	2	1	1											
4.40 - 4.49	1	1		2	1	1					3	1	1											
4.50 - 4.59		1		2	1			1			3													
4.60 - 4.69		2			1																			
n	18	25	15	16	18	24	9	15	10	16	78	20	87	38	18	27	4	13	6	4	2			2
M	3.79	4.14	4.06	4.15	4.00	3.92	3.82	3.75	3.67	3.78	3.84	3.95	3.64	3.71	3.64	3.52	3.58	3.49	3.45	3.70	4.05			4.05
SD	0.30	0.32	0.15	0.28	0.28	0.21	0.15	0.30	0.27	0.31	0.34	0.30	0.27	0.22	0.25	0.20		0.26						
SE	0.071	0.064	0.038	0.070	0.065	0.043	0.049	0.079	0.084	0.078	0.039	0.068	0.029	0.036	0.060	0.038		0.076						
MAX	4.4	4.6	4.3	4.5	4.6	4.4	4.0	4.5	4.0	4.4	4.5	4.4	4.4	4.1	4.0	4.2		4.2						
MIN	3.3	3.3	3.8	3.5	3.5	3.4	3.7	3.4	3.2	3.4	3.1	3.2	3.1	3.2	3.1	3.3		3.1						
RANGE	1.1	1.3	0.5	1.0	1.1	1.0	0.3	1.1	0.8	1.0	1.4	1.2	1.3	0.9	0.9	0.9		1.1						

Fig. 9. The averages and standard deviations of the lens thickness of the normal male eyes on the aging.

Ages

The lens thickness

女子水晶体厚の平均値と標準偏差

年令 / 水晶体厚 (mm)	MONTHS 0-1	1-3	3-6	6-12	YEARS 1	2	3	4	5	6	7	8	9	10	11	12	13	14	15	16	17	18	19	20
3.10 - 3.19														1	1	1								
3.20 - 3.29							2			1	1	1	3	1		1			1					
3.30 - 3.39					1	1		1	1		2		3	1	17	5	1	2						
3.40 - 3.49	3				1			2	2	1	4	1	14	2	9	2		2						1
3.50 - 3.59						1	2	2		2	9	3	10	6	10	1		1	2					
3.60 - 3.69	4				1	1	1	3		2	6	4	14	10	7	4	2		1					
3.70 - 3.79	3					4	3	3		4	17	3	10	10	2	4	2	1	2					
3.80 - 3.89	2		1	2	1	2	2	3	1	1	7	7	4	8	1	3								
3.90 - 3.99	5	1	1		5	2	3	3	1	2	15	5	5	6	1				4					
4.00 - 4.09	4		6	2	7	4	3	1	4	1	10	6	4	4	3	3								
4.10 - 4.19					5	3	5		3	1	2	1	1	6	1	1								
4.20 - 4.29			2			2	4	1	3	1	3	1		1	1	1								
4.30 - 4.39					4		1			1	3	1		3										
4.40 - 4.49			1				2				1					1								
4.50 - 4.59			1								3					1								
4.60 - 4.69							1																	
n	21	1	12	4	25	20	29	19	15	17	83	33	68	59	43	28	5	6	10					1
M	3.75	3.95	4.08	3.90	3.97	3.87	3.96	3.70	3.91	3.48	3.81	3.80	3.59	3.76	3.54	3.68	3.58	3.83	3.68					3.45
SD	0.20		0.20		0.25	0.24	0.36	0.23	0.30	0.26	0.28	0.24	0.21	0.26	0.24	0.36			0.23					
SE	0.045		0.059		0.050	0.054	0.066	0.052	0.079	0.070	0.031	0.041	0.026	0.034	0.037	0.068			0.074					
MAX	4.0		4.5		4.3	4.2	4.8	4.2	4.2	4.1	4.5	4.3	4.1	4.3	4.2	4.5			3.9					
MIN	3.4		3.8		3.3	3.3	3.2	3.3	3.3	3.1	3.2	3.2	3.2	3.1	3.1	3.1			3.2					
RANGE	0.6		0.7		1.0	0.9	1.6	0.9	0.9	1.0	1.3	1.1	0.9	1.2	1.1	1.4			0.7					

Fig. 10. The averages and standard deviations of the lens thickness of the normal female eyes on the aging.

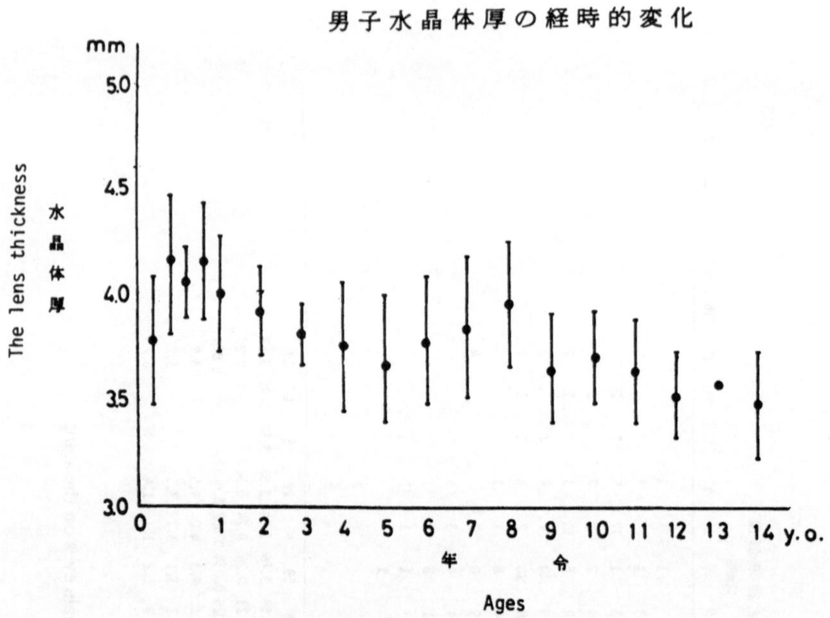

Fig. 11. **The growth curve of the lens thickness of the normal male eyes on the aging.**

noted. The average of the axial length of the eyes of newborn infants is 18.01 mm in boys and 17.32 mm in girls. Thus, it increases by an average of 3.75 mm in boys and 3.93 mm in girls during the first year after birth. On the other hand, the average of the axial length is 23.35 mm in seven-year-old boys and 22.81 mm in seven-year-old girls, thus increasing by an average of 1.58 mm in both sexes during the six years between one and seven. In every age group except for the eight-year-olds, the axial length of boys was significantly longer than that of girls. The difference ranged from 0.30 mm to 2.67 mm.

Figure 5 and 6 shows the average and standard deviations of the anterior chamber depth in each age group for boys and girls. Figure 7 and 8 also shows annual changes obtained by plotting the average and standard deviations. The anterior chamber depth increases rapidly up to the age of one. After that, it increases mildly. The anterior chamber depth was significantly greater in boys than in girls in each age group.

Figure 9 and 10 shows the average and standard deviations of the antero-posterior measurement of the lens in each age group and changes by year. The anteroposterior measurement is slightly long up to the age of one and after that, decreases slightly. Later, a marked decrease is hardly ever observed (Figure 11 and 12). The anteroposterior measurement was slightly longer in boys than in girls in each age group.

Figure 13 and 14 shows the average and standard deviations of the axial length of the vitreous body in each age group and the changes by year. The axial length of the vitreous body increase rapidly to the age of one (Figure 15 and 16). Its average in newborn infants is 11.28 mm in boys and 10.79 mm in girls. The average is 14.19 mm in one-year-old boys and 14.10 mm in one-year-old girls. Thus, one year after birth, it has increased rapidly by an average of 2.91 mm in boys and 3.31 mm in girls. It increases mildly by an average of 1.66 mm in boys and 1.39 mm in girls between one and seven. A more mild increase in the growth curve is noted during the period between seven and 15. Thus, we can observe clearly the increase in the axial length in proportion to growth and can divide its growth curve into three stages. The length was significantly, 0.17 mm–1.39 mm, longer in boys than in girls in subjects aged eight or more.

We also studied the relationship between the body height and the axial length of the eyes as presented in Figures 17 and 18. The subjects were 379 eyes of 192 boys and 406 eyes of 206 girls. The correlation coefficient of the body height and the axial length is 0.923 in boys and 0.852 in girls, indicating a significantly positive correlation in both sexes.

In addition, we studied the relationship between the body weight and the axial length as presented in Figure 19 and 20. The subjects were 375 eyes of 190 boys and 406 eyes of 206 girls. The correlation coefficient of the body weight and the axial length of the eye is 0.818 in boys and 0.730 in girls, indicating a significantly straight-like correlation in both.

We can postulate a significant correlation between the body length and the axial length and between the body weight and the axial length in the develop-

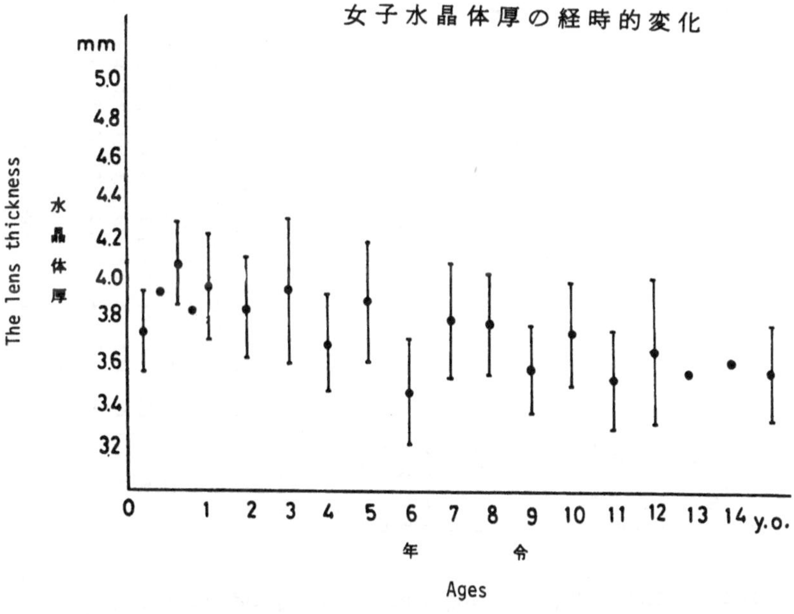

Fig. 12. The growth curve of the lens thickness of the normal female eyes on the aging.

男子硝子体長の平均値と標準偏差

Ages

The antero-posterior diameter of the vitreous body

年令 / 硝子体長 (mm)	MONTHS 0-1	1-3	3-6	6-12	YEARS 1	2	3	4	5	6	7	8	9	10	11	12	13	14	15	16	17	18	19	20
10.00 - 10.49																								
10.50 - 10.99	5																							
11.00 - 11.49	7	1																						
11.50 - 11.99	4	7																						
12.00 - 12.49	2	10	1																					
12.50 - 12.99		3	2	1																				
13.00 - 13.49		3	7	2		1																		
13.50 - 13.99		1	5	7	4	7																		
14.00 - 14.49				2	10	4	1	5	1															
14.50 - 14.99				2	4	5	2	5		1	7	1												
15.00 - 15.49				2		7	6	5	3	5	13	7	4											
15.50 - 15.99									3	7	24	6	17	14		3				1				1
16.00 - 16.49									3	3	25	3	27		4	1				3				
16.50 - 16.99											5	3	31	15	3	2		4	5		2			1
17.00 - 17.49											3		8	8	9	11		2	1					
17.50 - 17.99																6		7						
18.00 - 18.49														1	1	3	2							
18.50 - 18.99															1	1	1							
19.00 - 19.49																								
19.50 - 19.99																								
n	18	25	15	16	18	24	9	15	10	16	78	20	87	38	18	27	4	13	6	4	2			2
M	11.28	12.28	13.12	13.94	14.19	14.43	15.00	14.70	15.61	15.61	15.79	15.69	16.34	16.47	17.04	17.23	18.35	17.34	16.92	16.23	16.75			16.15
SD	0.47	0.58	0.59	0.72	0.31	0.65	0.42	0.47	0.60	0.39	0.61	0.58	0.51	0.71	0.70	0.70		0.39						
SE	0.111	0.116	0.149	0.180	0.074	0.133	0.141	0.122	0.191	0.099	0.069	0.130	0.054	0.115	0.164	0.138		0.110						
MAX	12.0	13.6	13.6	15.3	14.8	15.4	15.4	15.3	16.4	16.3	17.2	16.8	17.3	18.2	18.6	18.7		17.9						
MIN	10.5	11.2	12.4	12.8	13.7	13.4	14.4	14.0	14.4	14.7	14.0	14.8	15.3	15.5	16.0	15.8		16.8						
RANGE	1.5	2.4	1.2	2.5	1.1	2.0	1.0	1.3	2.0	1.6	3.2	2.0	2.0	2.7	2.6	2.9		1.1						

Fig. 13. The averages and standard deviations of the anteroposterior diameter of the vitreous body of the normal male eyes on the aging.

Ages

The anteroposterior diameter of the vitreous body

女子硝子体長の平均値と標準偏差

年令 / 硝子体長 (mm)	MONTHS 0-1	1-3	3-6	6-12	YEARS 1	2	3	4	5	6	7	8	9	10	11	12	13	14	15	16	17	18	19	20
10.00 - 10.49	6																							
10.50 - 10.99	9																							
11.00 - 11.49	3																							
11.50 - 11.99	3	1	6																					
12.00 - 12.49				2	1																			
12.50 - 12.99			4	1				3																
13.00 - 13.49			2	1	8			1	1															
13.50 - 13.99					2	3	2	1		2			3											
14.00 - 14.49					3	10	9		7				1		4	3				4				
14.50 - 14.99					5	7	3	6		3	13		1	4		1								
15.00 - 15.49					4		8	7	5	8	29	3	13	7	1	2	1							
15.50 - 15.99					2		4	1	2	4	24	10	9	8	12	1	4							
15.00 - 16.49							3				13	20	27	15	9	6		4						
15.50 - 16.99											3		8	17	7	9		2	4					
17.00 - 17.49											1		5	5	5	6			2					
17.50 - 17.99														2	3									
18.00 - 18.49													1	1	2									1
18.50 - 18.99																								
19.00 - 19.49																								
19.50 - 19.99																								
n	21	1	12	4	25	20	29	19	15	17	83	33	68	59	43	28	5	6	10					1
M	10.79	11.55	12.31	12.55	14.10	14.32	14.90	14.53	14.66	15.06	15.49	15.95	15.94	16.25	16.24	16.26	15.62	16.35	15.86					18.25
SD	0.52		0.62		0.95	0.30	0.70	0.96	0.76	0.58	0.51	0.34	0.82	0.77	0.96	0.94			1.38					
SE	0.113		0.179		0.189	0.007	0.131	0.219	0.195	0.140	0.056	0.059	0.100	0.101	0.146	0.178			0.438					
MAX	11.9		13.1		15.7	14.9	16.2	15.8	15.9	15.7	17.1	16.4	18.2	18.4	18.3	17.5			17.4					
MIN	10.0		11.5		12.0	13.8	13.9	12.8	13.4	13.5	14.5	15.0	13.9	14.7	14.0	14.3			14.2					
RANGE	1.9		1.6		3.7	1.1	2.3	3.0	2.5	2.2	2.6	1.4	4.3	3.7	4.3	3.2			3.2					

Fig. 14. The averages and standard deviations of the anteroposterior diameter of the vitreous body of the normal female eyes on the aging.

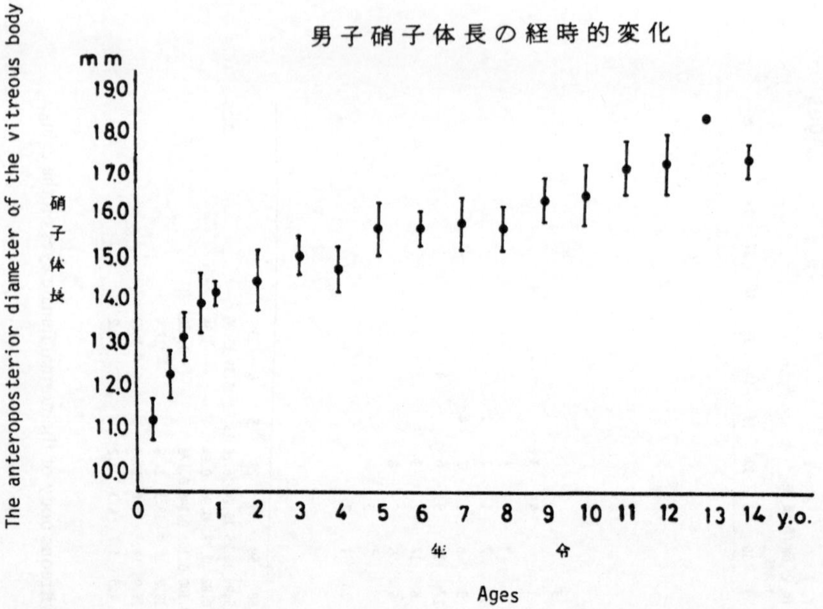

Fig. 15. The growth curve of the anteroposterior diameter of the vitreous body of the normal male eyes on the aging.

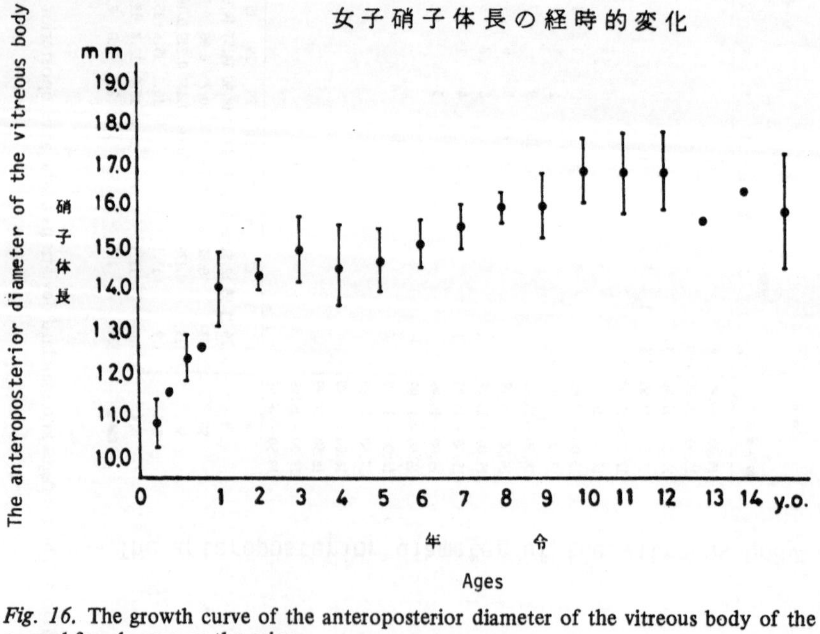

Fig. 16. The growth curve of the anteroposterior diameter of the vitreous body of the normal female eyes on the aging.

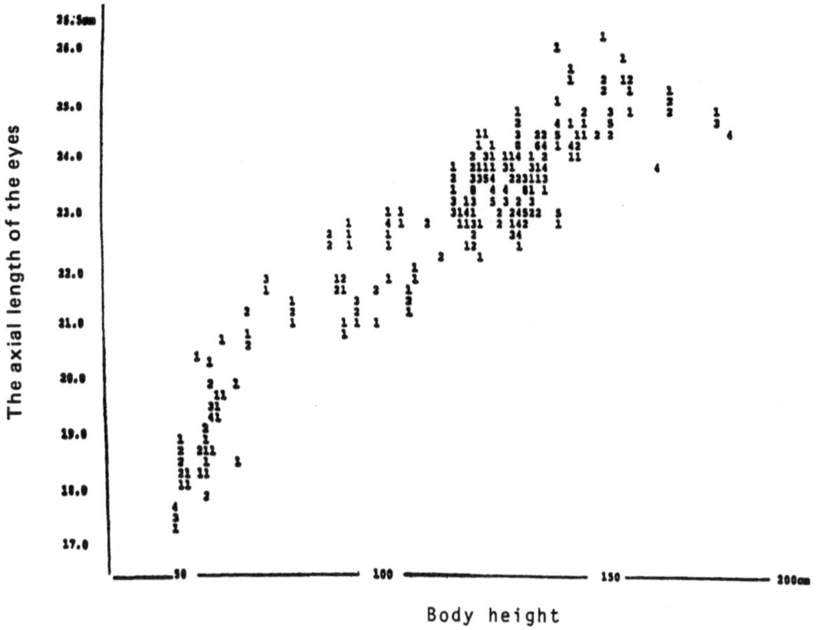

Fig. 17. The correlation between the axial length of the eyes and the body height in boys in the aging.

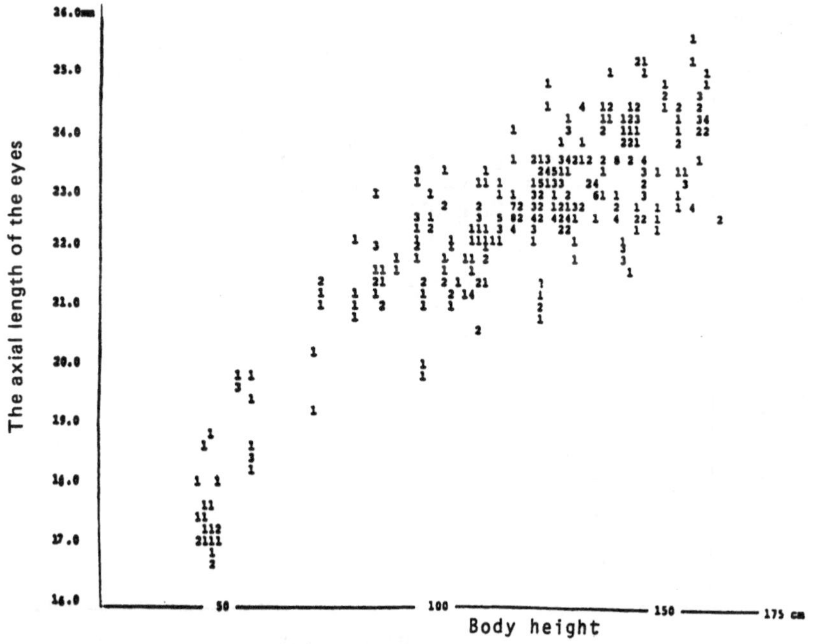

Fig. 18. The correlation between the axial length of the eyes and the body height in girls in the aging.

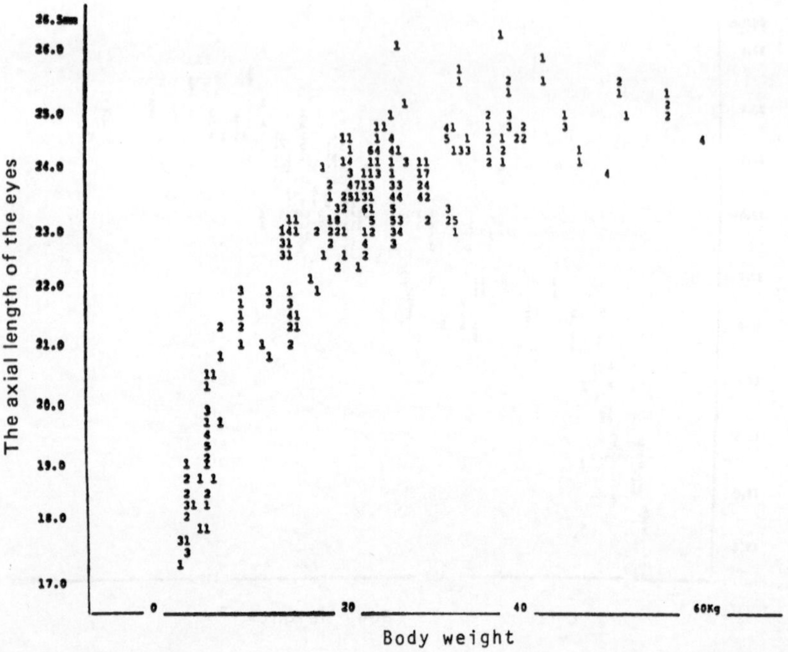

Fig. 19. The correlation between the axial length of the eyes and the body weight in boys in the aging.

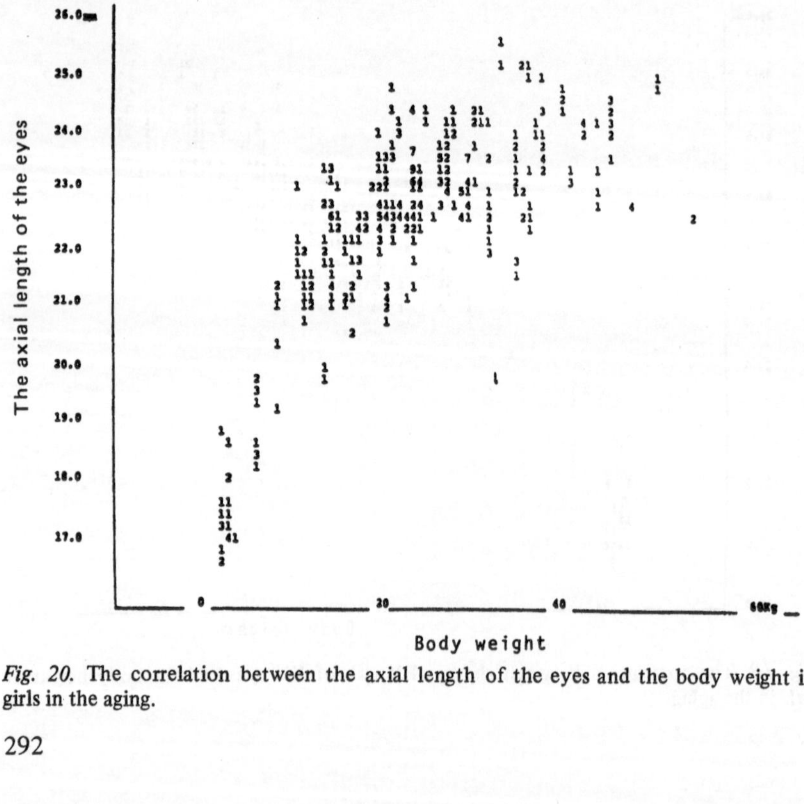

Fig. 20. The correlation between the axial length of the eyes and the body weight in girls in the aging.

mental stages of infants and children. However, we believe that the relationship is not always noted in adults.

CONCLUSION

We measured the total axial length of the eye and its refractive components of 964 normal eyes of Japanese subjects aged up to 20, 465 eyes of 239 boys and 499 eyes of 254 girls, and observed their growth process. We obtained the following results.

(1) A significantly positive correlation was present in changes according to the year between age and the axial length of the vitreous body and between age and the total axial length of the eye. The growth rate of the axial length of the vitreous body and the total axial length of the eye could be divided into three growth curves; up to the age of one, from one to seven and from seven to 14.

(2) All components were significantly longer in boys than in girls in each age group.

Author's address:
Department of Ophthalmology
St. Marianna University
School of Medicine
2095 Sugao
Miyamae-ku
Kawasaki-shi
Kanagawa-ken 213
Japan

BIOMETRY OF THE EYE DURING ACCOMMODATION

J. K. STOREY and E. P. RABIE
(Manchester, England)

ABSTRACT

A-scan biometry was performed on 9 near emmetropic and 5 highly myopic subjects with 2.00 dioptre changes in the stimulus to accommodation. The crystalline lenses of highly myopic eyes were found to be less efficient and moved back further from the cornea during accommodation than the lenses of near emmetropic eyes. Vitreous and total eye lengths of highly myopic eyes altered more than near emmetropic eyes.

INTRODUCTION

Many authors have used optical means to explore refractive changes in the eye during accommodation, but few have employed ultrasound as the principal tool. With A-mode ultrasonography we have not been able so far to determine curvatures accurately. In this study biometry during accommodation is confined to measurement between principal refractive surfaces.

Coleman, Wuchinich and Carlin (1969) and Coleman (1970) explored this subject. Their approach was to measure the eye at rest and then with about 6.5 dioptres of accommodation. They found that the vitreous might lengthen, shorten or remain unchanged in dimension without regard to the presence or absence of myopia. In our study, we have tried to quantify accommodation further by performing biometry with 2.00 dioptre changes in the stimulus to accommodation.

METHOD

The Kretz 7200 MA ultrasonoscope was used with a 10 MHz transducer. A calibration device immersed in a constant temperature water tank was used to verify the reliability of the Kretz system. The crystal calibration trace was adjusted before measurements were taken. A headband trial frame was adapted for monocular use. One eye was chosen at random for measurement. The appropraite distance spectacle prescription was taped into the back cells

Hillman, J.S./Le May, M.M. (eds.) Ophthalmic Ultrasonography

ISBN 978-94-009-7280-3.

and a +3.00 dioptre lens inserted loosely in the front cell, so that accommodation would be virtually at rest. Normal saline at near body temperature was used in the eye cup and the transducer dipped into this at least 5 mm from the eye, which avoided near field effects. Adjustments in the position of the transducer were made to achieve 'clear' echoes, with the corneal echo as high as possible followed in decreasing order of height by the anterior and posterior lens echoes and the echo off the vitreo-retinal interface. This gave some guarantee of centration over the optic axis of the eye and approximated the visual axis.

In the supine position, the contralateral eye focused on a word of the smallest type which was supported at 33 cm from the eye on a stand with suitable illumination. The print had to be clear before a photograph was taken. Photographs were taken with a Nikon camera and macro lens after each 2 dioptre change in the front lens of the trial frame. The sequence of lenses was +3.0, +1.0, −1.0, −3.0, and −5.0 dioptres. Negatives were measured on a travelling microscope which was read to an accuracy of 0.01 mm.

Although consensual accommodation was accepted here and Campbell (1960) has shown it to be representative of actual accommodation, an attempt has been made by Storey (1982) to construct a contact lens which permitted fixation along the ultrasound beam. This contact lens supported a microscope cover glass plate at 45 degrees to both the transducer and the eye. The ultrasound beam was reflected off the glass plate into the eye and back along the same route. Very thin glass plates like this avoid loss of sound in the same manner as very thin plastic membranes. When in use, the cornea was covered by saline, so a +16.0 dioptre lens at 35 mm vertex distance was needed on average to offset its neutralisation. An excellent A-scan was obtained, but subjects found it difficult to see well through such a strange optical path and this hindered worthwhile measurements on accommodation.

Subjects with a corrected visual acuity of 6/6 in each eye were drawn from students, members of staff and children, whose ages ranged from 14 to 30 years. The subjects were divided into two groups. Group 1 included 9 emmetropic and slightly myopic cases with an equivalent spherical refraction of plano to −2.50 dioptres and Group 2 included 5 highly myopic subjects with an equivalent spherical refraction of −4.00 to −11.0 dioptres.

RESULTS

The repeatability of the results was determined by performing the measurements five times for each accommodative step on five subjects. The average standard deviations were 0.07 mm for anterior chamber depth, 0.08 mm for lens thickness, 0.09 mm for vitreous length and 0.09 mm for total length. These were approximately equal for all accommodative steps.

The mean values for the main sagittal dimensions in the two groups at each stage of accommodation are presented in Tables 1 and 2. It can be seen that as accommodation increases there is a gradual reduction in anterior chamber depth and an obvious increase in lens thickness. Vitreous length and

Table 1. Mean ocular dimensions for 9 emmetropic and slightly myopic subjects. (Group 1: plano to −2.50 dioptres)

Stimulus to Accommodation (Dioptres)	A.C. (mm)	Lens (mm)	Vit. (mm)	Total Length (A.C. + Lens + Vit.) (mm)
0	3.85	3.74	16.74	24.36
2	3.79	3.86	16.78	24.44
4	3.67	3.97	16.70	24.35
6	3.62	4.02	16.61	24.38
8	3.49	4.17	16.70	24.36

Table 2. Mean ocular dimensions for 5 highly myopic subjects (Group 2: −4.00 to −11.00 dioptres)

Stimulus to Accommodation (Dioptres)	A.C. (mm)	Lens (mm)	Vit. (mm)	(A.C. + Lens + Vit.) (mm)
0	3.82	3.84	18.72	26.41
2	3.75	4.00	18.76	26.51
4	3.63	4.13	18.70	26.48
6	3.47	4.31	18.58	26.40
8	3.41	4.45	18.41	26.33

axial length altered more in Group 2 than Group 1. The changes in Group 2 are illustrated in Figure 1.

In Figure 2, the anterior chamber depth reduces at a greater rate in Group 2 where the slope is −0.055 ($r = -0.990$ and $p < 0.001$) than Group 1 where the slope is −0.044 ($r = -0.991$ and $p < 0.001$). In Figure 3, the crystalline lens increases in sagittal thickness more per dioptre of accommodation in the highly myopic eye, in other words it is less efficient than the lens in the near emmetropic eye. The slope for Group 1 was +0.051 ($r = +0.991$ $p < 0.001$) and for Group 2 was +0.076 ($r = +0.999$ $p < 0.001$).

Anterior chamber depth and lens thickness were added together to obtain the position of the posterior surface of the lens as shown in Figure 4. With accommodation a greater change was found in Group 2 than in Group 1. The slope for Group 1 was +0.006 ($r = +0.761$ and $0.10 > p > 0.05$) and for Group 2 was +0.021 ($r = +0.950$ and $p < 0.05$).

DISCUSSION

Coleman (1970) found a decrease in anterior chamber depth and an increase in lens thickness with accommodation. Coleman, Wuchinich and Carlin (1969) had found that there were axial length changes during accommodation, but the response varied. Some eyes lengthened whilst others shortened and this applied also to vitreous length. In this study Group 2 showed changes in axial length and especially in vitreous length with increasing accommodation. It is shown in Figure 4 that the posterior surface of the lens moves

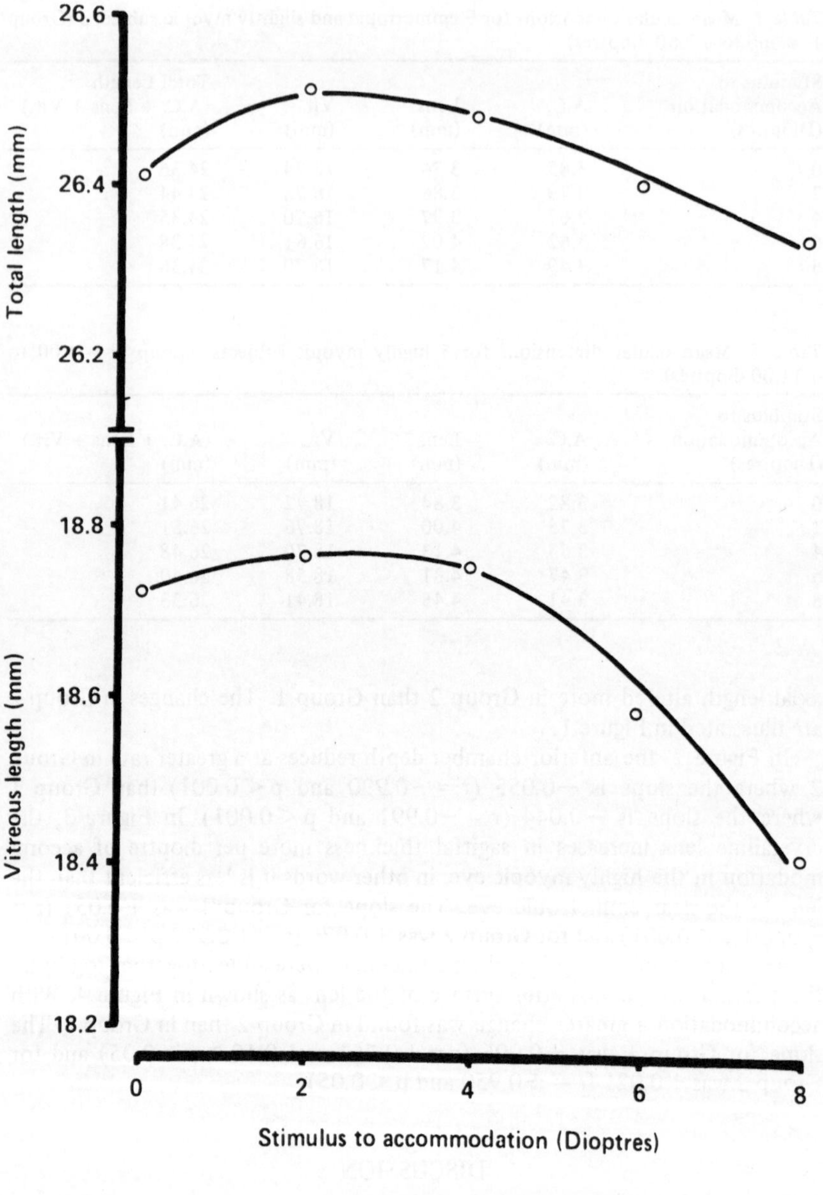

Fig. 1. Vitreous length (mm) and total length (mm) for 5 highly myopic subjects (Group 2: −4.00 to −11.00 dioptres) plotted against the stimulus to accommodation.

progressively backwards with respect to the cornea on accommodation, especially in Group 2. With two dioptres of accommodation there is a slight increase in vitreous length despite this backwards movement of the lens. If

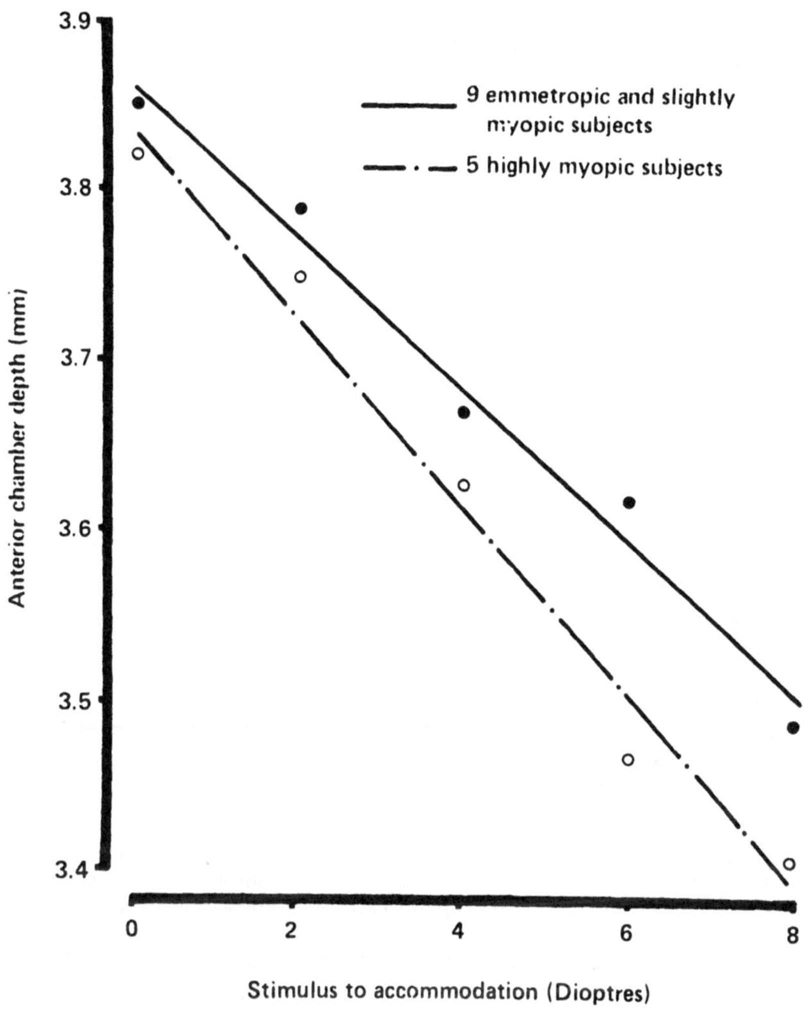

Fig. 2. Anterior chamber depth (mm) for emmetropic and slightly myopic subjects (Group 1: slope $= -0.044$ $r = -0.991$ $p < 0.001$) and for 5 highly myopic subjects (Group 2: slope $= -0.055$ $r = -0.990$ $p < 0.001$) plotted against the stimulus to accommodation.

this observation is valid, it would be compatible with Coleman's theory of accommodation as discussed by Bell (1980).

Subjects were examined supine in this study. Storey and Phillips (1973) showed that the lens gravitates towards the posterior pole in this position. So measurements in the erect position might yield slightly different results.

Brown (1973) showed with slit lamp photography that lens thickening during accommodation was due entirely to sagittal expansion of the nucleus with no change in cortical thickness. It is possible that a difference exists

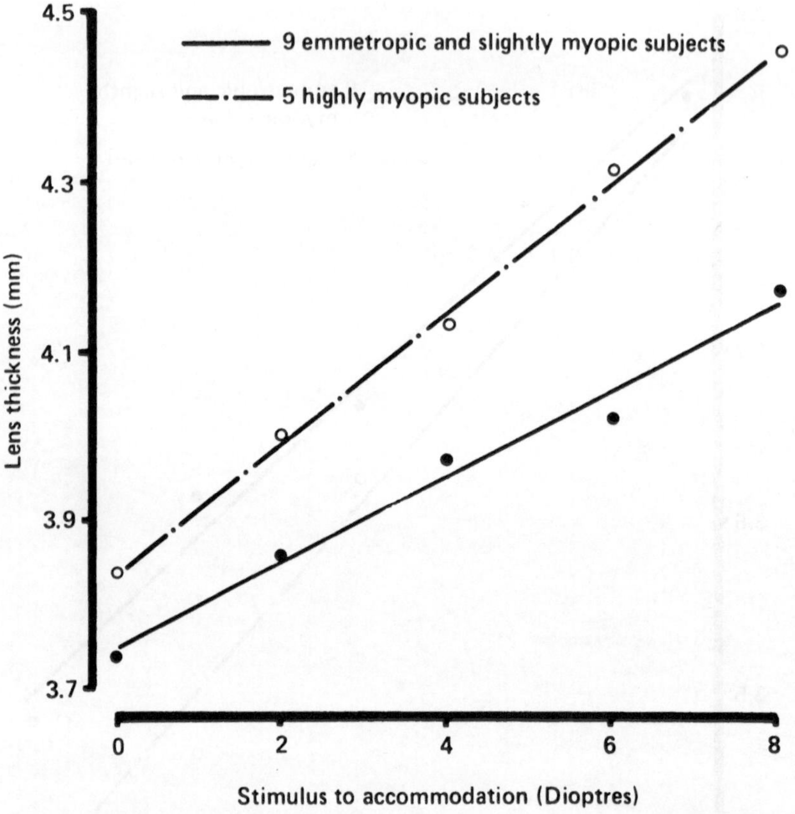

Fig. 3. Lens thickness (mm) for 9 emmetropic and slightly myopic subjects (Group 1: slope = + 0.051 r = + 0.991 $p < 0.001$) and for 5 highly myopic subjects (Group 2: slope = + 0.076 r = + 0.999 $p < 0.001$) plotted against the stimulus to accommodation.

between the velocity of ultrasound in the cortex and the nucleus, but we have been unable to obtain echoes from within the non-cataractous lens. If it is assumed that the velocity is greater in the nucleus, then an underestimate of lens thickening results. Vitreous length and anterior chamber depth would not be affected, although total axial length would be underestimated. However, this error is likely to be small.

REFERENCES

Bell G. R. (1980) The Coleman theory of accommodation and its relevance to myopia, J. of the Am. Optom. Assn. 51 (6) 582–588.

Brown N. (1973) The change in shape and internal form of the lens of the eye on accommodation, Exp. Eye Res. 15, 441–459.

Campbell F. W. (1960) Correlation of accommodation between the two eyes, J. Opt. Soc. Am. 50 (7) 738.

Coleman D. J. (1970) Unified model for accommodative mechanism, Am. J. Ophth. 69

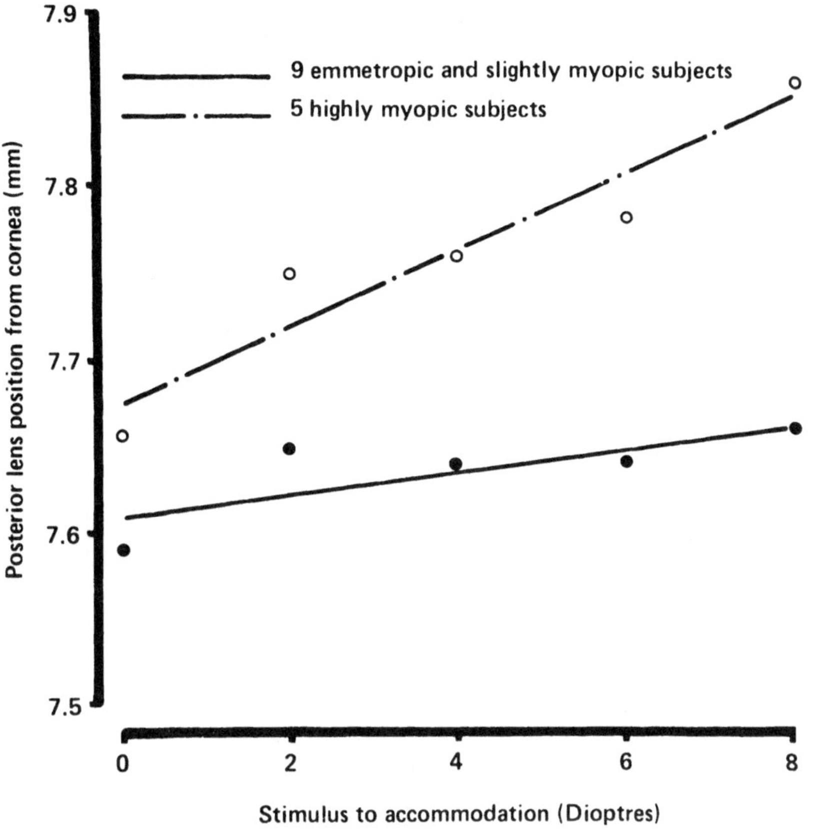

Fig. 4. The position of the posterior surface of the lens from the anterior surface of the cornea (mm) for 9 emmetropic and slightly myopic subjects (Group 1: slope = + 0.006 r = + 0.761 0.1 > p > 0.05) and for 5 highly myopic subjects (Group 2: slope = + 0.021 r = + 0.950 p < 0.05) plotted against the stimulus to accommodation.

(6) 1063–1079.

Coleman D. J., Wuchinich D. and Carlin B. (1969) Accommodative changes in the axial dimension of the human eye, In Gitter (1969) Ophthalmic Ultrasound. St. Louis, Mosby, 134–141.

Storey J. K. (1982) Measurement of the eye with ultrasound, Ophth. Optician 22 (5) 150–160.

Storey J. K. and Phillips C. I. (1973) Ultrasonic investigations on mobility of crystalline lens, SIDUO IV Centre National D'ophthalmologie des Quinze-Vingts, Paris, 261–264.

Authors' address:
Manchester Royal Eye Hospital
Oxford Road
Manchester M13 9WH
UK

COMPARISON OF AXIAL OCULOMETRY BY ULTRASOUND AND BY SLIT-LAMP PHOTOMETRY, A NEW MEASURING METHOD

H. C. FLEDELIUS, B. KROGSAA, J. LARSEN and H. LUND-ANDERSEN
(Copenhagen and Hillerød, Denmark)

ABSTRACT

During vitreous fluorophotometry an intra-ocular axial fluorescence profile is recorded (intensity on y-axis, sagittal slit-lamp movement on abscissa). Marks are now made on the graph when observing the focal plane of the slit-light on 1) macula, 2) and 3) lens surfaces, and 4) corneal inner surface. From classical physiological optics conversion factors are calculated for the three eye compartments, and a computer program has been designed to give recorded slit-lamp movements as axial eye distances.

The measuring method is compared with ultrasound oculometry in 11 observation sets. Except for anterior chamber depth, there seems to be a fair agreement between methods.

INTRODUCTION

A comparison is made between axial eye measurements performed by ultrasound (TAU) and by slit-lamp photometry. The latter technique has been developed in connection with vitreous fluoro-photometry research.

Having access to modern ultrasound oculometry there should be no need for reviving optical measuring methods – which has not been the principal aim of the present study either. In vitreous fluorometry, however, an estimate of vitreous volume is required for calculating the amount of intravenously injected fluorescein having leaked from the blood vessels of the eye. A built-in size estimate is therefore highly practical because all needed parameters are then collected in one examining procedure.

Being presented in more detail elsewhere (Krogsaa et al. 1982 a, b), the photometry method is given only in brief. Emphasis will be on the agreement of photometry results with those of the established method, ultrasound oculometry.

MATERIAL

Seven volunteering subjects (age 21–58 years, refraction −6.5 to +5.0 D) had one eye measured axially by both techniques, for a total of eleven measurements. Where one person had repeated measurements there was an

Hillman, J. S./Le May, M. M. (eds.) Ophthalmic Ultrasonography
©1983, Dr W. Junk Publishers, The Hague/Boston/Lancaster
ISBN 978-94-009-7280-3.

interval of weeks between examinations, which were all performed in mydriasis (after topical Mydriacyl ® 0.5% and Metaoxedrine 10%).

METHODS

(a) *Ultrasound oculometry (time-amplitude ultrasonography)*

The method is considered standard (Fledelius 1970, 1976), using a slightly focused 10 Mc transducer (Ultrasonolux) in a contact glass placed against the perilimbal sclera (patient supine) with Methocel ® 2% as coupling vehicle. Out of several equipments at disposal, the veteran ultrasound apparatus Kretztechnik 7000 was chosen due to its high level of reproducibility of measuring results. Eye distances are calculated from equipment units, based on the velocities of 1532 m/sec for aqueous and vitreous body, and 1641 m/sec for the lens (Jansson 1963).

The first ultrasound reflection being from the acoustic interface between precorneal Methocel and anterior corneal surface (vertex), the anterior chamber depth (ACD) is usually given with central corneal thickness included. In the present context this is not done for the sake of comparing the results of the two methods, because in slit lamp photometry the corresponding anterior reference point is inner (posterior) corneal surface. In the following a standard mean central corneal thickness of 0.52 mm (Kruse Hansen 1971) is thus subtracted from ultrasound ACD recordings, giving an ACD proper.

(b) *Oculometry by slit-lamp photometry*

The basic principle is that of assessing the intraocular shift of the focal plane from sagittal slit-lamp movement during monocular slit-lamp microscopy, using a Rodenstock RD 2000.

The blue slit-light is placed e.g. to the left (Fig. 1), and the exact position of the focal plane in the eye is marked (under visual control) by the shadow, or contour, of a fiber optic light probe placed in the right ocular, which is used for inspection during examination. The main objective of the light probe is to measure vitreous fluorescence, a possibility not necessarily exploited during the oculometry procedure. Regarding further technical details, cf. Krogsaa et al. 1983a.

For oculometry, the focal plane is placed first on the macular region of the retina, then – moving the slit-lamp axially towards the examiner – on the posterior and anterior lens surfaces, and finally on inner corneal surface. At each such position, a foot switch is activated (Fig. 2) to make a mark on the x-y paper-recording used for registering the actual slit-lamp movement during the procedure.

Converting such paper-recorded data to relevant intraocular shifts of the focal point (i.e. axial eye distances in mm) some conversion factors are necessary (Fig. 2). Empirically this could be achieved by comparing a sufficient number of results with those of other measuring principles (ultrasound in particular, but also Haag-Streit ACD pachymetry). It was, however,

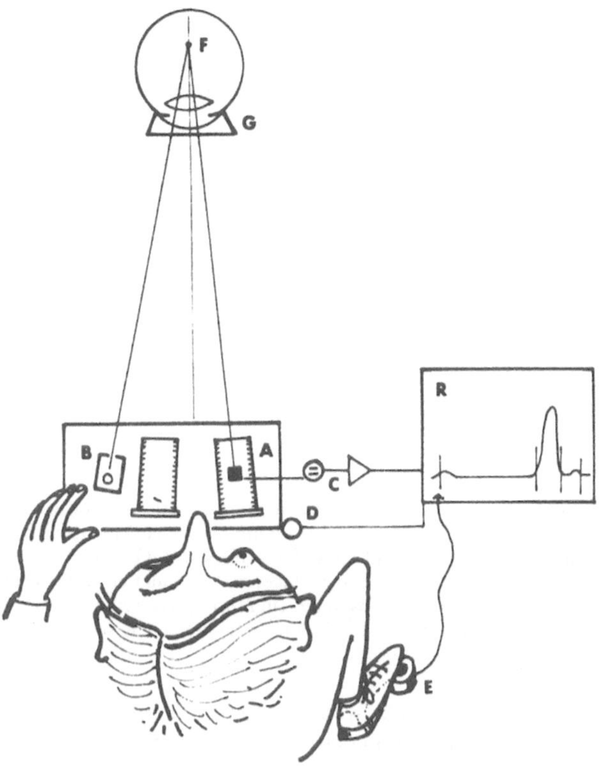

Fig. 1. Slit lamp equipment for fluorophotometry. A) Right ocular of slit-lamp with fiber optic probe. B) Blue slit-light beam, here placed to the left while measuring the left eye of the subject. For right eye measurement the fiber optic probe i placed in the left ocular and the blue slit-light to the right. C) Photomultiplier with amplifier. D) Potentiometer with amplification 1:12.1. E) Foot-switch activated marker mechanism. R) Recording, x-y on paper. F) focal point in the vitreous. G) Goldmann fundus contact lens.

preferred to test the method by keeping to its optical preconditions, and classical data regarding physiological optics (curvature radii, refractive indices, and axial distances between ocular structures) were entered into a model for calculation (BK). Later this has been transformed into a computer program (BK and JL, cf, Krogsaa et al. 1982a).

RESULTS

Table I gives measurement results by the two oculometry techniques, from eleven examinations in seven individuals. The main objective is to assess the overall agreement within observation sets, for which purpose Wilcoxon's matched pairs signed ranks test is considered suited. Mean values are also shown, and it is further possible, quite roughly, to estimate reproducibility

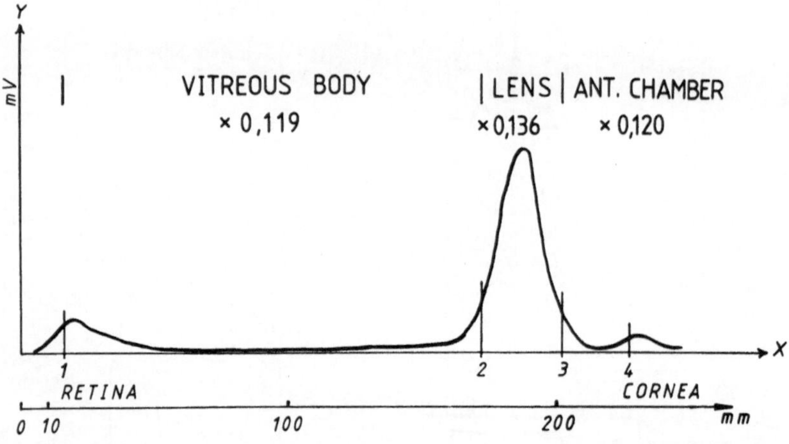

Fig. 2. Fluorophotometric concentration profile, with intensity of fluorescence on y-axis and movement of the recorder-pen (sagittal slit-lamp movement) on abscissa. The marker lines on the x-axis are to signify slit-lamp focal plane on 1) retina (macular region), 2) anterior lens surface, 3) posterior lens surface, and 4) inner corneal surface. Abscissa distances are converted to axial eye distances (in mm) by the factors 0.119 for vitreous, 0.136 for lens, and 0.120 for anterior chamber (aqueus). Their sum make up the axial length (minus central corneal thickness).

of results in those individuals who had repeated measurements. Finally, parametric within-set correlation coefficients are shown.

DISCUSSION

As estimated from Wilcoxon's test there is good agreement between measuring results. A significant difference is found regarding anterior chamber depth only, with shallower chambers (mean difference 0.17 mm) measured by ultrasound.

Considering the mean values of Table I, lens thicknesses are identical (difference 0.02 mm), and vitreous lengths almost identical (difference 0.12 mm). The overall result is that axial length appears somewhat shorter as assessed by ultrasound (averaging 0.27 mm), however, without reaching 0.05 significance level by the non-parametric Wilcoxon test.

Regarding the single sets of measurements, some within-set differences amount to less acceptable levels. In ACD and lens thickness recordings the extreme differences are thus about 0.7 mm. This is a deviation of about 25% if one of the methods be taken as correct. Correspondingly, a parametrical within-set correlation coefficient level (r) of about 0.7 is not quite satisfactory. Probably it is explained by a certain methodological error which manifests itself unduly where short target distances are to be measured.

Concerning the much longer vitreous and axial length distances, within-set differences amounting to about 1 mm are not equally disturbing. Not

Table 1. Eleven oculometric observation sets as measured by ultrasound and slit-lamp photometry, further presenting mean values and standard deviations of the three eye compartments (ACD, lens thickness and vitreous length). Results are shown of Wilcoxon matched pairs signed ranks test; n.s. = non significant, 5% level. At bottom, parametric correlation coefficients within observation sets

	Anterior chamber depth (mm)		Lens thickness (mm)		Vitreous length (mm)		Axial length (mm)	
	Ultrasound	Photometry	Ultrasound	Photometry	Ultrasound	Photometry	Ultrasound	Photometry
1.	3.03	3.03	3.76	3.99	16.28	16.16	23.07	23.18
2.	3.15	3.34	3.92	3.97	16.19	16.33	23.26	23.64
3.	2.42	3.16	4.66	3.99	13.23	13.23	20.31	20.38
4.	3.00	3.27	3.92	3.58	16.13	16.25	23.05	23.10
5.	3.58	3.54	3.64	3.47	17.74	18.58	24.96	25.59
6.	3.19	3.22	4.27	4.29	19.06	18.31	26.52	25.82
7.	3.12	3.09	3.75	3.73	15.75	15.70	22.62	22.52
8.	2.71	3.03	4.61	4.55	14.66	15.42	21.98	23.00
9.	3.03	3.32	3.76	3.95	16.09	15.86	22.88	23.13
10.	2.66	2.78	4.28	4.67	13.18	13.26	20.12	20.71
11.	3.19	3.24	3.71	3.88	16.20	16.68	23.10	23.80
x	3.01	3.18	4.03	4.01	15.86	15.98	22.90	23.17
SD ±	0.313	0.200	0.368	0.372	1.728	1.681	1.815	1.667
Wilcoxon test	$P < 0.02$		N.S.		N.S.		N.S.	
Correlation coefficient	0.69		0.68		0.97		0.97	

unexpectedly, the peak value is found in an eye with excessive myopia. Possible lacks in the whole set of optical preconditions – or merely undue large ranges in less well-defined parameters – may exert more influence, the longer the axial eye distance. Analysing optical oculometry based on phakometry, a similar conclusion was arrived at in a previous study by Sorsby et al. (1961). In this context, it may surprise that even some very short eyes show numerically important within-set differences, also regarding anterior eye segment structures. The rather small number of observation sets, however, must be taken into consideration.

Immediately, the basic physics of an axial ultrasound beam appear more simple to handle, and with less vague presuppositions. Blurring equipment factors are however well-known, and to remain open-minded it may be hard to tell, which of the two principles is in fact the more reliable.

Repeated measurements might give a clue hereto. Observation sets 1, 4, 9 are from one person, and the same holds for 2, 11 and for 3, 10. In general, agreement is fair in intra-individual recording sets, with only a suggested tendency of larger deviations by slit-lamp oculometry, but not systematically so.

Returning to the only statistically valid difference between methods – that implying ACD – a brief reference is made to a comparative ultrasound oculometry study reported on at an earlier SIDUO conference (Fledelius and Alsbirk 1975). Out of the three instruments tested then, the Kretztechnik 7000 (also used during the present investigation) gave ACD values about 0.1 mm lower than measured by the two other ultrasound instruments.

Comparing the actual ACD measurements with optical Haag-Streit ACD pachymetry, we found a closer match for photometry results. In this context, however, plain methodological factors may exert some influence. The optical methods are both performed with the subject sitting upright, while he is supine during ultrasound oculometry. If contrary, gravitational shifts of lens position might have explained the ACD differences actually found.

CONCLUSION

All considered, the study has shown a fair agreement between classical ultrasound oculometry and measurements performed by slit-lamp photometry. Regarding accuracy, the new optical method may still be questioned where decimals are concerned, but for the purposes of fluoro-photometry it is considered satisfactory. During the examination a built-in axial eye size estimate is required for subsequent calculation of amount of fluorescein having leaked into the vitreous. Supplementary ultrasound oculometry may thus be omitted, making the total procedure easier for patient and examiner.

REFERENCES

Fledelius, H. Ultrasound (A-mode) in a case of nasal posterior scleral ectasy. Acta ophthalmol. (Kbh.) 48:502–507 (1970)

Fledelius, H. Prematurity and the Eye. Thesis. Acta ophthalmol. (Kbh.) Suppl. 128 (1976)

Fledelius, H and Alsbirk, P.H. Comparative ultrasound oculometry. TAU-measurements of thirty eyes with three standard equipments. Bibl. ophthal., No 83 pp. 263–268. Karger, Basel (1975)

Jansson, F. Measurements of intraocular distances by ultrasound. Acta ophthalmol. (Kbh.) Suppl. 74 (1963)

Krogsaa, B., Fledelius, H., Larsen, J. and Lund-Andersen, H. Photometric oculometry I. Analysis of the optics in slit lamp fluorophotometry. Acta ophthalmol. (Kbh.) submitted for publ. (1983,a)

Krogsaa, B., Fledelius, H., Larsen, J. and Lund-Andersen, H. Photometric oculometry II. Measurement of axial eye distances by slit lamp photometry, clinical application. Acta ophthalmol. (Kbh.) submitted for publ. (1983,b)

Kruse Hansen, F. A clinical study of the normal human central corneal thickness. Acta ophthalmol. (Kbh.) 49:82–89 (1971)

Sorsby, A., Benjamin, B. and Sheridan, M. Refraction and its components during the growth of the eye from the age of three. Med. Res. Counc. spec. ser. no. 301, London (1961)

Author's address:
Department of Ophthalmology
Frederiksborg County Hospital
DK-3400 Hillerød
Denmark

INFLUENCE OF BIOMETRIC PARAMETERS ON SQUINT SURGERY

P. ROSSI, M. ZINGIRIAN, G. P. FAVA, A. RIVARA, C. BERTOLINI*
and A. POLIZZI
(Genoa, Italy)

SUMMARY

A geometrical analysis of the influence of the eye and orbit sizes on the effect of a rectus muscle recession is presented. The established relationship is checked comparing the results of surgery on monocular, amblyopic squints and the echographically established eye size.

The amount of muscle displacement needed for surgical squint correction, is usually based on the sensorimotor features of the deviation, whereas eyeball and orbit size is generally disregarded as having only a minor influence on the outcome of surgery.

The purpose of this study is to evaluate the influence of biometric features of the eye and orbit, particularly of the contact arc, on the outcome of surgery on the rectus muscles.

MATERIAL AND METHOD

Geometric evaluation

In a simplified model (Fig. 1), the eyeball is assumed to have a perfectly round shape, the scleral insertion of a rectus muscle being 10 mm from the anterior pole of the eye and its orbital insertion lying on the anteroposterior axis of the eye.

The eyeball rotations (PP′) caused by muscle recessions of different extent (R) has been calculated for eyeballs with diameters of 18; 24 and 30 mm respectively.

The influence of the size of the orbit is assessed evaluating the shift of the posterior end point (T) of the contact arc when the orbital insertion of the muscle moves between the points C and C′.

Biometric assessment

The latero-lateral axis of 19 subjects operated for a monocular squint with

*Istituto Elettrotecnica. Università di Genova

Hillman, J. S./Le May, M. M. (eds.) Ophthalmic Ultrasonography
©1983, Dr W. Junk Publishers, The Hague/Boston/Lancaster
ISBN 978-94-009-7280-3.

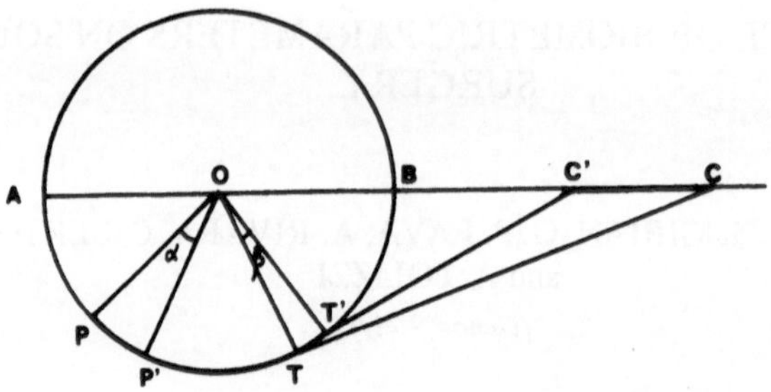

$$R = 2 \times \underbrace{\left[\arcsin \left(\frac{\overline{PP'}}{AB} \right) \right]}_{\alpha} + \underbrace{\left[\arccos \frac{\overline{AB}}{2.\overline{OC}} - \arccos \frac{\overline{AR}}{2.\overline{OC'}} \right]}_{\beta}$$

Fig. 1. Geometric pattern of the eye and orbit.

amblyopia was measured by means of A-Scan ecography, and the amount of angle reduction for 1 mm of muscle displacement was plotted against the size of the eye.

RESULTS

Table 1 reports the eyeball rotations calculated for muscle displacements of different extent performed on eyes of different diameters.

Table 2 reports the angular shift of the T point calculated according to the eyeball and orbit sizes.

Fig. 2 reports the squint reduction corresponding to a 1 mm muscle displacement obtained in operated eyes of different sizes.

COMMENT

The previous measurements allow some considerations:

(1) *Influence of eyeball size on surgery outcome*

The geometrical analysis shows that a given amount of muscle displacement brings about quite different eye rotations according to the size of the eye: a 1 mm recession causes a 6.37° rotation on a 18 mm eye, a 4.77° and 3.82 rotation on eyes with 24 and 30 mm diameters, respectively.

If percentage changes are considered, the same amount of muscle recession performed on eyes with diameters of 24 and 30 mm leads to a rotation that is 25% and 67% smaller than that obtained when the diameter is 18 mm.

These results were confirmed by the biometric measurements: the mean effect of muscle displacement progressively decreases with increasing eye sizes (Fig. 2).

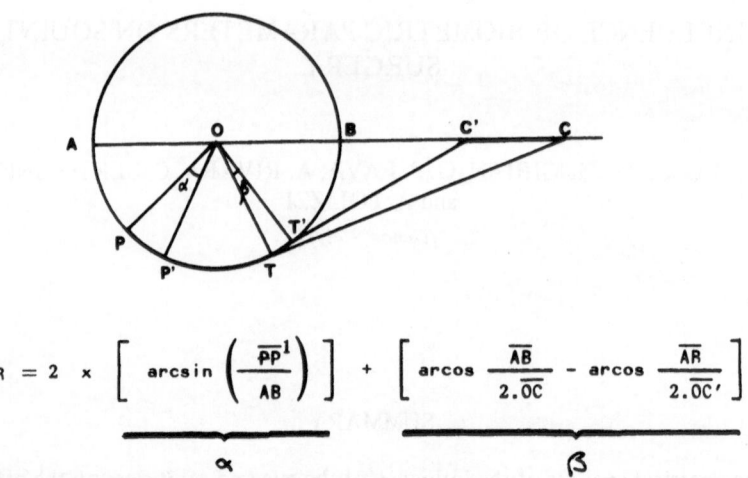

Table 1. Results: Eyeball rotation according to the amount of muscle recession and eye diameter. Maximal recession limited to the point where muscle insertion reaches the t. point (see Fig. 1)

Muscle displacement (mm)	Contact arc reduction (degrees)		
1	3.82204	4.77805	6.37217
2	7.64834	9.56442	12.76413
3	11.48319	14.36758	19.19625
4	15.33099	19.19625	25.69003
5	19.19625	24.05957	32.26887
6	23.08367	28.96726	38.95889
7	26.99820	33.92986	
8	30.94509	38.95889	
9	34.92995	44.06724	
10	38.95889	49.26945	
11	43.03856	54.58228	
12	47.17628	60.02537	
13	51.38028		
14	55.65980		
15	60.02537		
16	64.48915		
17	69.06540		
	30	24	18
		Eye diameter (mm)	

Scattering of the measurements is explained considering that surgical muscle displacement changes the viscoelastic properties and strength of a muscle. The proprioceptive input from intrafusal fibers, too, is altered. Finally, the anatomical alterations of a muscle that take place in older squinting people influence the outcome of surgery. However, inasmuch as surgery represents a merely mechanical way of coping with a neurophysiological problem, the influence of the eyeball size should be taken into account, especially when surgery is performed on very small or large eyes. Our work suggests that the amount of surgery dictated by experience and by the sensorimotor features of the squint should likely be varied according to the size of the eyeball.

(2) *Influence of the size of the orbit*

A very loose influence of orbit depth on the position of the endpoint of the contact arc was shown by the geometrical evaluation. A significant influence can be shown only when an actual displacement is present between the eye and the orbit. On purely geometric considerations, therefore, the orbit depth can be anticipated as having a negligible influence on the results of surgery in 'normal' squinting people.

Table 2. Result: Angular changes of the contact arc for different orbit depth (OC-OC′: see Fig. 1), according to the eye size

Orbit depth changes (mm)		Contact arc reduction (degrees)	Eye diameter (mm)
OC	OC′		
26	25	1.63617	
26	24	3.44923	
26	23	5.47359	30
26	22	7.75473	
26	21	10.35464	
26	20	13.36160	
32	31	0.74997	
32	30	1.55452	
32	29	2.42005	
32	28	3.35404	
32	27	4.36532	
32	28	3.35404	24
32	20	8.18795	
25	21	6.16710	
25	22	4.37217	
25	23	2.76474	
25	24	1.31516	
35	34	0.44907	
35	33	0.92641	
35	32	1.43484	
35	31	1.97751	
35	30	2.55808	18
25	24	0.92451	
25	23	1.93631	
25	22	3.04884	

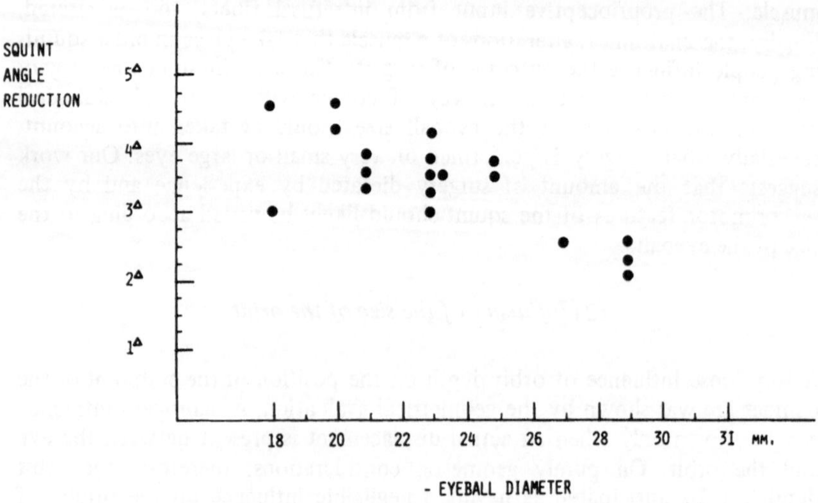

Fig. 2. Squint reduction corresponding to a 1 mm recession according to eye diameter.

CONCLUSIONS

Both the geometrical analysis and the biometric evaluation show that the size of the eyeball should be taken into account when surgery for squint is performed on very small or myopic eyes.

An echographic evaluation of the eye size should be performed especially when a monocular squint with amblyopia is concerned, as a fairly good outcome of surgery can be expected.

The orbit depth, in contrast, does not greatly influence the results of surgery and can thus be disregarded in normal people.

ACKNOWLEDGEMENT

This work was supported by a grant from the Consiglio Nazionale Delle Ricerche, Italy.

Authors' address:
University Eye Clinic
Viale Benedetto XV 5
I-1654 Genova
Italy

ULTRASONIC STUDY OF AXIAL LENGTH CHANGES AFTER ENCIRCLING OPERATION IN APHAKIC EYES

Y. BABA and A. SAWADA
(Miyazaki, Japan)

ABSTRACT

Encircling operation with a tightness of 15% was performed in aphakic rabbit eyes six months after the lens was removed by KPE. Refractive power, axial length and the radius of corneal curvature changed immediately after the encircling operation. Thereafter the variation was minimum. Correlation among these three factors at three months after encirclement was significant. Variation in these factors in aphakic eyes was quite different from those in phakic eyes, which was considered to be due to absence of the lens.

INTRODUCTION

It is very interesting to study changes in the refractive state developed after an operation for retinal detachment. The quality of changes depends on the kind of procedure used. In a previous study axial length and the length of ocular dimensions were ultrasonically measured for six months in adult pigmented eyes after the encircling operation. Immediately after encircling, myopia in proportion to the degree of tightness of encirclement was produced. Those results were presented in the Third International Conference on Myopia in Copenhagen and in the 8th SIDUO Congress in Nijmegen in 1980. (Baba and Sawada, 1981). In that study the effect of lens as one of refractive factors remained unsolved. To study the effect of the lens the same procedures were performed in aphakic eyes of adult non-pigmented rabbits in which the lens had been previously removed by Kelman phacoemulsification and aspiration (KPE). After the encircling operation axial length as an axial factor, and the radius of corneal curvature as a refractive factor were measured for three months. There has been no report in which changes in refractive state after encirclement in artificial rabbit eyes were investigated.

MATERIALS AND METHODS

Adult non-pigmented rabbit eyes were used for the experiments because the lens is pigmented rabbit eyes was so hard that it took much time to be emulsified and aspirated.

Hillman, J. S./Le May, M. M. (eds.) Ophthalmic Ultrasonography
©1983, Dr W. Junk Publishers, The Hague/Boston/Lancaster
ISBN 978-94-009-7280-3.

Six months after the lens was removed by KPE, the encircling operation with a tightness of 15% was performed. The tightness of encirclement was decided by the length of a silicone rod fixed on the sclera at the equator and tightened. The tightness of 15% means that the eye ball was encircled by a silicone rod with 85% of the length of the total circumference.

Before, immediately after and periodically for three months after the encircling operation, changes in refractive power, axial length and the radius of corneal curvature were studied. The refractive power was measured with Rodenstock's refractometer after fitting the specially made hard contact lens. The contact lens was + 20 diopters in the refractive power, 11 mm in diameter and 7.2 to 9.0 mm in the base curve. Axial length and the length of ocular dimensions were measured with the Digital Biometric Ruler 300 (Sonometrics). The propagation velocity of ultrasound was set at 1639 m/sec for the cornea and at 1532 m/sec for the anterior chamber and the vitreous. The radius of corneal curvature was measured with Bausch-Lomb's keratometer.

RESULTS

The average and standard deviation of the refractive power, the axial length and the radius of corneal curvature in seven non-pigmented rabbit eyes six months after the lens removal by KPE are shown in Table 1. These values were used as preoperative values for the encircling operation. Table 2 shows those values three months after the encircling operation. The changes at intervals of these three values are shown in Fig. 1-3.

Table 1. Average and statistical analysis of refractive power, axial length and radius of corneal curvature before encircling operation (6 months after KPE)

	$\bar{X} \pm$ S.D.
refractive power [D]	+ 27.86 ± 1.85
axial length [mm]	17.60 ± 0.56
radius of corneal curvature [mm]	8.15 ± 0.34

n = 7

Table 2. Average and statistical analysis of refractive power, axial length and radius of corneal curvature 3 months after encircling operation

	$\bar{X} \pm$ S.D.
refractive power [D]	+ 25.21 ± 1.51
axial length [mm]	18.69 ± 0.59
radius of corneal curvature [mm]	8.09 ± 0.32

n = 7

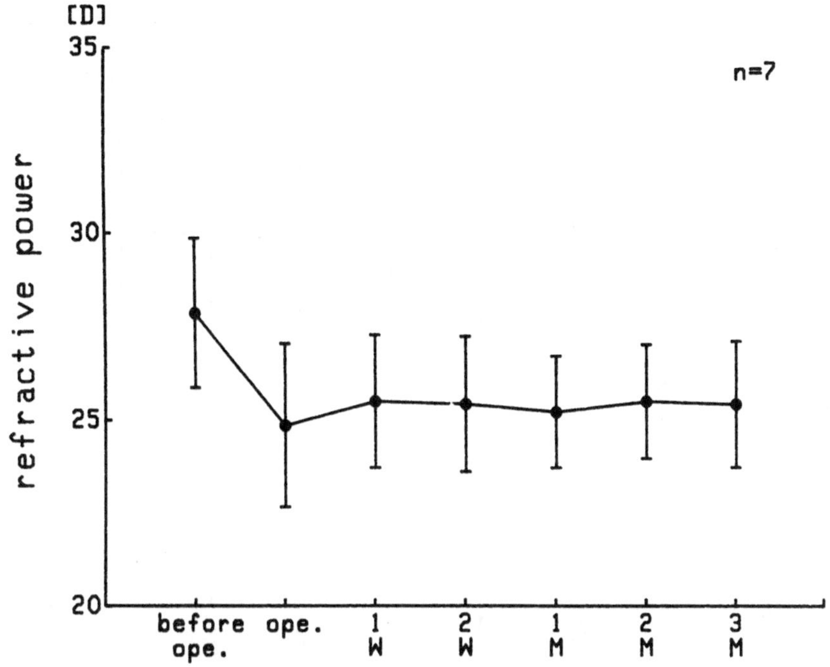

Fig. 1. Changes in refractive power after encircling operations.

CHANGE OF EACH VALUES

(1) Refractive power (Fig. 1)

The refractive power reduced from + 27.86 ± 1.85 (D) to + 24.86 ± 2.19 (D) immediately after the encircling operation. Thereafter the refractive power showed no marked change, and reached + 25.21 ± 1.51 (D) at three months after the encircling operation.

(2) Axial length (Fig. 2)

The axial length changed from 17.60 ± 0.56 (mm) to 18.42 ± 0.68 (mm) immediately after the encircling operation. Thereafter the axial length showed no marked change, and reached 18.69 ± 0.59 (mm) at three months after the encircling operation.

(3) Radius of corneal curvature (Fig. 3)

The radius of corneal curvature changed from 8.15 ± 0.34 (mm) to 8.09 ± 0.33 (mm) immediately after the encircling operation. Thereafter the radius showed no marked change, and reached 8.09 ± 0.32 (mm) at three months after the encircling operation.

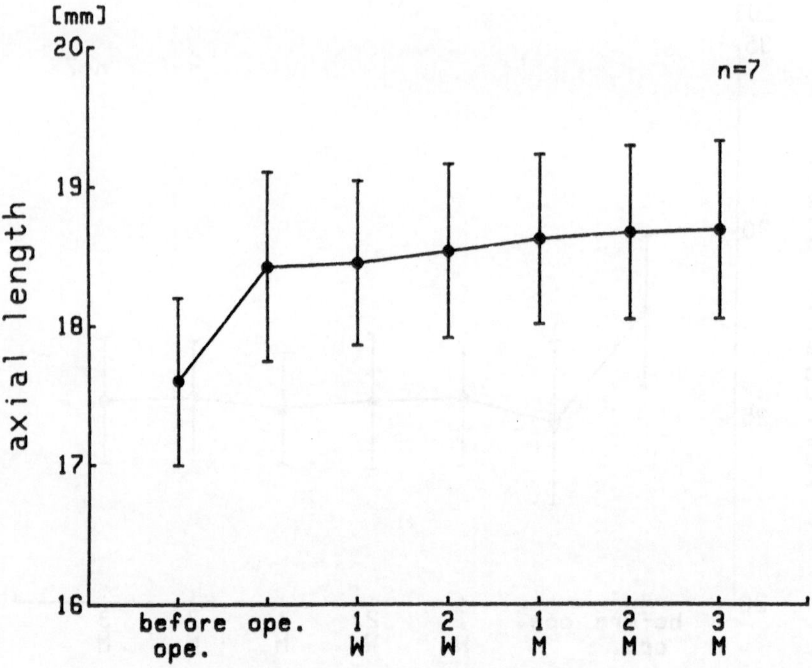

Fig. 2. Changes in axial length after encircling operations.

Correlation between the values

At three months after the encircling operation, the amount of changes in these three factors was found to be correlated.

Between changes in refractive power and those in axial length at three months after the encircling operation a strong correlation was proved, as shown in Fig. 4. The correlation coefficient was − 0.94.

Between changes in the radius of corneal curvature and those in refractive power at three months after the encircling operation a strong correlation was proved, as shown in Fig. 5. The correlation coefficient was 0.68.

Between changes in the radius of corneal curvature and those in axial length at three months after the encircling operation a strong correlation was proved, as shown in Fig. 6. The correlation coefficient was − 0.63.

DISCUSSION

Myopia or increase in myopia after an encircling operation for retinal detachment has been controversial. To clarify the true character of induced or increased myopia, changes in refractive power, axial length and the radius of corneal curvature were studied for six months after encircling operation with different tightness of 10%, 15% and 20% in adult pigmented rabbit

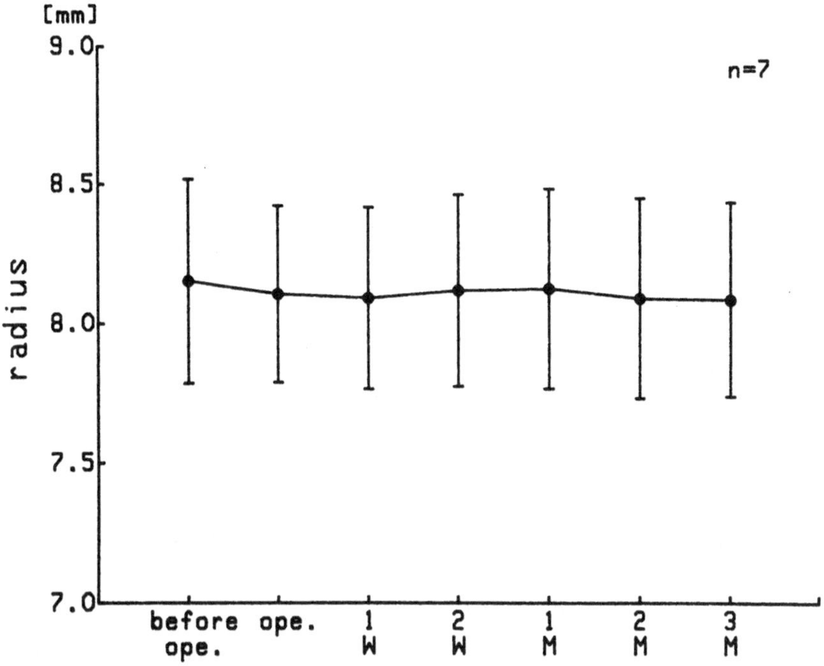

Fig. 3. Changes in radius of corneal curvature after encircling operations.

eyes. (Baba and Sawada, 1981). In those experiments, myopia developed markedly in proportion to the tightness of encirclement immediately after the operation, reduced with a relative rapidity during the first two weeks, thereafter, started to increase again and stopped increasing at two months. These changes were more pronounced in eyes in which the encirclement was more tightly done.

Changes in axial length showed almost the same variation as those in refractive power. Axial length is composed of corneal thickness, anterior chamber depth, lens thickness and vitreous length. From the results of changes in these components, it was suggested that forward shift of the lens after the encircling operation had some influence on changes in refractive power, while the radius of corneal curvature is the other important factor in deciding the refractive power.

To clarify the effect of lens in producing and increasing myopia, changes of refractive power, axial length and the radius of corneal curvature after encircling operation in artificial aphakic eyes were studied.

Changes in refractive power were observed immediately after the encircling operation. These changes were almost maintained at three months. (Fig. 1) Postoperative elongation of the axial length was most marked immediately after encirclement. The resulting changes were the same as in those in refractive power. (Fig. 2) The radius of corneal curvature was slightly reduced immediately after encirclement. Thereafter it did not vary. (Fig. 3)

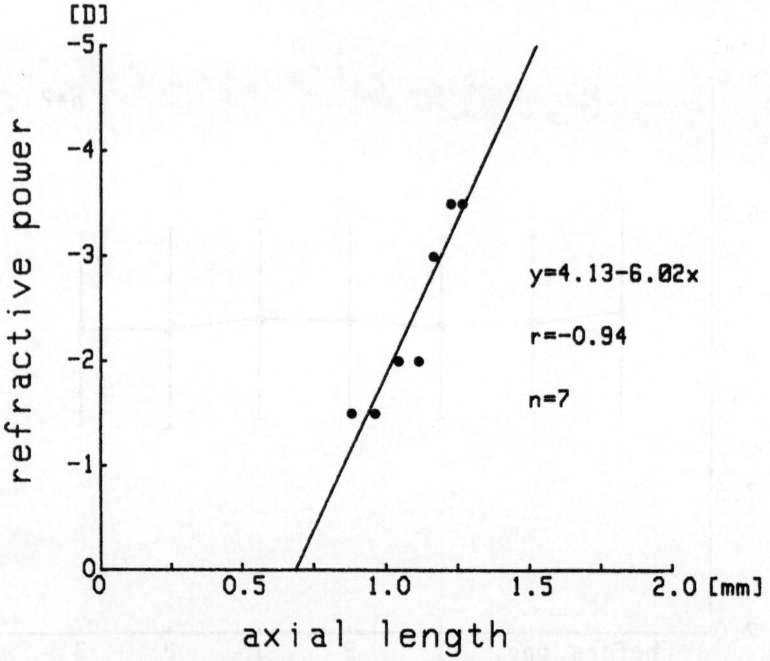

Fig. 4. Correlation between changes in reflective power and those in axial length three months after encircling operations.

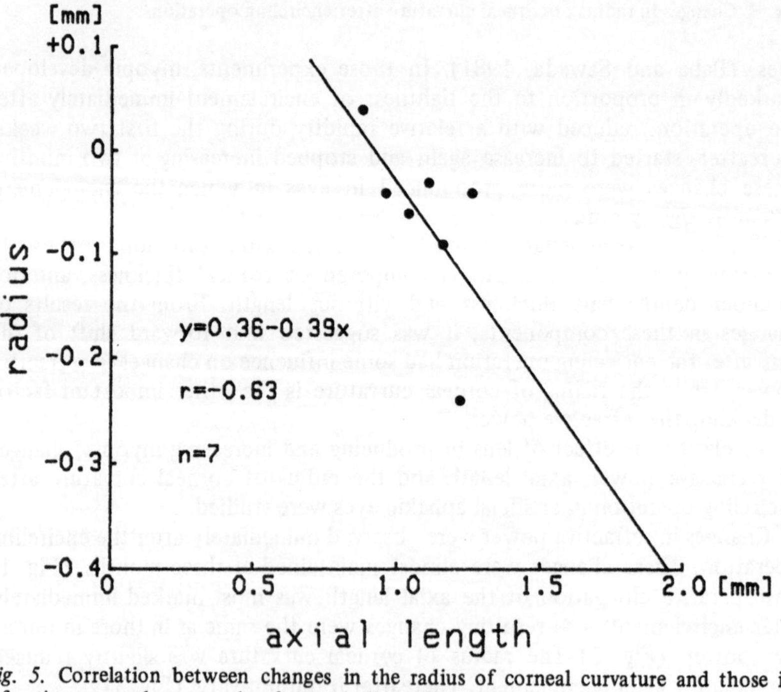

Fig. 5. Correlation between changes in the radius of corneal curvature and those in refractive power three months after encircling operations.

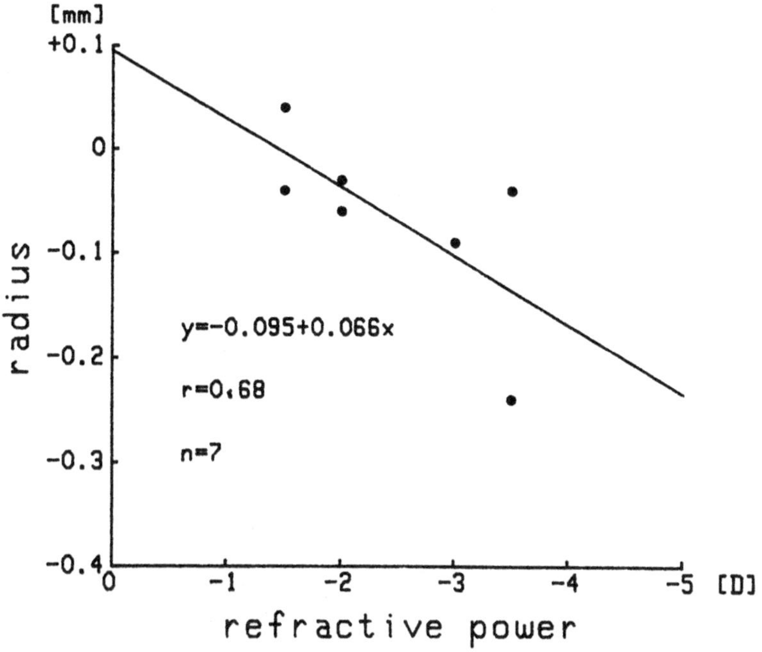

Fig. 6. Correlation between changes in ther radius of corneal curvature and those in axial length three months after encircling operations.

Changes in refractive power, axial length and the radius of corneal curvature in artificial aphakic eyes were quite different from those in phakic eyes, which were previously reported. Such differences are considered to result from the absence of the lens.

REFERENCES

Baba, Y. and Sawada, A. A study of experimental myopia after encircling operation. Doc. Ophthal. Proc. Series, Vol. 28, Third International Conference on Myopia (ed. Fledelius, H.C., Alsbirk, P.H. and Goldschmidt, E.) p. 177–185, Dr W. Junk, The Hague, 1981

Baba, Y. and Sawada, A. Ultrasonic study of axial length changes after encircling operation. Doc. Ophthal. Proc. Series, Vol. 29, Ultrasonography in Ophthalmology (ed. Thijssen, J.M. and Verbeek, A.M.) p. 197–203, Dr W. Junk, The Hague, 1981

Authors' address:
Department of Ophthalmology
Miyazaki Medical College
5200 Kihara
Kiyotake
Miyazaki 889-16
Japan

BIOMETRIC EVALUATION OF EYEBALL VOLUME CHANGES AFTER ENCIRCLING PROCEDURES

M. ZINGIRIAN, P. ROSSI, G. P. FAVA and A. POLIZZI
(Genova, Italy)

SUMMARY

By means of computer assisted analysis of B-scan images, the eyeball volume changes after encircling procedures are compared with the results obtained with an immersion non-echographic technique. The results and the reliability of the echographic measurements are discussed.

Echographic studies of the biometric eye parameters after surgery for retinal detachment have been previously reported (Baba et al., 1981; Burton et al., 1977; Clayman et al., 1981; Coleman, 1979; Fava et al., 1980; Fiore et al., 1970; Grignolo et al., 1973; Larsen et al., 1979; Levada et al., 1982) but disagreement exists among the findings.

The purpose of this work is to evaluate eyeball volume reductions obtained with cerclages of decreasing diameter and to check the reliability of "in vivo" echographic measurements after encircling procedures.

MATERIAL AND METHOD

The vitreous chamber of three calf eyes was filled with water using a vitreous infusion-suction-cutter system connected to a computerized unit for the automatic control of the I.O.P. (Surgikon-Optikon) (Fig. 1).

An equatorial cerclage was applied by means of a 4-0 silk thread, and the eyeball circumference was progressively reduced by 1 cm. steps, while keeping the I.O.P. at a steady level of 18 mmHg.

The eyeball volume was measured by two methods:

(1) Immersion, non echographic method.

The eyeball is immersed in a beaker containing 100 cc. of water. The eyeball volume is deduced by the amount of water needed to raise the liquid level to 200 cc.

Each measurement is repeated five times and the arithmetical mean is calculated.

Hillman, J. S./Le May, M. M. (eds.) Ophthalmic Ultrasonography

ISBN 978-94-009-7280-3.

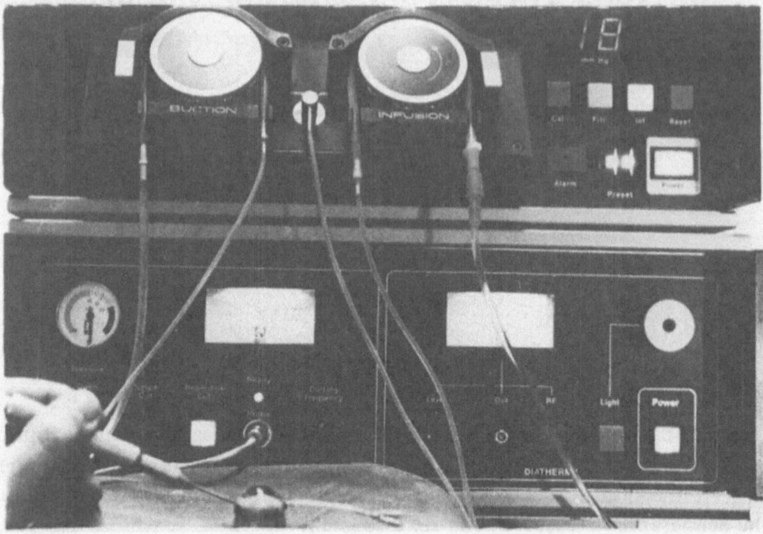

Fig. 1. **The infusion – suction system for the automatic control of the I.O.P.**

(2) Echographic method.

By means of an Ocuscan 400 an antero-posterior B-scan of the eye is obtained. The eyeball volume is evaluated by processing the echographic pattern using a digital image analyser (UDC 501 TESAK connected to a PDP 11/34 computer).

This device breaks down every image into many small squares and evaluates the mean luminance of each square. It is possible to know the number of squares whose mean luminance is included in any given interval. As the normal eyeball cavity is acoustically silent, except for the iris and the lens borders, the eyeball volume was calculated by the number of squares with a mean value between 0 and 5 in an arbitrary luminance scale (Fig. 2).

Five separate scans for each cerclage length in each eye were obtained and processed; the arithmetical mean and the percentage volume changes were calculated.

RESULTS

The eyeball volumes calculated with both the immersion and the echographic methods for cerclages of different lengths are presented in Fig. 3 and the corresponding measurements are also reported in Table 1.

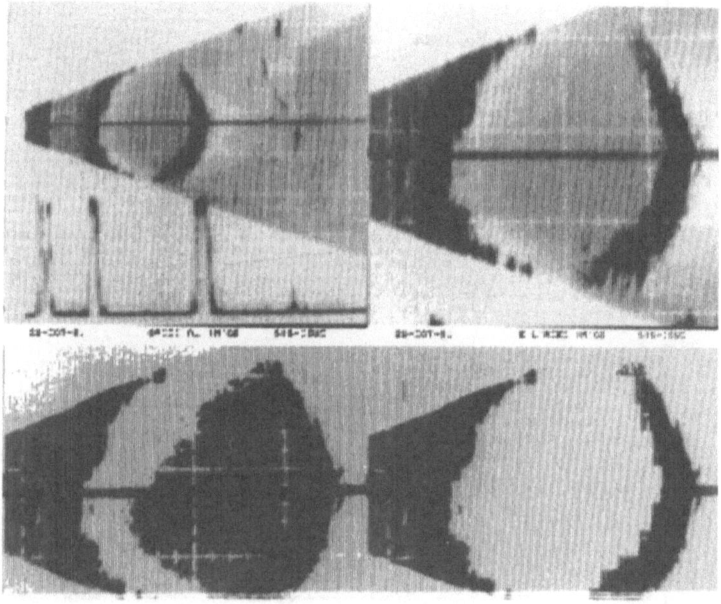

Fig. 2. The processing steps of the echographic image.

Table 1. The mean value of the eye volume corresponding to equatorial circumferences of different lengths are reported (volume expressed in c.c.). The volumes estimated with the echographic method (volume expressed as the number of low luminance squares) is reported in brackets

	INITIAL CIRCUMFERENCE (I.C.)	I.C. −10 MM.	I.C. −20 MM.	I.C. −30 MM.	I.C. −40 MM.
1ST EYE	26.4 ±3.1 (726)	24.2 ±2.9 (668)	19.3 ±2.0 (531)	15.6 ±1.6 (415)	14.1 ±1.5 (381)
2ND EYE	23.1 ±2.9 (631)	21.1 ±1.8 (576)	18.1 ±1.6 (489)	13.9 ±1.9 (380)	12.5 ±1.1 (321)
3RD EYE	25.1 ±2.1 (691)	23.9 ±2.1 (631)	16.9 ±1.1 (482)	13.5 ±2.1 (381)	12.1 ±1.4 (321)

CONSIDERATIONS

The data presented suggest some observations on the influence of equatorial cerclages on the eyeball volume and on the reliability of the echographic measurements.

1-Influence of cerclages on the eyeball volume

Progressive tightening of an equatorial cerclage results in a progressive reduction in eyeball volume. The most efficient volume reduction is achieved with

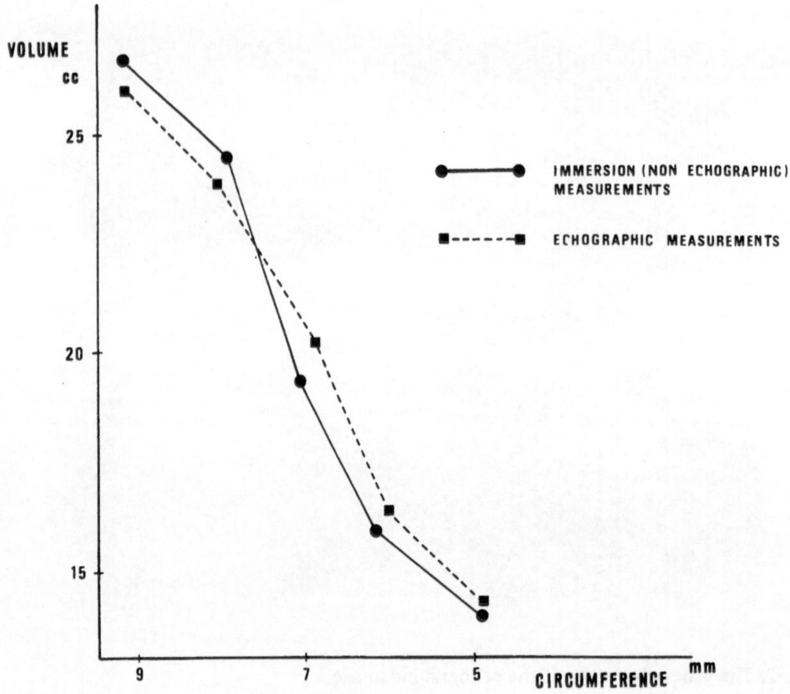

Fig. 3. A comparison of echographic and immersion (non-echographic) measurements of eye volume changes after different amounts of cerclage.

initial tightening: maximal effectiveness is obtained when the eyeball circumference is reduced to about 3/4 of its original length. Further tightening of the cerclage causes progressively decreasing volume reductions.

2-Reliability of echographic measurements

The computer-assisted digital analysis of the B-scans was used to obtain a percentage assessment of the eyeball volume changes, not to calculate its actual volume.

In this respect, echographic measurements were found to be quite reliable and the estimated changes of the eyeball volume correlated well with those obtained with the immersion method, differences being usually less than 5%. Therefore, computerized analysis of B-scans can be used for "in vivo" estimations of eyeball changes after encircling procedures.

CONCLUSIONS

Equatorial cerclages attain their greatest effect on eyeball volume when the eyeball circumference is reduced to about 3/4 of its initial value: further tightening of the cerclage leads to progressively decreasing volume reductions.

Computerized analysis of a B-scan of the eyeball allows for a fairly reliable method of estimating "in vivo" percentage reductions in eyeball volume.

ACKNOWLEDGEMENT

This work was supported by a grant from the Consiglio Nazionale Delle Ricerche, Italy.

REFERENCES

1. Baba, Y.; Sawada, A. Ultrasonic study of axial length changes after encircling operation. Doc. Ophthalmol. Proc. 29–197–203, 1981.
2. Burton, T. C.; Herron, B. E.; Ossoinig, K. C. Axial length changes after retinal detachment surgery. Am. J. Ophthalmol. 83:59, 1977.
3. Clayman, H. M.; Jaffe, N. S.; Light, D. S.; Jaffe, M. S.; Cassady, J. C. Intraocular lenses, axial length, and retinal detachment. Am. J. Ophthalmol. 92:778–780, 1981.
4. Coleman, D. J. Ultrasonic measurement of eye dimensions. Int. Ophthalmol. Clin. 19(4):225–236, 1979.
5. Fava, G. P.; Rossi, P. L.; Ciurlo, G.; Zingirian, M. Valutazione ecografica delle variazioni biometriche conseguenti ad intervento per distacco di retina. Atti 5° Congr. Naz. S.I.S.U.M. Milano, 1980, pp. 265–270.
6. Fiore, J. V. Jr.; Newton, J. C. Anterior segment changes following the scleral buckling procedures. Arch. Ophthalmol. 84:284–287, 1970.
7. Grignolo, A.; Rivara, A.; Zingirian, M. Evaluation of errors of optical and ultrasound methods employed in ocular biometry. 2nd World Congress on Ultrasonic in Medicine. Amsterdam, 1973.
8. Larsen, J. S.; Syrdalen, P. Ultrasonographic study on changes in axial eye dimensions after encircling procedure in retinal detachment surgery. Acta Ophthalmol. 57: 337–343, 1979.
9. Levada, A.; Blumenkranz, M. S. Biometric alterations in the globe following scleral buckling. Invest. Ophthalmol. Visual Sci. 22 (suppl. ARVO):53, 1982.

Authors' address:
University Eye Clinic
Viale Benedetto XV 5
16132 Genova
Italy

REAL-TIME IMAGING OF BLOOD VESSELS WITHIN OCULAR TUMORS AND THE ORBIT

ALAN L. SUSAL
(Stanford, USA)

ABSTRACT

Blood vessels and vascular pulse phenomena within the eye and the orbit can now be imaged in real-time. A newly-developed electronically-scanned array system enables the vascular observations to be made at 60 frames per second with the results viewed on a television screen. Within the orbit the ophthalmic artery and its major branches are imaged in A- and B-modes. Regions of orbital inflammation are highlighted by the increased vascular pulsatile appearance they exhibit. Blood vessels within ocular tumors can also be viewed with the new equipment. The number, size and distribution of the vessels aids in determining a more accurate ultrasonic tumor diagnosis.

INTRODUCTION

It is now possible to image ocular arteries and veins with real-time ultrasound. The imaging of ocular vessels and associated regions of vascular pulsations has clinical applications in the detection of tumors, identification of ocular tissue types and the localization of regions of orbital inflammation. These studies are possible as a result of newly-developed, electronically-scanned ultrasonic systems which possess higher sensitivity and greater picture stability compared to contemporary apparatus.

METHODS

Electronically scanned, multiple transducer array systems (Fig. 1) enable ocular blood vessels to be imaged in-vivo on a television display and the examination to be directly recorded on videotape. (Susal et al. 1980) By electronically switching 35 elements in a linear array transducer, a 60 frame-per-second image is produced without any of the instability associated with mechanically-scanned single transducer apparatus. The stable display (also without scanning flicker) provides a television image which allows ocular vessels to be viewed in A- and B-modes (Fig. 2).

Hillman, J.S./Le May, M.M. (eds.) Ophthalmic Ultrasonography

ISBN 978-94-009-7280-3.

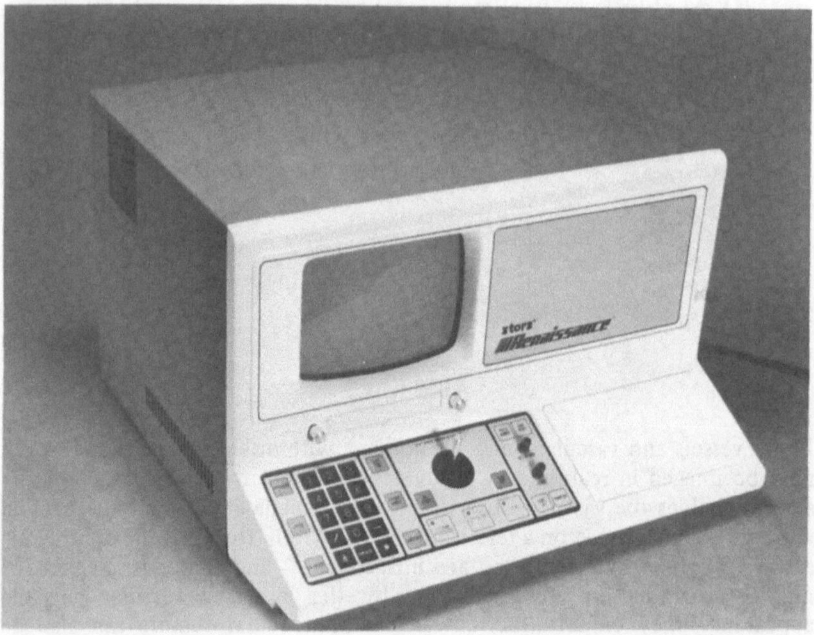

Fig. 1. Computer controlled, electronically-scanned ultrasonic system used for making real-time vascular observations. Simultaneous A- and B-mode images are presented on the 22 cm television display.

For blood vessel studies, it is important to hold the transducer as steady as possible in relation to the patient's eye. The patient is also told to hold his eye still while the physician studies the real-time display. Any extraneous movement distracts from observing the subtle pulsations of the blood vessels. We usually employ a water-immersion bath to provide greater sensitivity with blood vessel studies but have found contact scanning on the closed eyelids or direct transducer contact on the cornea or sclera will also image these vessels.

A valsalva maneuver is used to detect abnormal venous channels while performing the real-time sonography. (Dadd et al 1978) The valsalva maneuver will balloon out abnormal veins and vessels associated with A-V fistulas. It may also cause a noticeable compression of the orbital fat in venous dependent pathology.

RESULTS

The larger orbital arteries can be directly imaged as expanding and contracting tubular structures on the real-time display. The 7.2 MHz operating frequency of the linear-array transducer gives an axial resolution of better than 0.5 mm. The dynamic lateral resolution of the system is approximately

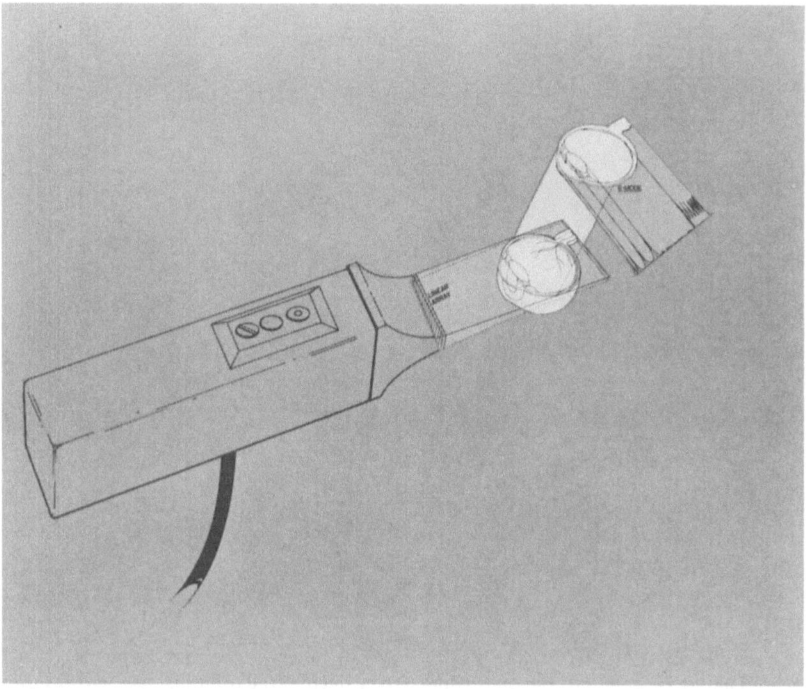

Fig. 2. Schematic representation of the hand-held probe with a 35 element transducer which is electronically switched to give 60 independent ultrasonic images per second in both A- and B-modes.

1.0 mm making it easier to detect vessels with a path perpendicular to the optic nerve. The ophthalmic artery and some of its immediate branches are usually well imaged (Fig. 3) as they cross over the optic nerve from the lateral to the nasal orbit.

Small vessels are identified by the expansile pertubations they cause in surrounding ocular tissues. These surrounding tissues are normally quiescent making it easy to identify the concentric expansion and contraction that small vessels cause in them. These pulsations are noted to by synchronous with the pulse. Even small vessels, such as the posterior ciliary arteries, arterial arcades of the lid and blood vessels within ocular neoplasms are identified in this manner. (Susal 1981)

Areas of orbital inflammation cause an enhanced vascular pulse phenomenon where the pulsations of the larger vessels are transmitted throughout a region of normally quiescent orbital fat or muscle. Thus, a region affected with orbital inflammation will be easily highlighted and outlined using real-time ultrasound (Fig. 4). It will appear to pulsate en-mass as compared to the static surrounding orbital tissue. This is probably due to inflammatory edema which permeates the inflamed tissues and (being incompressible) transmits pulsations from active blood vessels in the affected region to the infiltrated tissues.

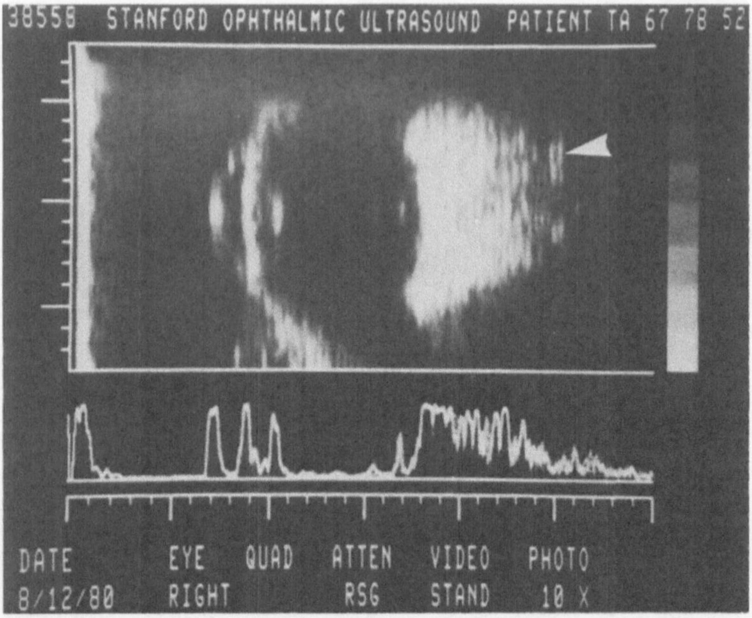

Fig. 3. The arrow points to the ophthalmic artery deep in the orbit just as it crosses over the optic nerve. Pulsations from the artery were readily distinguished on the real-time display.

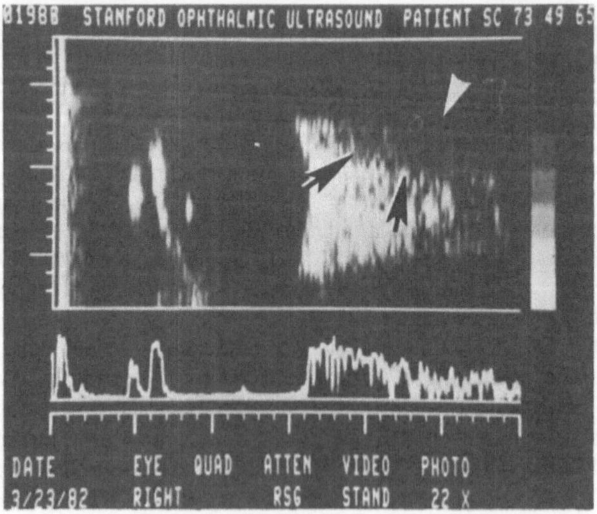

Fig. 4. The arrows point to regions of inflammatory infiltration of the orbit demonstrating transmitted vascular pulsations (thyroid ophthalmopathy).

DISCUSSION

We now have the ability to detect the number and distribution of blood vessels within ocular tumors to help us determine a more accurate tissue diagnosis. A better differential diagnosis is possible by noting the vascular activity in the tumor. For example, fibrotic lesions tend to be quiescent and display little vascularity (Fig. 5). Orbital neoplasms exhibit a variable degree of vascular activity with malignant melanomata and retinoblastomas occasionally showing small active vessels from their interior (Fig. 6). Thus, it has been possible to differentiate malignant melanomata from solid, elevated disciform macular lesions and to distinguish retinoblastomas from inflammatory-gliotic lesions by noting the presence or absence of blood vessels within the tumors. In cavernous hemangiomas, the active vessels within the tumor make this neoplasm particularly identifiable with real-time imaging.

Real-time sonography also enables us to detect rapid growing new blood vessels. These vessels appear primarily in metastatic lesions. The interior of these tumors gives a continuous changing, writhing appearance which may be out of synchrony with the cardiac cycle. These observations are thought to be due to the presence of active vascular channels. Dyssynchronous pulsations are particularly associated with rapid growing neoplasms and are presumed to be simultaneous observations of arterial and venous blood channels as well as delayed pulse phenomenon from elastic new blood vessels.

Orbital inflammation has been easier to detect and evaluate with real-time ultrasound due to the enhanced vascular pulsatile phenomenon demonstrated in the affected region. This enables the sonographer to identify orbital fat and muscle involvement in thyroid ophthalmopathy, orbital myositis, and orbital pseudotumors. It also makes it easier to detect optic neuritis and posterior scleritis where localized regions of abnormal vascular pulsations exist adjacent to the affected tissues.

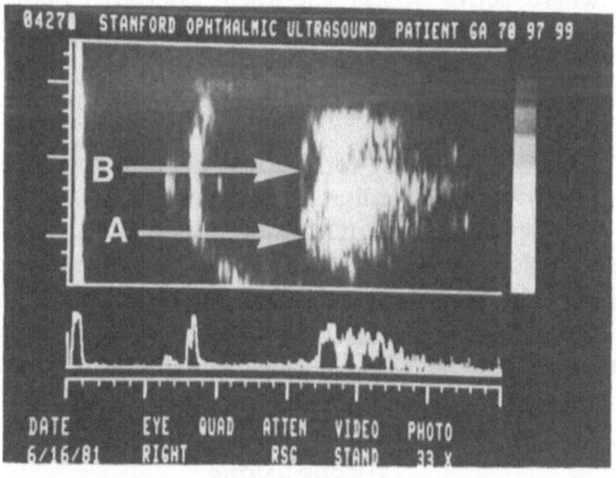

Fig. 5. Solid elevated inflammatory macular lesion (A) with adjacent posterior vitreous hyaloid detachment (B) No vessels were seen in the interior of this mass. It resolved spontaneously.

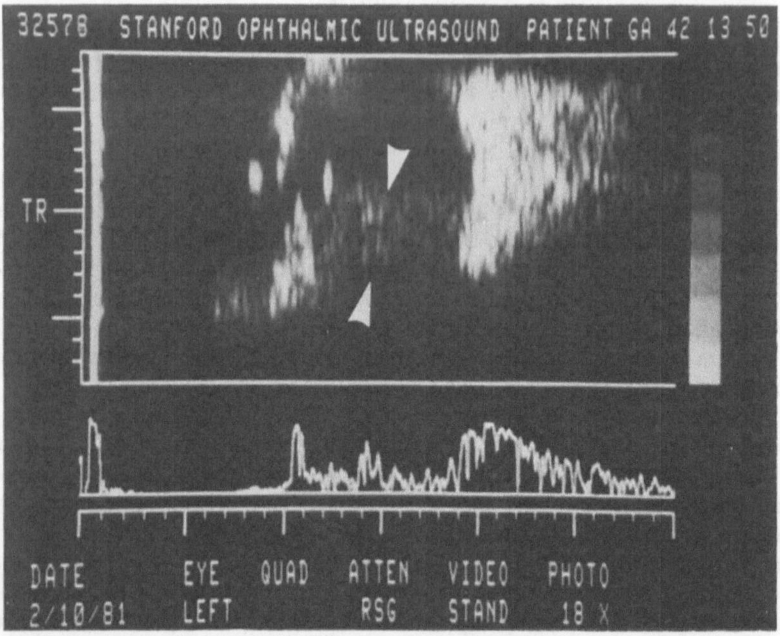

Fig. 6. Solid intraocular neoplasm. This malignant melanoma showed a few small arteries in its interior which helped to distinguish its neoplastic nature.

Identification of the ophthalmic artery and its branches helps to localize orbital pathology and gives a better understanding of the physiology of the orbital region. Computerized tomography, although complementary to ocular ultrasound, does not possess the powerful advantage of real-time sonography where active vessels and their associated pulse phenomenon can be used to gain more comprehensive clinical information.

CONCLUSION

The ability to detect and study for the first time the presence of small and large blood vessels and their pulsatile phenomenon in ocular tissues opens a new vista in diagnostic ultrasound. New ultrasound apparatus employing advanced electronic technology enables the sonographer to study and dynamically record observations of blood vessels in several ocular tissues. Although a definitive tissue diagnosis cannot be made with real-time sonography alone, these techniques will enhance our ability to provide an accurate noninvasive assessment of the condition.

REFERENCES

Dadd, M.; Hughes, H.; Kossoff, G.: Ultrasonic examination of orbital vasculature. Jour. Clin. Ultrasound 6:36–40, 1978

Susal, A.L.; Walker, J.T. and Meindl, J.D.: Small organ dynamic imaging system. Jour. Clin. Ultrasound 8:421–426, 1980.
Susal, A.L.: Vascular studies of the orbital cavity. Ophthalmol. 88:6:548–551, 1981.

Authors' address:
Division of Ophthalmology A-227
Stanford University Medical Center
Stanford, CA 94305
USA

ULTRASONIC IMAGING OF ORBITAL TUMORS

SONG GUO-XIANG
(*Tianjin, China*)

Since the early sixties, the technique of ultrasonic imaging has been employed in the diagnosis of orbital tumors (Baum and Greenwood 1960). In the seventies, many kinds of special ophthalmic instruments became available and have been widely used in ophthalmology. Because this technique can provide a tomographic picture of orbital soft tissue, it has already become indispensable in the diagnosis of orbital tumors.

MATERIALS AND METHODS

From July, 1979 to December, 1981, 183 cases of orbital tumors were scanned in our hospital by the ultrasonic imaging technique and were later confirmed by pathological examination. The diagnosis and ultrasonic findings are shown in table 1.

Table 1. Diagnosis and ultrasonic findings in 183 cases of proved orbital tumors

Diagnoses	No. of cases	Ultrasonic findings	
		Abnormal	Normal
Hemangioma and lymphangioma	32	32	–
Pseudotumor and other granulomas	30	30	–
Secondary tumors	19	18	1
Dermoid cyst	14	14	–
Mucocele	14	14	–
Neurilemmoma	13	12	1
Lacrimal gland epithelial tumors	13	13	–
Hematoma	9	9	–
Metastatic cancers	9	8	1
Varix	8	8	–
Primary meningioma	6	6	–
Fibrous histiocytoma	4	4	–
Optic nerve glioma	3	3	–
Other tumors	9	9	–
Total	183	180	3

Hillman, J. S./Le May, M. M. (eds.) Ophthalmic Ultrasonography

ISBN 978-94-009-7280-3.

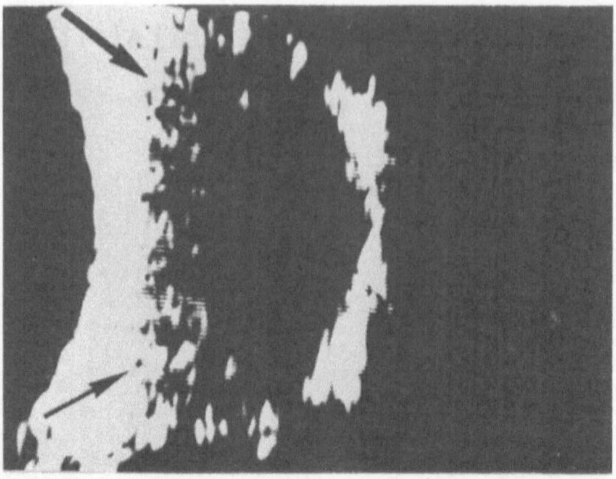

Fig. 1. **B-scan ultrasonogram of a neurilemmoma located in the muscle cone, demonstrating a comparatively poor echo area in the rectrobulbar echo pattern.**

Ophthalmic contact B-scan ultrasonography is used with a 10 MHz transducer. The patient is supine, with the eye naturally closed. Liquid paraffin or methylcellulose is used as contact medium. When the scanner is held in contact with the patient's eyelids, a tomographic image of the orbit is displayed on the screen of the monitor. The scanner is then moved upwards and downwards, changing the angle of incidence simultaneously. After sagittal scanning, the scanner is put on the patient's eyelid transversely to obtain a cross-section of the orbit. As soon as the lesion is found, it is advisable to examine this area from different sites, to recognise the location, shape, size, border, internal echoes and sound transmission of the lesion and secondary changes such as deformation of the eyeball and displacement of the optic nerve etc can be noted. The scanner is then pressed upon the globe in order to apply pressure indirectly on the lesion, and to observe any change in shape of the tumor. In patients with exophthalmos, in the absence of any space-occupying lesion, attention must be paid to changes in the extraocular muscles and orbital vessels, since orbital inflammation or vascular malformations can cause the similar clinical features.

In addition to conventional B-scan examination, it is important to compare examination with the contralateral orbit, with A-scan ultrasonography and with the information resulting from other examinations.

RESULTS

In the 183 cases of our series, space-occupying lesions were displayed by B-scan ultrasonography in 180 cases (98.4%), there were three false negatives in which tumors were situated in the apex of the orbit or on the orbital bony wall. Of all the positive findings, three basic echo patterns could be seen: (1) a comparatively weak or echo-free area in the retrobulbar echo pattern, representing a mass lesion in the muscle cone (Fig. 1); (2) A deformed

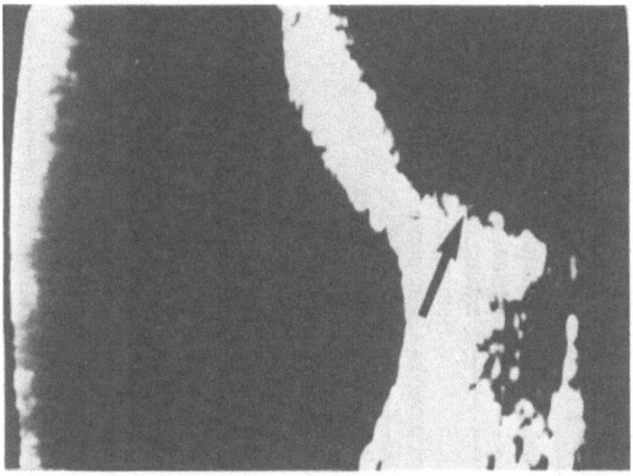

Fig. 2. B-scan ultrasonogram of an osteoma outside the muscle cone showing the deformation of the orbital echo pattern.

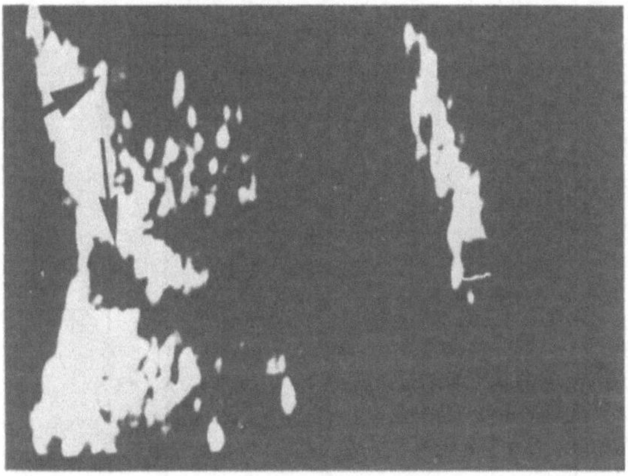

Fig. 3. B-scan ultrasonogram of a lacrimal gland adenocystic carcinoma demonstrating displacement of the optic nerve downward.

orbital echo pattern, usually due to tumor outside the muscle cone (Fig. 2); (3) deformation or displacement of the normal orbital structures, such as flattening of the posterior pole of the globe, enlargement of the extraocular muscle or displacement of optic nerve (Fig. 3). Each group of tumors has its special characteristic pattern as shown in table 2.

DISCUSSION

Most intraorbital tumors are situated behind the eyeball. In the early stages no symptoms and signs are present except unilateral exophthalmos. X-ray is

Table 2. Echo patterns of 180 cases of orbital tumors

Pattern	Shape	Border	Internal echoes	Sound transmission	Compressibility	Other ultrasonic information	Diagnoses
			More and strong	Fair	Medium	In muscle cone	Cavernous hemangioma
				Fair	Strong	upper part of the orbit	Dermoid cyst
			Fair	Fair	Poor	In lacrimal fossa	Lacrimal gland mixed tumor
		Clear-cut and smooth					Neurilemmoma
			Poor	Fair to good	Poor		Hemangiopericytoma
						Enlargement of optic nerve	Optic nerve glioma
						Defect of bone wall	Mucocele
	Round or oval					Upper part of orbit	Dermoid cyst
Mass lesion			None to poor	Good	Strong	Traumatic history	Hematoma
							Simple cyst
						In lacrimal fossa	Lacrimal gland carcinoma
		Irregular	Poor	Weak	None	Surrounded the optic nerve	Primary orbital meningioma
							Fibrous histiocytoma
							Pseudotumor
			Poor	Weak	None	Defect of bone wall	Secondary carcinoma
	Irregular	Irregular				Cancer history	Metastatic cancers
			Echo-free cavity	Good	Very strong	Pulsating echo-free cavity	Cirsoid hemangioma
						Positional	Varix
							Osteoma
	Display anterior margin	Clear-cut	None	None	None	Strong reflectivity	Psammomatous meningioma

of diagnostic significance only at the later stage. Although examination with contrast medium and angiography can demonstrate early mass lesion, these investigations are painful and harmful. The orbital examination technique has been improved by the application of B-scan ultrasonography. This technique causes no pain with a diagnosis rate up to 88% (Lloyd 1977). In our series, all the 183 cases except three gave positive results (98.4%).

At the present time, ultrasonic imaging can only reveal the gross texture of the lesion and does not show the histologic picture. According to the morphology and sound transmission of the lesion, Coleman (1972) classified orbital mass lesions into 4 categories: solid tumor; cystic tumor; angiomatous tumor; and infiltrative tumor. On the basis of an analysis of the echo patterns of 180 patients with orbital tumors in our study, considering the shape, border, internal echoes, sound transmission, compressibility and location of the tumors, it is believed that the ultrasonic differential diagnosis can be further improved as shown in table 2.

Although B-scan is able to reveal the nature of a mass lesion to some extent, the condition is complex. The echo pattern is affected by many factors.

The shape of the lesion is of some value in distinguishing the nature of the tumor. A benign tumor is enlarged in all directions equally within the orbit where little restriction is present. On echo pattern it may be exhibited as a round or oval image. Conversely, a malignant neoplasms or pseudotumors are expanded in a non-uniform fashion and the echo pattern can be irregular in shape. In a vascular lesion such as a varix no definite contour is formed. In practice it is possible to meet with some difficulties in judging the shape of mass lesions. Because of the limited scanning field, we are unable to get a complete view on sectioning. In some tumors the sound energy is absorbed in the anterior layers and is unable to penetrate through them to show the posterior margin. Under such circumstances, it is impossible to demonstrate the accurate shape of the tumor. The demonstrable shape of a tumor should not be regarded as the main diagnostic feature, but only regarded as a reference in differential diagnosis of orbital tumors.

Two types of tumor border are identified: sharp or unclear; smooth or irregular. A benign tumor is encapsulated with a fibrous membrane which has a markedly different sound impedence from the surrounding orbital fat. On ultrasonography, it exhibits a sharp and smooth border. Malignant tumors and pseudotumors show an infiltrative edge. There is no clear-cut boundary between the tumor and normal tisses on echo pattern.

The internal echoes represent the sound structure of the lesion, that is the number, size, orientation and distribution of the reflection interfaces, as well as the strength of ultrasonic reflection of the tumor. For example, a cavernous hemangioma is composed of many blood sinuses which can cause strong reflection, therefore, its internal echoes are strong and plentiful (Fig. 4). On the contrary, a mucocele which is filled with fluid has no internal reflective interface, showing as an echo-free area (Fig. 5). Besides the acoustic nature of the tumor itself, the internal echo of the lesion is influenced by other factors, such as the resolution and sensitivity of the apparatus, the scanning location, incidence angle, the depth in which the tumor lies and the sound

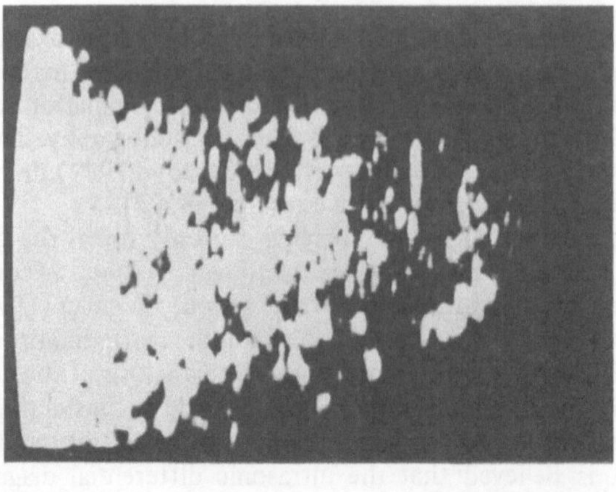

Fig. 4. **B-scan ultrasonogram of a cavernous hemangioma showing strong internal echoes.**

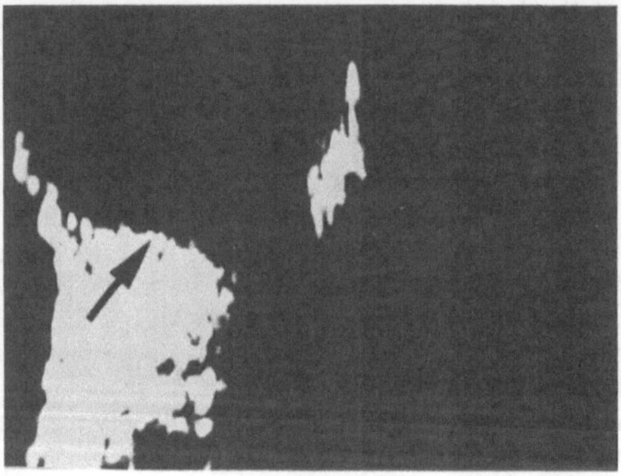

Fig. 5. **B-scan ultrasonogram of a mucocele showing no internal echo.**

absorption taking place between the scanner and the tumor. The higher the resolution and sensitivity of the apparatus, the more plentiful and stronger the echoes. The deeper the tumor is located and the more sound absorption there is between the scanner and tumor, the poorer are the internal echoes. Using the same instrument to examine similar tumors at similar depths; in a patient with severe old trachoma, with a cavernous hemangioma in his orbit, the internal echoes of the tumor were very poor because the sound energy was greatly absorbed by the heavily scarred eyelid.

Sound transmission at identical frequencies is mainly determined by the nature and fashion of the structure of the lesion. A tumor containing a greater amount of fibrous tissues without regular arrangement may absorb

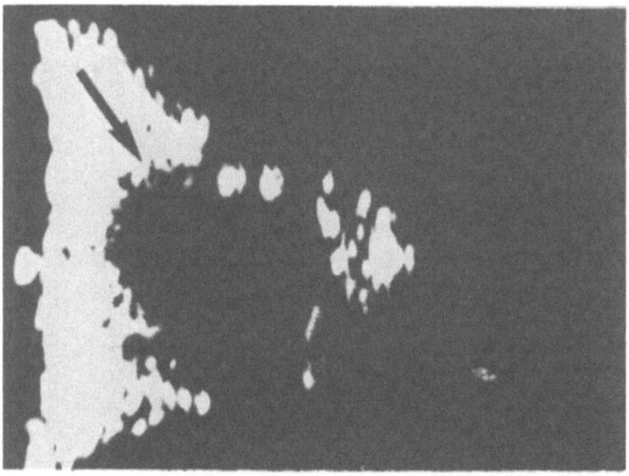

Fig. 6. B-scan ultrasonogram of an optic nerve glioma showing that the tumor is the optic nerve itself.

a lot of sound energy and the sound transmission is poor, while a fluid-containing cyst has good sound transmission. In an osteoma or psammomatous meningioma, owing to the marked difference of the sound impedance between adjacent tissues, the majority of ultrasound is reflected back and hence only the anterior margin of the tumor may be shown.

A test of compressibility of the tumor will aid much in evaluating the consistency of the tumor. Cysts and varices alter markedly as the scanner presses upon the globe. Pressure seems to have little effect upon the contour of hard growths, such as carcinoma, meningioma and pseudotumor.

On analysing echo patterns, attention should be paid to the location of the tumor and its relation to normal structures. For instance, optic nerve glioma is a tumor originated from the involved nerve itself (Fig. 6); growths in the lacrimal fossa often arise from lacrimal gland; cystic tumors of the upper orbit are mostly a dermoid cysts.

SUMMARY

An analysis of the echo patterns of 183 cases or orbital tumors with discussion on various factors affecting the echo pattern is presented in this paper. Positive ultrasonic findings were obtained in 180 cases (98.4%). In another three cases, the tumors were situated in the apex of the orbit or on the orbital bony wall.

REFERENCES

Baum, G. and Greenwood, I. Ultrasound in ophthalmology. Am. J. Ophthalmol. 49:249 (1960).

Lloyd, G. A. S. The impact of CT scanning and ultrasonography on orbital diagnosis. Clin. Radio. 28:583 (1977).
Coleman, D. J. Reliability of ocular and orbital diagnosis with B-scan ultrasound. Am. J. Ophthalmol. 74:704 (1972).

Author's address:
Dept. of Ophthalmology
Teaching Hospital of Tianjin Medical College
Tianjin
People's Republic of China

STANDARDIZED ECHOGRAPHY IN THE DIAGNOSIS OF HEMANGIOENDOTHELIOMA

SANDRA FRAZIER BYRNE
(Miami, USA)

Standardized echography (combined standardized A-scan – Kretztechnik 7200MA, contact B-scan, and Doppler instrumentation) is a highly useful modality for the detection and characterization of orbital lesions [7]. Approximately seventy entities or groups of lesions may be differentiated, ten of which are vascular neoplasms or malformations [8]. The rarest of these vascular entities is a group comprising capillary hemangioma, hemangiopericytoma, hemangioendothelioma, angiofibroma and angiosarcoma, which echographically cannot be distinguished one from another [8]. This paper specifically addresses one case of hemangioendothelioma and its acoustic characteristics.

CASE REPORT

A 49 year old white female was referred to Bascom Palmer Eye Institute for evaluation. For the past year she had complained of right upper lid ptosis, lid swelling and epiphora. On examination, visual activity was 20/20 in both eyes and Hertel exophthalmometry yielded 1.5 mm. of right proptosis. Two millimeters of right ptosis was present and ocular motility was full.

CT EXAMINATION

High resolution CT scan views of the orbits (with contrast media) were performed using the GE 8800. Coronal sections demonstrated a localized, enhancing mass of non-specific nature in the superior, nasal aspect of the right orbit (Fig. 1). Axial CT sections failed to display the mass adequately.

STANDARDIZED ECHOGRAPHIC EVALUATION

Prior to excision, the patient was referred for a preoperative evaluation with standardized echography. The mass was quickly detected with standardized A-scan basic examination techniques. 'Special examination techniques'

Hillman, J. S./Le May, M. M. (eds.) Ophthalmic Ultrasonography
© 1983, Dr W. Junk Publishers, The Hague/Boston/Lancaster.
ISBN 978-94-009-7280-3.

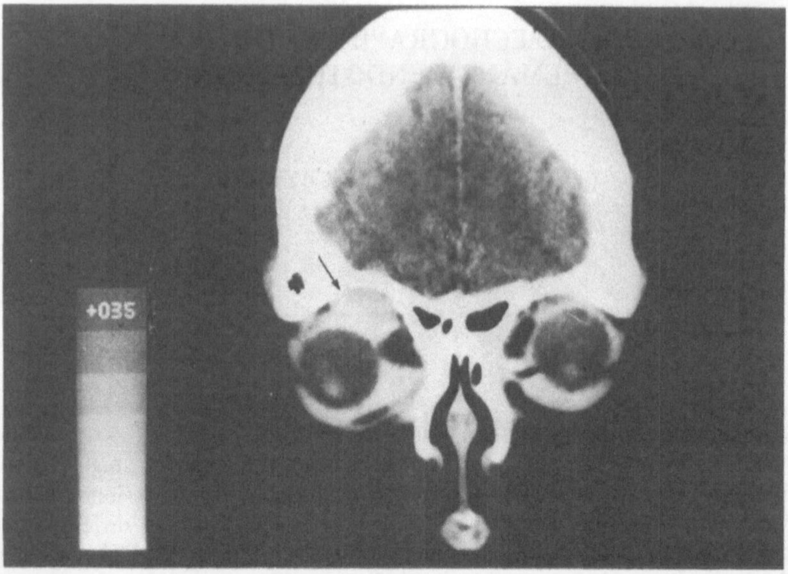

Fig. 1. **Coronal CT scan of lesion in the right orbit (arrow). The mass is enhanced by contrast medium.**

Table 1. **Special examination techniques for orbital diagnosis**

Acoustic information	Equipment used*
Internal Structure	A
Internal Reflectivity	A
Sound Attenuation	A
Location	A·B
Shape	B·A
Border Type	A
Consistency	A
Vascularity	A·D

*A: *Standardized* A-scan (Kretztechnik 7200 MA)
B: Contact B-scan
D: Doppler instrumentation

This Table details the acoustic information necessary for making reliable differential diagnoses. Standardized A-scan, contact B-scan and Doppler instrumentation should be used as listed above to achieve optimal results.

[1, 2, 6] (quantitative, topographic, and kinetic echography) were applied for lesion differentiation (Table 1).

SPECIAL EXAMINATION TECHNIQUES

Using the 'tissue sensitivity setting' [5, 9] of the standardized A-scan, quantitative echography demonstrated a regularly structured, homogeneous mass of low internal reflectivity (uniform, low spikes) (Fig. 2). The angle kappa, defined as the angle formed by an imaginery line drawn through the peaks

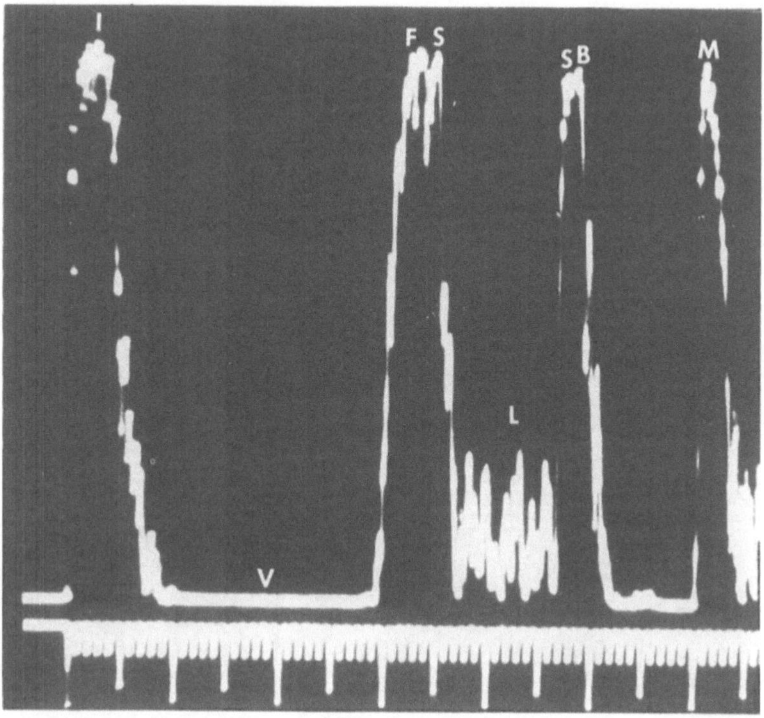

Fig. 2. Transocular A-scan of tumor at the tissue sensitivity setting. I = initial spike corresponding to probe tip, V = vitreous, F = fundus signals, S = tumor surfaces, L = internal lesion spikes, B = bone spike, M = multiple reverberation (artifact).

of the internal lesion spikes and its intersection with the baseline, was low (less than 30 degrees).

Topographic techniques were next applied for determination of location, shape and border type. Both the transocular approach (sound beam through globe) and paraocular orientation (sound beam next to globe) were utilized. The A-scan sound beam was directed through the superior orbital tissues, demonstrating the mass between 11:30 and 1:30 o'clock, in the more anterior orbit. By combining the lesion's maximal width of 9 mm. (transocular) with its maximal depth of 22 mm. (paraocular), the A-scan method revealed its ovoid shape. B-scan was applied for documentation of these findings (Fig. 3).

Evaluation of border type was achieved with the standardized A-scan using the paraocular approach. This orientation was essential in obtaining perpendicular anteroposterior beam exposure to the lesion's posterior surface (thus avoiding spike confusion with the orbital roof). With this technique, a smooth, relatively high, double peaked surface spike was displayed, indicating a well outlined mass (thin capsule)(Fig. 4). Cysts produce a more steeply rising, higher posterior surface spike with wide double peak [6].

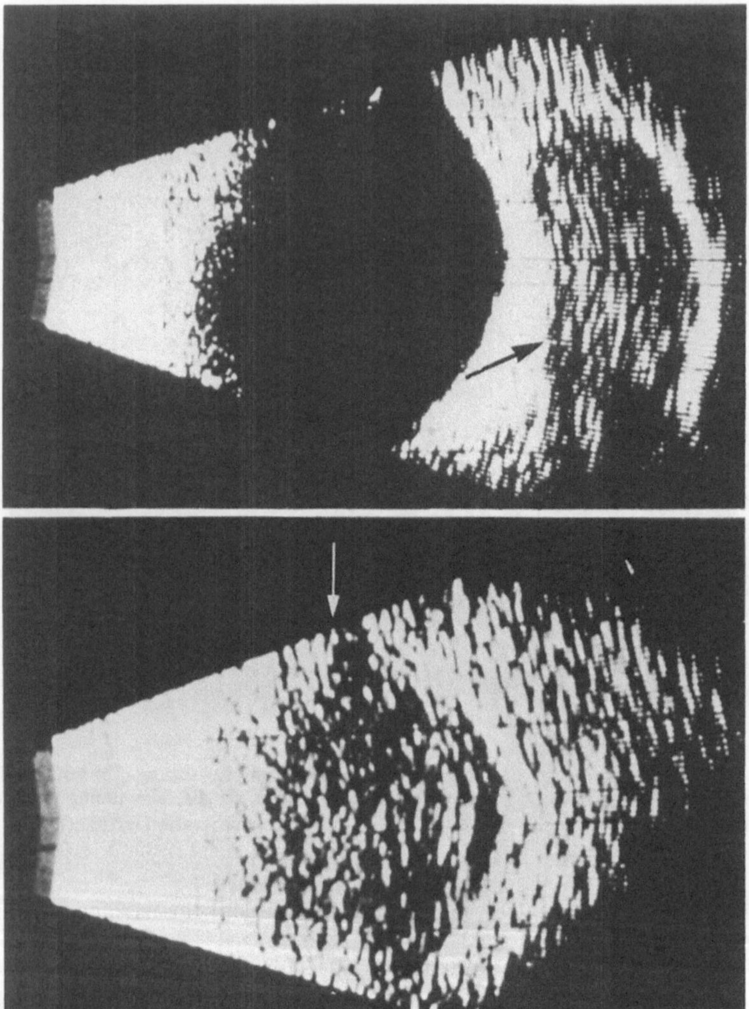

Fig. 3. B-scans of transocular (top) and paraocular (bottom) views of lesion. The transocular section shows its oval shape horizontally and the paraocular its rounded shape in anteroposterior section.

The final aspect of the differentiation process was kinetic evaluation to determine consistency (compressibility) and vascularity (blood flow). The consistency of the mass was evaluated with the standardized A-scan by the transocular method. The lesion was first displayed in its maximal width by directing the sound beam through its center. Pressure was then exerted by the probe against the globe and in turn against the lesion. Only minimal decrease in lesion width was noted during this maneuver, indicating firm consistency. With soft lesions, the lesion pattern narrows during compression testing while hard lesions show no narrowing of the pattern (Fig. 5).

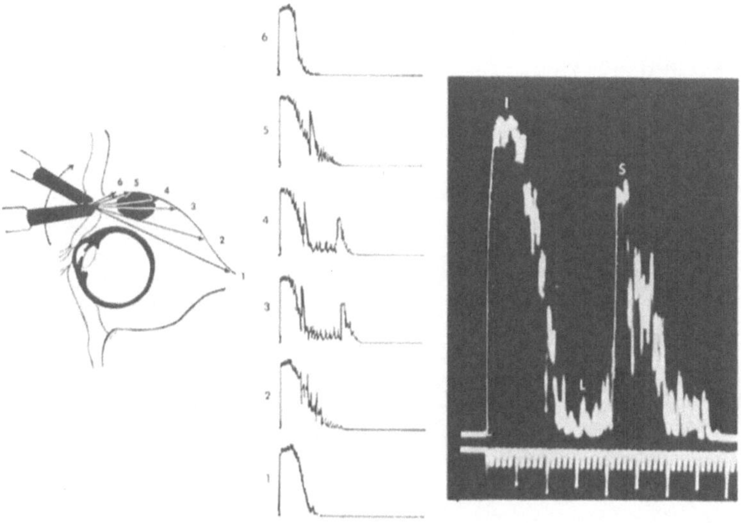

Fig. 4. Left, schematic representation of paraocular approach and the scanning technique used to obtain perpendicular exposure to the lesion's posterior surface. View #3 shows optimal (perpendicular) alignment with posterior surface. Right, paraocular echogram of the mass with beam directed perpendicular to its posterior surface (note steeply rising surface spike). I = normal anterior orbital tissue spikes superimposed over initial spike, L = internal lesion spikes, S = posterior lesion surface (double peak indicates capsule).

Proof of the lesion's vascular nature was the presence of marked internal blood flow. A fast, low amplitude flickering was noted from the internal lesion spikes on the standardized A-scan oscilloscope. Doppler instrumentation was then applied which confirmed this vascular component [6, 7].

DOCUMENTATION OF FINDINGS

Echograms were documented with polaroid photographs of the A and B-scan screen displays. Blood flow detected with the audio Doppler instrument was recorded on cassette tape. An orbital drawing was then made to provide the surgeon with a pictorial display for surgery, including a summary of the main differential criteria and lesion measurements (Fig. 6). Once all data obtained with the special examination techniques were assimilated, the final echographic diagnosis was notated as 'angiomatous tumor' with characteristics distinct from the more familiar, cavernous hemangioma of the adult type.

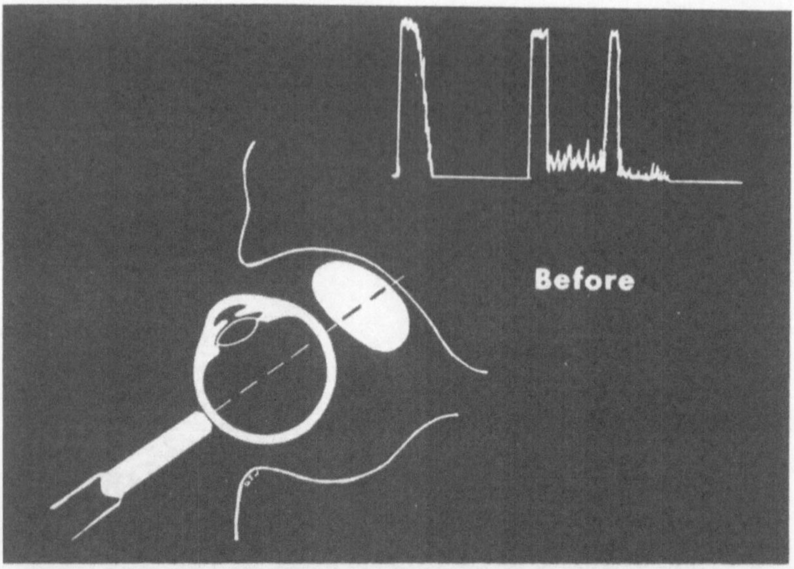

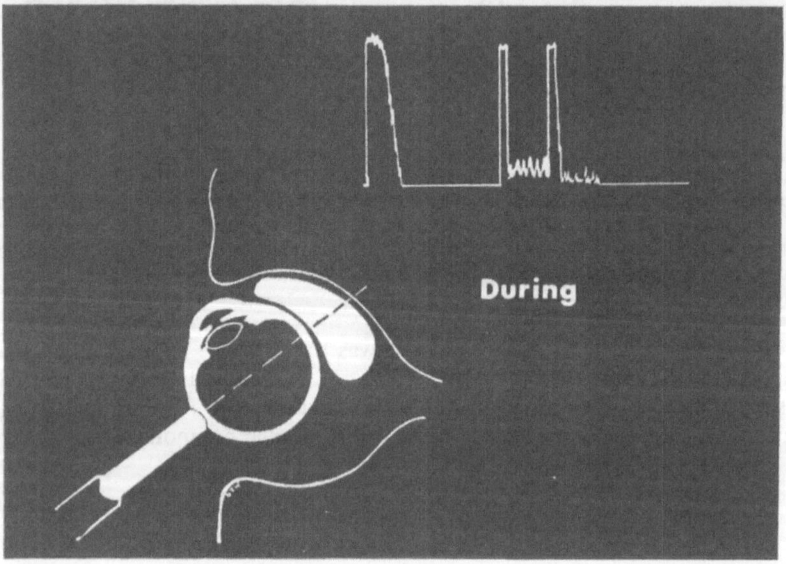

Fig. 5. Technique for performing compression testing to determine consistency of a lesion. Top, the lesion is displayed in its maximal width before exerting probe pressure. Bottom, during the test, the lesion and its echogram decrease in width proving its soft consistency.

Cavernous hemangiomas are usually located in the muscle cone below and temporal to the optic nerve. They typically produce echograms of regular, heterogeneous (honeycomb-like) internal structure, high reflectivity and medium angle kappa (Fig. 7). They are rounded, encapsulated and

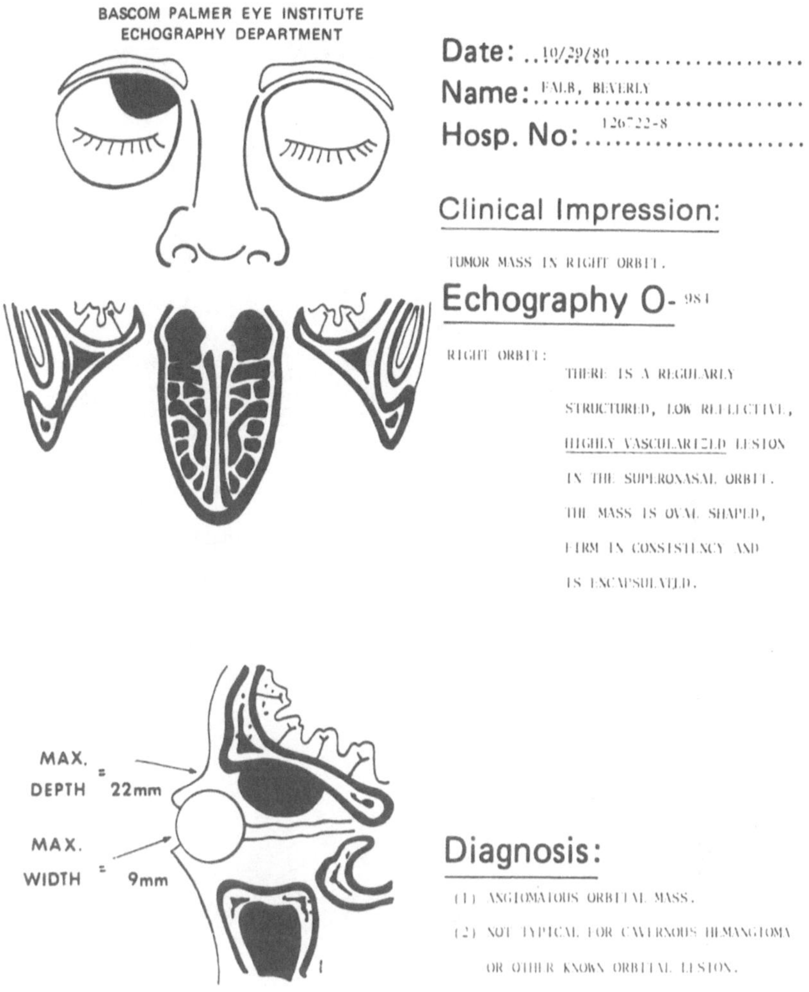

BASCOM PALMER EYE INSTITUTE
ECHOGRAPHY DEPARTMENT
Date: 10/29/80
Name: FALB, BEVERLY
Hosp. No: 126722-8
Clinical Impression:
TUMOR MASS IN RIGHT ORBIT.
Echography O- 981
RIGHT ORBIT:
THERE IS A REGULARLY
STRUCTURED, LOW REFLECTIVE,
HIGHLY VASCULARIZED LESION
IN THE SUPERONASAL ORBIT.
THE MASS IS OVAL SHAPED,
FIRM IN CONSISTENCY AND
IS ENCAPSULATED.
MAX. DEPTH = 22mm
MAX. WIDTH = 9mm
Diagnosis:
(1) ANGIOMATOUS ORBITAL MASS.
(2) NOT TYPICAL FOR CAVERNOUS HEMANGIOMA
OR OTHER KNOWN ORBITAL LESION.

Fig. 6. **Preoperative orbital drawing indicating echographic findings.**

nonvascularized. Compression testing on an interrupted basis over a period of 30 seconds shows significant decrease in lesion width as the stagnant blood within the cavernous spaces is slowly forced out of the smaller feeder vessels, a unique kinetic finding specific for this lesion [6, 7].

The lesion was easily excised with capsule intact. Microscopic examination revealed spindle shaped cells with foamy appearance, fibrous tissue, multiple and small endothelized vascular channels (Fig. 8). The final histologic diagnosis was read out as hemangioendothelioma, although several examiners felt that the lesion might actually be a hemangiopericytoma.

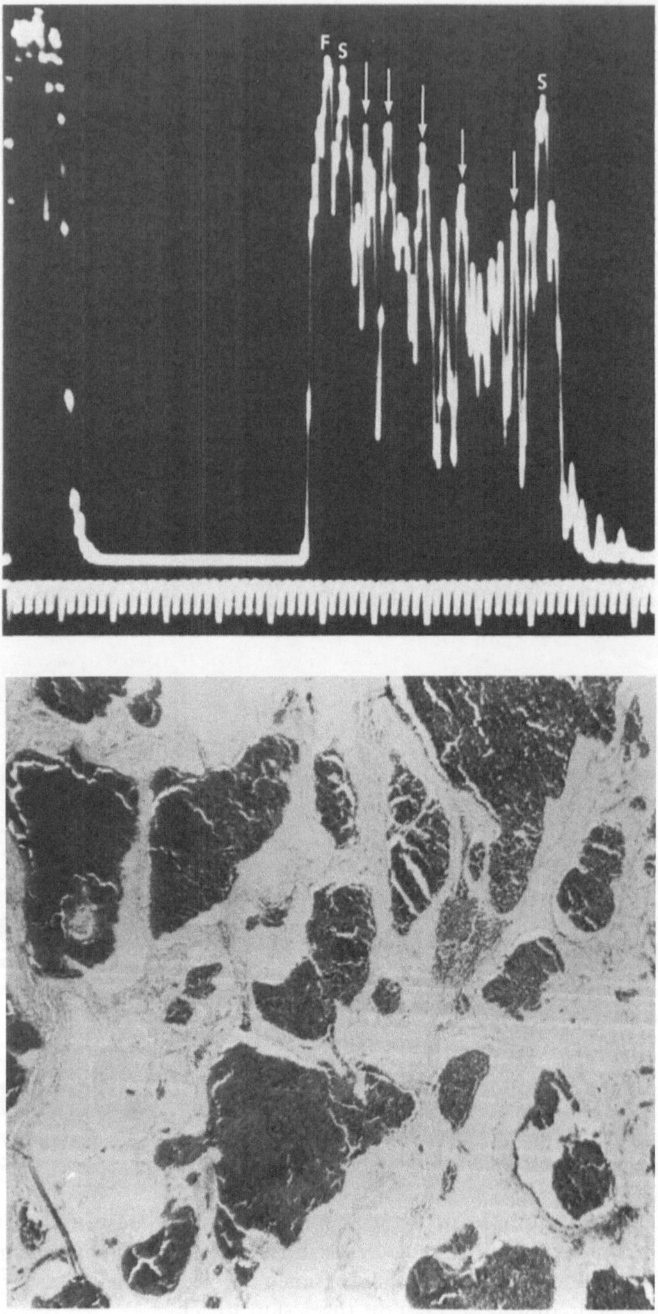

Fig. 7. Transocular A-scan and accompanying histologic section of typical cavernous hemangioma of the adult type. The high internal reflectivity and spike appearance denote a honeycomb, cavernous structure. Arrows = surface of the cavernous spaces. Lower spikes between arrows are produced by stagnant blood within these large vascular channels. F = fundus, S = surfaces of the tumor.

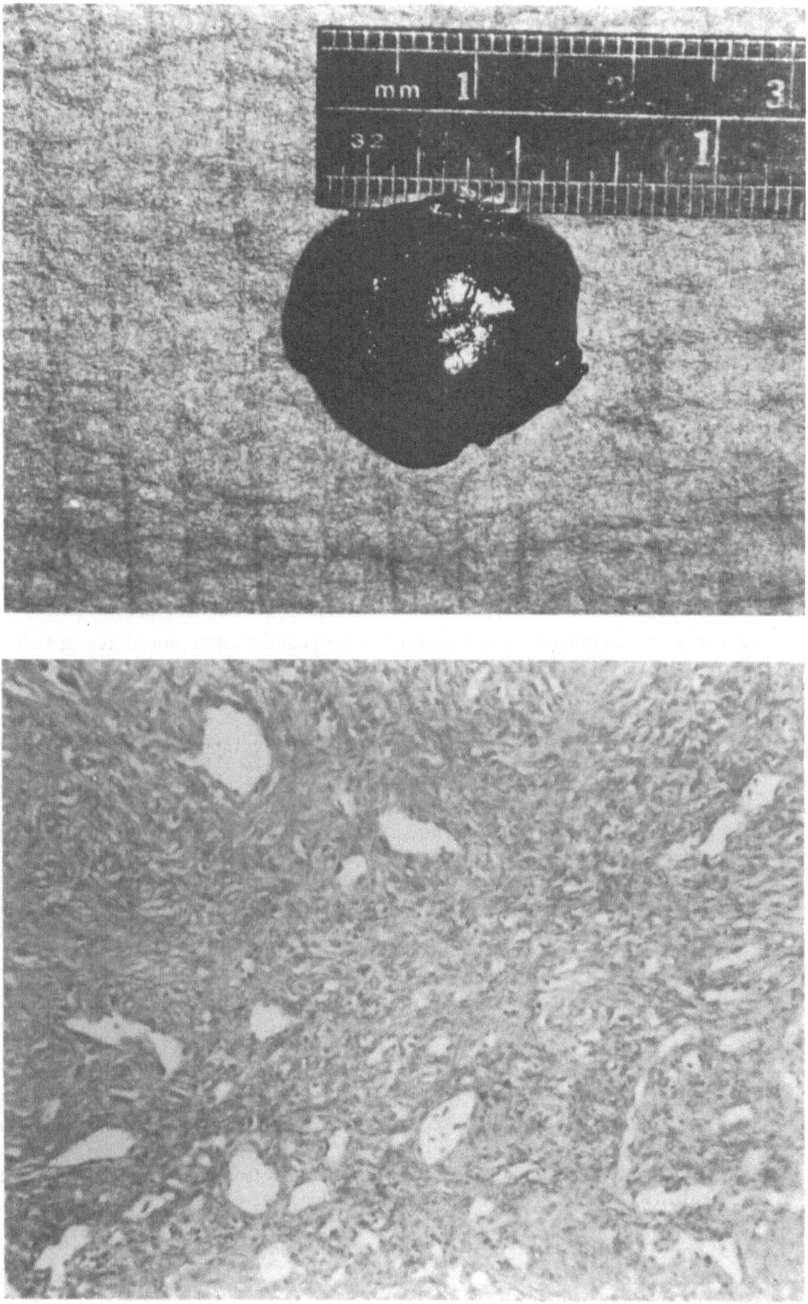

Fig. 8. Top, excised tumor. Bottom, representative histologic section diagnosed as hemangioendothelioma.

CONCLUSION

Standardized echography is the method of choice for distinguishing vascular from nonvascular masses in the orbit. This hemangioendothelioma, although echographically not distinguishable from capillary hemangioma, hemangiopericytoma, angiofibroma or angiosarcoma, presented echograms distinctly different from cavernous hemangioma of the adult type and other vascular orbital lesions which have been described by Ossoinig [7, 8]. The application of dynamic kinetic echography is essential in characterizing the vascular nature of these lesions, and thus provides the orbital surgeon with invaluable preoperative information.

ACKNOWLEDGMENTS

The author wishes to thank Trish Feally for typing this manuscript as well as Debbie Weinstein, Randy Hughes, Susan Eswine, and Keith Siegel for the graphics.

REFERENCES

1. Byrne, S. F.: Standardized echography: A-scan examination procedures, in Dallow, R. L. (ed): Int Opthal Clin, 19/4. Boston: Little Brown & Co, 1979, pp. 267–281.
2. Byrne, S. F. and Saclarides, E.: Standardized ophthalmic echography and the health care professional. Jont, 1/1, 1982, pp. 19–27.
3. Coleman, D. J.: Reliability of ocular and orbital diagnosis with B-scan ultrasound: II. Orbital diagnosis. Am J Ophthalmol, 74: 704, 1972.
4. Ossoinig, K. C. and Patel, J. H.: A-scan instrumentation for acoustic tissue differentiation: II. Clinical significance of various technical parameters of the 7200 MA unit of Kretztechnik, in White, D. and Brown, R. E. (eds): Ultrasound in Medicine, 3B. New York: Plenum, 1977, pp. 1949–1954.
5. Ossoinig, K. C. and Patel, J. H.: A-scan instrumentation for acoustic tissue differentiation: III. Testing and calibration of the 7200 MA unit of Kretztechnik, in White, D. and Brown, R. E. (eds): Ultrasound in Medicine, 3B. New York: Plenum, 1977, pp. 1955–1964.
6. Ossoinig, K. C.: Echography of the eye, orbit and periorbital region, Arger, P. H. (ed): Orbital Roentgenology, New York: Wiley, 1977, pp. 224–269.
7. Ossoinig, K. C.: Standardized echography: Basic principles, clinical application and results, in Dallow, R. L. (ed): Int Ophthal Clin, 19/4. Boston: Little Brown & Co, 1979, pp. 127–210.
8. Ossoinig, K. C.: Echographic differentiation of vascular tumors in the orbit in Thijssen, J. M. and Verbeek, A. M. (eds): Documental Ophthalmol, 29. The Hague: Dr. W. Junk, 1981, pp. 283–291.
9. Till, P.: Solid tissue model for the standardization of the echo-ophthalmograph 7200 MA (Kretztechnik). Documental Ophthalmol, 41 (2): 205, 1976.

Author's address:
Department of Echography
Bascom Palmer Eye Institute
P.O. Box 016880
Miami, FL 33101
USA

ULTRASONOGRAPHIC AND CLINICAL FINDINGS IN CAVERNOUS ORBITAL HAEMANGIOMA

F. GOES
(Ghent, Belgium)

Over the last 12 years we have examined 204 cases of unilateral exophthalmos of at least 2 mm and the diagnosis was verified in 161 cases.

Dysthyroid orbitopathy was responsible for 20% of the verified cases and exophthalmos was the first manifestation of the disease in over 50% of these (Table 1). *Orbital pseudotumour* was responsible for 12% of the cases in which important associated clinical signs were: anterior segment irritation (80%), pain (60%) and ocular motility disturbances (70%). 14% of the exophthalmos cases were *non-tumoural* lesions – 10% being vascular (Aneurysm, varyx, haematoma) and 4% non-vascular (Inflammatory). *Tumoural lesions* were responsible for 54% of the exophthalmos cases and within this group the numbers of malignant tumours (26%) and benign tumours (28%) were almost equal.

Table 1. Aetiology of 161 cases of unilateral exophthalmos

Unilateral Exophthalmos: 161		
Non tumoural		: 46%
	Endocrine	: 20%
	Pseudotumour	: 12%
	Vascular	: 10%
	Other	: 4%
Tumoural		: 54%
	Benign	: 28%
	Malignant	: 26%

Among the benign tumours we made the diagnosis of *cavernous orbital haemangioma* in 9 cases (Table 2) and this was the fourth most common tumour after mucocele (21) metastatic carcinoma (17) and orbital sarcoma (10). All of these cases were verified histologically. The mean age of patients with cavernous orbital hemangioma was 40 years (range 3–66 years) and the mean exophthalmos reading was 6 mm (range 3–10 mm). The mean dimension of the tumour was 10 mm (range 5–20 mm). The onset of the exophthalmos was usually rather fast (6/9 shorter than 4 months) and motility disturbance was present in only one case. Signs of anterior eye disturbance (eyelid hematoma, subconjunctival bleeding) were present in only two cases and a

Hillman, J. S./Le May, M. M. (eds.) Ophthalmic Ultrasonography

ISBN 978-94-009-7280-3

Table 2. Nature of 87 orbital tumours

Orbital tumours: 87	
Mucocele	: 21
Metastatic Carcinoma	: 17
Cavernous Haemangioma	: 9
Sarcoma	: 10
Sinus Carcinoma	: 9
Meningioma	: 5
Lacrimal gland carcinoma – neurinoma – M. lymphoma – B. lymphoma – Epithelioma – Ep. Cyst	: 2
M. Myeloma – Fibrous bone dyspl. – Lacrymal sac. ca. – Fibrolipoma	: 1

case in a 3 year old girl was complicated by a significant eyelid haematoma. The tumour was situated on the Right side in 3 cases and on the Left in 6 cases. With a single exception, the tumours were all situated within the muscle cone and an inferior localisation was most frequent (6/9: 3/9 nasally, 3/9 temporally).

The most striking clinical phenomenon in this group was the presence of signs of *posterior pole compression* with peripapillary choroidal folds (Fig. 1), papilloedema and resulting visual loss which were present in 7 cases out of 9. In 2 cases there was no posterior pole compression but one of these tumours was extra-conal and could be palpated in the inferior temporal region. Significant visual loss (visual acuity reduced to 0.2 or less) was present in 5 of the 7 cases. In one case uncorrected visual acuity was 0.05 but improved to 0.9 after correction of the 6 Dioptre hypermetropia. Significant shortening of the globe which could amount to more than 2.0 mm (Fig. 2) with resulting hypermetropia as a consequence of posterior pole compression was demonstrated echographically in 4 cases (Table 3). This hypermetropisation was only partly reversible on surgical excision of the tumour and usually only after a long period. In one case, a 3 Dioptre hypermetropisation persisted 2 years after surgery. The papilloedema usually disappeared 6 weeks to 3 months after treatment but the choroidal folds could last much longer and in one case choroidal folds were still clearly visible 2 years after surgery and they were complicated by pigment epithelium changes in the macular region. In the cases with longstanding posterior pole compression and choroidal folds the visual acuity remained impaired after treatment because of these secondary retinal changes. We, therefore, advise early surgical treatment of this benign orbital lesion – especially when there are signs of posterior pole compression.

In 5 groups of orbital lesions in our series *involvement of the posterior pole* of the eye was present in more than 20%, but the accompanying clinical signs of these lesions were very different and in none of these cases could a similar shortening of the eye-length be observed.

In the *peri-orbital malignancy* group posterior pole involvement was present in 50% of the cases and in this group motility disturbances were frequently present (50%).

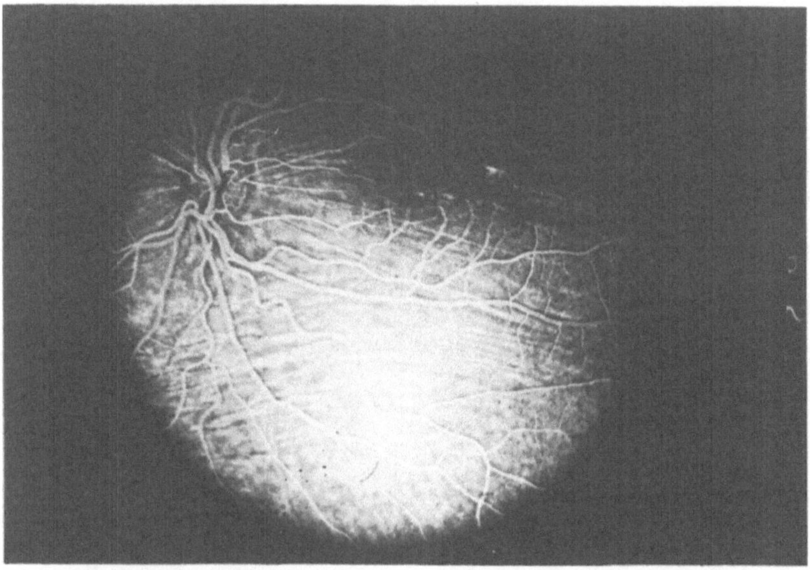

Fig. 1. Choroidal folds in cavernous orbital haemangioma.

The *metastatic carcinoma* group had rather frequent posterior pole involvement (35%) also with almost always a fast onset (acute in 4/17) and almost always motility disturbances (14/17) with complete immobilisation of the eye in 4 cases. *Vascular non-tumour* lesions caused posterior pole involvement in 36% cases but in this group there were usually signs of anterior segment irritation (80%: chemosis, haemorrhage, congestion), motility disturbances (75%) and also a fast onset (14/16 acute).

The *sarcoma* and *pseudotumour* groups had posterior segment involvement in 20% of cases but these were fast developing tumours and in addition the pseudotumours often caused motility disturbances (65%) and anterior eye irritation (85%).

The A-scan echogram of cavernous haemangioma has been described in detail by Ossoinig et al (1981) and we summarise the following characteristics (Fig. 3):

(1) The tumour is characterised by a chain of alternately high and low echo spikes caused by the large, smooth highly reflective surfaces of the cavernous vascular spaces and the stagnant non-coagulated blood within the spaces giving a heterogenous honeycomb internal structure.

(2) High reflectivity: 80–95% of display height.

(3) Strong sound attenuation: Angle kappa 45° (Fig. 4).

(4) Well-defined border echoes (surface spikes).

(5) Delay compressibility – the echogram shortens with prolonged pressure of 30 to 60 seconds duration.

Also, the tumour is usually situated within the muscle cone and usually on the temporal side with a round to oval shape. Because of the presence of stagnant blood there is no detectable fast blood flow on the screen and

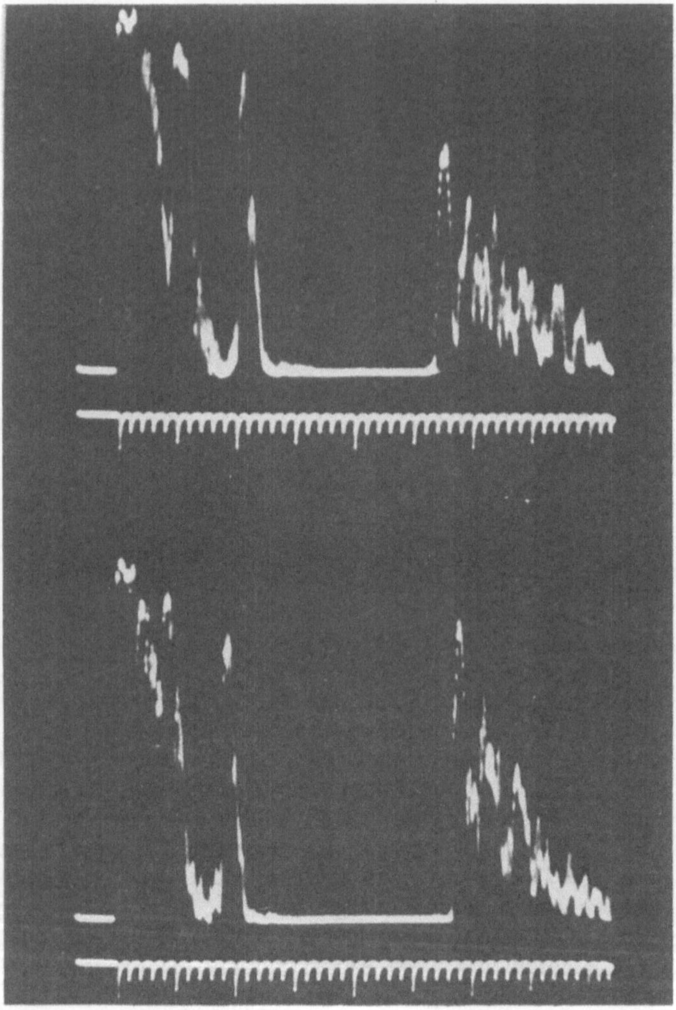

Fig. 2. **Biometry of the normal side (lower) and involved side (upper) showing significant shortening on the exophthalmos side.**

because of the hard consistency of the lesion there is no spontaneous movement.

On comparing the orbital echograms of the other groups with frequent posterior pole compression we find them all very different from the cavernous haemangioma echogram:

Peri-orbital malignancy which has an irregular internal structure gives as a consequence an irregular and mostly large echogram in which high and low spikes alternate and are often separated by short base lines. The irregular structure is confirmed by angling the probe when the echogram changes quickly. This tumour is usually situated extraconally and often has associated bone defects.

Table 3. Vitreous shortening and hypermetropisation in 4 cases of cavernous orbital haemangioma

Vitreous Shortening	Hypermetropisation
	+ 2.25
1.1 mm	+ 3.0
2.3 mm	+ 6.0
1.7 mm	+ 4.5

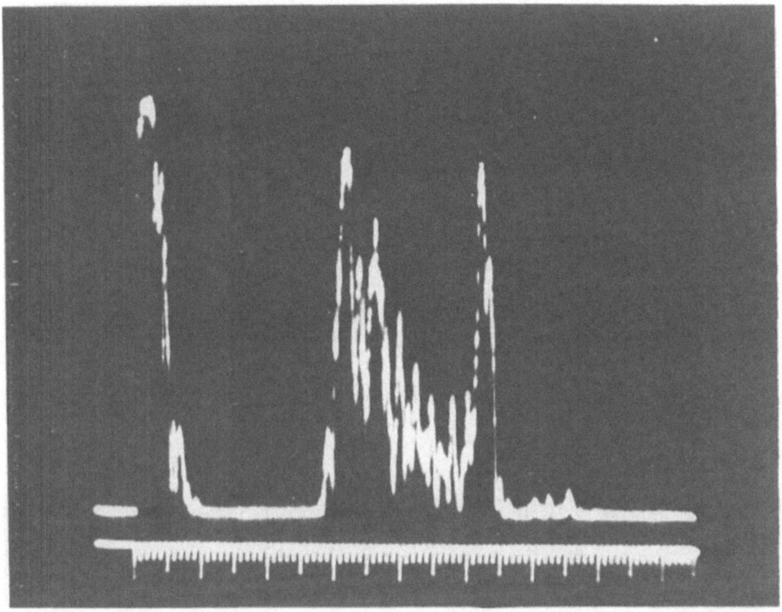

Fig. 3. A-scan ultrasonogram of orbital haemangioma.

Orbital carcinomas give a highly reflective immobile echogram which is poorly outlined indicating infiltrative growth and also of hard consistency (Fig. 5)(Ossoinig, 1975).

The *sarcoma-lymphoma* group which give low reflective echograms may be difficult to separate when the tumour is larger with a denser centre.

Vascular non-tumour lesions (varyx, haematoma, fistula, thrombosis) usually give characteristic echograms with fast vertical movements of all spikes in an A–V fistula and a cystic homogeneous low amplitude echogram in haematoma and varyx.

A comparison of the diagnostic accuracy of the examination techniques in this small haemangioma series shows that Radiology (8/8) and Gammagraphy (4/4) always gave a tumour-positive result (Table 5). Angiography, however, demonstrated the presence of a vascular mass lesion in only 2 cases and in the other 3 cases only indirect signs of ophthalmic artery compression were visible. C.T. Scan diagnosed the presence of a vascular tumour in one case and gave a wrong differential tumour diagnosis in 3 other cases.

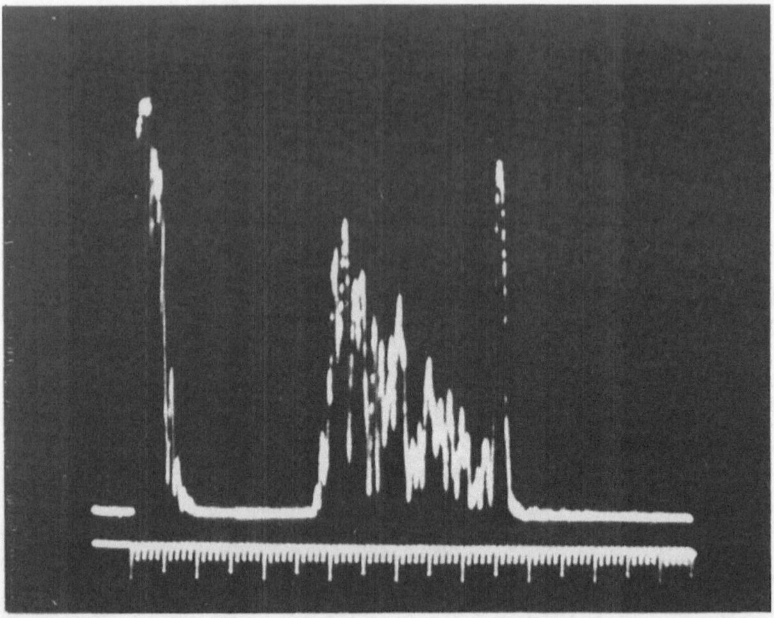

Fig. 4. A-scan of cavernous orbital haemangioma with strong sound attenuation and border echoes.

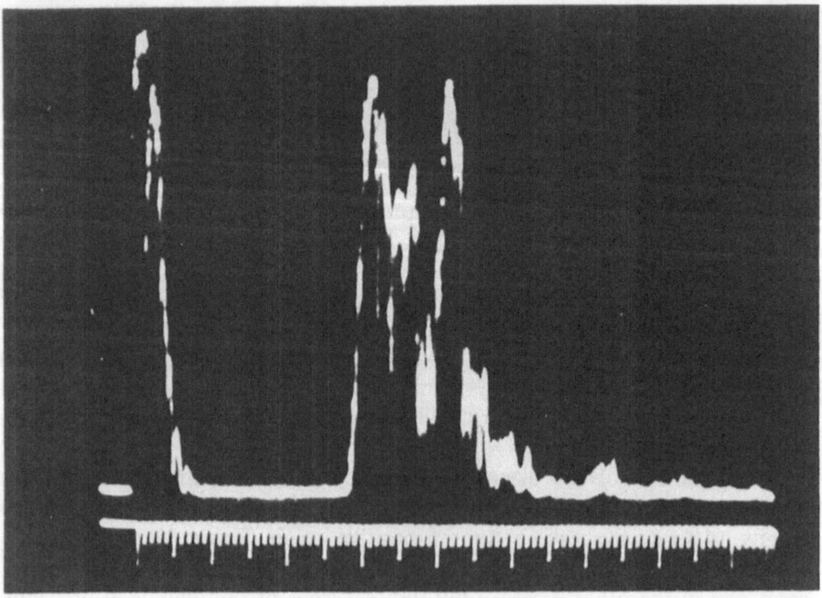

Fig. 5. A-scan of metastatic orbital carcinoma showing high reflectivity and hard consistency.

Table 4. Associated signs in 5 orbital pathology groups with frequent posterior pole compression

	N	Onset	Post. Segment	Vision	Motility	Ant. Segment
peri-orbital malignancy	9	slow	50%	55%	50%	10%
metastatic carcinoma	17	fast	35%	35%	85%	50%
vascular non-tumoural	16	fast	36%	40%	75%	80%
sarcoma	10	fast	20%	20%	30%	40%
pseudotumour	20	fast	20%	15%	65%	85%

Table 5. Positive technical examinations in the 8 cases of orbital cavernous haemangioma

Positive Technical Examination in Cavernous Haemangioma	
Radiology	0/8
Gammagraphy	0/4
Angiography	5/5
C.T.	4/4
Ultrasound	9/9

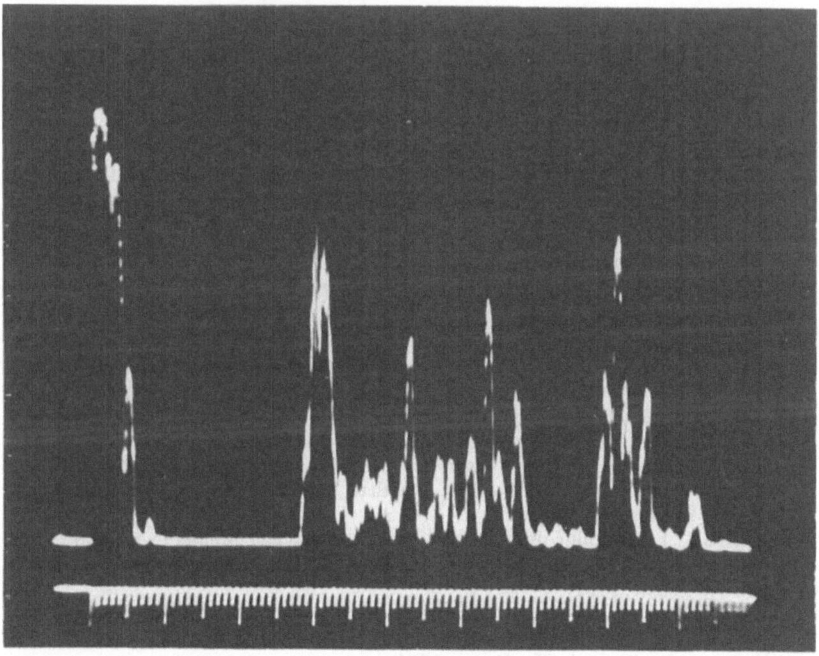

Fig. 6. A-scan of periorbital malignancy with irregular ultrasound appearance and bone defects.

Ultrasound consistently diagnosed the presence of a solid tumour but differential diagnosis was possible in only 4 cases out of 9. In our whole exophthalmos series of 161 cases ultrasound gave a positive diagnosis in 94% and this diagnostic rate was followed by C.T. Scan (75%), then Angiography

(60%), Radiology (37%) and Gammagraphy (36%). Similar diagnostic results were obtained if we consider only the orbital tumours (Table 6). Gammagraphy had a good diagnostic rate only in the meningioma group, Radiology gave a good accuracy only in detecting bone lesions and Angiography had a high accuracy in vascular lesions. C.T. Scan examination approached the diagnostic rate of ultrasound, especially in the orbital tumour group, but was only used in a limited number of cases (28 orbital tumours).

Table 6. Positive technical examinations in the exophthalmos cases

Positive Technical Examinations in Unilateral Exophthalmos		
161 : Total		87 : Orbital Tumours
Ultrasonography	: 94%	91%
C.T. Scan	: 75%	92%
Angiography	: 60%	69%
Radiology	: 37%	55%
Gammagraphy	: 36%	43%

Although Ossoinig et al (1975–1981) and also Till and Hauff (1981) who surveyed 422 orbital and peri-orbital tumours and pseudotumours were able to demonstrate 99% of the orbital lesions causing signs or symptoms and were able to differentiate 85% of the detected lesions in 28 different entities, we are convinced that not all ophthalmologists will achieve the same high score. We feel, therefore, that a knowledge of the typical associated clinical signs in an exophthalmos case is essential and will give invaluable information towards a final diagnosis. The association of clinical signs of posterior pole compression especially when accompanied by significant shortening of the eye with a typical echogram increases the diagnostic success rate in cases of cavernous orbital hemangioma.

REFERENCES

Ossoinig, K. C. Keenan, T. P. and Bigar, F. Cavernous Hemangioma of the Orbit. Ultrasonography in Ophthalmology, Bib. Ophthal. 83, 236–244. ed. Francois J. and Goes, F., Karger Basel, 1975.

Ossoinig, K. C. Echographic differential diagnosis of vascular tumors in the orbit. Doc. Ophthal. Proc. Series, 29, 283–291, ed. J. M. Thijssen and A. M. Verbeek, Dr. W. Junk. The Hague, 1981.

Till, P. and Hauff, W. Differential diagnostic results of clinical echography in orbital tumours. Doc. Ophthal. Proc. Series, 29, 277–282, ed. J. M. Thijssen and A. M. Verbeeck. Dr. W. Junk; The Hague, 1981.

Author's address:
Ophthalmological Clinic
University of Ghent
Ghent
Belgium

COMPARATIVE VALUE OF ULTRASOUND AND CT SCANNING IN ORBITAL OPTIC NERVE EVALUATION

HAROLD W. SKALKA and LANNING B. KLINE
(Birmingham, USA)

ABSTRACT

Ophthalmic ultrasonography and CT scanning represent our two useful methods of 'visualization' of the orbital optic nerve. The advantages and relative value of each of these modalities are considered, beginning at the optic disc, and continuing back to the orbital apex. As a diagnostic technique, ultrasonography is clearly superior for evaluation of the most distal portion of the optic nerve (disc and anterior muscle cone area), while CT scanning offers unique advantages as the orbital apex is approached. In appropriate cases, the combination of these modalities allows for optimal diagnostic evaluation.

Evaluation of the orbital portion of the optic nerve has always been difficult. Until the development of ophthalmic ultrasonography and CT scanning, techniques were largely limited to evaluation of the disc in eyes with clear media, and the finding of prechiasmal field defects in eyes with no fundus pathology (along with less specific clinical signs such as pupillary responses). The advent of pattern ERG testing may provide some degree of ability to study ganglion cell function, but 'visualization' of the orbital optic nerve remains the province of echography and neuroradiology.

The relative advantages of the two techniques are well recognized. Ultrasonography involves no radiation, and is a dynamic technique which can be performed in real time under 'direct' visualization. It may be performed by the ophthalmologist caring for the patient, thus allowing an optimal examination tailored to the needs of the particular case and providing an 'immediate' report. Ultrasonography allows accurate biometry, and is relatively portable and economical. CT is a static technique, but CT scanners have improved greatly in a short number of years, and are now capable of imaging the entire intraorbital course of the optic nerve. In addition, multiple CT sections (coronal, axial, sagittal) can show the nerve in cross section and demonstrate its relationship to other orbital and periorbital structures at different orbital depths. The use of contrast enhancement is helpful in demonstrating the vascularity of lesions, and reformatted images enable reconstructions of the nerve to be created along selected planes.

Hillman, J. S./Le May, M. M. (eds.) Ophthalmic Ultrasonography

ISBN 978-94-009-7280-3

DISC

Other than direct visualization, ultrasonography is clearly the technique of choice in evaluation of the optic disc, and in some cases may even be superior to ophthalmoscopic examination (e.g. buried disc drusen). Drusen and disc edema, while perhaps demonstrable on appropriate CT views, are easily and clearly seen echographically, especially with B-scan techniques. Using B-scan, cupping of the disc may be demonstrated when the vertical cup/disc ratio exceeds 0.7, and the lamina cribrosa can often be evaluated regarding the presence or absence of posterior bowing (Fig. 1). This is useful in distinguishing glaucomatous cupping from a large physiologic cup. Colobomas and staphylomas may also be appreciated. Likewise, avulsion of the nerve from the globe can be demonstrated with ultrasound, while the retention of an intact dural sheath makes CT demonstration of this entity problematical at best. Small tumors on or adjoining the nervehead are obviously better appreciated and analyzed echographically.

MID ORBIT

In the anterior portion of the muscle cone, both techniques have significant value. A-scan echography is, of course, peerless for biometry, enabling us to make reproducible diametric measurements of the retrobulbar optic nerve proper, as well as of its enveloping cerebrospinal fluid and dura-arachnoid sheaths. Such perineural measurements have proven reliable in several studies, for example, as a means of monitoring response to therapy in patients with optic atrophy and chronic increased intracranial pressure without performing repeated lumbar punctures.

Both techniques are capable of demonstrating intrinsic nerve tumors in this area. CT scanning may provide a better overall 'view' of the size and shape of the lesion. Although quantitative A-scan ultrasonography remains superior in diagnosing the nature of the lesion, the list of possible diagnoses here is quite limited. Ultrasonography probably retains the advantage in differentiating 'extrinsic' (e.g. meningioma) from intrinsic (e.g. glioma) tumors.

Muscle cone lesions abutting the optic nerve are well-demonstrated by both techniques. Differential diagnosis is more accurate with echography; but the use of contrast enhancement, finer matrices, and multiple projections have enabled CT scanning to achieve increasing reliability in this regard.

POSTERIOR ORBIT

Sound attenuation, refraction of the sound beam through additional tissues of varying acoustic properties, and reflections from the converging orbital walls make posterior orbital structures difficult to visualize and evaluate with ophthalmic ultrasound techniques. Here, CT scanning offers definite advantages. For example, coronal CT sections can clearly show the massive posterior

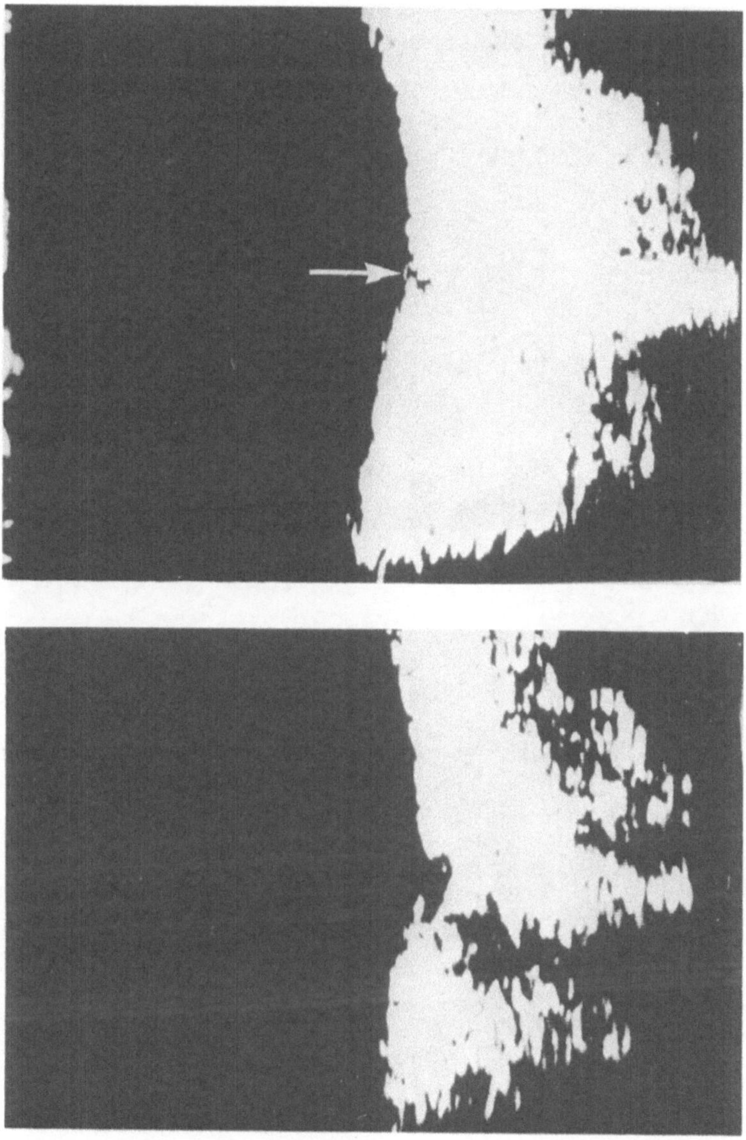

Fig. 1. Contact B-scans of cupped disc. Probe placed vertically on temporal sclera. Upper photo at 80 Db sensitivity, showing suggestion of cupping at disc (arrow); lower photo at 70 dB, demonstrating cupping and posterior bowing of the lamina cribrosa.

orbital extraocular muscle thickening seen in some cases of endocrine orbitopathy (posterior to the region most accurately measured echographically), allowing better understanding of the embarrassment of optic nerve function in specific cases, as well as more accurate estimates of the potential usefulness of orbital decompression procedures in individual cases (Fig. 2).

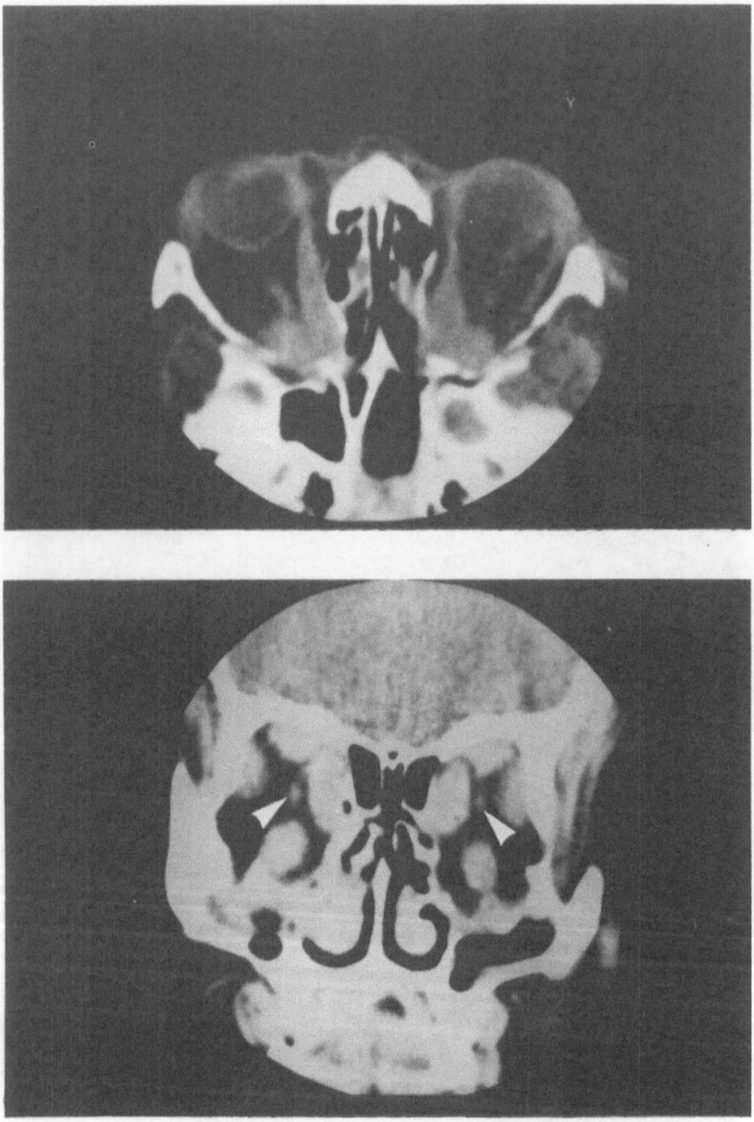

Fig. 2. Axial (above) and coronal (below) CT views of extraocular muscle thickening in the posterior orbits of a patient with endocrine orbitopathy. Coronal view shows optic nerves (arrowheads) surrounded by enlarged rectus muscles in posterior orbits.

As the orbital apex is approached, CT scanning assumes greater importance in the evaluation of the orbital optic nerve. The posterior extension of lesions is better seen with CT, and one can determine, for example, if an optic nerve tumor is resectable in the orbit, or extends into (or beyond) the optic canal (Fig. 3). Apical bone defects and extension of lesions into, or out of, the orbit can more reliably be shown by advanced CT techniques.

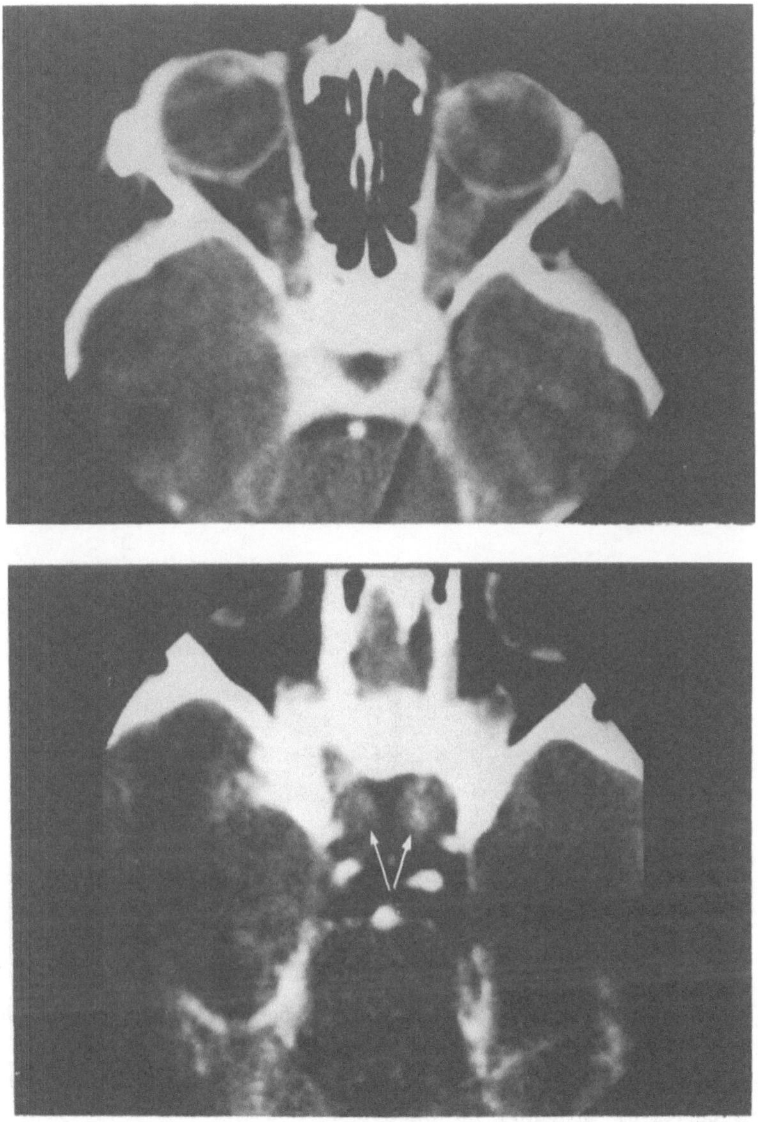

Fig. 3. CT scans of patient with bilateral optic nerve gliomas. Upper view demonstrates thickened optic nerves in both orbits; lower view demonstrates bilateral intracranial involvement (arrows).

CONCLUSION

In general, the relative value of ultrasonography decreases, and that of CT scanning increases, as we evaluate the orbital optic nerve from the disc back to the foramen of the optic canal (Fig. 4). While individuals particularly

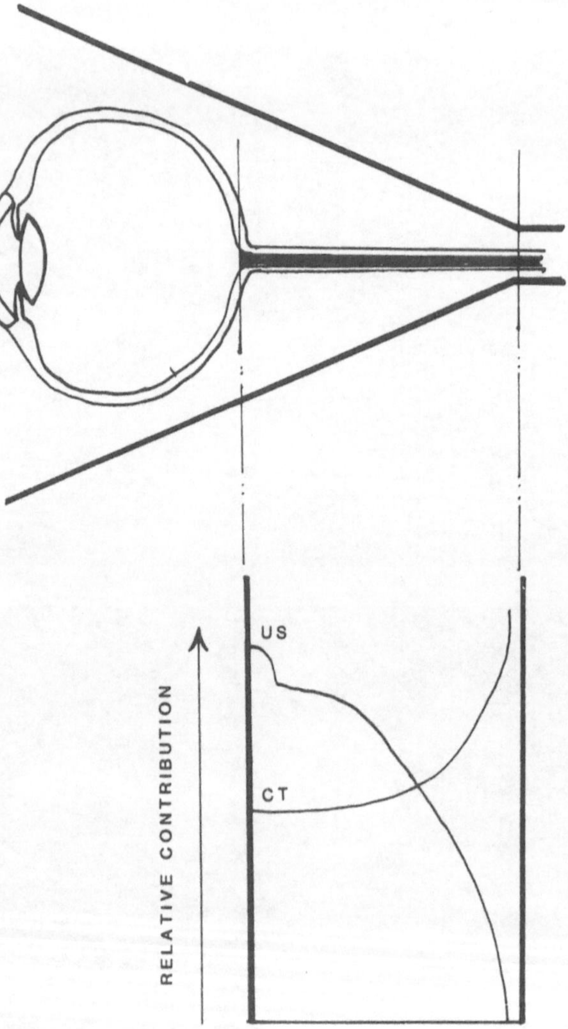

Fig. 4. Relative diagnostic contributions of ultrasonography and CT scanning along course of orbital optic nerve, from disc to optic foramen.

expert with either of these diagnostic modalities may be capable of skewing these curves by extracting information and making diagnoses beyond the capabilities of the average competent examiner, the majority of diagnosticians (whether ophthalmologists or neuroradiologists) should be aware of the strengths and weaknesses of both techniques, and proceed accordingly. The judicious combined use of ophthalmic ultrasonography and CT scanning can often enable us to answer even the most difficult diagnostic questions.

Authors' address:
The Eye Foundation Hospital
1720 University Boulevard
Birmingham, AL 35233
USA

ECHOGRAPHY, VECP AND COMPUTERIZED TOMOGRAPHY IN TUMOURS OF THE OPTIC NERVE

W. BUSCHMANN, W. HAIGIS and P. SOLIS-REDON
(Würzburg, W. Germany)

INTRODUCTION

The early clinical symptoms of optic nerve tumours are visual field defects (sometimes of irregular shape) and diminished visual acuity. The disc may appear normal but in other cases papilledema, sometimes in combination with atrophy, optico-ciliary shunt vessels and choroidal folds may be found. Usually, the diagnosis of neuritis or vascular obstruction is made at this stage. With or without corresponding treatment, the visual acuity may improve during the following weeks and months before it drops again permanently.

The exophthalmos is minimal in early stages of the disease. Ultrasound exophthalmometry, nevertheless, may prove it whilst Hertel's exophthalmometry remains within the error range.

Correct diagnosis of optic nerve and optic nerve sheath tumours depends on B- and A-scan ultrasonography, analysis of the visually evoked cortical potentials, and on computerized tomography.

ULTRASONOGRAPHIC TECHNIQUE FOR OPTIC NERVE EXAMINATION

1. Reproducible, measurement-based examination conditions

Reliability of ultrasonography depends on reproducible examination conditions and on the examiner's knowledge of some more important data of the equipment used. We strictly recommend to use equipment checks which are in accordance with the IEC and AIUM drafts on measurement of equipment data in diagnostic ultrasonography. We developed a set of simple devices which allow to get these measurements done by an ultrasound technician under hospital conditions. Details were given at the previous SIDUO congresses.

2. Routine procedure of optic nerve ultrasonography

We prefer to start with real time B-scan, using a narrow-band-width 10 MHz transducer probe. An additional 5 MHz examination may be helpful especially

Hillman, J. S./Le May, M. M. (eds.) Ophthalmic Ultrasonography

ISBN 978-94-009-7280-3

for lesions in the posterior part of the orbit. The gap in the orbital fat echogram caused by the optic nerve is first studied in straight gaze position using horizontal and vertical scans. This gap is normally V-shaped. The posterior enlargement of the diameter is an acoustic artefact caused by the shadowing effect of the normal bends of the optic nerve in this gaze direction. The echograms are taken at maximum sensitivity of our Ocuscan 400 which corresponds to 52 dB above the standard echo of the W38 test reflector. It may be necessary to reduce this sensitivity by 10 dB for detailed examination of the disc and the optic nerve part adjacent to the sclera. Exudate in Tenon's space, for example, may be visualized better this way.

Then, the movements of the optic nerve in the orbital fat are studied, especially in horizontal scans, whilst the patient is changing the gaze direction from left to right and vice versa (Figs. 1, 2). The sensitivity is readjusted to the higher level. Finally, the longitudinal and cross section echograms of the optic nerve are studied. For this purpose, the patient looks to the temporal

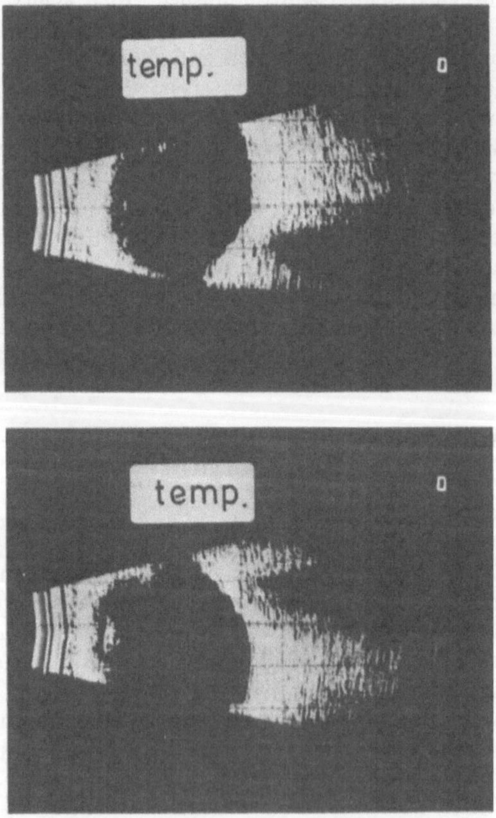

Figs. 1 and 2. **Movement of optic nerve in the orbit, right eye, change of gaze direction from right (Fig. 1) to left (Fig. 2). Real time B-scan, Sonometrics Ocuscan 400, working frequency 9.7 MHz, Δv(W38) = 52 dB.**

side, so that the optic nerve is stretched nearly parallel to the medial orbital wall. For the longitudinal scan, the probe is held in the horizontal plane but is turned around the bulbus centre for about 80° to the temporal side to get optimal adjustment of the sound beam axis to the optic nerve sheath. Then, the scan axis is turned to the vertical direction with the transducer probe in the same position, to demonstrate cross section views of the optic nerve. Some tilting of the transducer probe enables several sections to be obtained. However, we have to admit that the posterior third of the optic nerve in the orbit is poorly shown in ultrasonographic A- and B-scans, due to the unfavourable angle of incidence onto the normal structures in the orbital apex area.

RESULTS OF ULTRASONOGRAPHY

The incidence of echographic findings in a group of optic nerve or sheath tumours is shown in Table 1.

The most reliable criteria were: a sharply outlined mass lesion (Figs. 3, 4) with structure echo amplitudes lower than fat echoes in the area of the optic nerve; U-shaped or wide-angled anterior end of the optic nerve gap in the orbital fat echo pattern; and movement of the lesion with the optic nerve.

Table 1. Echographic B-scan findings in optic nerve tumours

(4 sheath meningiomas, 1 spongioblastoma, 2 sheath neurofibromas)	
Mass lesion in optic nerve area	7
well outlined	7
U-shaped or wide-angled at sclera	7
Pathol. echoes from lesion area (negative in 2 sheath meningiomas)	pos. 5
Echo chains parallel to optic nerve (negative in 2 sheath meningiomas and in 1 neurofibroma)	pos. 4
Impression of posterior globe wall (2 only slightly, 1 neurofibroma negative)	pos. 4
Disc elevated (negative in 2 neurofibromas)	pos. 5
Ultrasound attenuation in lesion area less than in normal orbit (1 slightly less, 2 sheath meningiomas and the spongioblastoma negative)	pos. 3
Mass moves with optic nerve (not tested in 2)	pos. 5
Exudate in Tenon's space slightly (negative in 4)	pos. 3

Echo chains in the nerve sheath area are no proof for sheath meningioma. They may occur in inflammatory lesions as well, and also in tumours of the optic nerve itself like in this spongioblastoma (Fig. 5).

Pathological echoes from the area of the optic nerve can be diagnosed only from scan *series.* They must be differentiated from normal findings at the margins of the nerve.

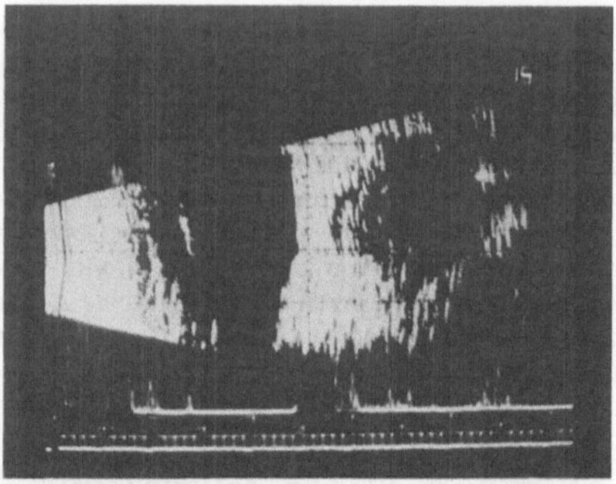

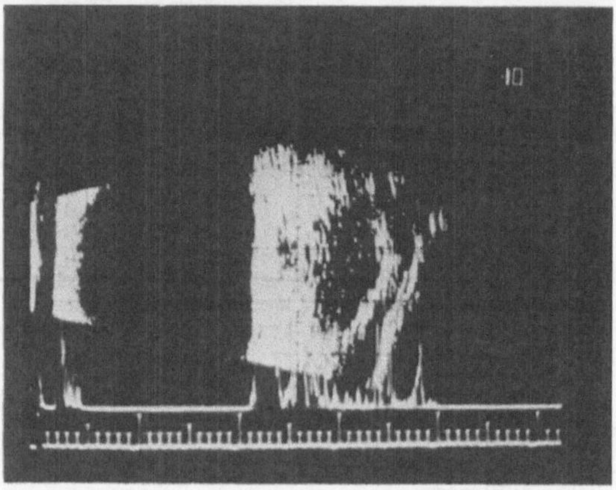

Figs. 3 and 4. **Optic nerve sheath meningioma. Ocuscan 400, vertical scans.**
Fig. 3. **Straight gaze direction, working frequency 4.9 MHz, Δv(W38) = 52 dB.**
Fig. 4. **Scan plane tilted 60° to temporal side, gaze direction temporal, working frequency 9.7 MHz, Δv(W38) = 44 dB.**

ULTRASOUND ATTENUATION IN THE LESION AREA

A rough estimation can be achieved considering the echoes from structures behind the lesion area. The ultrasound attenuation in solid tumour tissues ca ben lower or higher than in normal orbital fat. If it is lower, fat and other normal structures (e.g. orbital wall), located behind the tumour mass in a depth of the orbit from which normally at this frequency no echoes can be detected, may reflect well-recognizable echoes (Figs. 3, 4).

In cysts and mucoceles, the sound attenuation is even less. The use of 2 different frequencies (5 and 10 MHz and/or different sensitivity settings may be helpful in this examination, as well as the comparison with the other (healthy) orbit.

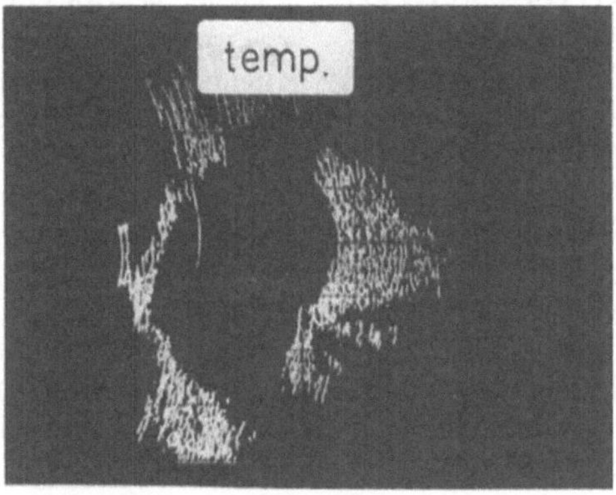

Fig. 5. Optic nerve spongioblastoma. Horizontal immersion scan (Ophthalmoscan), 5 mm above plane of optical axis, nom. frequency 10 MHz.

A more precise evaluation of attenuation can be derived from the analysis of lesion structure echo amplitudes in A-scans. Visual evaluation of the amplitude decrease in single or several A-scans failed ('angle kappa'). It proved necessary to use echogram series and computerized averaging, previously described (Haigis and Buschmann 1983). In one A-scan echogram of an intraocular melanoblastoma the amplitude decrease at 8.3 MHz was 2.50 dB/μsec; the averaging of 4 echograms brought this figure down to 2.05 dB/μsec, and many more echograms must be averaged before we get reliable figures.

We averaged 128 normal orbital fat echograms and found an attenuation of 0.13 dB/(μsec MHz), which is, at the 9.6 MHz working frequency used, equivalent to 1.26 dB/μsec.

A similar number of echograms must be averaged for the determination of the amplitude *range* of pathologic structure echoes. Based on a small number of echograms, Ossoinig and Bigar reported that the structure echoes of optic nerve sheath meningiomas, in their technique with the KRETZ 7200 MA, would be between 40 and 60% of maximum echo amplitude on the screen. According to their description of the amplifier characteristics, this corresponds to an amplitude variation of only 6 dB. Structure echoes of such meningiomas should then be found only in the amplitude range of 50 to 56 dB above the standard echo of our test reflector W38.

This range is too small, also with regard to histopathologic variability. We found in a group of echograms of one patient (A. K.) 48 ± 3 dB above the test reflector W38 standard echo at a working frequency of 6.2 MHz. In another, much larger sheath meningioma (R. H.) we found 62 ± 2 dB at 7.6 MHz working frequency and 48 ± 6 dB at 10.9 MHz working frequency.

We were also able to measure structure echoes from the healthy optic nerve at 6.2 MHz working frequency, which were 65 ± 2 dB above the test reflector echo. Many more of such measurements are needed before reliable figures for the amplitude ranges in these tissues could be given.

VISUALLY EVOKED CORTICAL POTENTIALS

These potentials were evaluated in 12 patients with optic nerve compression due to optic nerve or sheath tumours or adjacent orbital tumours. 2 checkerboard stimuli of different size were used. Comparing the results with the control group, we found increased latency (statistically significant, especially for P_3 with large checkerboard) and reduced amplitudes (mainly P_1) in all cases. Comparison with the patient's other (healthy) eye proved increased latency (P_2, P_3) as well, but no significant amplitude differences. Similar pathologic alterations of the VECP were found in patients with Papillitis. In one case (sheath meningioma) we got no VECP with the checkerboard stimulus, but only flash-VECP's from the affected side (visual acuity 0.8, nearly 'hemianopic' field defect).

X–RAY AND COMPUTERIZED TOMOGRAPHY

Native X-ray photographs of the optic canal should be taken. Huber prefers – despite the radiation dose – polytomographic series from this area. The results of Rhese's technique, however, should not be over-emphasized. False positive findings with unilateral enlargement and lacking extension of the optic nerve tumour into the canal do occur as well as false negative findings with equal configuration of the canal and its walls on both sides, and neurosurgically proven tumour extension through the canal (Wright et al. 1980).

Computerized tomography contributes significantly to optic nerve tumour diagnosis, especially since high resolution scanners became available and scan planes other than the axial ones can be examined or reconstructed. Coronal scans proved much more suitable than the axial scans, and planes exactly vertical to the optic nerve may be even better. Examination in such scan planes, however, can be handicapped badly by metallic tooth-crowns, and reconstruction from axial scans can be connected with loss of resolution.

The main criteria in optic nerve tumours are optic nerve diameter, respectively areas of increased density involving the optic nerve, and contrast enhancement. Enlargement of the diameter due to congestion or inflammation could not always be differentiated from tumour-induced enlargement in CT-scans, but safely in combined evaluation of ultrasonographic and CT results.

Results of computerized tomography in our group of patients

Enlargement of the optic nerve diameter, respectively an area of high density involving the optic nerve, was found in accordance with the ultrasonic findings in 6 of the 7 patients (Figs. 6, 7 and 8). Axial CT-scans only were performed in 1 spongioblastoma case and failed; we insisted, with regard to the clinical symptoms and echographic results in this patient, to get coronal scans, and these stated thickening of the optic nerve.

Combined evaluation of ultrasonic and CT findings also proved helpful in an alcoholic patient with bilateral optic neuritis caused by vitamin-B-deficiency.

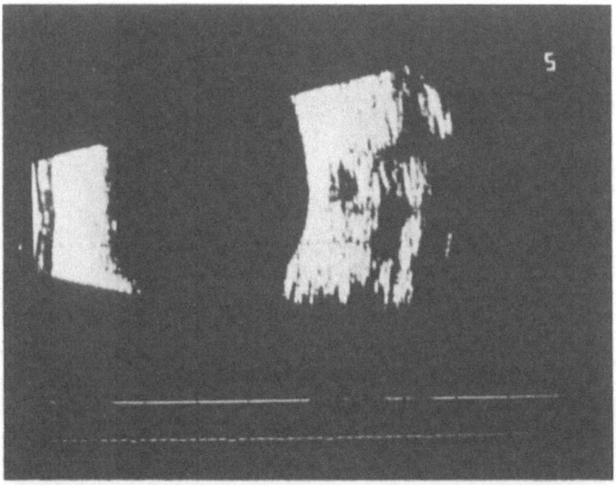

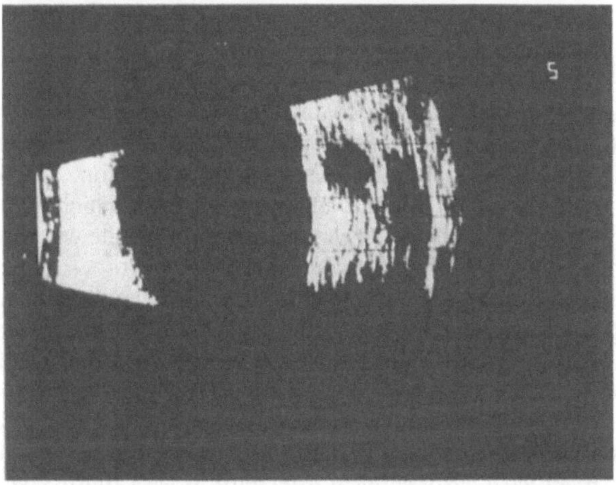

Figs. 6 and 7. **Optic nerve cross section views, gaze direction to temporal side, vertical scans (Ocuscan 400) from temporal side. Working frequency 9.7 MHz, Δv(W38) = 48 dB.**
Fig. 6. **Normal findings, right eye and orbit.**
Fig. 7. **Optic nerve diameter enlarged (sheath meningioma), left orbit.**

Ultrasound showed diameter enlargement and pronounced sheath echoes, whilst CT – at the window settings chosen – demonstrated reduced nerve diameters.

CONCLUSION

In case of suspected optic nerve tumour, ultrasound exophthalmometry, B- and A-scan ultrasonography, visually evoked responses, and computerized tomography proved very helpful and are now mandatory for diagnosis as well as for follow-up studies.

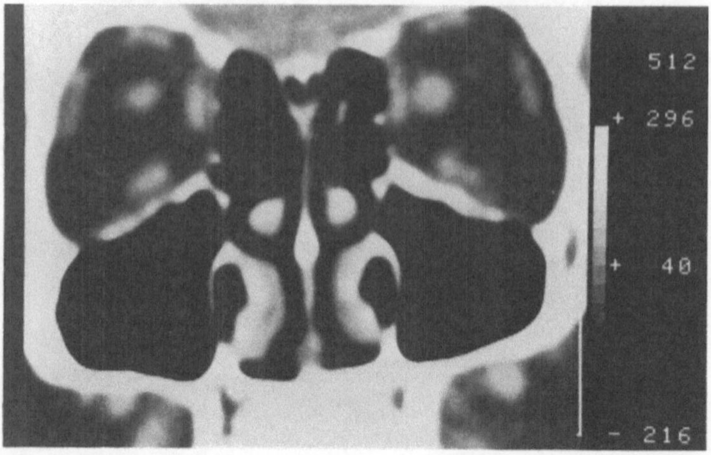

Fig. 8. Coronal CT-scan, case shown in Fig. 6 and 7.

Generally, it is not possible to differentiate echographically optic nerve tumours (e.g. gliomas) safely from meningiomas of the optic nerve sheath. Concentric growth of the meningioma is an exception. The tumour mass usually is much larger on one side of the optic nerve, which makes it difficult to identify the optic nerve in the echogram and to decide whether the tumour arises from the sheath or from the nerve itself.

Regarding CT, it is not sufficient to have good equipment available. The examining doctor must have profound knowledge in the special techniques of computerized tomography of the orbit as well as of the specific pathology and anatomy of this area.

No clinical decision should be based on the results of only one of the methods described. Combined evaluation improves the preoperative diagnosis markedly. Even with early surgical intervention we cannot save vision but at best a blind eye. However, we can save the patient's life which may be in danger even in non-malignant tumours of the optic nerve and its sheath.

REFERENCES

Abramson, D. H., Coleman, D. J. and Franzen, L. A.: Ultrasonography of Optic Nerve Lesions. In: Francois, J. and Goes, F.: Ultrasonography in Ophthalmology, Karger, Basel 1975, S. 231–235.

Babel, J., Stangos, N., Korol, S. and Spiritus, M.: Ocular Electrophysiology, Georg Thieme Verlag, Stuttgart 1977.

Behrens, M. M.: Neuro-Ophthalmic Aspects of Orbital Tumors. In: Jacobiec, F. A., 1978 (see below), S. 863.

Bigar, F. H., Spiess and Bosshard, C.: Standardized A-scan Echography and Computerized Tomography for Evaluation of Orbital Disease. In: Bleeker, G. M., 1978 (see below), p. 141.

Bleeker, G. M., (ed.): Proceedings of the 3rd International Symposium on Orbital Disorders, Dr. W. Junk Publishers, Den Haag 1978.

Buschmann, W.: Zu Diagnostik und Therapie von Optikus-Tumoren/On Diagnosis and

Treatment of Optic Nerve Tumors. Paper for the 79th Conference of The DOG, Heidelberg 1981.
Coleman, D. J., Dallow, R. L. and Smith, M. E.: Immersion Ultrasonography – Simultaneous A-Scan and B-Scan. In: Dallow, R. L. (ed.) (see below), 1979, p. 67, 211.
Dallow, R. L. (ed.): Ophthalmic Ultrasonography – Comparative Techniques, Little, Brown & Co., Boston 1979.
Grove, A. S.: Coronal Computer Tomography of the Orbit, In: Jacobiec, F. A., 1978 (see below), p. 271.
Haigis, W. and Buschmann, W.: Performance measurements and quantitative echography. In: Hillman, J. S. and Le May M. M. (eds.), Docum. Ophthal. Proc. Series vol. 38. The Hague: Dr. W. Junk Publishers, 1983, pp. 433–443.
Halliday, A. M., Halliday, E., Kriss, A., McDonald, W. T. and Mushin, J.: The Pattern-Evoked Potential in Compression of the Anterior Visual Pathways, Brain 99, 1976, 357–374.
Huber, A.: Diagnosis and Treatment of Optic Nerve Tumors. In: Orbit, Vol. 1, No. 2, p. 75–83.
Jacobiec, F. A. (ed.): Ocular and Adnexal Tumors. Aesculapius Publishing Co., Birmingham/Alabama 1978.
Kazner, E., Wende, S., Grumme, T., Lanksch, W. and Stochdorph, O.: Computertomographie intrakranieller Tumoren aus klinischer Sicht. Springer, Heidelberg 1981.
Oksala, A., Hadidi, M. A. and Jääslahti, S. L.: Experimental Observations on the Echograms of the Optic Nerve and on the Effects of Some Tissues upon them. Acta Ophthalm. Vol. 50, 1972, p. 360–366.
Ossoinig, K. C.: The Role of Clinical Echography in Modern Diagnosis of Orbital and Periorbital Lesions. In: Bleeker, G. M., 1978 (see above), p. 496.
Ossoinig, K. C.: Standardized Echography – Basic Principles, Clinical Application and Results. In: Dallow, R. L., 1979 (see above), p. 127.
Schroeder, W.: Ultrasonography of the Optic Nerve. In: Bleeker, G. M., 1978 (see above), p. 71.
Skalka, H. W.: Ultrasonography of the Optic Nerve. In: Neuro-Ophthalmology Up-date, J. L. Smith, ed., Massoon Publishing USA 1977a.
Skalka, H. W.: Ultrasonography of the Optic Nerve. In: Neuro-Ophthalmology 1981, Vol. 1, No. 4, pp. 261–272.
Wright, J. E., McDonald, W. I. and Call, N. B.: Management of Optic Nerve Gliomas, Brit. J. Ophthalmol. 64, 1980, pp. 545–552.

Authors' address:
University Eye Hospital
Josef-Schneider-str. 11
D-8700 Würzburg
Federal Republic of Germany

MYOSITIS OF EXTRAOCULAR MUSCLES DIAGNOSED WITH STANDARDIZED ECHOGRAPHY

KARL C. OSSOINIG and VERNON M. HERMSEN
(Iowa City, USA)

Disorders of extraocular muscles are a frequent cause underlying signs or symptoms of orbital disease, such as exophthalmos or double vision. In the Echography Service of the Department of Ophthalmology at The University of Iowa, 1321 patients with exophthalmos or other signs of orbital disease were examined during a 5-year period between February 1978 (date of first echographic diagnosis of orbital myositis) and February 1983. In 468 (35.4%) of the patients, a thickening of one or more extraocular muscles was the only or main cause of the orbital signs and symptoms. The majority of these cases had Graves' disease. In 45 cases (3.4% of all orbital cases, 9.6% of the cases with thickened muscles), a myositis was diagnosed and treated.

The 45 cases diagnosed as orbital myositis were spread over a wide spectrum, ranging from very mild cases (7), which did not require any treatment and were only followed until the signs and symptoms disappeared, to severe cases with total paresis of the affected muscle(s)(11) that required extended, intensive treatment; they ranged from cases in which only one muscle was diseased (21) to patients who suffered from myositis of all (straight and oblique) extraocular muscles in both orbits (5). Some of the patients displayed typical clinical symptoms, but in the majority of cases, standardized echography was needed to clearly diagnose orbital myositis.

Early diagnosis and intensive medical therapy (usually high doses of Cortisone given systemically) are the keys to a quick and complete cure of orbital myositis. It is very important to continue treatment after the clinical symptoms have ceased, until the diseased muscle(s) is(are) fully normalized. Standardized echography provides not only a prompt, reliable and accurate diagnosis of extraocular myositis; it also monitors the progress made during therapy and clearly indicates the time when a diseased muscle has returned to normal and the medication can be safely tapered or stopped. When standardized echography is used to monitor the treatment or extraocular myositis, it is possible to avoid otherwise frequent reoccurrences of the condition that are difficult and time-consuming to treat and cause prolonged morbidity of the patient.

Standardized A-scan (7200 MA of Kretztechnik) is performed to detect and measure thickening of extraocular muscles, and to differentiate the type of muscle disorder. Contact, real-time B-scan (e.g., Ocuscan 400 of Sonometrics Systems, Inc.) is used to evaluate and document the topography of

Hillman, J. S./Le May, M. M. (eds.) Opthalmic Ultrasonography

ISBN 978-94-009-7280-3

the diseased muscle(s). The examination techniques used to measure thickening of straight and oblique extraocular muscles have already been described in detail (1–3). Because of its finer histological structure, normal extraocular muscles produce clearly weaker echoes than the surrounding fat tissues with their large and highly reflective connective-tissue septa. The surfaces of the muscle sheaths produce particularly strong, short echoes, provided that those surfaces are reached by a perpendicular sound beam. Since the surface signals are so strong and contrast very well with the internal muscle echoes, which are relatively weak, it is easy to measure the thickness of a muscle. Because of refraction of the sound beam that occurs somewhere between the ocular wall and the surface of the muscle sheaths, such a perpendicular sound-beam approach can be achieved in the anterior two-thirds to three-fourths of the straight extraocular muscles and the superior oblique muscle, and at all portions of the inferior oblique muscle. Near the orbital apex, the sound beam will always be oblique to the muscle surface; there the measurements are less accurate, but still reliable when the corresponding muscles in both orbits of a patient are compared with each other.

The measured muscle thicknesses are either compared to tables that have been compiled for normals (Table 1), or, more accurately, are compared directly to the thicknesses of the corresponding muscles in the fellow orbit of a patient: differences of 0.3 mm (or more) at the muscle belly and of

Table 1. **Maximum rectus-muscle sizes in normal population**

Muscle	Percentile*	Value in microseconds	Value in millimeters
Superior Rectus	100	7.8	6.1
	95	7.0	5.4
	90	6.0	4.7
Lateral Rectus	100	7.2	5.6
	95	6.8	5.3
	90	6.5	5.0
Inferior Rectus	100	6.0	4.7
	95	5.5	4.3
	90	5.0	3.9
Medial Rectus	100	8.7	6.7
	95	6.9	5.4
	90	6.7	5.2

*Percentage of normal population with a muscle thickness of less than value indicated.

0.15 mm (or more) at the insertion between the maximum thicknesses of corresponding muscles in both orbits clearly indicate that one of the muscles (usually the thicker one) is abnormal. Basically, all sections of a muscle can be measured. But only a muscle's maximum thickness at the muscle belly and at the insertion of its tendon into the globe can be compared reliably and accurately between the two orbits and in follow-up examinations at different times. The evaluation of extraocular muscles is a dynamic procedure. It is the appearance of the muscle patterns in the display of orbital echograms that indicates whether an adequate sound-beam alignment has been achieved or not. The dynamic examination also assures that the maximum thicknesses, which are the only comparable values, are obtained.

Besides the degree and location of thickening of a muscle, its internal acoustic reflectivity and structure are of great importance for the *differential diagnosis*; these muscle properties are best evaluated with standardized A-scan (Fig. 1). Thickened muscles in Graves' disease show a heterogeneous and highly reflective internal structure (Table 2). All other disorders of extraocular muscles, in particular myositis (Table 3), show a lower than normal reflectivity and a pronounced homogeneity of the diseased muscle (see Figs. 2 and 3). This different acoustic behavior of thickened muscles, which provides indications of the different underlying conditions, is explained by their histopathological structure: in Graves' disease, the thickened muscle contains large amounts of fluid that more effectively separate the muscle fibers from each other and from vessels embedded in fat tissues than is the case in normal muscles. This results in an enhancement of the acoustic interfaces that reflect strongly and explains the increased reflectivity and the more heterogeneous internal structure seen in Graves' orbital myopathy. By contrast, the acoustic interfaces in muscles with dense cellular infiltration (e.g., in pseudotumor, lymphoma or metastatic carcinoma) are washed out or destroyed entirely so that a lower reflectivity and more homogeneous internal structure results. This latter histopathology can also be postulated to exist in myositis although no histopathological sections have been obtained from such muscles up to the present to prove it.

In cases of acute myositis, the entire muscle is lower in reflectivity and more homogeneous in structure than a normal muscle. But the inserting tendon of the muscle is most involved and shows most of the thickening (Fig. 4), while more posterior sections of the muscle may be only slightly thickened. This finding clearly separates myositis from other cellular infiltration, i.e., tumors; in these, the muscle bellies are most involved and show marked and sometimes nodular thickening.

It is extremely important to evaluate the reflectivity of an extraocular muscle in its most anterior third (see Figs. 2 and 3) since there sound attenuation by the globe is minimal, and the spike height of the muscle pattern directly indicates the reflectivity of the muscle. More posterior sections of a muscle can be examined only in sound-beam directions that are so oblique toward the ocular wall that a major portion of the energy is totally reflected and never reaches the muscle. Since the same situation holds true for the returning echoes, echo signals from posterior sections of the muscles are always much weaker (the more posterior the section examined is, the weaker the returning echoes are; see *bottom* echograms in Fig. 3). This makes the evaluation of the reflectivity of muscle tissues unreliable or impossible in their posterior two-thirds. While the sound attenuation mentioned also affects the evaluation of heterogeneity of the muscle tissues, marked heterogeneity can be detected even in posterior sections of a muscle.

Because of the pronounced homogeneity and low reflectivity of inflamed extraocular muscles (conditions that are evaluated best with standardized

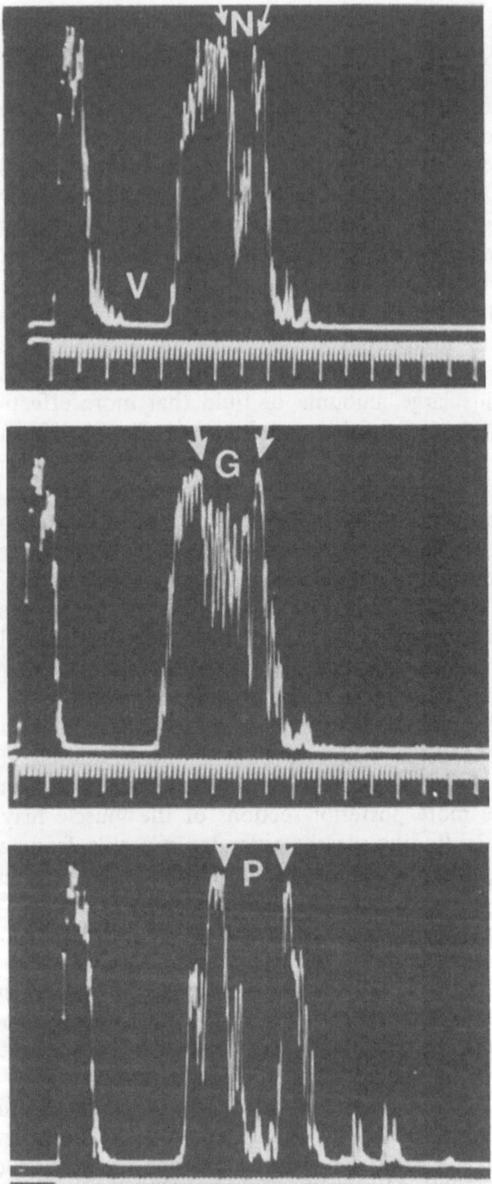

Fig. 1. Standardized A-scan echograms displaying cross-sections of a normal medial rectus muscle (*N*), a markedly thickened medial rectus muscle in Graves' disease (*G*) and a large medial rectus muscle in a case of pseudotumor (*P*). *V* vitreous cavity; *arrows* point at lateral (*left*) and medial (*right*) muscle sheaths. Note the high reflectivity of the thickened muscle in Graves' disease in contrast to the very low reflectivity of the inflamed muscle.

Table 2. Acoustic signs of Graves' disease

1) Absence of orbital tumor.
2) Diffuse enlargement of orbital soft tissues that show coarser than normal structures (changes mostly in anterior and temporal orbit).
3) *Several extraocular muscles thickened*, at least two in one orbit. Thickness must be measured in mid-orbit (muscle belly).

   Thickening is:
   *bilateral in 90% of cases
   *affecting mostly posterior portions of muscles
   *rarely affecting inserting tendon
   *variable over time in regard to type and degree of muscles involved.

4) *Increased reflectivity and more irregular internal structure* of thickened muscles (must be evaluated in anterior 1/3 to 1/2 of muscle only).
5) Irregular thickening of muscle sheaths.
6) Very often thickening of optic-nerve sheaths (overall thickness [sheaths and nerve] of optic nerve above 6 μsec indicates optic neuropathy).
7) Often thickening of periorbit.
8) Occasionally enlargement of lacrimal gland.

Table 3. Acoustic signs of extraocular myositis

1) Marked thickening of inserting tendon (> 100%).
2) Mild to moderate thickening of muscle belly (10%–50%).
3) Markedly decreased internal reflectivity of muscle.
4) More homogeneous internal structure of muscle (often V-shaped muscle echogram).
5) Sometimes episcleritis near muscle insertion.
6) Muscle thickening minor, but functional loss major (and immediate) as compared to other muscle disorders.
7) Stretching of thickened (diseased) muscle (attempt at extreme gaze shift in direction opposite to muscle function) causes (increased) discomfort or pain.

A-scan; see Table 3), particularly clear B-scan patterns of the muscles are obtained in myositis (Figs. 5 and 6). B-scan echograms of extraocular muscles are displayed with a technique similar to that employed in A-scan examinations. The probe is positioned (with the exception of the inferior oblique muscle) on the globe opposite the muscle to be examined. The acoustic section is placed across as well as along the muscle through transverse and longitudinal examinations respectively. Often, it is sufficient for documentation to photograph a longitudinal and a transverse (cross-sectional) echogram. A dynamic examination of cross-sections of the muscle is particularly helpful in clarifying the topography; it involves continuous sweeping of the acoustic section from the inserting tendon anteriorly to the orbital apex for the display of straight extraocular muscles (Fig. 6), from the trochlear area to the orbital apex for the display of the superior oblique muscle, and along the course of the inferior oblique muscle.

In the majority of the 45 cases of orbital myositis that have been seen at The University of Iowa, the diagnosis was based only or primarily on the echographic findings. The clinical course or the complete morphological and functional restoration of the muscles following steroid therapy appeared to confirm the echographic diagnosis. The echographic picture observed in the 45 cases and discussed above is obviously specific for this condition;

Fig. 2.

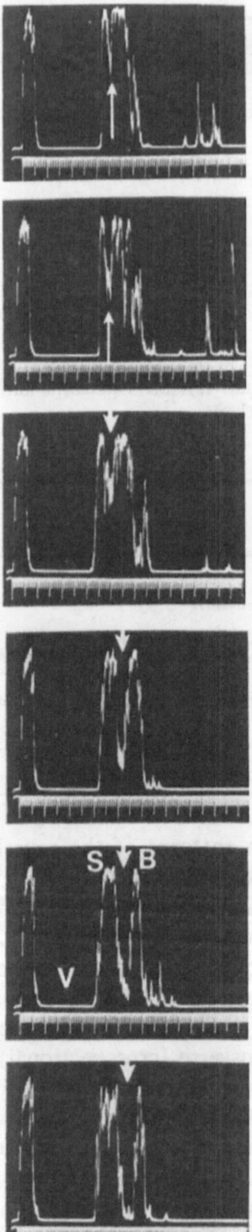

Fig. 3.

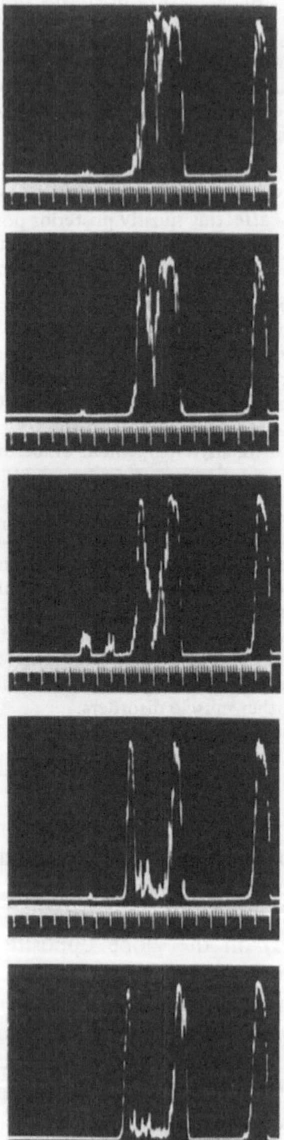

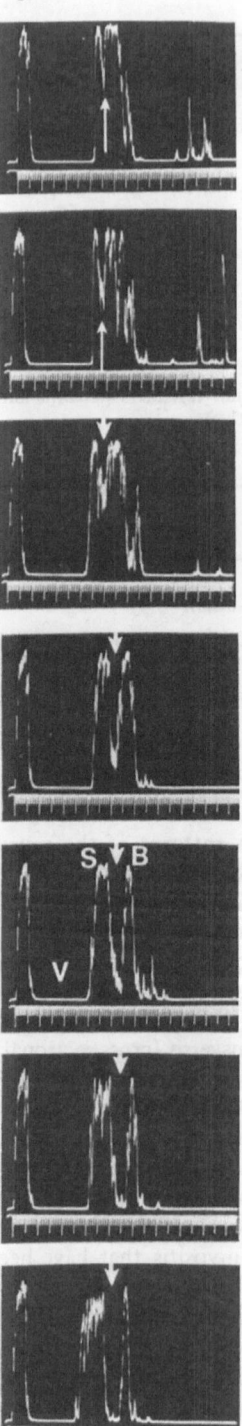

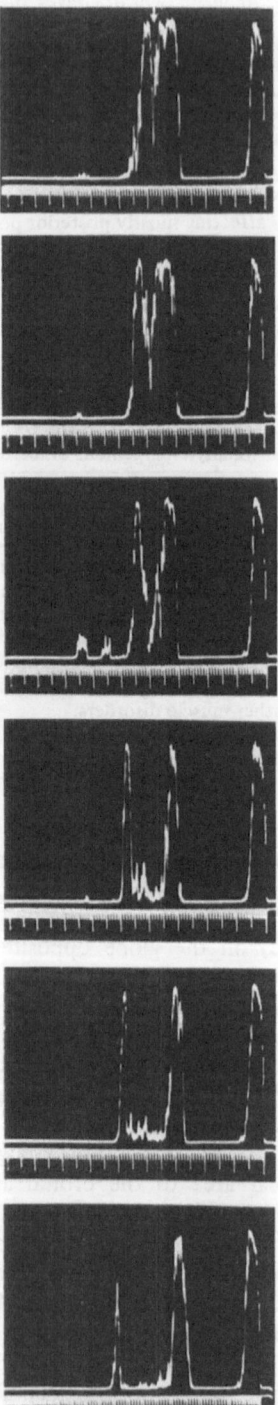

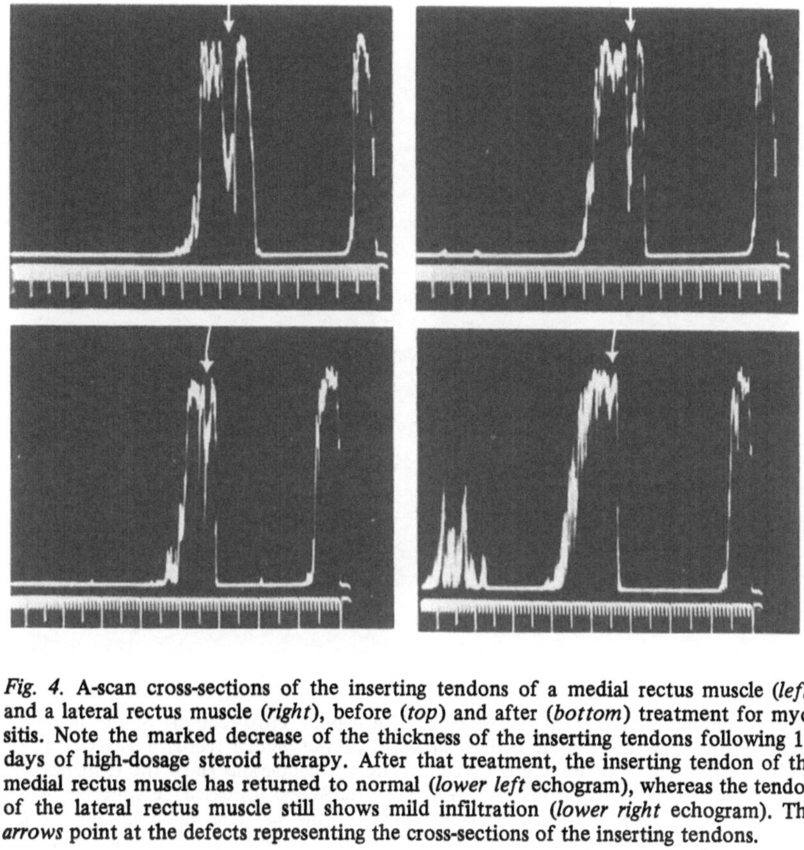

Fig. 4. A-scan cross-sections of the inserting tendons of a medial rectus muscle (*left*) and a lateral rectus muscle (*right*), before (*top*) and after (*bottom*) treatment for myositis. Note the marked decrease of the thickness of the inserting tendons following 10 days of high-dosage steroid therapy. After that treatment, the inserting tendon of the medial rectus muscle has returned to normal (*lower left* echogram), whereas the tendon of the lateral rectus muscle still shows mild infiltration (*lower right* echogram). The *arrows* point at the defects representing the cross-sections of the inserting tendons.

Fig. 2. Series of standardized A-scan echograms showing cross-sections of a thickened medial rectus muscle (myositis) obtained during dynamic scanning from its insertion into the globe (*top*) to near the orbital apex (*bottom*). The *arrows* point at the defects in spike height that represent the diseased muscle in the echograms. *V* vitreous cavity; *S* sclera; *B* bone spike next to the medial surface signal of the muscle. Note the low reflectivity and homogeneity of the internal muscle structures (best evaluated in the anterior one-third of the muscle, which is represented by the *top* five echograms). The thickening of the muscle (as compared to the normal muscles) is more pronounced in the area of the inserting tendon. Also note that the muscle defect in the pattern shifts from the sclera to the bone (typical for a straight extraocular muscle) as the sound beam is shifted through the orbit from anterior to posterior.

Fig. 3. Series of standardized A-scan echograms from markedly thickened superior oblique muscle. Like the medial rectus muscle thickened because of myositis as shown in Fig. 2, this metastatic carcinoma growing extensively within the muscle sheaths of the superior oblique muscle shows low reflectivity and increased homogeneity. The reflectivity of the muscle's internal structure is best evaluated in the *top* four echograms, which correspond to the anterior one-third of the muscle. In contrast to myositis, the muscle belly is markedly thickened in metastatic carcinoma (see lower three echograms). Unlike the medial rectus muscle, the defect representing the superior oblique muscle in the echograms stays with the bony orbital wall, even anteriorly (just behind the trochlea; see *arrow*). This acoustic behavior clearly indicates a superior oblique muscle.

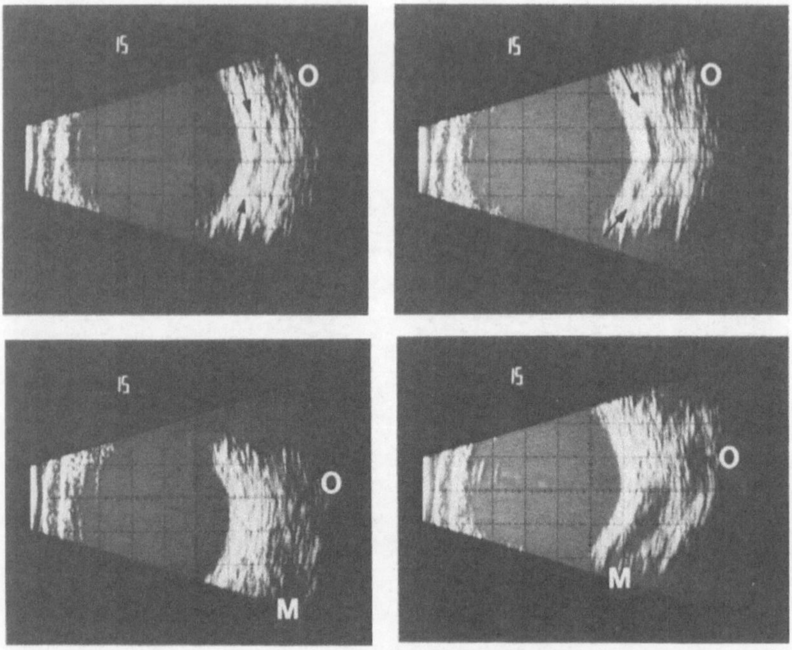

Fig. 5. Contact, real-time B-scan echograms displaying cross-sections of the inserting tendons (*top*) and the muscle bellies (*bottom*) of the medial rectus muscles in both orbits of a patient with unilateral myositis. The *left* echograms show the right normal muscle; the *right* echograms display the slightly thickened (diseased) left muscle. Note the marked difference in clarity and thickness of the patterns between the normal and abnormal tendons of the medial rectus muscles (between *black arrows*), and the difference in clarity between the patterns of the normal and abnormal muscle bellies (left superior oblique muscle also affected). *M* medial rectus muscle; *O* superior oblique muscle.

it was not detected in any other disorder. It should, however, be mentioned that in 3 cases of Graves' orbitopathy, the echographic signs of acute myositis (together with the clinical symptoms of inflammation such as pain) were detected. After treatment with high doses of steroids, the inflammatory signs and symptoms disappeared and a picture typical of Graves' ophthalmopathy evolved. It may be that these cases represent the extreme end of the spectrum of Graves' disease with extremely dense cellular infiltration, or that these patients suffered from two different conditions. It is also quite common in cases of episcleritis or scleritis that the tendons of inserting muscles in the area of the inflammation are involved and show some thickening and lower reflectivity. However, in these cases (which were not included in our statistics on myositis), the inflammatory changes in the muscles were restricted to the most anterior portions of the inserting tendons.

In summary, standardized echography is an important tool for the diagnosis of orbital myositis. By providing echograms specific for myositis, it helps to differentiate this condition from all other disorders of the extraocular muscles and from tumors. Echography is particularly suited for follow-up treatment since it alone indicates the effect of the treatment on the muscles themselves, and not just on clinical signs and symptoms such as lid swelling, double vision and pain. To achieve permanent results and avoid otherwise frequent reoccurrences that are difficult to control and require more intensive and prolonged treatment, it is of paramount importance to use standardized A-scan to monitor progress during steroid therapy and taper or stop the treatment only after the involved muscles have assumed normal thickness and reflectivity.

Fig. 6.

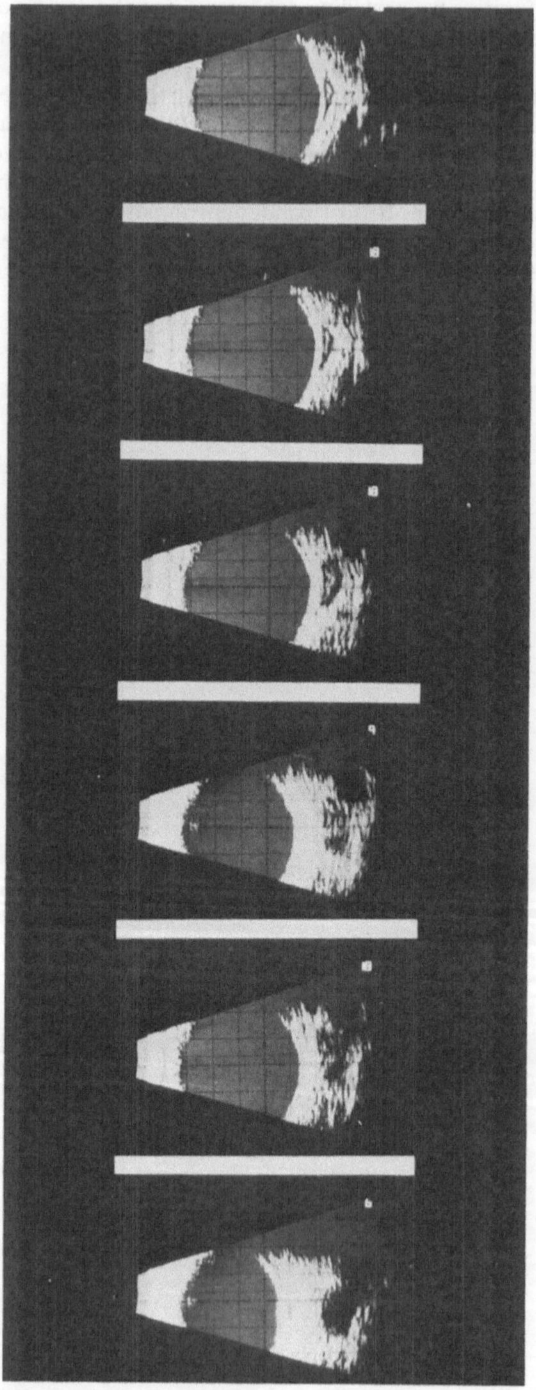

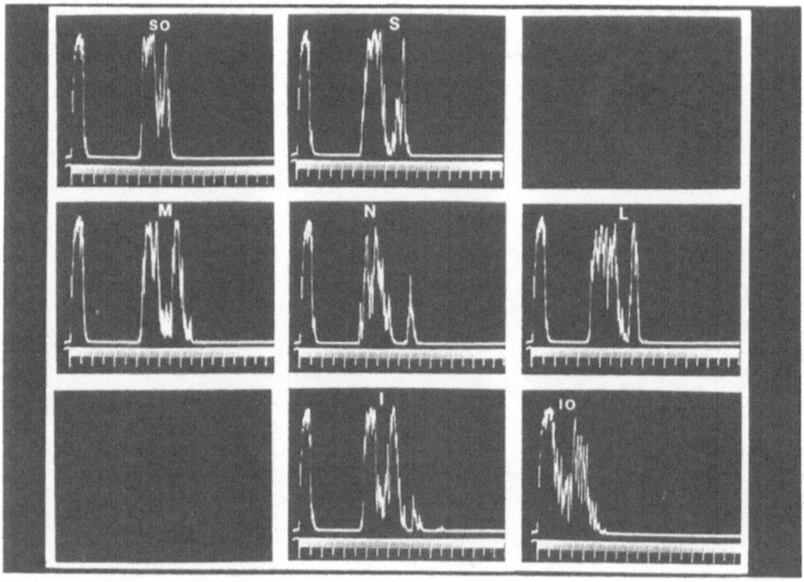

Fig. 7. A-scan documentation of maximum thicknesses of the extraocular muscles in the left orbit of a patient with myositis. The echograms are so arranged that they represent the muscles as the examiner sitting opposite the patient would see them: The optic-nerve thickness is shown in the *center* (*N*). Representative echograms of the superior rectus muscle (*S*), the superior oblique muscle (*so*), the medial rectus muscle (*M*), the lateral rectus muscle (*L*), the inferior rectus muscle (*I*), and the inferior oblique muscle (*io*) are all shown in their appropriate positions. Note the low reflectivity and homogeneous internal structure of the thickened muscles. The straight muscles and the superior oblique muscle were obtained by placing the probe opposite the muscle body on the globe and displaying their cross-sections in a transocular examination. The inferior oblique muscle was displayed by placing the probe on the skin of the lower lid in the 5 o'clock meridian and aiming the beam in a sagittal direction (below the globe) through the belly of the muscle. Compare these echograms with the normal sizes and reflectivities of these muscles after treatment (high dosage systemic steroid therapy) as shown in Fig. 8.

Fig. 6. Series of contact, real-time B-scan echograms obtained during a dynamic scanning of a thickened medial rectus muscle in a case of myositis. The cross-section of the inserting tendon is shown in the *top* picture, that of the muscle belly is displayed in the *bottom* picture. The echograms in between show increasingly more posterior cross-sections of the muscle (from *top* to *bottom*). In the *lower* three echograms, note the additional defect caused by the equally thickened superior oblique muscle (on top of the defect caused by the medial rectus muscle). Also note the clarity of the muscle patterns which is typical of myositis (low reflectivity and pronounced homogeneity of the muscle).

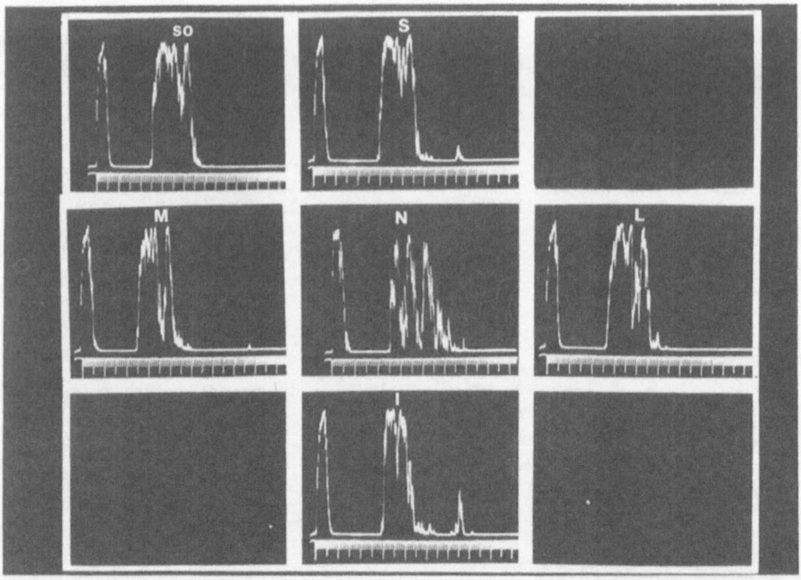

Fig. 8. A-scan documentation of maximum thicknesses of extraocular muscles in the left orbit of the same case depicted in Fig. 7 after the patient was treated for left orbital myositis (for details, see Fig. 7). Note the decreased (normalized) thicknesses of all the muscles. Except for the medial rectus muscle, all muscles have assumed normal reflectivity at this point. The inferior oblique muscle had shrunk to the point that it was impossible to document this muscle adequately after the treatment.

REFERENCES

1. McNutt, L. C., Kaefring, S. L. and Ossoinig, K. C.: Echographic Measurement of Extraocular Muscles. In: Ultrasound in Medicine (White, D. and Brown, R. E., eds.), 3A:927–932. Plenum, New York, 1977.
2. Ossoinig, K. C.: Standardized Echography: Basic Principles, Clinical Applications and Results. In: Ophthalmic Ultrasonography: Comparative Techniques (Dallow, R. L., ed.). Int. Ophthalmol. Clin., 19/4: 127–210. Little, Brown & Co., Boston, 1979.
3. Ossoinig, K. C.: The Technique of Measuring Extraocular Muscles. In: Diagnostica Ultrasonica in Ophthalmologia (Gernet, H., ed.), 166–172. Remy, Münster, 1979.
4. Ossoinig, K. C.: Ein neues echographisches Merkmal zur verlässlichen Differentialdiagnostik des endokrinen Exophthalmus. Klin. Monas. tbl. Augenheilk., 180: 189–197, 1982.

Authors' address:
Department of Ophthalmology
University of Iowa
Iowa City, IA 55242
USA

B-SCAN ULTRASONOGRAPHY OF ORBITAL VARICES

SONG GUO-XIANG AND XIAO LI-HUA
(Tianjin, China)

SUMMARY

Twenty three cases of orbital varices were revealed by contact B-scan ultrasonography, among which 19 were of the primary type and 4 were secondary. This paper describes the special echo patterns seen in primary and secondary orbital varices by the pressure test. The clinical pictures of orbital varices and the key points of the ultrasonic diagnosis are discussed.

Orbital varices can be divided into two types: primary and secondary. The former is a congenital venous malformation, and the latter is caused by either intracranial or intraorbital arteriovenous communication. Orbital venography is employed in the diagnosis of primary varices, while carotid angiography is used to demonstrate secondary varices. Both procedures are painful, although they are effective in detecting the malformed vessels. In our study, 23 cases with suspected intraorbital varices were examined with B-scan ultrasonography. Positive results were obtained in all cases. As a nonpainful method ultrasonography has advantages, as compared with the conventional painful procedures.

METHODS

An ophthalmic contact B-scan ultrasound system with a 10 MHz transducer has been used in our study. The scanner touches the patient's eyelid for routine examination in order to rule out any orbital space-occupying lesions. In patients with intermittent exophthalmos, the head of patient should not be lowered to the degree to cause proptosis. A sphygmomanometer cuff is wound around the patient's neck to exert pressure during the examination. After the initial scanning, the cuff is inflated raising the pressure to 20–40 mm Hg. Now, the patient begins to show exophthalmos and the change of orbital echo pattern can be identified. In patients with pulsating exophthalmos, the examiner should pay more attention to scanning in the upper and lower orbit in order to visualize the superior and inferior opthalmic veins as echo-free cavities. Once these veins are identified, the scanner should

Hillman, J. S./Le May, M. M. (eds.) Ophthalmic Ultrasonography

ISBN 978-94-009-7280-3

be pressed upon the patient's eyeball or pressure applied with fingers upon the ipsilateral carotid artery. When the pressure exceeds the intra-arterial pressure, the echo-free cavities will disappear as well as the pulsation.

RESULTS

During the period from July 1979 to June 1982, we examined 23 cases of orbital varices. Among them 19 were primary and 4 secondary. All these patients presented some characteristic ultrasonic findings, however, the acoustic pictures of these two types differ markedly.

Primary orbital varices. Among the 19 patients with primary varices, 9 underwent surgical operation and the diagnosis was established by histologic examination. The others all presented typical clinical features. The echo patterns were nearly identical in all 19 cases. In patients without any exophthalmos, the orbital echo patterns were normal; in other words, the retrobulbar fat pattern was displayed as a W- or V-shaped acoustically opaque (white) area (Fig. 1). Now inflating the bag of the sphygmomanometer to increase the pressure upon the patient's neck the retrobulbar echo pattern enlarges, and echo-free cavities appear (Fig. 2). Each acoustic cavity represents a tomographic picture of the abnormal vessel.

Secondary orbital varices. There were 4 cases of secondary varices. All of them were proved to be carotid-cavernous sinus fistulas by carotid angiography and/or surgery.

During ultrasonic examination, the scanner was placed on the center of the eyelid for sagittal scanning. A circular echo-free cavity was shown above the optic nerve. When the scanner handle was held downward obliquely, this circular cavity was elongated and a handlike echo-free cavity appeared just below the superior rectus (Fig. 3). With the scanner placed horizontally on the lower lid, a circular echo-free cavity appeared too (Fig. 4). These were the acoustic tomographic images of the dilated superior ophthalmic vein from different angles and positions. With proper sound beam incidence it is possible to detect the pulsation of this cavity which is synchronized with the heart beat. In the pressure test, the echo-free cavity changed in shape and then completely closed. Before closure, the pulsation became more marked. With the scanner held on the upper lid, the inferior ophthalmic vein was examined in the same way. This vessel was visualized in only one of the four cases.

In addition to vascular changes, the retrobulbar fat pattern was enclarged and the extraocular muscles were thicker with more internal echoes than normal.

TYPICAL CASE REPORTS

Case 1. A 26-year-old woman was admitted to hospital on September 8, 1979 with a complaint of intermittent exophthalmos associated with pain

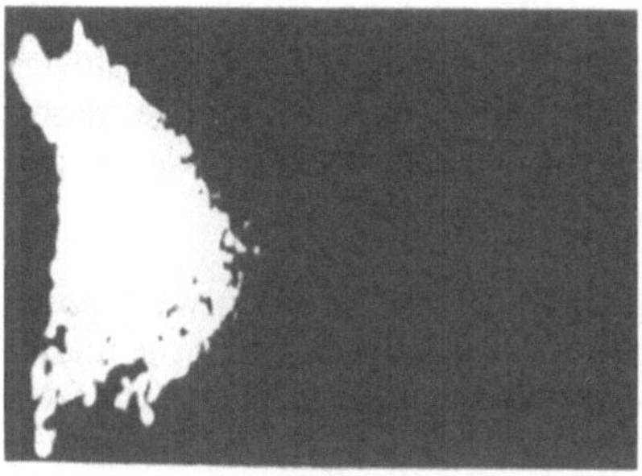

Fig. 1. B-scan ultrasonogram of a primary orbital varix before pressing on patient's jugular vein, showing a normal orbital fat pattern.

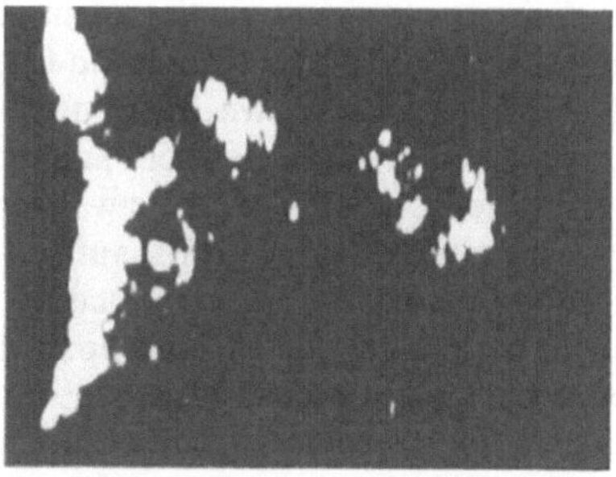

Fig. 2. The same patient as in Fig. 1, after pressing on the jugular vein, showing some echo-free cavities in the orbital fat echo pattern.

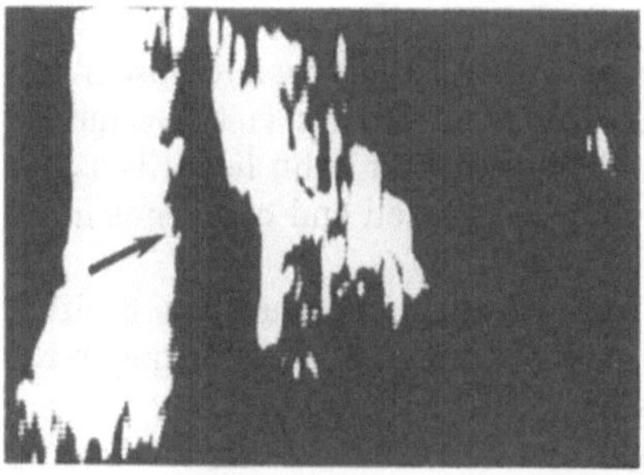

Fig. 3. B-scan ultrasonogram of a secondary orbital varix showing the dilated superior ophthalmic vein as a echo-free band on sagittal tomography.

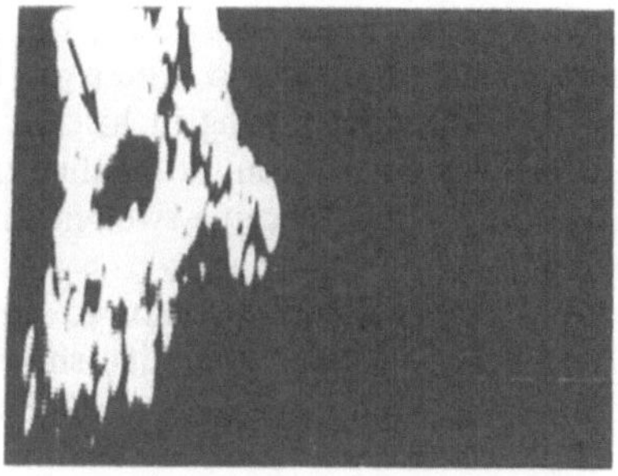

Fig. 4. B-scan ultrasonogram of a secondary orbital varix showing the dilated superior ophthalmic vein as a circular echo-free cavity on transversable section (the same patient as to Fig. 3).

and nausea for one and half years. In 1978, as she was bending, her right eye protruded, accompanied with pain in the orbital area, nausea and blurring of vision. When she returned upright, her eye gradually replaced to its original position and the symptoms disappeared. Since then such attacks recurred whenever the patient bent her head to work or carry a heavy load. It had become more frequent before admission. Sometimes the orbital pain wakened her. She had been in good health before 1978.

On admission, her general condition was good. No abnormal vessels could be found in her head, neck or any body surface elsewhere. Vision of both eyes was 1.5. Slight right enophthalmos was evident in the upright position, the orbit felt empty on palpation. The fundus was normal and the globe moved freely. The left eye was normal. In the upright position, the protrusion of the right eye was 13 mm, and that of the left 15 mm. With her head bending, the right eye protrusion measured 20 mm and the left 15 mm. X-ray examination of the orbit demonstrated 2 phleboliths in the right orbit.

Ultrasonic examination. In the supine position with the head slightly elevated, the B-scan ultrasonogram of the right orbit showed a normal pattern (Fig. 1). During the pressure test, the retrobulbar opaque area became enlarged rapidly and a number of connected echo-free cavities were visualized (Fig. 2). Moving the scanner slowly, we found that all the cavities were within the muscle cone. They were closed on pressure to the eyeball with the scanner and reappeared when the pressure was removed.

Diagnosis: primary orbital varix.

The operation was performed on September 25, 1979. When we exposed the muscle cone and pressed upon the patient's neck, we saw that the muscle cone enlarged and many tortuous dilated vessels appeared within it. The fatty tissues which enclosed the vessels were normal. This appearance is similar to the echo pattern shown. In order to preserve visual function, we only removed a part of the malformed veins, dissecting and destroying the remaining ones by forceps and pressing them with gelatin sponge.

Case 2. A 37-year-old man was admitted on April 9, 1981 with a complaint of a head injury 3 months previously and exophthalmos for 2 and a half months. On January 30, 1981, the patient fell from a high place with his face touching the ground. There was bleeding from his left ear and nose. After the accident, the hearing in his left ear decreased and his face became expressionless. Since then, he has had trouble with a bruit in his head. Ten days later, the left eye became swollen, the globe protruded and could not move freely.

Physical examination showed the patient was conscious and healthy. The heart, lungs and abdomen showed no abnormalities. The hearing in the left ear was poor, bone conduction being better than air conduction.

Eye examination showed that the right eye was normal. The visual acuity of the left eye was 0.1 and proptosis was noted with a 5 mm prominence compared with the right eye. On slit lamp examination, a slight pulsation of the globe was noticeable. In the orbital and temporal region, a vascular bruit was heard, but it disappeared when the ipsilateral carotid was pressed. The eyelid was swollen with severe edema and congestion of the bulbar conjunctiva which protruded from the palpebral fissure. The pupil diameter was 6 mm and both direct and indirect light reflex was absent. Ophthalmoscopic examination showed that the optic disc margin was blurred and elevated. The retinal veins were tortuous and dilated. Extraocular muscle movement was impaired in all directions.

Carotid angiography. In the arterial phase, the cavernous sinus was seen to be markedly enlarged, with dilated superior and inferior ophthalmic veins.

Ultrasonic examination. The right orbit was normal. The echo pattern of the left orbital fat was enlarged and the 4 rectus muscles were all slightly swollen with more echoes than normal. There was a echo-free zone below the superior rectus. On sagittal section it was band-like (Fig. 3) while a transverse scan demonstrated a circular echo-free cavity (Fig. 4). There was pulsation synchronized with the heart beat. Pressing the scanner upon the globe or fingers on the ipsilateral carotid made the echo-free cavity disappear as well as the pulsation. A similar echo-free cavity was also found in the lower part of the orbit, but it was less marked.

Diagnosis: Secondary orbital varix due to carotid-cavernous fistula.

Exploration of the cavernous sinus was performed by the neurosurgeons on May 16, 1981 and eye condition was improved after surgery.

DISCUSSION

Primary varix represents a congenital malformation with proliferation and dilation of the orbital veins. Any increase of jugular intravenous pressure can result in exophthalmos including bending the head, pressure on the jugular veins, coughing, forced expiration, crying or laughing. This brings on stasis in the orbital veins, increases the intraorbital venous pressure and then the eye-ball protrudes. Sudden increase of intraorbital pressure will also bring about pain, nausea and visual blurring. Symptoms will disappear seconds, minutes or hours after the venous pressure is decreased. X-ray examination demonstrated phleboliths in some, which is valuable for diagnosis. Final diagnosis is often made by orbital venography. However, this method has its disadvantages. a. The malformed vessels do not necessary communicate with the superior ophthalmic vein, or the latter may be thrombosed, so injection of contrast media into the angular vein may fail to display the abnormal vessels. b. The images are overlapped and it is difficult to identify the minute structure of the lesion. c. In about half of our cases, puncture of the angular venous system is unsuccessful. d. The examination is painful.

Primary orbital varices can be easily demonstrated by B-scan ultrasound. By pressure test, we have detected the lesions in all 19 cases. Otherwise, this technique also obtains the following information. 1. Whether the anomaly is a single venous dilation or is composed of numerous malformed vessels. 2. The location, scope and distribution of the lesion. 3. The relationship between the malformed vessels and the optic nerve as well as the extraocular muscles. All this information plays an important role in deciding the treatment and selecting the surgical approach.

CT can also be used to detect primary orbital varices. In our study 7 cases were examined by this technique and all demonstrated a mass lesion in the affected orbit, but it can not display the internal texture of the lesion either. According to our personal experience, of these three diagnostic techniques, the real time B-scan is the best method in evaluating primary orbital varices.

Secondary orbital varices are usually caused by an arteriovenous communication either intracranially or intraorbitally. All 4 cases in our series are due to a carotid-cavernous sinus fistula caused by trauma. Carotid rupture allows direct escape of arterial blood at high pressure into the cavernous sinus and ophthalmic veins. The intravenous pressure in markedly increased, which causes dilatation and tortuosity of the veins. In such a case, the varices are normal expanded veins. These can be shown by carotid angiography, but this method is painful and has poor patient tolerance. In a recent examination of 4 cases by ultrasonic examination, we assumed the presence of ateriovenous communication on the basis of the superior and inferior ophthalmic veins dilation and pulsation, though we could not directly demonstrate the arteriovenous fistula itself.

In our ultrasonic laboratory we also found 2 other pulsatile orbital lesions,

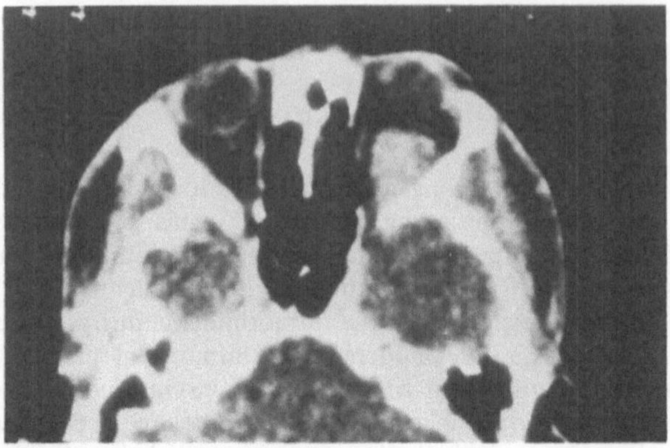

Fig. 5. Primary orbital varix on CT scanning showing a mass lesion in the left orbit.

one was a cirsoid hemangioma, and the other an intraorbital encephalocele. Cirsoid hemangioma is composed of masses of thickened tortuous vessels and capillaries. When the sound beam passes through the lesion, pulsatile echo-free cavities can be discerned in the acoustic pictures. But they differ from those found in secondary orbital varices. The pulsatile cavities have no fixed location in the former and have other characteristics seen in space-occupying lesions, while the latter have a definite location, because they are the superior and inferior ophthalmic veins themselves. Intraorbital encephalocele is common in neurofibromatosis. The defect of the orbital bone allows the frontal and temporal lobes to bulge into the orbit. The ultrasonic picture shows pulsation without echo-free cavities.

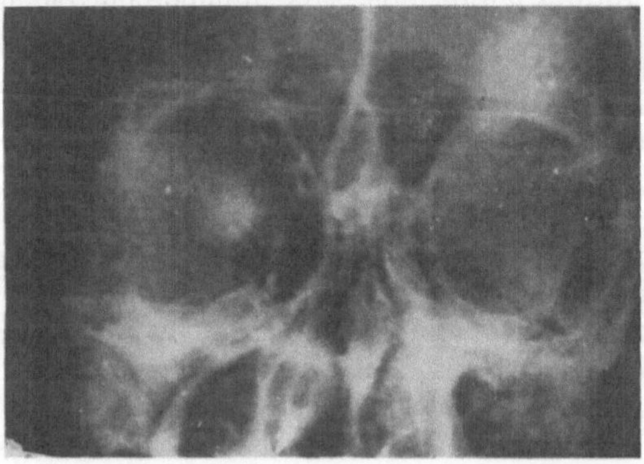

Fig. 6. Venogram of a primary orbital varix showing the abnormal vessels filled with contrast medium.

Authors' address:
Department of Ophthalmology
Teaching Hospital of Tianjin Medical College
Tianjin
People's Republic of China

ECHOGRAPHY IN CAROTID-CAVERNOUS FISTULAS

W. HAUFF AND P. TILL
(Vienna, Austria)

SUMMARY

Carotid-cavernous fistulas involving the internal carotid artery are fast-draining, high-pressure shunts. The dural-cavernous fistulas are low-flow, low-pressure shunts caused by the rupture of thin-walled, small-caliber arteries in the wall of the cavernous sinus. Very seldom congenital arterio-venous shunts can be observed.

Even when clinical signs are missing with standardized echography all types of carotid-cavernous fistulas are reliably diagnosed and differentiated. During the last 8 years 19 carotid-cavernous fistulas were diagnosed. 8 high-pressure fistulas were caused by frontal trauma, only one by the rupture of an internal carotid aneurysm. In one case clinical signs were bilateral. In 9 patients spontaneous, low-draining, low-pressure fistulas were detected; in a three months old infant a congenital arterio-venous shunt was observed.

The intracranial dura receives its blood supply from the internal carotid, the external carotid and the vertebral arteries. Abnormal communication with the cavernous sinus may be supplied by any combination of these sources. In a study clarifying the relationship of the afferent vessels in dural arteriovenous malformations in 89% the external carotid artery was involved; in cases of malformations of the cavernous sinus alone in 75% vessels arose from the internal carotid artery. Supply from the vertebral artery is uncommon (Newton, T. H., Hoyt, W. F. 1970). When the main blood supply originates from the external system, the middle meningeal artery is the most frequently involved branch communicating with the venous sinus.

In one quarter of patients with carotid-cavernous fistulas spontaneous dural-cavernous shunts are caused by the rupture of thin-walled, small-caliber arteries in the wall of the cavernous sinus. Congenital defects in the media, small congenital aneurysms or atherosclerotic changes are responsible. Most of these patients are middle aged women. The dural-cavernous fistulas are low-flow, low-pressure shunts and the symptoms may be transient. The lower venous pressure is the reason, that bilateral venous engorgement caused by intracavernous communication is less likely to occur in these shunts than in those originating in the internal carotid artery. Proptosis is not severe and

Hillman, J. S./Le May, M. M. (eds.) Ophthalmic Ultrasonography

ISBN 978-94-009-7280-3

because of this flow bruits occur in only 50% of the patients (Biglan, A. W. and others 1981).

Trauma is responsible for about three-quarters of the carotid-cavernous fistulas (Walsh, F. B., Hoyt, W. F. 1969). These posttraumatic internal carotid-cavernous fistulas occur especially in young patients after frontal head trauma on the same side of the fistula. Penetrating orbital injuries in the direction of the orbital apex or complications after transspenoidal operations may be other reasons.

The rupture of the carotid artery or its branch in the cavernous sinus causes a markedly increased venous pressure. Fistulas involving the internal carotid artery are high-flow, high-pressure shunts. The increased pressure in the cavernous sinus causes the dilatation of entering veins and a reverse blood flow in these vessels. Arterial blood escaping into the cavernous sinus finds several exit channels. The drainage into the superior ophthalmic vein is the most common pattern of venous outflow, followed by drainage into the inferior ophthalmic vein, the petrosal sinuses and the clival plexus (Newton, T. H., Hoyt, W. F. 1970). The arterial blood may also flow from one cavernous sinus to the other via a system of intracavernous or portal veins. This may produce clinical signs in the opposite orbit and eye.

Dilatation of arterialized orbital veins and congestion in the orbital tissues account for the proptosis and swelling of the eyelids. The tortuous arterialized vessels pulsate and thus impart pulsation to the eyeball itself. Features common to both types of carotid-cavernous fistulas include unilateral headache, ipsilateral retro-orbital pain, dilated episcleral and concunctival vessels and increased tearing. Paralysis of oculomotor and abducens nerve, glaucoma, neovascular changes on the peripheral iris, cataract, folds in the Descemet's membrane and corneal opacification can be observed. In the fundus choroidal detachment, distended retinal veins, retinal hemorrhages, exudates and papilledema occasionally can be seen. Loss of visual acuity may be caused by decreased retinal perfusion resulting from narrowing of the arteriovenous pressure gradient secondary to increased venous pressure.

For diagnosis and differentiation of orbital lesions standardized echography with a combination of A-scan unit 7200 MA Kretztechnik, a contact B-scan Bronson-Turner and a Doppler ultrasound instrument Minivason 9 is used. In the echographic department of 2nd University-Eye Clinic during the last eight years in 19 patients the diagnosis of a carotid-cavernous fistula was verified. During this time we detected 8 carotid-cavernous fistulas caused by frontal trauma. One young man developed a fast-draining spontaneous carotid-cavernous fistula caused by the rupture of an internal carotid aneurysm. In one case clinical and echographical findings were bilateral (Fig. 1). 8 of total 9 patients with low-draining spontaneous dural-cavernous fistulas were middle aged women. We examined a three month old infant with unilateral proptosis of the globe and detected a high-flow, high-pressure shunt originating from the external carotid artery.

Arterio-venous fistulas that drain through the orbit widening the superior ophthalmic vein and pushing the blood through this vein into facial anastomoses, produce echograms pathognomonic of this condition. Echographical criteria are the regular structure, the very low reflectivity and weak sound

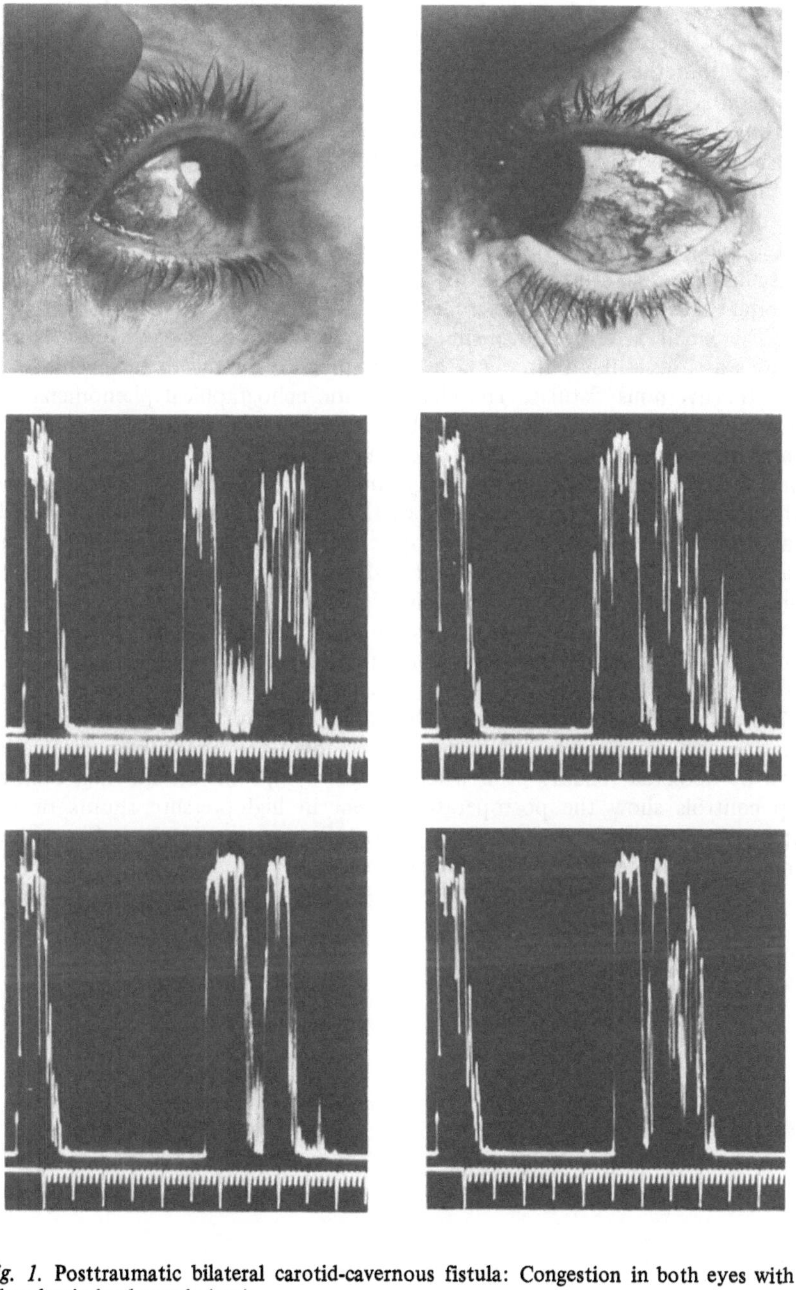

Fig. 1. Posttraumatic bilateral carotid-cavernous fistula: Congestion in both eyes with dilated episcleral vessels (top).
Transocular A-scan echograms demonstrate the pathognomonic acoustic criteria in both orbits: sharply outlined orbital defects, regular structure, very low reflectivity, fast flickering movements of the blood spikes (center and bottom).

attenuation (Ossoinig, K. C. 1979). The fast flickering movement of the blood spikes within the sharply outlined orbital defect confirm the diagnosis (Fig. 2). The movements of the blood spikes indicating arterialized blood flow within the vessels are often better seen when a greater horizontal expansion is used. B-scan echograms show the dilated superior vein as a sharply outlined orbital defect (Fig. 3) of meandering shape curving from anterior nasal to temporal posterior in the superior orbit. The dilated orbital vessel is mobile and shifts with eye movements. During kinetic echography with compression by the probe the dilated arterialized orbital vein shows the phenomenon of a delayed, sudden compressibility. After overcoming intravascular pressure and exhausting the compressibility of surrounding soft orbital tissues increasing pressure leads to sudden collapse (Ossoinig, K. C.).

The small arterio-venous shunt in spontanous dural-cavernous fistulas causes a slower blood flow and a lower pressure in the dilated veins as in carotid-cavernous fistulas. The characteristic echographical phenomena can also be seen in this type of shunts. Usually the orbital veins drain posteriorly into the sinuses. Congestion in the orbital tissues by blocking the orbital vessels is typical. A-scan echography shows that all extraocular muscles are thickened. The maximum thickness of the optic nerve is increased by sheathing signs indicating swelling of the optic nerve sheaths. The episcleral venous pressure is raised. Dilated episcleral and conjunctival vessels with chemosis and increased tearing may be misinterpreted as conjunctivitis, episcleritis, iritis or glaucoma and treated over months unsuccessfully. Standardized echography can clarify that in a few minutes.

Orbital vascular malformations are easily and reliably diagnosed and differentiated with standardized echography. Regarding the pathognomonic criteria fast-draining carotid-cavernous and low-flow dural-cavernous fistulas can be detected reliably even when clinical symptoms are missing. Follow-up controls show the postoperative effect in high-pressure shunts or the spontanous regression of low-draining fistulas and save patients from other invasive and more dangerous examinations.

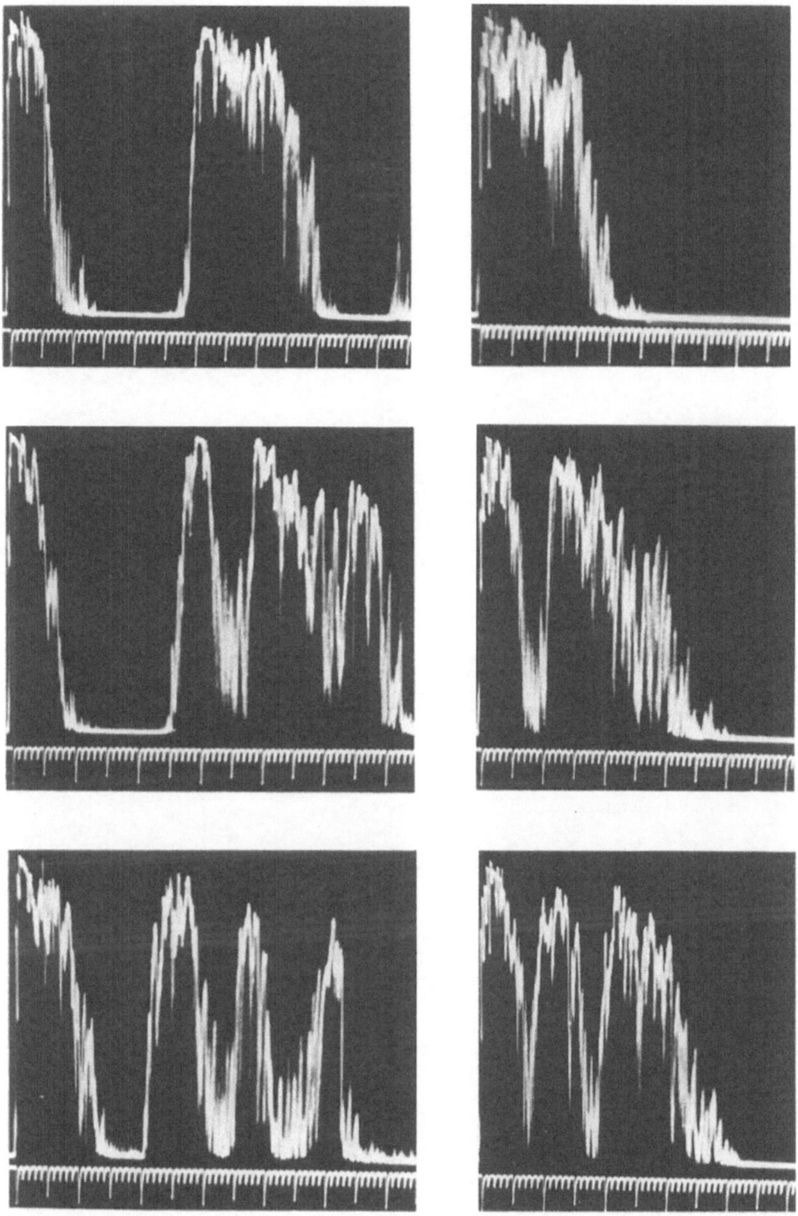

Fig. 2. Posttraumatic unilateral fistula: Transocular (left) and paraocular (right) A-scan echograms of normal orbital tissue (top), fast-draining carotid-cavernous fistula (center) and oblique section through the meandering dilated superior ophthalmic vein (sound beam aimed through the afferent and efferent portions of the meandering vessel) (bottom).

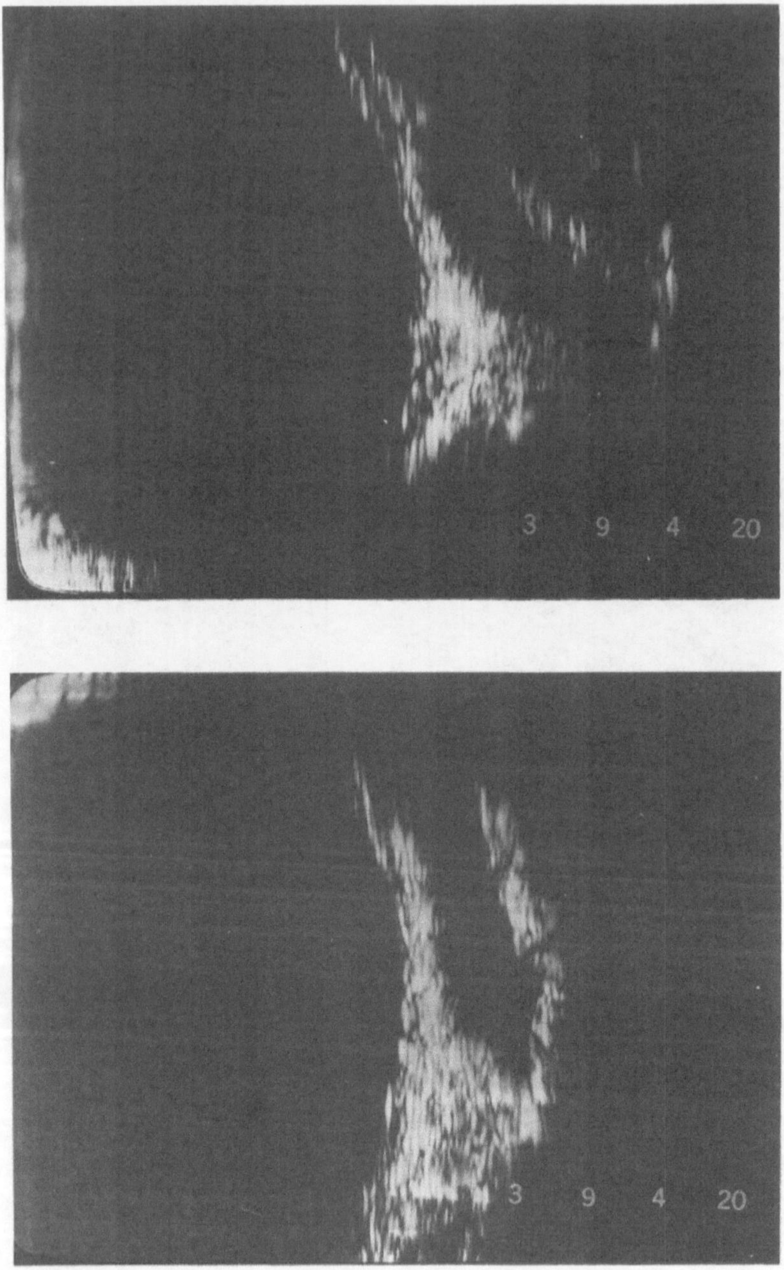

Fig. 3. **B-scan echograms show the dilated superior ophthalmic vein curving from anterior nasal to temporal posterior in the superior orbit: vertical section (top) horizontal section (bottom).**

REFERENCES

Biglan, A. W., Pang, D., Shuckett, E. P. and Kerber, C.: External carotid-cavernous fistula in an infant. Amer. J. Ophthal. 91:351 (1981).

Costin, J. A., Weinstein, M. A., Berlin, A. J., Hardy, R. W. G. and Gutman, F. A.: Dural arterio-venous malformations involving the cavernous sinus: a case report. Brit. J. Ophthal. 62:478 (1978).

Harbison, J. W., Guerry, D. and Wiesinger, H.: Dural arteriovenous fistula and spontaneous choroidal detachment: new cause of an old disease. Brit. J. Ophthal. 62: 483 (1978).

Henderson, J. W. and Schneider, R. C.: The ocular findings in carotid-cavernous fistula in a series of 17 cases. Amer. J. Ophthal. 48:585 (1959).

Ossoinig, K. C.: Preoperative differential diagnosis of tumors with echography: IV. Diagnosis of orbital tumors. Current Concepts in Ophthalmology 4:313 (1974).

Ossoinig, K. C.: Standardized echography: basic principles, clinical applications, and results. Ophthalmic Ultrasonography: Comparative Techniques. International Ophthalmology Clinics: 19 (4):127 (1979).

Ossoinig, K. C.: Echography of orbital disorders. Clinical Handbook of Ultrasound (M. de Vlieger, ed.). New York: Wiley, p. 881 (1978).

Ossoinig, K. C.: The role of clinical echography in modern diagnosis of periorbital and orbital lesions. Proc. 3rd Int. Symp. on Orbital Disorders (C. Bleeker, ed.) The Hague: Junk, p. 496 (1978).

Newton, T. H. and Hoyt, W. F.: Dural arteriovenous shunts in the region of the cavernous sinus. Neuroradiology 1:71 (1970).

Sanders, M. D. and Hoyt, W. F.: Hypoxic ocular sequelae of carotid-cavernous fistulae. Brit. J. Ophthal. 53:82 (1969).

Walsh, F. B. and Hoyt, W. F.: Clinical Neuroophthalmology. Vol. 2:1714 (The Williams and Wilkins Company, Baltimore)(1969).

Authors' address:
II. Universitäts-Augenklinik
Alserstrasse 4
A-1090 Wien
Austria

THE DIAGNOSIS OF ORBITAL MUCOCELES AND PYOCELES WITH STANDARDIZED ECHOGRAPHY

G. HASENFRATZ and K. C. OSSOINIG
(Iowa City, USA)

Among the periorbital lesions that affect and secondarily invade the orbit, benign mucoceles and pyoceles of the paranasal sinuses play a prominent role. The incidence of these orbital 'Muco(pyo)celes' among all orbital tumors ranges between 3% and 10%; they are the cause of unilateral proptosis in 3% to 15% of the cases (1–4, 6, 11, 12, 14). Orbital mucoceles usually originate in the frontal and adjacent ethmoidal sinuses; a mucocele rarely invades the orbit from the sphenoidal or maxillary sinuses. Therefore, an orbital mucocele is clinically suspected in a case of unilateral proptosis in which the globe is displaced mostly temporally and inferiorly rather than anteriorly, and in which a smoothly outlined mass can be palpated in the superonasal anterior orbit. Diplopia, pain and headaches may occur, and patients with this condition frequently give a typical history of chronic rhinological problems or severe head injury (skull fracture) long before the onset of the displacement of the globe.

Since the first alarming sign of an orbital mucocele is usually the displacement of the globe, most patients with this disorder are first seen by an ophthalmologist. If standardized echography is used as the screening method for the orbit, it will be the first diagnostic method to detect and identify or confirm the presence of an orbital mucocele or pyocele.

Table 1 lists the 10 acoustic criteria that are determined with standardized echography and usually clinch the diagnosis (3, 8, 9). While most or all acoustic criteria are needed to make a safe diagnosis, some of the criteria are more significant than others. A regular internal structure combined with a low reflectivity, a sharp outline with cyst wall and the typical location clearly separate orbital muco(pyo)celes from other periorbital lesions. If these key criteria are present, echograms can be considered 'pathognomonic for' orbital mucoceles. If one of these key criteria is not clearly present, a mucocele can still be diagnosed with echography, but the echograms are then called 'consistent with' this type of lesion. Echographically, it is impossible at this time to differentiate between a mucocele and a pyocele. Occasionally, the presence of a pyocele can be suspected from the inflammatory changes accompanying the lesion; usually, however, the diagnosis includes both the possibilities that the cyst is filled with mucous or with pus.

Figures 1–5 illustrate the typical clinical and echographic findings in

Hillman, J. S./Le May, M. M. (eds.) Ophthalmic Ultrasonography

ISBN 978-94-009-7280-3

Table 1. The acoustic criteria that are diagnostic for an orbital mucocele or pyocele, as evaluated with standardized echography

I. Quantitative echography	1. Regular Internal Structure [A*] 2. Extremely-Low to Low Reflectivity (2%–40% spike height; the surface spikes are excluded from this evaluation) [A] 3. Mostly Weak Sound Attenuation (angle kappa may vary between 10° and 40°) [A]
II. Topographic echography	4. Large, Regularly Outlined, Total Bony Defect [A(B)] 5. Sharply Outlined Borders (steeply rising surface spikes with very few high-frequency nodules at the ascending limb; surface spikes are double-peaked indicating cyst wall) [A] 6. Roundish Shape with Scalloped Margins Superiorly and Medially [B, A] 7. Location Most Frequently in the Superonasal Anterior Orbit (frontal mucocele) or Nasally (ethmoidal mucocele); Inferonasally Anteriorly (maxillary mucocele) or Nasally Far Posteriorly (sphenoidal mucocele) [A, B]
III. Kinetic echography	8. Avascular [A] 9. Immobile [A] 10. Usually Hard (particularly large mucoceles with very large bony defects may be minimally compressible [firm]) [A]

*A = determined with standardized A-scan; B = determined with contact, real-time B-scan.

a fronto-ethmoidal mucocele. Note the very steep rise of the surface spikes at tissue sensitivity seen in the transocular and paraocular A-scan echograms in Fig. 2. Although the slight sound attenuation, as seen from the angle kappa (the angle between the baseline and a line through the centers or peaks of the echo spikes excluding the surface signals), can be seen in most echograms at tissue sensitivity, an exact evaluation of this angle is only possible at medium spike height (9)(see bottom echogram in Fig. 3, which was obtained at 7 decibels above tissue sensitivity). The presence of a large bony defect (in the superonasal anterior orbital wall in this case) can be determined in several ways (3, 8, 9, 13). By placing the probe on the medial aspect of the upper lid and aiming the sound beam toward the frontal sinus, the examiner can quickly detect the fact that much of the echogram is recorded from outside the orbit. This is particularly obvious when a comparison is made with the same area in the normal fellow orbit. If it is proven that at least part of the echogram is obtained from outside the orbit, then the maximum height of the remote surface signal obtained at tissue sensitivity determines whether there is a bony defect (100% high, overloaded surface spike) or not (lower than 100% high surface spike; see Fig. 4A). A more elegant and sophisticated way of determining a bony defect is to sweep the ultrasonic beam across the area in several directions and observe the

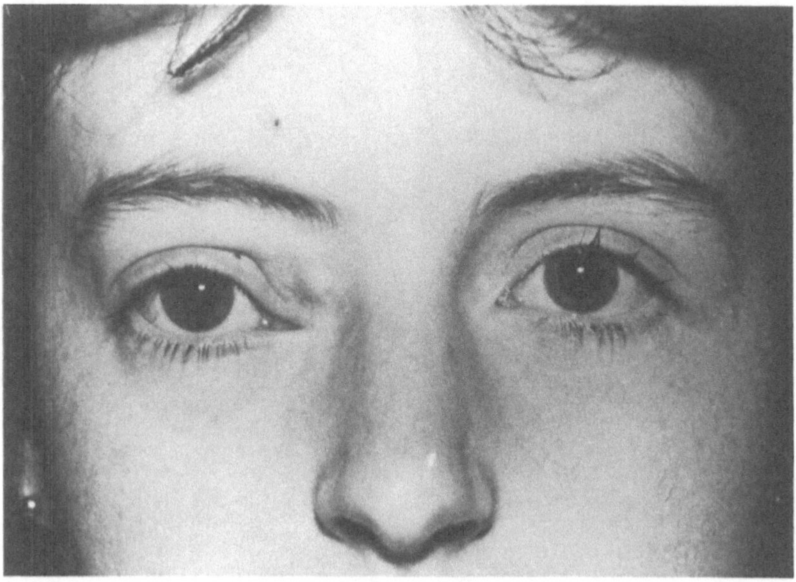

Fig. 1. 24-year old white female who presented with a displacement of the right globe inferiorly and laterally and with a palpable mass in the anterior superonasal quadrant of the orbit.

behavior of the surface spike (6)(part *B* in Fig. 4): a see-saw movement of two surface spikes during this procedure indicates a step in the bony outline and, with sufficient distance between the two surface spikes, a bony defect. The scalloped appearance of the borders of a mucocele in B-scan echograms (see Fig. 5) may stem from an acoustic cut across the margin of the bony defect or, more frequently, is due to the corresponding shape of the sinus walls. While B-scan is helpful in determining the topography of a mucocele, the essential acoustic information is obtained with standardized A-scan. Standardized A-scan also permits the accurate measurement of the dimensions of the mucocele.

Tables 2 and 3 present the results obtained with standardized echography (in the diagnosis of orbital mucoceles and pyoceles) during an 11-year period in the Echography Service of the Department of Ophthalmology at The University of Iowa. As can be seen from these tables, the *sensitivity* of standardized echography (i.e., the number of correct echographic diagnoses as a percentage of all histologically and/or surgically proven mucoceles and pyoceles) is 97.6%. There was only one false-negative diagnosis among the 41 cases in the study. The echograms for the great majority of the orbital mucoceles and pyceles (i.e., 85% of all correctly diagnosed cases) were classified as 'pathognomonic for' muco(pyo)celes. The *reliability* of standardized echography (i.e., the number of the correctly made echographic diagnoses as a percentage of all such diagnoses of orbital muco(pyo)celes) is also 97.6% overall. When the echograms were called 'pathognomonic for' muco(pyo)cele,

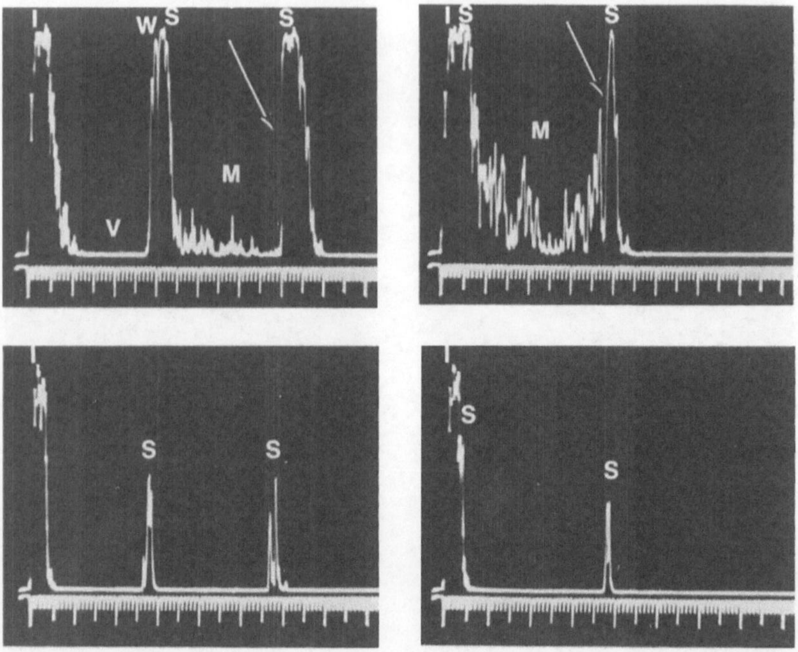

Fig. 2. Standardized A-scan echograms from right fronto-ethmoidal mucocele found in patient shown in Fig. 1. *Left* transocular echograms obtained in the 1:30 meridian from the most anterior orbit and the frontal sinus. *Right* paraocular echograms recorded from the same area with the probe placed at the inner end of the upper lid and with the beam aimed toward the frontal sinus. *Top* echograms were recorded at 'tissue sensitivity'; *bottom* echograms at markedly reduced 'measuring sensitivity'. *I* initial spike indicating the surface of the probe as placed on the globe or upper lid; *V* clear vitreous cavity; *W* ocular wall signals; *S* surface spikes of mucocele (steeply rising or falling at tissue sensitivity, double-peaked at measuring sensitivity). *M* echo signals from mucoid contents of the cyst. Note that the diameter of the mucocele as measured with the electronic scale (calibrated in microseconds) in the beam direction described above is larger than the diameter of the globe. Also note the particularly steep rise of the ascending limb of the right surface spikes at tissue sensitivity indicating the smooth epithelialized inner surface of the mucocele (*arrows*).

the reliability was 100%. When the echograms were called only 'consistent with' orbital muco(pyo)cele, the reliability was 85.7%, since there was one false-positive echographic diagnosis in this latter group. On the basis of these results, an echographic diagnosis 'pathognomonic for' orbital muco(pyo)cele can be considered to have a probability of almost 100%, whereas the echographic diagnosis 'consistent with' orbital muco(pyo)cele has a probability of about 85%.

It should be mentioned that in three additional cases, no confirmation of an echographic diagnosis of muco(pyo)cele was obtained (no surgery was performed so far), and that in three more cases, standardized echography suggested the possibility of an 'atypical' muco(pyo)cele among other diagnostic alternatives. The atypical appearance in all three cases was caused by a location next to or entirely separate from the paranasal

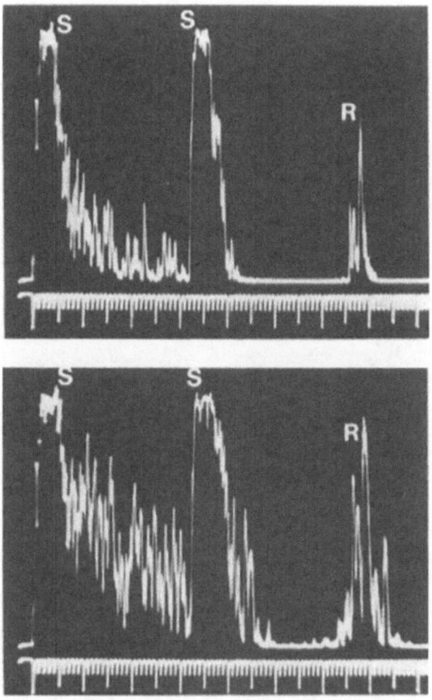

Fig. 3. Standardized A-scan echograms recorded with a paraocular beam (probe placed at the inner end of the upper lid and beam directed toward frontal sinus). The *top* echogram was obtained at 'tissue sensitivity' showing low spike height. The *bottom* echogram was recorded at a 6 decibels higher sensitivity setting of the instrument in order to produce medium spike height (medium height of the echo spikes representing the mucoid contents of the mucocele). At this medium spike height, the angle kappa (i.e., the angle between the baseline and a line through the centers or the peaks of the spikes) is about 40° indicating slight to moderate sound attenuation within the mucocele. *S* surface spikes; *R* reverberation signals from the remote wall of the mucocele indicating the particularly high reflectivity of this wall (echo pulses were reverberating twice between the probe and the opposite wall of the mucocele).

sinuses with an atypically located bony defect in the orbital wall. In all three cases, a lesion different than a muco(pyo)cele was found histologically and/or surgically: in two of the cases, an aneurysmal bone cyst and in the third, an eosinophilic granuloma. In one of the aneurysmal bone cysts, echography had indicated 'cholesteatoma' as an alternative possibility to atypical mucocele.

Standardized echography is the method of choice in detecting or confirming orbital muco(pyo)celes because of its excellent results (see Tables 2 and 3), for the fact that it will usually (where available) be performed first and because of other advantages over X-ray examination procedures, in particular CT-scans (see Table 4). A positive diagnosis by ultrasound carries a particularly high reliability (100%) when the echographic findings can be classified as 'pathognomonic for' a muco(pyo)cele (i.e., when the acoustic key criteria are clearly and completely present); this is often the case (in > 80% of all cases). Echography is also very helpful in the detection of

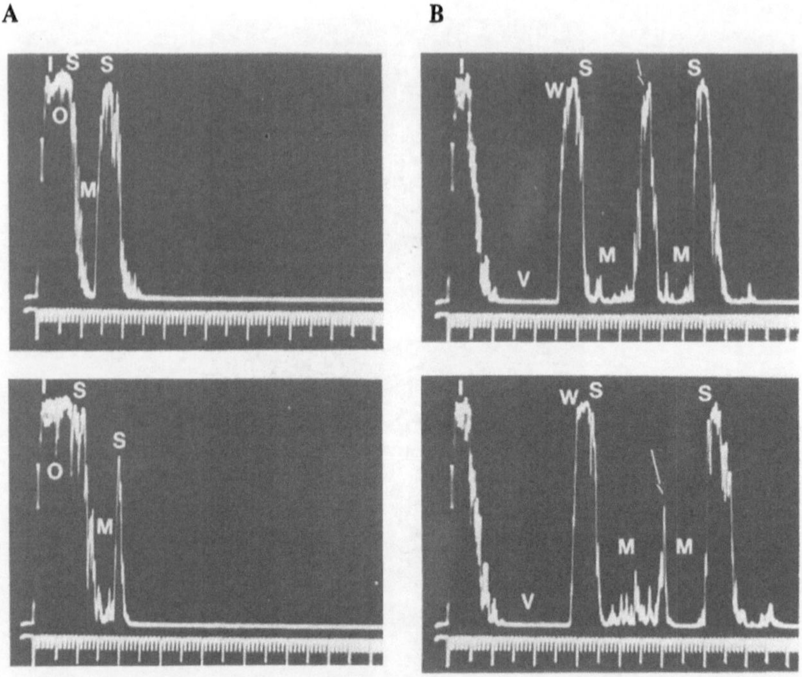

Fig. 4. Echographic proof of total bony defect in the orbital wall area of the mucocele. *A* paraocular echograms from areas with total bony defect (above) and with intact bone or bony shell (below). Both echograms represent the frontal sinus which is devoid of air. Note the 100% high overloaded broad spike from the sinus roof obtained through the bony defect whereas the same surface appears as an 80% high narrow spike as most of the ultrasonic energy is absorbed by the intact bony orbital wall or a bony shell covering in the other area. *B* transocular echograms which were obtained when the beam was half intercepted by the orbital wall and half entering the frontal sinus (above) and when most of the beam was entering the sinus and only the beam periphery was intercepted by the orbital wall to a very small degree (below). *I* initial spike representing the surface of the probe where it was placed on the skin surface (*A*) or globe surface (*B*); *O* normal subcutaneous or orbital tissues; *V* clear vitreous cavity; *W* ocular wall signals; *S* surface spikes representing the anterior (inferior) wall of mucocele next to normal subcutaneous tissues (on the left side of mucocele echograms) and indicating the epithelialized mucocele wall at the roof of the sinus (on the right). *Arrows* point at orbital roof next to bony defect, which is reached by half the ultrasonic beam (*top* echogram in *B*) and by the beam periphery only (*bottom* echogram in *B*) respectively. *M* mucoid contents of mucocele. Note the steeply rising right surface spikes corresponding to the epithelial lining of the mucocele wall.

bilateral mucoceles which, at least on plain X-ray films, may be difficult to diagnose due to the lack of a comparison with normal fellow orbits and sinuses. Whenever the echograms are unduly irregular in internal structure, a solid tumor, usually a carcinoma of the sinuses, should be suspected. If the location of the tumor and the bony defect is atypical for a sinus lesion, other cysts such as a dermoid cyst, an aneurysmal bone cyst or an eosinophilic granuloma should be considered.

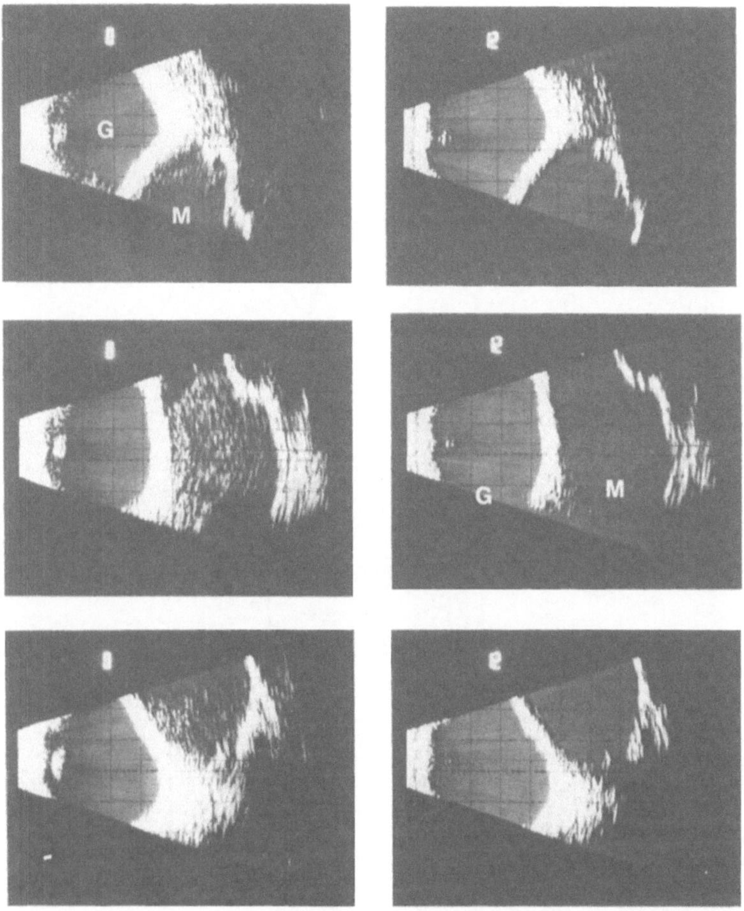

Fig. 5A. The transocular B-scan echograms were obtained with transverse sections (acoustic sections that are aligned perpendicular to ocular meridians) across the 12:30 (*top* patterns), 1:30 (*central* echograms) and 4 o'clock meridians (*bottom* echograms). The 12:30 pictures show the temporal edge, whereas the 4 o'clock echograms illustrate the inferonasal edge of the mucocele. Note the scalloped appearance of the right surface line in the central echograms which is typical of a mucocele. Also note that the globe is clearly indented by the tumor. *G* globe; *M* mucocele.

Table 2. Results of standardized echography in diagnosing 41 consecutive cases of histologically and/or surgically proven orbital muco(pyo)celes (Echography Service, Department of Ophthalmology, The University of Iowa, 1972–1982)

All cases	Correct diagnoses (Sensitivity of Standardized Echography)		Incorrect diagnosis (False-Negative)
41 (100%)	40 (97.6%)		1 (2.4%)
	'pathognomonic for' 34 (85%)	'consistent with' 6 (15%)	

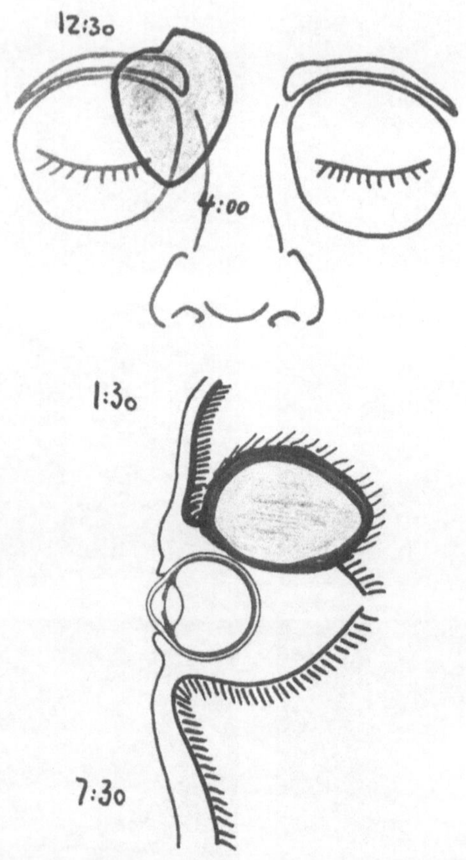

Fig. 5B. Frontal view (*top*) and sagittal section (*bottom*) through mucocele indicating the affected meridians and the dimensions of the tumor and the bony defect. The drawings are based on the A-scan and B-scan findings, and are part of the echographic report of the case illustrated in Fig. 1.

Table 3. Final results (histological and/or surgical proof) in 41 consecutive cases in which standardized echography diagnosed an orbital muco(pyo)cele (Echography Service, Department of Ophthalmology, The University of Iowa, 1972–1982)

	Correct Diagnoses (Reliability of Standardized Echography)	Incorrect diagnoses (False-Negative)
Total 41 (100%)	40 (97.6%)	1 (2.4%)
'pathognomonic for' 34 (82.9%)	34 (100%)	– (0%)
'consistent with' 7 (17.1%)	6 (85.7%)	1 (14.3%)

Table 4. Clear advantages of standardized echography in diagnosing orbital mucoceles or pyoceles

*	Echography, used as a screening method for the orbit, will easily and quickly detect orbital and periorbital tumors.
*	Superior sensitivity of standardized echography in differentiating orbital and periorbital tumors.
*	Superior reliability of standardized echography in differentiating orbital and periorbital tumors.
*	Great accuracy of standardized echography in the measurement of orbital and periorbital tumors.
*	Mobile, relatively inexpensive equipment.
*	Completely harmless procedure.

REFERENCES

1. Babel, J., Psilas, K., Soriano, H. and Houber, J. P.: Differential diagnosis of orbital tumors by echography A. Clinico-pathological study of 54 cases. In: Orbital Disorders (Proc. of 2nd Int. Symp. on Orbital Disorders, Amsterdam, 1973, Bleeker, G. M. et al., eds.). Mod. Probl. Ophthalmol., 14:254–264. Karger, Basel/New York, 1975.
2. Harrison, D. F.: The ENT surgeon looks at the orbit. J. Laryngol. Otol., 3 (Suppl.): 1–43, 1980.
3. Hauff, W. and Till, P.: Echographic findings in orbital mucoceles. In: Diagnostica Ultrasonica in Ophthalmologia (proc. of SIDUO VII, Münster, 1978, Gernet, H., ed.), 151–154. Remy, Münster, 1979.
4. Henderson, J. W.: Orbital Tumors, 96–105. Thieme-Stratton, New York, 1980.
5. Moss, H. M.: Expanding Lesions of the Orbit. Am. J. Ophthalmol., 54:761–770, 1962.
6. Ossoinig, K. C. and Blodi, F. C.: Preoperative Differential Diagnosis of Tumors with Echography. Part IV. Diagnosis of Orbital Tumors. In: Current Concepts in Ophthalmology (Blodi, F. C., ed.), 4:313–341. C. V. Mosby, St. Louis, 1974.
7. Ossoinig, K. C. and Till, P.: Ten-Year Study on Clinical Echography in Intraocular Disease. In: Ultrasonography in Ophthalmology (Proc. of SIDUO V, Ghent, 1973, Francois, J. and Goes, F., eds.). Bibl. Ophthalmol., 83:49–62. Karger, Basel/New York, 1975.
8. Ossoinig, K. C.: The Role of Clinical Echography in Modern Diagnosis of Periorbital and Orbital Lesions. In: Proc. of 3rd Int. Symp. on Orbital Disorders (Bleeker, G. M., ed.), 496–540. Dr. W. Junk, Amsterdam, 1978.
9. Ossoinig, K. C.: Standardized Echography: Basic Principles, Clinical Applications and Results. In: Ophthalmic Ultrasonography: Comparative Techniques (Dallow, R. L., ed.). Int. Ophthalmol. Clin., 19/4:127–210. Little, Brown & Co., Boston, 1979.
10. Ossoinig, K. C.: Diagnostic Ultrasound. In: Neuro-Ophthalmology Volume 2/1982 (Lessell, S. and van Dalen, J. T. W., eds.), 373–388. Excerpta Medica, Amsterdam, 1982.
11. Palmer, B. W.: Unilateral Exophthalmos. Arch. Otolaryngol., 28:415–424, 1965.
12. Silva, D.: Orbital Tumors. Am. J. Ophthalmol., 65:318–339, 1968.
13. Till, P.: Echography in Rhinogenic Orbital Conditions. In: Orbital Disorders (Proc. 2nd Int. Symp. on Orbital Disorders, Amsterdam, 1973, Bleeker, G. M. et al., eds.). Mod. Probl. Ophthalmol., 14:273–277. Karger, Basel/New York, 1975.
14. Zizmor, J., Fasano, C. V., Smith, B. and Rabett, W.: Roentgenographic Diagnosis of Unilateral Exophthalmos. JAMA, 197/5:343–346, 1966.

Authors' address:
Department of Ophthalmology
University of Iowa,
Iowa City, IA 55242
USA

ECHOGRAPHIC PATTERNS OF PERIPHERAL NERVE TUMOURS

V. MAZZEO, R. SCORRANO, L. RAVALLI and M. SPETTOLI
(Ferrara, Italy)

SUMMARY

Neurofibroma, neurofibromatosis, schwannoma and paraganglioma are the benign types of peripheral nerve tumour, the last two of which have also a malignant form. Neurofibroma and schwannoma originate from the neuroglia, neurofibromatosis, (von Recklinghausen's disease), originates from astrocyte proliferation.

All those forms are not frequent, so in the echographic literature rather few cases are reported. For this reason it is clearly difficult to find out a pathognomic echopattern; in fact many authors found very contrasting characteristics. Our cases and the pertinent literature are discussed in order to improve our recognition of this pathology.

Peripheral nerve tumours have been discussed in the past because of their various and often personal classifications (Henderson 1973). Only recently Zimmerman and Sobin in a WHO publication (1980) have revised the international histological classification, subdividing them into: traumatic neuroma, neurofibroma/plexiform neuroma, neurofibromatosis, schwannoma and paraganglioma. The last two also have a malignant form.

This confusion has caused many Authors to classify case reports in different ways. This is also true of the echographic literature where there are very few cases of each kind of tumour. After reviewing the pertinent literature some cases we have dealt with are discussed below.

Rootman et al. (1982) have described seven clinical pictures of primary orbital schwannomas. They report ultrasonographic patterns without mentioning the equipment they used. Three out of the four cases they examined with ultrasound had intraconal masses: 'All were described as encapsulated solid lesions with a well demarcated anterior border. Within the mass were a number of tissue interfaces which attenuated dramatically. A posterior border could not be detected'.

Previous Authors had already described the echopattern of these neurogenic tumours. Ossoinig (1975), using the so-called 'standardized A.scan', reported these lesions as highly reflective, variable in consistency (hard to

Hillman, J. S./Le May, M. M. (eds.) Ophthalmic Ultrasonography

ISBN 978-94-009-7280-3

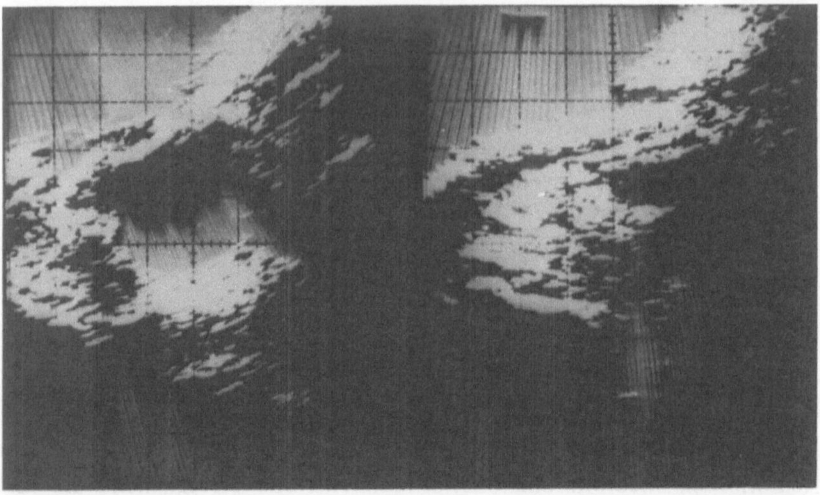

Fig. 1. **Neurofibromatosis. Gray scale immersion B-scans (5 MHz). Right: temporal to the globe a real echogenic mass is seen. Left: cutaneous mass just outside the lateral orbital wall.**

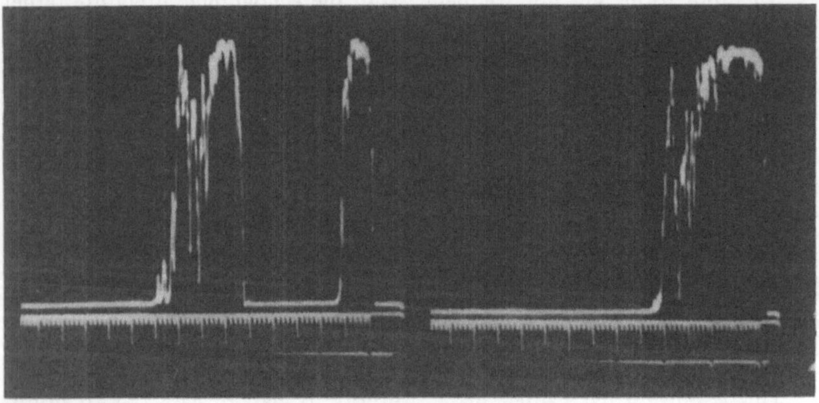

Fig. 2. High reflective neurofibroma.

soft), strong attenuating, from poorly outlined to diffuse and mobile. No other author reports A-scan echo patterns, which can, however, be inferred indirectly as being extremely variable (Janev, et al. 1979; Till and Hauff 1981).

Coleman, et al. (1977) describe neurilemmomas and neurofibromas as poorly encapsulated or not encapsulated, and showing a poor sound transmission (i.e. infiltrative type of ultrasonic pattern on the B-scan). Schroeder (1979) classifies the neurogenic tumours as well delimited. Restori, et al. (1978) and Restori (1979) report the following characteristics for neurilemmomas: '. . . . . rounded echo-free mass, but give rise to medium amplitude echoes throughout the lesion or in part of the lesion'.

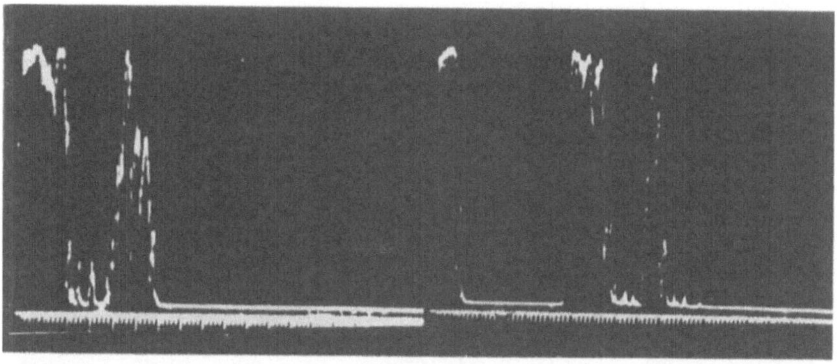

Fig. 3. Neurofibroma. Left: paraocular, right: transocular. Very low reflective well delimited mass.

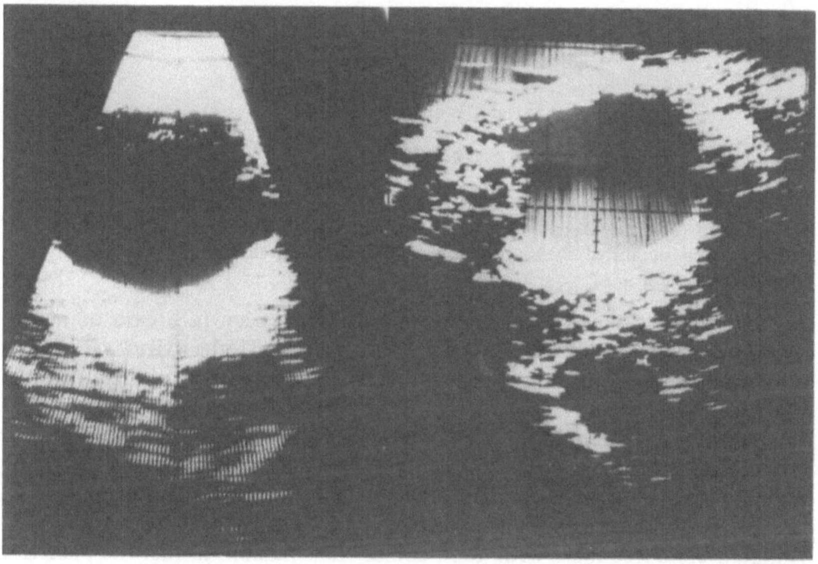

Fig. 4. Neurofibroma. Right: contact B-scan (7.5 MHz), left: immersion gray scale B-scan (5 MHz). Well delimited echo-free mass; the presence of posterior limit indicates good sound transmission.

Two cases of neurofibromatosis and four cases of neurofibromas have undergone echography over the past five years. A Kretztechnik 7200 MA with an 8 MHz probe and a Sonometrics Ophthalmoscan 200 were used.

The two cases of neurofibromatosis were found in a 10 year old boy and a 4 year old girl. The boy showed marked facial asymmetry. In this first case the orbital A-scan echo trace was rather poor, while the immersion B-scan clearly revealed the high reflective mass just outside the lateral orbital wall (Fig. 1). No definite mass but only an increased reflectivity of the whole orbital content was found in the girl.

The histological structure explained the different echo traces found in

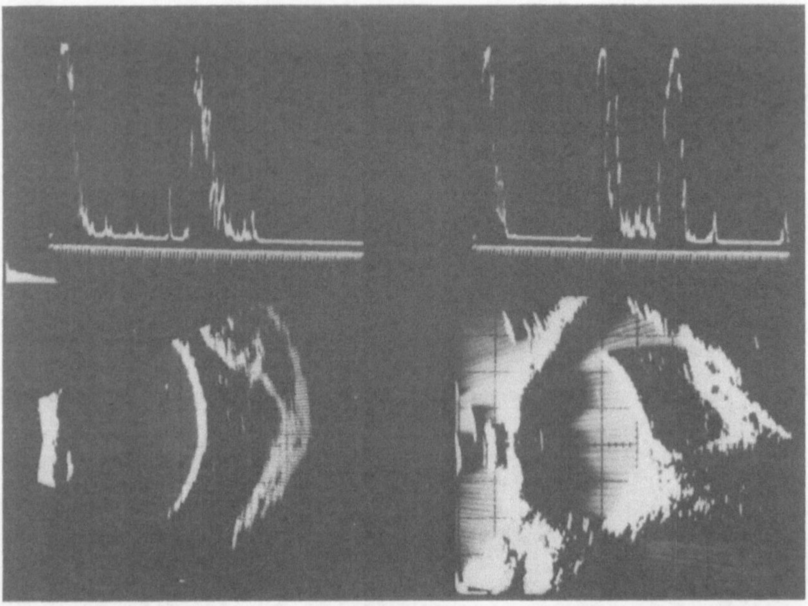

Fig. 5. Lymphoma. Top (A-scan echo traces): well delimited low reflective solid areas. Bottom left (contact B-scan, 7.5 MHz) bottom right (gray scale immersion B-scan. 10 MHz): well delimited mass, very low echoes diffused throughout the lesion, good sound transmission.

the four adult cases. The highest reflectivity was seen in a case of neurofibroma showing calcified areas (Fig. 2). Medium reflectivity was shown by a vascular neurofibroma (Gallenga P. E., et al. 1980). Very low internal reflectivity was found in the other two cases (Fig. 3). The tumour areas were always well delimited. We prefer not to use the term 'encapsulated' when referring to well delimited lesions, but to use it only when describing lesions which have real double-peaked wall echoes (Mazzeo, et al. 1981). The B-scan showed nearly the same echopattern as the A-scan i.e. a well delimited echo-free mass with good sound transmission, in fact the posterior limit of the lesion was clearly visible (Fig. 3).

All things considered one could say that a 'characteristic' echo pattern of all peripheral nerve tumours does not exist. The differential diagnosis is extremely difficult because it changes in relation to each echo trace found.

We found it very difficult to differentiate between isolated forms of peripheral nerve tumours and those showing a 'sarcoma-lymphoma-pseudotumour' pattern (Figs. 4 and 5).

REFERENCES

Coleman D. J., Lizzi F. C., Jack R. L.: 'Ultrasonography of the eye and orbit'. Philadelphia, Lea and Febiger (1977).

Gallenga P. E., Mazzeo V., Scorrano R., Rossi A.: 'Misinterpretation in orbital diagnosis'. In: Investigative Ultrasonography. 2 Clinical Advances (C. Alvisi, C. R. Hill eds.), Bath, Pitman Press (1981) p. 312.

Henderson J. W.: 'Orbital tumors'. Philadelphia, Saunders Co. (1973).
Janev K. G., Ossoinig K. C., Frazier S. W., Fish G.: 'Ultrasound in diagnosis of orbital diseases'. In: Diagnostica Ultrasonica in Ophthalmologia, (H. Gernet ed.) Münster, R. A. Remy (1979) p. 159.
Mazzeo V., Ravalli L., Scorrano R.: 'L'ecografia nei tumori dell'Orbita'. In: Clinica dei tumori dell'occhio e dell'orbita. (A. Rossi ed.); LXI S.O.I. Cong., Roma (1981) p. 455.
Ossoinig K. C.: 'A-scan echography and órbital disease'. In: Orbital Disorders, (G. M. Bleeker et al. eds.) Basel, Karger (1975) p. 203.
Restori M.: 'Ultrasound in orbital diagnosis'. Trans. Ophthal. Soc. U.K. 99:223 (1979).
Restori M., Wright J. E., McLeod D.: 'B-scan and C-scan imaging in the orbit'. In: 3rd. International Symposium on Orbital Disorders. The Hague, W. Junk (1978) p. 43.
Rootman J., Goldberg C., Robertson W.: 'Primary orbital schwannomas' Brit. J. Ophthalmol. 66:194 (1982).
Schroeder W.: 'Zur Unterscheidung von infiltrativen und expansiven Raumforderungen in der Orbita'. In: Diagnostica Ultrasonica in Ophthalmologia, (H. Gernet ed.) Münster, R. A. Remy (1979) p. 173.
Till P., Hauff W.: 'Differential diagnostic results of clinical echography in orbital tumors'. In: Ultrasonography in Ophthalmology (J. M. Thijssen, A. M. Verbeek eds.) The Hague, W. Junk (1981) p. 277.
Zimmerman L. E., Sobin L. H.: 'Histological typing of tumours of the eye and its adnexa'. Int. hist. class. of tumours. Geneva, WHO (1980).

Authors' address:
Clinica Oculistica
Università di Ferrara
corsa Giovecca, 203
1–44100 Ferrara
Italy

ULTRASOUND INTERACTION IN THE EYE

MARIE RESTORI, SIDNEY LEEMAN and JOHN WEIGHT
(London, England)

INTRODUCTION

It is indicated how pulsed fields from transducers, as used for imaging and echo analysis, are quite different in practice from the continuous fields described in most text books. The propagation of pulses within the eye is discussed with particular emphasis on scattering and reflection. Some tissue characterisation methods are also discussed.

A video film will be shown to demonstrate the propagation and scattering of short pulses of sound.

PULSED FIELDS

Many of the descriptions in text books place great emphasis on fields produced by a transducer activated with a sinusoidal voltage; the emitted sound field is called a continuous wave field. In practice however, most medical applications employ transducers which are transiently excited to produce a short pulse of ultrasound. The generated acoustic pulse is a localised three dimensional package of ultrasonic energy which travels from the transducer through a medium at a velocity determined by the latter. Outside this small energy packet there is virtually no ultrasonic energy in the medium. As it travels the shape of the pulse will change. If a sensor, which can convert acoustic pressure to voltage, is placed on the acoustic axis of the pulse, its output is typically as shown in Fig. 1a; this is called the axial pressure pulse. It is important to realise that the axial pulse shape changes with distance from the transducer. If, at some distance from the transducer face, the sensor is moved perpendicularly to the acoustic axis and some characteristic feature of the measured voltage trace (such as its peak value) is plotted against distance from the axis, the so called beam profile (Fig. 1b) is obtained. This is a somewhat more loosely defined entity than the axial pulse shape, since its precise form depends on the characteristic feature selected. The beam profile also varies with distance from the transducer. The axial pressure pulse and beam profile are often used to describe the three dimensional form of the pulse.

An understanding of the way in which the form of the pulse varies

Hillman, J. S./Le May, M. M. (eds.) Ophthalmic Ultrasonography

ISBN 978-94-009-7280-3

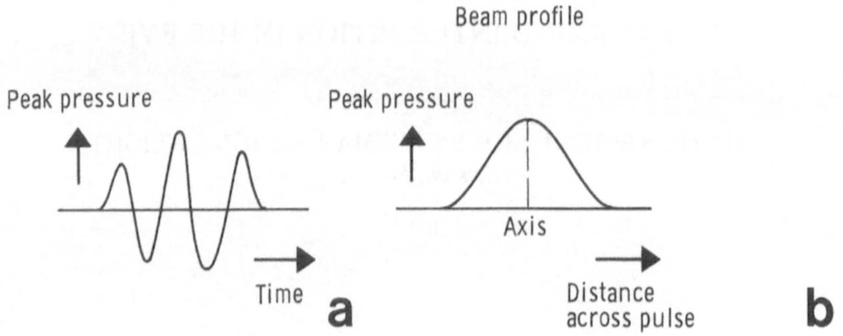

Fig. 1. (a) Axial pulse. (b) Beam profile.

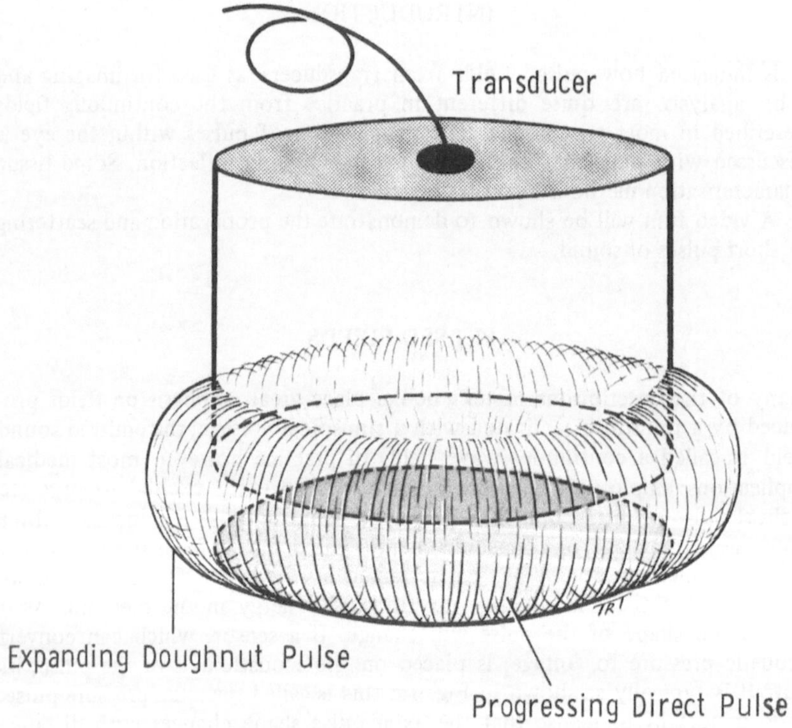

Fig. 2. Direct and Edge pulse (3 dimensional representation).

throughout the medium is of importance in appreciating the limitations of ultrasonic pulse-echo imaging techniques and the above description for a propagating pulse is inadequate for many purposes. Consider a planar, uniformly excited, circular transducer (Figs. 2 and 3), on shock excitation it produces a progressing circular planar pulse with the same diameter as the activated area of the transducer (direct pulse) and the circular periphery of the transducer element generates an expanding toroidal or 'doughnut-shaped'

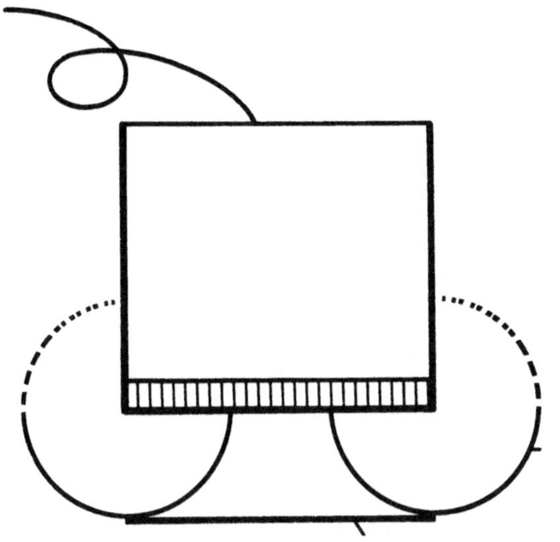

Fig 3. Direct and Edge pulse (2 dimensional representation).

pulse, (the edge pulse). The former travels away from the transducer face without expanding whereas the toroidal pulse expands out in all directions into the medium; its cross-sectional radius is equal to the distance of the direct wave from the transducer (Fig. 3).

A detailed description of the direct and edge pulses is given by Weight and Hayman (1978) and only a few features need to be noted here. An important point is that, on axis, irrespective of range, the direct and edge pulse have equal amplitude and opposite polarity, (close to the transducer the direct and edge pulse can be time separated; further away they increasingly superimpose one another). Although, for uniform excitation, the direct pulse has constant amplitude, the toroidal pulse is non-uniform. In practice, when the activation is not impulsive, the actual durations of the direct and toroidal pulse are determined by that of the transducer excitation. It can easily be appreciated that the range resolution on an image can be much poorer than implied by the duration of the DIRECT pulse emitted.

At very large distances from the transducer the fusion of the direct and edge pulses produces a spherical outgoing pulse with intensity falling off according to the inverse square law. Even for continuous wave emission, the plane and edge wave structure is still present in the field but is totally masked by the strong interference which occurs between them. The conventional separation of the field into near and far field zone is not so appropriate for pulsed fields.

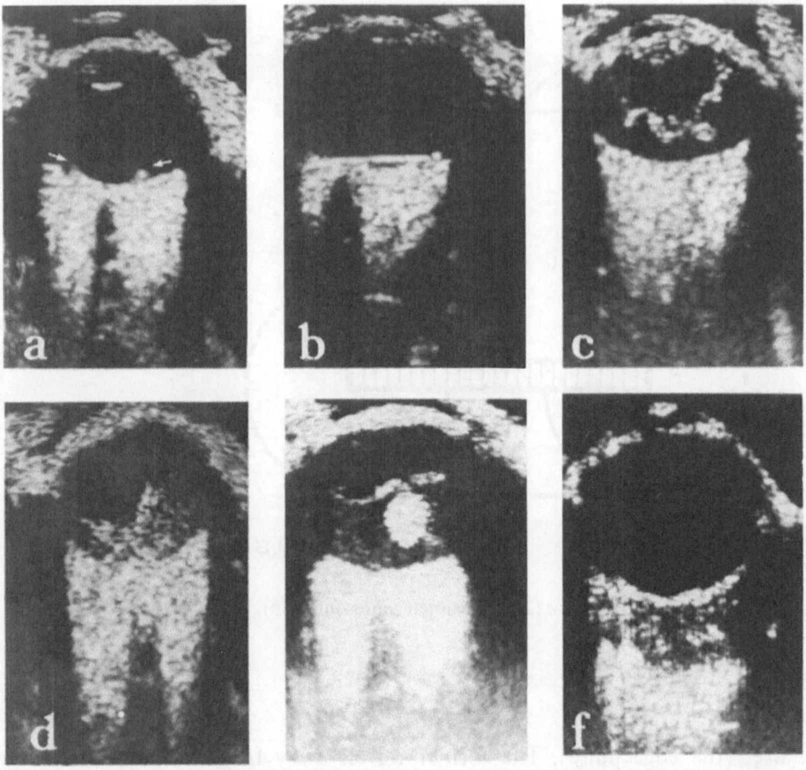

Fig. 4. **Horizontal linear B-scan sections. (a) Baum's bumps (arrows) on retina. (b) Blood fluid level (specular reflector) in retrohyaloid space. (c) Total retinal detachment. (d) Retrohyaloid haemorrhage. (e) Sub-retinal haemorrhage and malignant melanoma. (f) Orbital lymphoma lying directly behind the globe.**

REFRACTION

Refraction of sound occurs when an ultrasonic pulse traverses the boundary between two media with different sound velocities. Refraction through the lens of the eye is considered to be responsible for 'Baum's bumps' on the retina (Fig. 4a). Refraction is a familiar and relatively well understood phenomenon and is not considered at greater length here.

SCATTERING

Scattering is the re-radiation of ultrasonic energy from the site of interaction into many different directions. When the conditions are such that the scattered field is re-radiated into a dominantly single (non-forward)

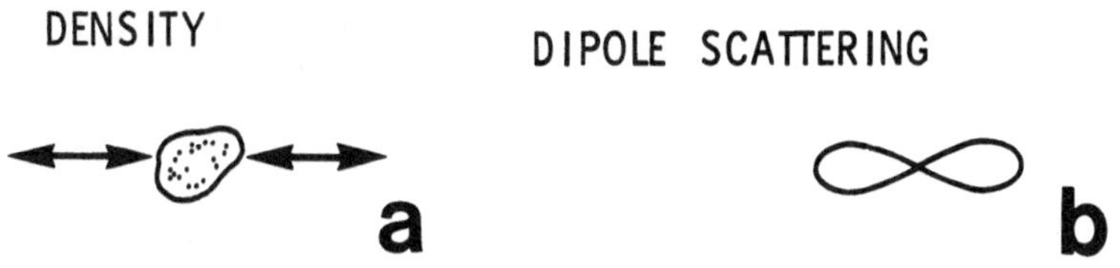

Fig. 5. (a) Density fluctuation. (b) scatter directivity pattern.

direction only, it is conventional to call the process specular reflection (see below and Fig. 4b).

For diagnostic pulse-echo work, the echoes represent that portion of the incident field which is back-scattered – i.e. re-radiated at close to 180° to the direction of forward propagation of the incident pulse.

There are basically two types of situation in which scatter can occur. The first situation is that of reflection from rough boundaries: for example, most pathological membranes, such as the detached retina, (Fig. 4c).

The second situation occurs when a pulse traverses an inhomogenous medium. Typical ophthalmological examples of such scattering media are normal orbital fat (Figs. 4a, 4b, 4c), vitreous haemorrhage (Fig. 4d) intraocular tumours (Fig. 4e) and orbital tumours (Fig. 4f).

Such scatter-generating inhomogeneties arise in tissue because of variations in density, elasticity and absorption. In order to understand this physically it should be remembered that an ultrasound field may be regarded as either a region of pressure variation or equivalently, a region of local displacement of the particle within the medium.

A small density fluctuation, in an otherwise homogenous medium, when exposed to a pulse of ultrasound will exhibit a different displacement amplitude to the other surrounding elements in the medium. Such a relative motion is equivalent to an oscillating particle in a stationary medium; that is a dipole source of sound scattering (Fig. 5), showing a non-isotropic directivity scatter pattern (compare the directivity of sound produced by a tuning fork).

A small elasticity fluctuation in an otherwise homogenous medium, would expand or contract differently to the surrounding medium particles. Its behaviour could be described as being equivalent to a pulsating object in a stationary medium that is as a monopole source of isotropic scatter (Fig. 6).

A small fluctuation in absorption within the medium changes the local amplitude of the pulse of sound. This is equivalent to a vibrating membrane within an otherwise stationary medium (Fig. 7) and produces a complicated scatter directivity pattern.

In most medical applications we are concerned with the back and forward scattering only. The back-scattering to a first approximation is determined by a combination of density and elasticity fluctuations which is identical to acoustic impedance. The forward scattering depends predominantly on velocity fluctuations. In some tissues bulk scattering from absorption fluctuations is weak and can be neglected.

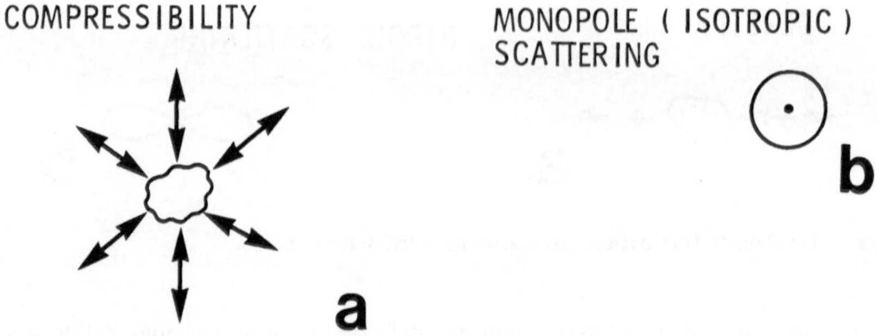

Fig. 6. (a) Elasticity fluctuation. (b) scatter directivity pattern.

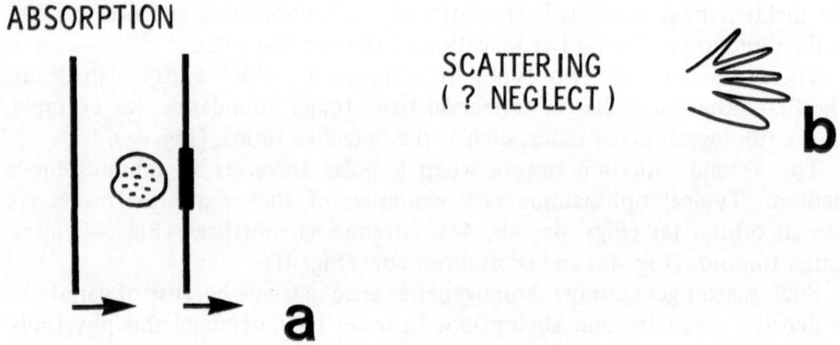

Fig. 7. (a) Absorption fluctuation. (b) scatter directivity pattern.

SPECULAR REFLECTION

The distinction between reflection and scattering is largely conventional and the two processes are identical physically. When the scattering structure is very smooth (on a scale of the order of a wavelength) and large compared to the beam profile the scattering conspires to produce a reflected pulse, that is, one travelling in a well defined direction only.

Pathological specular reflectors in the eye are rare, one example, however, is that of a blood fluid level in the retrohyaloid space, (Fig. 4b) in proliferative diabetic eye disease.

As most biological reflecting interfaces are unlikely to be as rigid as assumed in simple calculations, it can be expected that the incident pulse shape will be modified on reflection. It should also be noted that most treatments of a pulse traversing an interface assume that absorption can be neglected. However, if attenuation (which will be defined later) is included in the analysis it is found the reflection coefficient is dependent not only on characteristic impedance mismatch and the angle of incidence but also on frequency since scattering (reflection) by absorption fluctuations would also be frequency dependent (Leeman et al. 1979).

Table 1. Absorption coefficients in various media

Medium	Absorption coefficient (dB/cm at 1 MHz)
Air	12.00
Water	0.002
Aqueous/Vitreous	0.1
Lens	2.0
Fat	0.6
Bone	13.0

ABSORPTION

The dissipation of ultrasonic energy during the passage through a medium by conversion into heat is known as absorption. Some values of the linear absorption coefficient, for ocular tissues are given in Table 1. The lens has 20 times and (orbital fat 6 times) the absorption of the vitreous. In human soft tissues, the relatively few data that are available suggest that absorption has an approximately linear dependence on frequency. Absorption of ultrasound pulses decreases as the water content of the tissue rises and increases as the structural protein content increases. However, the exact physical mechanisms whereby tissues absorb ultrasound energy are yet to be described.

ATTENUATION

Attenuation is the removal of energy from the forward propagating pulse by both absorption and scattering. Most measurements of attenuation give a similar dependence on frequency to that of absorption (that is, approximately linear for most human soft tissues). Since scattering would be expected to exhibit a complicated and usually greater than linear dependence on frequency, these measurements suggest that scattering in tissues is rather weak.

TISSUE CHARACTERISATION

Tissue characterisation is an attempt to extract from ultrasound signals those quantitative parameters which are intrinsic to the tissue itself and useful medically. Ultrasound tissue characterisation is a rapidly expanding subject and many of the computational techniques now being employed are sophisticated so that it would be impossible to make more than a few introductory remarks here.

From a data acquisition point of view, tissue characterisation methods may be divided into two main classifications: those analysing echoes from a small region of tissue (local methods) and those looking at signals from a more extensive region (non-local methods). Clearly, the disease states to which the two methods are applicable are rather disjoint. It is useful to point out here, though, that an example of the former would be the analysis of echoes reflected from a thin membrane (Coleman et al. 1977) and an example of the latter would be the analysis of the ensemble of echoes present in an A scan taken through a region of pathology (Ossoinig, 1975).

From a data analysis point of view, tissue characterisation methods also fall into two main classes (Jones and Leeman, 1982). The first may be called 'structure tissue characterisation'. Here an attempt is made to apply signal processing methods to obtain some quantitative measure of the spatial arrangement and correlation of the scattering elements of tissues. The results of such methods may be heavily dependant on the instrumentation used, since the techniques are usually applied to signals which are already processed by the ultrasound equipment. Choice of scanning frequency, machine settings, transducer and scanner characteristics all influence echo patterns and may be expected to introduce artefacts, unless robust analysis techniques are employed. One example of a robust, (i.e. relatively independant of instrumental artefacts) structural (local) tissue characterisation method is the analysis of layer thickness, by spectral methods (Coleman et al, 1977). One way round the difficulties introduced by instrumental influences, is to apply structural tissue characterisation methods only to signals which have been processed to remove instrumental artefacts. That is, to apply tissue characterisation to the so-called 'impulse response' of tissues. This is not easy to carry out in practice and has yet to be applied to in vivo data.

The second and more promising class of tissue characterisation methods are the so-called 'parameter estimation' techniques. These involve attempts at quantitative measurements of tissue acoustical properties, such as impedance, attenuation and velocity. All of these may be expected to change with the pathological state of the tissue. This approach reflects the ultimate goal of extracting (and imaging) ultrasound/tissue interaction parameters (density, elasticity and absorption) from ultrasound signals. While density information can be determined by our modalities, elasticity and absorption are bound up with the mechanical and micro-structural properties of tissue and are not easily measured by other methods. For example, the echoes from an interface between two tissues types is modified by the impedance and absorption mismatches across that interface, as well as by the relative elasticities of the two tissues. In principle, information about all these tissue properties may be obtained by analysing the ultrasound echoes reflected from that interface. In practice, this local method had not been applied, probably because of the confusing effect of interface geometry on the results.

Attenuation and velocity tomographic images of the eye may be in principle obtained from transmission studies, somewhat akin to X-ray computerised tomography. Such 'quantitative' images would be the precursors to successful structural tissue characterisation methods. However, as yet, such methods are impracticable for ophthalmological investigations and interest has focused on techniques for extracting either attenuation or impedance values from back-scattered echoes only. Attenuation assessment is usually made by analysing the echo amplitude reduction in the depth (Ossoinig, 1977) or by the rather more robust technique of monitoring the reduction of mean frequency of the echoes from small regions as the pulse travels the tissue of interest (Jones and Leeman, 1982; Thijssen et al. 1981). Attempts to remove the influence of scanner characteristics are made in a technique such as impediography which estimates tissue impedance values from a knowledge of the incident pulse and measured reflection echo sequence. Impediographic techniques have already been applied to the eye and the initial results show some promise (Jones and Cole-Beuglet, 1980).

It is clear that tissue characterisation methods are of great interest ophthalmologically, but they demand an accurate knowledge of ultrasound/tissue interactions and require a careful specification of the propagating pulse. It is also for this reason that the description of the pulsed field in terms of direct and edge waves (given above) may turn out to be of more wide-ranging influence than its importance in imaging work.

CONCLUSIONS

A knowledge of the nature of the pulsed field and the study of the pulse propagation in tissue is important if ultrasound/tissue interaction mechanisms are to be understood. An understanding of such interactions potentially opens the door to tissue characterisation techniques which extract the basic parameters intrinsic to the physiological or pathological state of a tissue.

ADDENDUM

A video film of stroboscopic schlieren visualisation of short ultrasound pulses demonstrated the presence of plane and edge pulses in water; reflection and transmission of a pulse at perpendicular incidence to the boundary between two media; reflection and refraction at the same boundary; random and ordered scattering from an object; forward and backscatter as the pulse passes through a scattering object; regular scatter from a smooth cylinder in water, demonstrating that specular reflection does not occur even though the object is much larger than the acoustic wavelength (in water).

REFERENCES

Coleman D. J., Lizzi F. L. and Jack R. L. (1977) Ultrasonography of the Eye and Orbit. Lea and Febiger, Philadelphia. pp. 83–87.

Jones J. P. and Cole-Beuglet C. (1980) Acoustical Imaging, Vol 8 Ed H. F. Metherell, Plenum, New York.

Jones J. P. and Leeman S. (in press 1982) IEEE Transactions and Computers.

Leeman S., Leeks R., Sutton P. (1979) Information Processsing in Medical Imaging INSERM Vol 88 pp. 35–48.

Ossoinig K. C. and Till P. (1975) Bibl Ophthal No 83 pp. 200–216 (Karger, Basel).

Ossoinig K. C. (1977) Orbit Roentgenology. Edited by P. Arger. John Wiley and Sons. New York/Chichester/Brisbane/Toronto p 223–269.
Thijssen J. M., Cloostermans M. and Bayer A. L. (1981) Docum Ophthal Proc series Vol 29, ed by J. M. Thijssen and A. M. Verbeck. Dr W. Junk publ, The Hague
Weight J. P. and Hayman A. J. (1978) J Acoust Soc Amer, 63, 396

Authors' addresses:
Marie Restori
Ultrasound Department
Moorfields Eye Hospital
City Road
London EC1
UK

Sidney Leeman
Medical Physics Department
Hammersmith Hospital
London
UK

John Weight
Physics Department
City University
London
UK

PERFORMANCE MEASUREMENTS AND QUANTITATIVE ECHOGRAPHY

W. HAIGIS and W. BUSCHMANN
(Würzburg, W. Germany)

SUMMARY

It was demonstrated how serious malfunctions of diagnostic ultrasonic equipment can be detected with the help of simple acoustic and electronic performance measurements. Furthermore, the benefit of these measurements for computer-assisted A-scan signal analysis was shown. A low-cost minicomputer system could be used to gain additional tissue differentiation data. These were – to a certain degree of approximation – free from the individual characteristics of the ultrasound system used, thus making diagnostic findings easier to be compared and valid in a more general sense.

INTRODUCTION

Today, an increasing number of diagnostic ultrasonic instruments is being offered on the market. Lacking standardization, these instruments still differ in basic performance features. Since the image generated on the screen of an echograph is strongly affected by the unit's various performance parameters, it is essential to know 'what the system does to the signals'. This holds especially where quantitative echography is concerned.

Our working group as well as others (Buschmann et al. 1977, Haigis and Buschmann 1981, Haigis et al. 1981, Ossoinig and Patel 1977, Reuter et al. 1980, 1981, Trier 1969) have developed a number of simple performance measurement methods for diagnostic ultrasound systems mainly serving two purposes:

– to allow quick calibrational checks on the instrument,
– to provide data enabling a user to express his diagnostic findings – to a certain degree of approximation – independent of the particular instrument used.

In the following we shall first describe how –very quickly – serious fault conditions in ultrasound instruments can be detected using these measurement methods. The second part will deal with diagnostic A-scan signal

Hillman, J. S./Le May, M. M. (eds.) Ophthalmic Ultrasonography

ISBN 978-94-009-7280-3

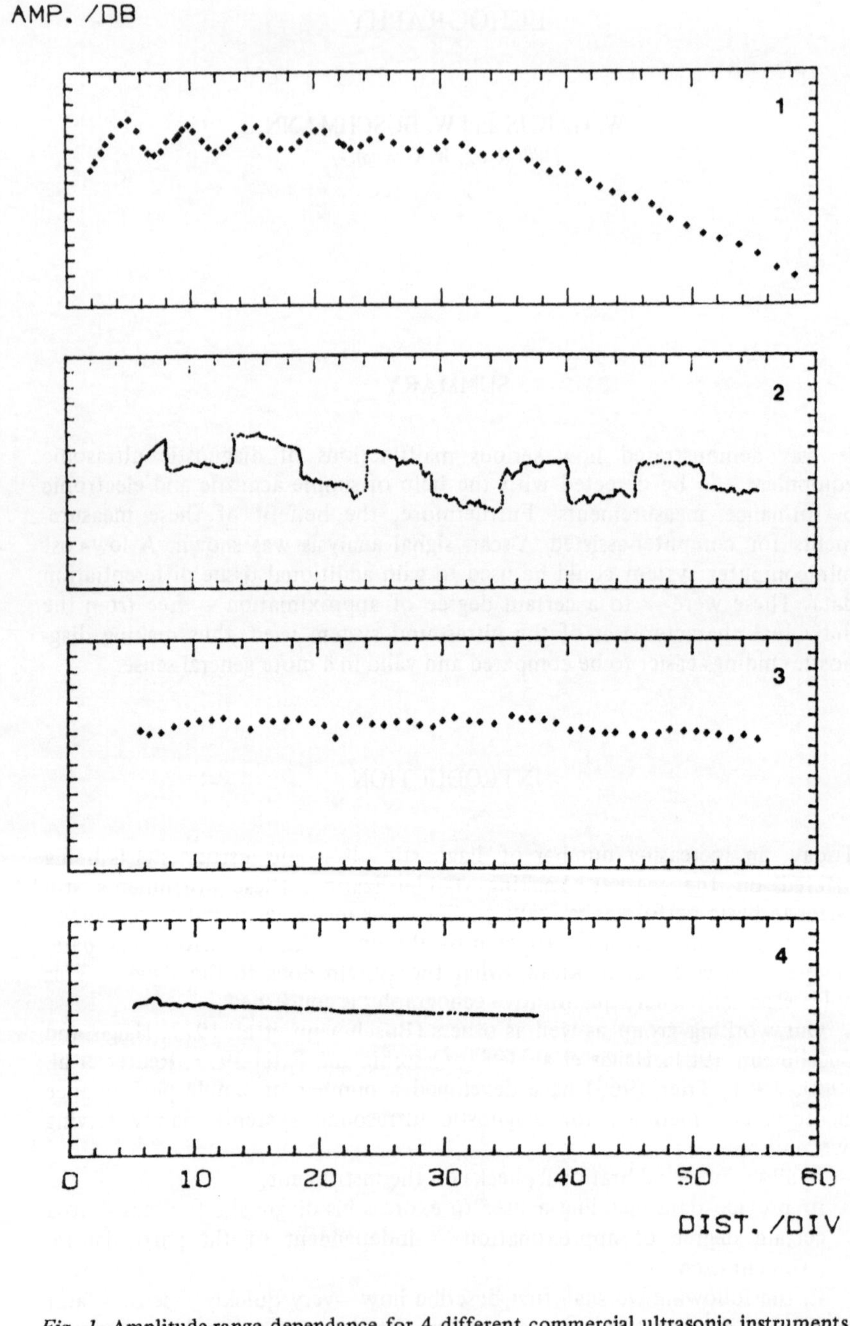

Fig. 1. Amplitude-range dependance for 4 different commercial ultrasonic instruments. Scaling: vertical 2 dB/div., horizontal 1 mm/div. Transducer frequencies: 10 MHz (nominal). Echo interface: W38 HEMA test reflector.

analysis which can be carried out by means of a small 'personal computer' on the basis of performance measurement data.

PERFORMANCE MEASUREMENTS

Calibration and performance measurements may be divided into acoustic (Haigis et al. 1981) and electronic (Reuter et al. 1981) measurements. Whereas the former use natural echoes of e.g. test reflectors or tissue phantoms, synthetic echoes are electronically generated in the latter case. An essential feature of acoustic measurements lies in the fact that the ultrasound system is tested in the very configuration in which it is operated diagnostically. Most electronic measurements usually comprise only subcomponents of the total system. Results of both methods, however, combine to give a comprehensive description of the overall performance of the ultrasound instrument under test.

As an example for results of an acoustic measurement, the amplitude-range-dependance for 4 ultrasonic instruments is depicted in Fig. 1. A W38 test reflector (Haigis et al. 1981), immersed in saline, served as a 'working standard plane echo interface' (International Electrotechnical Commission 1979). With the system gain kept constant, the amplitude of the W38 reflector echo was subsequently measured while increasing the distance between transducer and reflector.

This simple measurement procedure and set-up reveals serious technical defects in instruments no. 1 and no. 2, while no. 3 and no. 4 exhibit the normal amplitude-range-dependance which is to be expected from the laws of ultrasound physics. The origin of the periodic distortions observable in the plots for instrument no. 1 and no. 2 is not a physical, but an electronic one.

Any echogram taken with one of these ultrasonic devices will be affected in such a way as if the respective system gain were periodically varied – continuously in instrument no. 1, on-off-like in instrument no. 2. Obviously, this malfunction will cause e.g. wrong texture patterns in diagnostic echograms, and any attempt at quantitative echography will lead to erroneous results.

With respect to quantitative echography one system feature is essentially important: the amplifier (gain) calibration. Very often it has been found in commercial ultrasonic instruments that the dB-calibration was more or less faulty. Fig. 2 shows an example of an electronical dB-check. We used the ECHOSIMULATOR (Reuter et al. 1980) to feed synthetic test signals of different frequencies into the ultrasound system. The indicated attenuation settings necessary to maintain constant · amplitude were noted while the signal amplitudes were varied in calibrated steps. Frequency-dependent differences of up to 4 dB (equal to an error of 20%) were found between indicated and true attenuation values. Although, according to our experience, a de-calibration as shown in Fig. 2 has to be considered as relatively small,

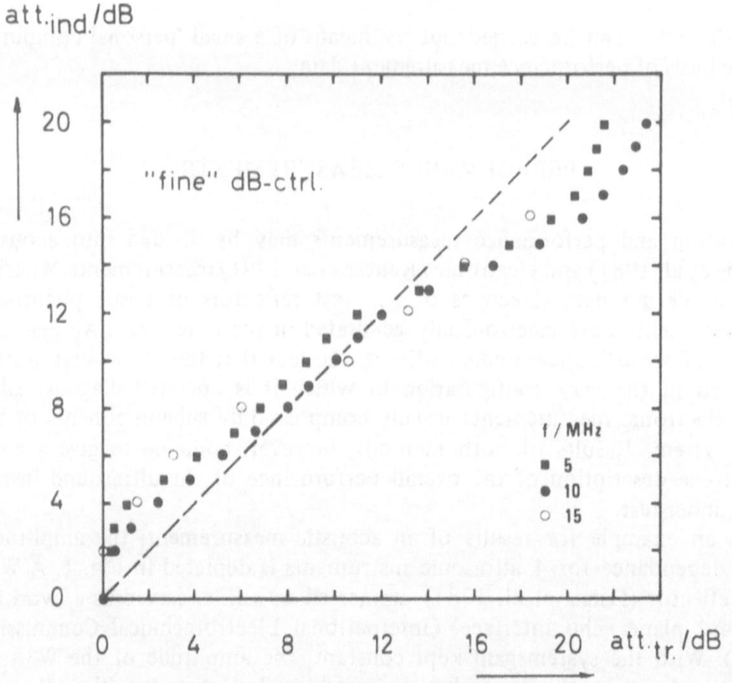

Fig. 2. **Comparison between indicated (att_{ind}) and true (att_{tr}) attenuation at different frequencies for a commercial diagnostic ultrasound instrument.**

this effect is likely to add to other system deficiencies, thus resulting eventually in serious errors.

Another typical application of an electronic performance measurement is illustrated in Fig. 3, showing amplifier characteristics of 3 different commercial ultrasound instruments for ophthalmic use. Whereas the Kretz characteristic is of the famous S-shape, it can be seen from Fig. 3 that the other two instruments rather use linear amplification until saturation is reached. In addition, there is quite a difference in maximum available screen amplitude. This holds especially for the Ultrascan and the Ocuscan, although both instruments are equipped with picture tubes of identical geometrical dimensions of the same make.

Since it is *inter alia* the amplifier characteristic which essentially determines how small, medium and high signals are displayed on the screen, it is quite obvious that an echo train arising from a given tissue structure will look completely different when processed by different types of amplifiers. Any attempt to express diagnostic findings in a more general way, i.e. free from the peculiarities of the particular instrument used, must therefore take this system feature into account.

Application to A-scan signal analysis

A number of working groups (e.g. Bonn/Stuttgart, New York, Nijmegen; references e.g. in Thijssen 1980) are engaged in the field of signal analysis

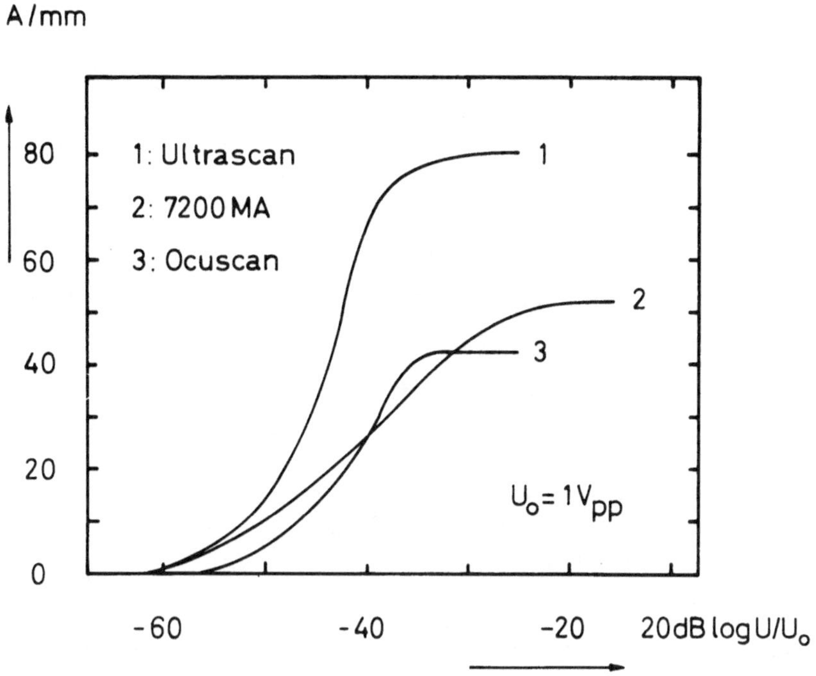

Fig. 3. Amplifier characteristics of 3 commercial instruments.

of ophthalmic echographic data for tissue differentiation. Various approaches to the problem have been chosen, starting either from RF- or from video-data. Having in mind that usually typical (A-scan) echograms are documented on photographic material and that a large number of clinical echograms is stored away in patient files we began to post-process these A-scan photos in order

- to extract numerical data such as amplitude means, distributions, specific attenuation values, which may serve as additional tissue differentiation parameters,
- to express these data as free as possible from technical characteristics of the instrument used.

The method applied is as follows:

The photographic negative of an A-scan echogram is projected onto the active area of a Hewlett Packard 9874 A Digitizer and subsequently digitized point by point. The data are transferred to a personal computer system consisting of a Commodore cbm 3032 main unit and a cbm 3040 dual floppy drive. Evaluation starts with rescaling the data via the amplifier characteristic of the instrument used. Fig. 4 shows the gain curve family of the Kretz 7200 MA unit for 5 different system gain settings. The measurement data for this plot were fed directly into the computer making use of a special interface (Haigis et al. 1982) to connect the ECHOSIMULATOR to the cbm 3032 main unit. The 0 dB-point of Fig. 4 is given by an electrical signal

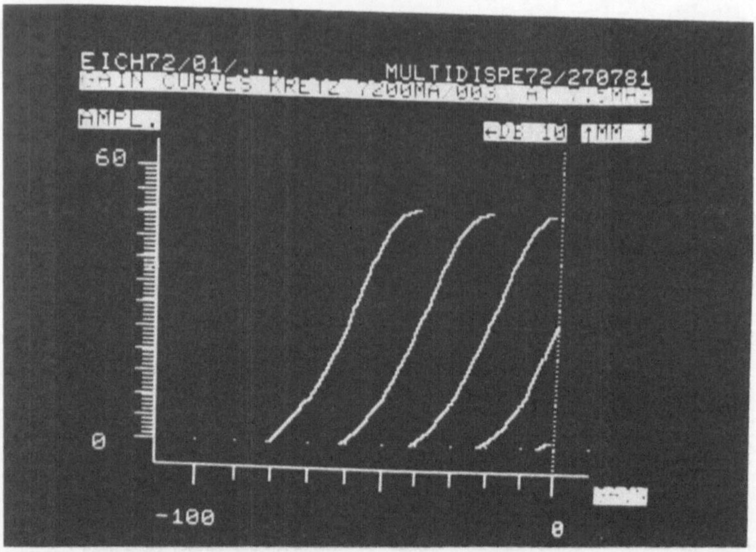

Fig. 4. Gain curve family for the Kretz 7200 MA, measured at 7.5 MHz. Instrument settings: Sw = 0, Sbg = 1. Nominal gain settings for individual curves from left to right: 80, 60, 40, 20, 0 dB. Scale factors: horizontal 10 dB/div. (input signal amplitude; 0 dB $\hat{=}$ 1 V_{pp} at 50 Ohms), vertical 1 mm/div. (screen amplitude).

signal amplitude of 1 V_{pp} at 50 Ohms. To make allowance for the acoustic (overall) sensitivity of the total ultrasound system, an 'acoustic 0 dB-point' has to be introduced as follows:

The gain setting necessary for a 10 mm echo amplitude of a W38/saline interface in a distance of 30 μsec from the transducer, the so-called W38-value, is a characteristic system parameter. The respective gain curve labelled by this value defines – for an amplitude of 10 mm – a dB-value on the abscissa of Fig. 4, which is then taken as an acoustic point of reference.

Thus, rescaling consists of two steps:

- to calculate the gain curve for the particular gain setting that was chosen to take the echogram,
- to compute the difference in dB to the acoustic point of reference for each signal amplitude,

using the performance data of Fig. 4 as well as the W38 value. As a result of the rescaling program, the echo amplitudes are now given in dB relative to the W38 reflectivity. Taking into account the reflectivity difference of – 17.4 dB between the W38 and the perfect reflector (Haigis et al. 1981), the amplitude data may very easily be related to the latter also.

Statistical analysis of the digitized and rescaled echogram is done by the computer main program, which outputs its results to a printer and an X-Y

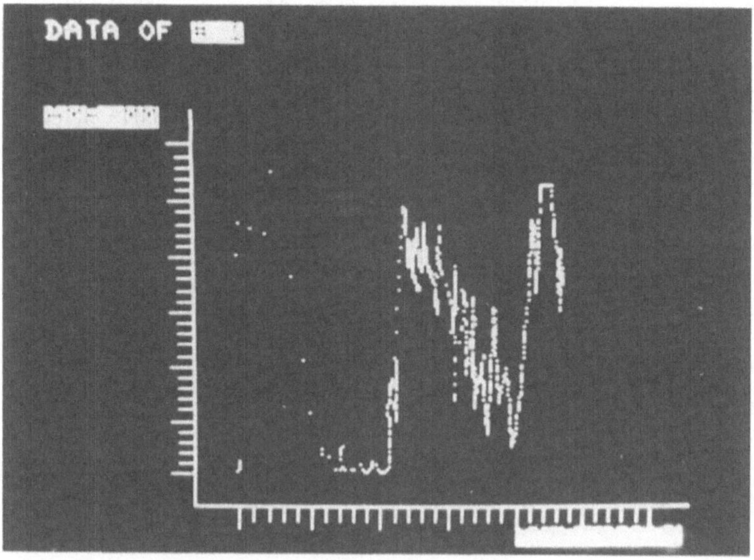

Fig. 5. Digitized echogram of a melanoma on the screen of the cbm 3032. Vertical axis: 7200 MA amplitude in mm; horizontal axis: time of flight in μsec. Statistical results for this echogram are given in Fig. 6 (cf. ID :1).

plotter. The overall resolution obtainable amounts to ± 0.1 dB for the amplitude axis and to 10–25 nsec for the time axis.

As an example for the above described method Fig. 5 shows a digitized echogram of a melanoma, as it is displayed on the computer's screen. The diagnostic device was a Kretz 7200 MA unit with a transducer working at 8.3 MHz.

Four echograms in this sound beam orientation were statistically evaluated leading to the print-out of Fig. 6. Calculated attenuation values range from − 1.65 to − 2.50 dB/μsec with correlation coefficients from 68.6% to 86.7%. The latter describe the quality of the regression line fit used to calculate the specific attenuation. Software-averaging of these 4 echograms results in the plots of Fig. 7, the regression line corresponding to a specific attenuation of − 2.05 dB/μsec. From the amplitude distribution, depicted on the right side of Fig. 7, additional information concerning texture and homogenity of the tissue can be gained.

Further results we have obtained so far with the method described are compiled in Table 1. It also contains additional statistical parameters such as mean amplitudes, standard deviations etc. and specifies computational data in more detail. It may be pointed out that a specific attenuation for normal orbital fat of − 1.26 dB/μsec (equivalent to − 1.65 dB/mm tissue)

```
DATE              13/07/82          MEAN AMPL.        -55.40 DB
ID                1                 STAND. DEV.        06.20 DB

WORK.FREQ.        8.3 MHZ           MAX. AMPL.        -46.00 DB
BANDWIDTH         3.0 MHZ           MIN. AMPL.        -71.20 DB
SOURCE            7200/DIG.

NR. OF SWEEPS     1                 CORR.COEFF.        86.70 %
NR. OF AMPL.      627               SPEC. ATT.        -02.29 DB/MICSEC
```

```
DATE              13/07/82          MEAN AMPL.        -59.10 DB
ID                0                 STAND. DEV.        05.10 DB

WORK.FREQ.        8.3 MHZ           MAX. AMPL.        -45.30 DB
BANDWIDTH         3.0 MHZ           MIN. AMPL.        -73.10 DB
SOURCE            7200/DIG.

NR. OF SWEEPS     1                 CORR.COEFF.        73.60 %
NR. OF AMPL.      538               SPEC. ATT.        -01.65 DB/MICSEC
```

```
DATE              13/07/82          MEAN AMPL.        -56.30 DB
ID                3                 STAND. DEV.        05.50 DB

WORK.FREQ.        8.3 MHZ           MAX. AMPL.        -42.80 DB
BANDWIDTH         3.0 MHZ           MIN. AMPL.        -74.80 DB
SOURCE            7200/DIG.

NR. OF SWEEPS     1                 CORR.COEFF.        68.60 %
NR. OF AMPL.      390               SPEC. ATT.        -01.93 DB/MICSEC
```

```
DATE              13/07/82          MEAN AMPL.        -59.20 DB
ID                4                 STAND. DEV.        07.20 DB

WORK.FREQ.        8.3 MHZ           MAX. AMPL.        -43.70 DB
BANDWIDTH         3.0 MHZ           MIN. AMPL.        -75.40 DB
SOURCE            7200/DIG.

NR. OF SWEEPS     1                 CORR.COEFF.        85.20 %
NR. OF AMPL.      530               SPEC. ATT.        -02.50 DB/MICSEC
```

Fig. 6. Print-out of statistical results for 4 echograms of a melanoma. The top data group contains results of the echogram of Fig. 5.

Table 1. Statistical tissue parameters. Nr. of sweeps = Nr. of single echograms used for averaging. Mean amplitude is expressed in dB relative to the reflectivity of the W38 test reflector. Tissue reflectivities may be related to the perfect reflector by adding − 17.4 dB. Working frequencies and − 3 dB-band-widths are stated for the transducers used. Apart from the orbital fat data, all results were gained with a narrow-band frequency response instrument.

Tissue examined	Nr. of sweeps	Nr. of amplit.	Mean ampl./dB	Stand. dev./dB	Correl. Coeff./%	Spec. att. /(dB/μsec)	Work. freq. /MHz	Band w. /MHz
orbit. fat	128	255	− 55.6	± 6.3	69.6	− 1.26	9.6	0.9
melanoma	4	753	− 57.9	± 6.1	86.0	− 2.05	8.3	3.0
optic nerve sheath meningioma	6	95	− 48.1	± 2.5	81.4	− 0.99	6.2	1.0
meningioma	4	45	− 47.5	± 6.0	84.5	− 1.27	10.9	5.0
optic nerve	5	114	− 64.8	± 1.7	93.4	− 0.84	6.2	1.0

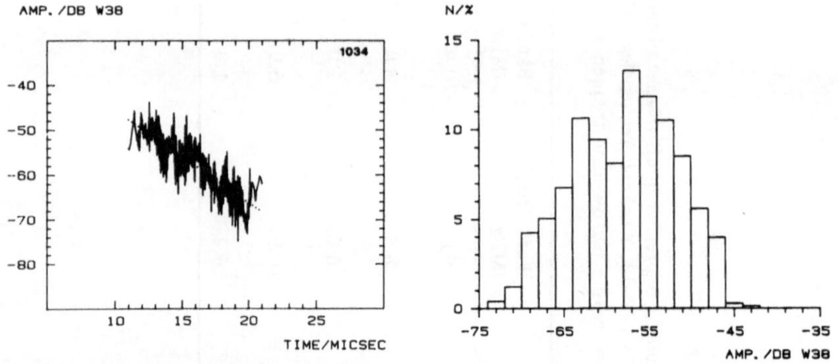

Fig. 7. Left: Averaged and time-spread echogram of the tumour region of Fig. 5. Four single echograms, the individual statistical results of which are compiled in Fig. 6, were used to generate this computer plot. Regression line fit yields a specific attenuation value of -2.05 dB/μsec for this melanoma. Right: Amplitude histogram of the averaged echogram on the left side.

compares very well to a value of -1.5 dB/mm reported by Thijssen (Thijssen and Verbeek 1981) if the higher frequency (9.6 MHz) we have been using is considered.

SUMMARY

It was demonstrated how serious malfunctions of diagnostic ultrasonic equipment can be detected with the help of simple acoustic and electronic performance measurements. Furthermore, the benefit of these measurements for computer-assisted A-scan signal analysis was shown. A low-cost mini-computer system could be used to gain additional tissue differentiation data. These were – to a certain degree of approximation – free from the individual characteristics of the ultrasound system used, thus making diagnostic findings easier to be compared and valid in a more general sense.

REFERENCES

Buschmann, W., Linnert, D. and Eysholdt, E. Measurement of Equipment Sensitivity in Diagnostic Ultrasonography. In: Ultrasound in Medicine, Vol. 3B. (D. White and R. Brown eds.) New York: Plenum Publishing Corp. (1977) p. 1925.

Haigis, W. and Buschmann, W. Klinisch anwendbare Methoden zur Überprüfung von diagnostisch relevanten Geräteparametern von Impuls-Echo-Geräten. In: Ultraschalldiagnostik in der Medizin, ed: G. Rettenmaier, E.-G. Loch, M. Hansmann, H. G. Trier, Georg Thieme Verlag, Stuttgart, New York (1981) p. 253.

Haigis, W., Reuter, R., Lepper, R.-D. Comparative Measurements on Different Pulse-Echo Systems Using Test Reflectors. In: Ultrasonography in Ophthalmology 8, Proc. of the SIDUO VIII Symposium, Nijmegen, 1980. J. M. Thijssen and A. M. Verbeek, eds., Doc. Ophthal. Proc. Series, Vol. 29. Junk, Den Haag (1981) p. 445.

Haigis, W., Schneider, S., Reuter, R. Halbautomatische, rechnergestützte Kalibrierungsmessungen an diagnostischen Ultraschallgeräten (1982), to be published
International Electrotechnical Commission, Tech. Comm. 29: Electroacoustics, Sub-Comm. 29D: Ultrasonics. Draft: Methods of measuring the performance of ultrasonic pulse-echo diagnostic equipment (1979).
Ossoinig, K. C. and Patel, J. H. A-Scan Instrumentation for Acoustic Tissue Differentiation. In: Ultrasound in Medicine, Vol. 3B (D. White and R. Brown, eds.) New York: Plenum Publishing Corp. (1977) p. 1955.
Reuter, R., Trier, H. G., Lepper, R.-D. Ein elektrisches Prüfverfahren und Prüfgerät für Ultraschalldiagnostik-Anlagen. In: Medizinal-Markt/Acta Medicotechnica, 28. Jahrgang, Nr. 2 (1980) p. 58.
Reuter, R., Lepper, R.-D. Haigis, W. Comparative Measurements on Ultrasonic Pulse-Echo Equipment with the ECHOSIMULATOR. In: Ultrasonography in Ophthalmology 8, Proc. of the SIDUO VIII Symposium, Nijmegen, 1980. J. M. Thijssen and A. M. Verbeek, eds., Doc. Ophthal. Proc. Series Vol. 29. Junk, Den Haag (1981) p. 463.
Thijssen, J. M. (ed.) Ultrasonic Tissue Characterization, Stafleu's Scientific Publishing Company, Alphen aan den Rijn/Brussels (1980).
Thijssen, J. M. and Verbeek, A. M. Computer analysis of A-mode echograms from choroidal melanoma. In: Ultrasonography in Ophthalmology 8, Proc. of the SIDOU VIII Symposium, Nijmegen, 1980, J. M. Thijssen and A. M. Verbeek, eds., Doc. Ophthal. Proc. Series Vol. 29. Junk, Den Haag (1981) p. 123.
Trier, H. G. Lichtdurchlässige, feststoffähnlich bearbeitbare Kunststoffe mit Schallgeschwindigkeiten unter 2000 m/sec. In: Proc. I. Weltkongress Ultraschalldiagnostik Med. und SIDOU III Vol. 2 (1969) p. 199.

Author's address:
University eye clinic
Würzburg
Federal Republic of Germany

ACOUSTIC PARAMETERS OF OCULAR TISSUES

J. M. THIJSSEN, H. J. M. MOL, M. J. T. M. CLOOSTERMANS,
W. J. M. VERHOEF, M. VAN LIESHOUT, M. R. TIMMER,
and A. M. VERBEEK
(Nijmegen, The Netherlands)

ABSTRACT

A survey is presented of literature data on acoustic parameters of healthy ocular tissues. These data are very rare, therefore, a new research effort, making use of modern signal processing techniques, has been undertaken. The clinical impact of the data, which include sound velocity, attenuation, and acoustic impedance, may be found in the possibility of an absolute estimation of these parameters of suspected tissues if in vivo the involvement of intermediate tissues can be predicted. The experimental techniques employed in this in vitro study are outlined and the accuracy limits are indicated. Some results on animal eyes (pig) are presented.

INTRODUCTION

The estimation of the acoustic parameters of biological tissues in general, and of ocular tissues in particular, was a topic in the first decade of medical ultrasound. Most research was devoted to the estimation of the sound velocity, which of course is very important for the application of echo techniques to the biometry of organs. The techniques employed range from sophisticated continuous wave interferometry to simple visual reading at the oscilloscope screen of an A-mode pulse-echo device. The measurement of the other two parameters was almost neglected, probably because of the technical difficulties inherent in the techniques available at that time. A comprehensive survey of velocity data may be found in Coleman et al. 1979, and some data both on velocity and on attenuation are found in Chivers and Parry, 1978, Goss et al. 1980.

SURVEY OF LITERATURE

The data are given in Table 1. The table comprises only data from human eyes, which have been estimated at body temperature. For the velocity the data of Araki (1961), Jansson (1961, 1962) Rivara and Sanna (1962),

Hillman, J. S./Le May, M. M. (eds.) Ophthalmic Ultrasonography
© 1983, Dr W. Junk Publishers, The Hague/Boston/Lancaster
ISBN 978-94-009-7280-3

Table 1. Acoustic properties of ocular tissues (literature)

	Cornea	humour	lens	retina	sclera
Velocity (m/s	1620 (± 12)	1530 (± 4)	1647 (± 3)	1565	1650 (± 10)
attenuation (dB/cm.MHz)		0.1	2.0	0.3	
impedance (10^6 kg/m^2 s)	1.55	1.54	1.85	1.61	1.61
thickness (mm)	0.55		4.0	0.2–0.4	0.5–1.

Table 2. Reflectivity (dB) relative to absolute maximum (1), and to humour/retina interface (calculated from Table 1)

	1	2
cornea/humour	– 50	– 17
humour/lens	– 20	+ 13
humour/retina	– 33	0
sclera/humour	– 33	0

of Nover and Glanschneider (1965), Tschewnenko (1965), Vanijsek et al. (1969) and Coleman et al. (1975) have been used. The figure between brackets gives the standard deviation of the mean of the data used. Attenuation data were found from Heuter and Bolt (1951), Begui (1954), Filipczinski et al. (1967). It may be remarked that the velocity and the attenuation in the retina were taken from measurements of the human brain, because no other evidence is available. The data on the acoustic impedance have been obtained from the book by Vanẏsek et al. (1969), but no details of the equipment or of the methods are known. The impedance of the retina happens to be identical to the value deduced by Thijssen et al. (1981) from known data of the human brain. The reflection coefficient at some anatomically significant transitions of human ocular tissues follow from the listed impedances. The reflection coefficient is defined as:

$$r = 20^{10} \log \quad (Z_2 - Z_1)/(Z_2 + Z_1) \quad _{\text{abs.}}$$

which formula yields the reflection strength in decibels relative to a perfect 100% reflecting boundary (absolute maximum) and relative to the reflection at the retina in situ. The direction of sound propagation is not relevant, because the absolute value that is taken of the difference of the impedances. It may be concluded that the reflection coefficients are not very realistic, since it is known that the cornea is a relatively strong reflector, and also that a 15 to 20 dB difference in reflectivity between the humour/retina interface and the choroid/sclera interface is observed.

Table 3. Experimental Values and standard deviation of acoustic parameters of animal eyes (pig) at room temperature. Literature values between brackets (Yamamoto et al. 1961; Araki, 1961; Janssen and Sundmark, 1961, Rivara and Sanna, 1962)

	cornea	humour	lens	sclera	retina
Velocity (m/s)	1555 ± 2 (1592)	1497 ± 1 (1521)	1651 ± 2 (1655)	1661 ± 2 –	1532 ± 4 –
Attenuation (dB/cm.MHz)		(0.1)	(2)	0.3	
Impedance (10^6 kg/m^2.s)	1.56 ± 1%	1.54	1.85	1.64	

EXPERIMENTAL TECHNIQUES

The equipment

The echoapparatus used is a broadband Panametrics 3052 PR (10 MHz) with a medium focused (f = 25 mm), ϕ 6 mm, 7.5 MHz transducer. The transducer is fixed in a stepmotor driven XYZ cross table with an adjustable housing. The adjustment allows for exact aiming of the sound beam perpendicular to the flat bottom of a water tank. The stepping is controlled by the digital computer (PDP 11/34) enabling automatic velocity measurements of liquids. The RF signal (15 MHz bandwidth) is digitized at a rate of 100 MHz with a transient recorder (Biomation 8100). The memory of the recorder is read by the digital computer.

The preparation of the eyes

Pig eyes are obtained fresh (a few hours) after slaughter. The anterior segment is removed completely, the lens is freed next and the iris is taken out from behind. The vitreous humour is removed carefully and then the retina is loosened and after completion cut at the optic disc. All parts are kept in physiological saline solution at room temperature. The tissues under measurement are placed on a small stand with a central hole of $\simeq$ 8 mm, which allows the sound beam to reach the bottom (1 cm below the stand) freely.

Estimation of velocity

The principle is sketched in Fig. 1. The velocity in the specimen, C_x, is obtained from three time measurements and the known velocity, C_o, in the surrounding fluid. If the specimen is very thin the accuracy, even with a 100 MHz sampling rate, of the computerized estimation of the velocity is not sufficiently high. For that reason the RF echograms are Fourier transformed to the spectral domain (Fig. 2) and the obtained phase spectra of two echograms are subtracted. This method (cf. Bayer and Thijssen, 1981) yields an optimum accuracy of the estimate of time differences and, therefore, of the velocity. The estimation of the sound velocity in the retina demands a still more subtle method, which is a combination of time

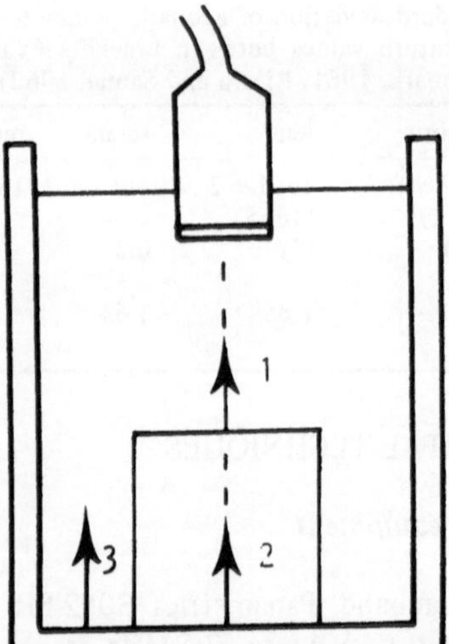

$$C_x = C_o \frac{T_3 - T_1}{T_2 - T_1}$$

Fig. 1.

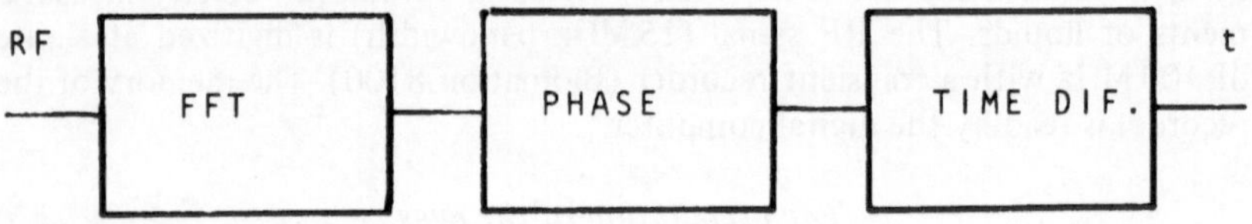

Fig. 2.

measurements as described and displacement of the transducer. The estimation of the velocity in the saline solution and the vitreous humour is performed according to the principle shown in Fig. 3 (cf. Verbeek et al. 1981). The XYZ table is stepped in vertical direction over distances which are known with a high accuracy (1 μm step of the table per drive pulse). The computer delivers a plot of distance (z) vs. time, the slope of which yields the velocity (accuracy $\simeq$ 0.1%). The attenuation is estimated by measuring the amplitude of the (2nd, or 3rd, order multiple reflection) bottom of the water tank with and without a specimen interposed. By this means the ultrasound passes 4 to 6 times through the relatively thin area, which greatly improves the measurement of the effect of attenuation. The measurement has to be corrected for the effect of reflection at the transitions with the surrounding fluid.

The estimation of the impedance is obtained by using the already obtained value of the velocity and subsequent measurement of the mass density. The latter measurement is performed by a volume substitution method with a small water filled cuvette and a high accuracy balance. The accuracy and reproduceability of these measurements is better than 1%.

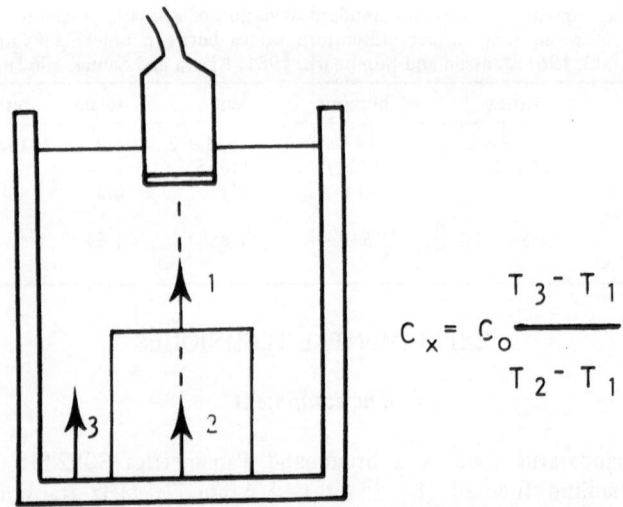

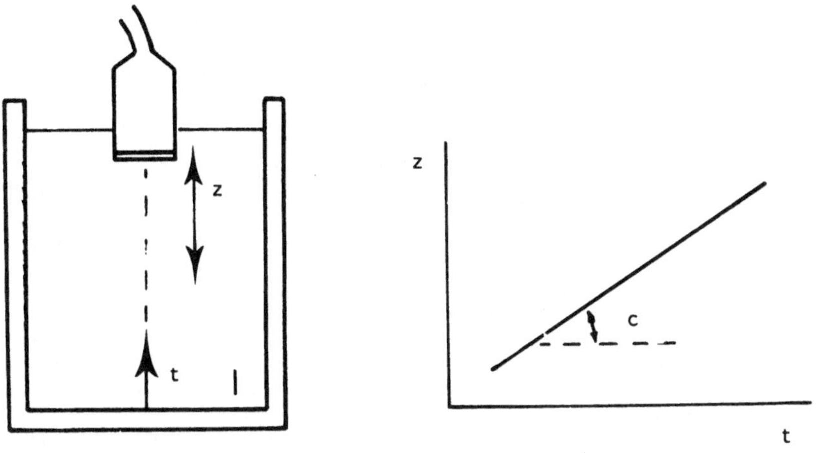

Fig. 3.

RESULTS

The first series of experiments has been performed with animal eyes (pig) and it may be considered as a pilot study for subsequent experiments with human eyes (also in vitro). The data are summarized in Table 3. The accuracy values that are presented are in indication of the accuracy of the employed analysis techniques. A larger series of eyes would be needed to obtain information on the biological variance of a single species. The estimation of the mass density is of the order of 1%, so the accuracy of the velocity estimates is far better ($\simeq$ 0.1%). The accuracy of the estimation of the impedance is, therefore, also of the order of 1%. The attenuation estimates are influenced by the reflections at the interfaces: if corrected for this effect by using the estimated impedances (as compared to water) the values would be in most instances approximately 10% lower.

CONCLUSION

We are now in the position to determine accurately the acoustic parameters of human ocular media.

REFERENCES

Araki, M. Studies on refractive elements of human eye by means of ultrasonic echogram. Jap. J. Clin. Ophthal. 15, 111 (1961).

Bayer, A. L. and Thijssen, J. M. In vivo characterization of intraocular membranes. In: 'Ultrasonography in Ophthalmology'. Eds. J. M. Thijssen and A. M. Verbeek, The Hague (1981). pp. 411–418.

Begui, Z. E. Acoustic properties of the refractive media of the eye. J. Acoust. Soc. Amer. 26, 365 (1954).

Chivers, R. C. and Parry, R. J. Ultrasonic velocity and attenuation in mammalian tissues. J. Acoust. Soc. Amer. 63, 940 (1978).

Coleman, D. J., Lizzi, F. L. and Jack, R. L. A determination of the velocity of ultrasound in cataractous lenses. In: 'Ultrasonography in Ophthalmology'. Eds. J. Francois and F. Goes. Bibliotheca Ophthal. 83. Karger, Basel 1975. Pp. 246–251.

Coleman, D. J., Lizzi, F. L., and Jack, L. R. 'Ultrasonography of the eye and orbit', Lea and Feibiger, Philadelphia, 1977.

Filipczinski, L. et al. Visualizating internal structures of the eye by means of ultrasonics. Proc. Vibr. Probl. 4, 357 (1967).

Goss, S. A., Johnston, R. L., and Dunn, F. Compilation of emperical ultrasonic properties of mammalian tissues II. J. Acoust. Soc. Amer. 68, 93 (1980).

Hueter, T. F. and Bolt, R. H. An ultrasonic method for outlining the cerebral ventricles. J. Acoust. Soc. Amer. 23, 160 (1951).

Jansson, F. and Sundmark, E. Determination of the velocity of ultrasound in ocular tissues at different temperatures. Acta Ophthal. 39, 899 (1961).

Nover, A. and Glanschneider, D. Untersuchungen Über die Fortpflanzungsgeschwindigkeit und Absorption des Ultraschalls im Gewebe. v. Graefes Arch. Ophthal. 168, 304 (1965).

Rivara, A., and Sanna, G. Determination of the speed of ultrasound in ocular tissues of humans and swine. Ann. Ottal. 88, 675 (1962).

Tschewnenko, A. Über die Ausbreitungsgeschwindigkeit des Ultraschalles in den Augengeweben. SIDOU i, Wiss. Z. Humboldt Univ. Berlin. Math. -Nat. R XIV, 67 (1965).

Vanysek, J., Preisová, J. and Obraz, J. 'Ultrasonography in Ophthalmology'. Czechoslovak Medical Press, London, Prague (1969).

Verbeek, A. M. Bayer, A. L. and Thijssen, J. M. Echographic diagnosis after intraocular silicon oil injection. In: 'Ultrasonography in Ophthalmology'. Eds. J. M. Thijssen and A. M. Verbeek. Junk, The Hague (1981). pp. 59–66.

Authors' address:
Biophysics Laboratory
Institute of Ophthalmology
University of Nijmegen
6500 HB Nijmegen
The Netherlands

ULTRASOUND INVESTIGATION OF THE CAROTID VESSELS

V. J. MARMION, M. ALDOORI, J. P. WOODCOCK and E. J. SHEDDEN
(Bristol, England)

SUMMARY

Twenty consecutive patients with transient ischemic attacks, or resolved strokes, have been examined using Doppler Ultrasound evaluation of carotid perfusion. The common internal and external vessels have been examined by Duplex scanning. The incidence of demonstrable stenosis is high (90%). The presence of bilateral lesions is commented upon and the effect of beta blockade on flow is noted. Comments are made on the comparability of ultrasound lesions with defects which could be demonstrated by angiography.

The occurrence of an attack of Amaurosis Fugax is of practical clinical importance to an ophthalmologist because of both the local and systemic implications. Traditionally the further investigation of these attacks has been with ophthalmodynamometry or its further refinements and arteriography.

The development of the Doppler Ultrasound technique of Satomura (1959) into a standardised clinical examination has taken place over the past ten years, Woodcock (1980). The Doppler Flowmeter permits the resolution of direction of flow, an analysis of the blood-velocity/time wave form can be made at specific sites along the vessel, and the detection of stenosis and its degree estimated, Spencer and Reid (1979). Vessels can also be examined using a real-time ultrasound scanner and the presence of plaques, stenosis and calcification can be readily demonstrated. The system used in this study, is a combination of real-time scanner with an attached pulsed Doppler Flowmeter, is non-invasive, and rarely causes discomfort to the patient. This technique should therefore be a suitable system for the evaluation of patients experiencing Amaurosis Fugax.

MATERIALS AND METHODS

Twenty patients who had more than one attack of Amaurosis Fugax of a classical type were investigated. The mean age, sex ratio and laterality of the lesions are shown in Fig. 1. Five patients had suffered a stroke with hemiplegia, after the attacks of amaurosis fugax. In ten patients satisfactory

Hillman, J. S./Le May, M. M. (eds.) Ophthalmic Ultrasonography

ISBN 978-94-009-7280-3

TRANSIENT ISCHEMIC ATTACKS. (20 Cases)	
Mean Age	68
M/F Ratio	10/10
Side R/L	11/9
Hemiplegia	5 cases

Fig. 1.

OPHTHALMODYNAMOMETRY (10 Cases)	
Affected	38.5
Non-affected	39.0

Fig. 2.

ULTRASOUND SCAN OF INTERNAL CAROTID.

	Affected	Non-affected
PLAQUE	15	6
FLOW DISTURBANCE	3	7
NO ABNORMALITY	2	7

Fig. 3.

diastolic ophthalmodynametric readings were obtained. The mean diastolic pressure on the affected and other side are shown in Fig. 2. All twenty patients were examined with the Advanced Technology Laboratories 5 MHz range gated Duplex Scanner which combines a B Scan capability with a flow meter. Lesions present around the Carotid bifurcation were classified as: no abnormality, Flow disturbance, and, plaques, which were subsequently graded.

RESULTS

Fig. 3 shows the strong pre-disposition, in this group to the development of plaque formation. It is of interest to note that in three instances there were plaques in the common, as well as the internal carotid and, in one case, the external carotid on the same side showed a significant occlusion. There was a high incidence of bilateral plaques – six out of twenty. Two patients have shown an increased incidence of amaurosis fugax while on Beta Blockers.

DISCUSSION

The results from ophthalmodynamometry, in retrospect, were disappointing. It would seem that the Duplex Scanner is more likely to give a satisfactory demonstration of underlying pathology which correlates with the clinical picture. The incidence of bilateral lesions in the internal carotid is not inconsistant with the clinical observation of bilateral amaurosis fugax. The inability to demonstrate lesions in two out of the twenty patients, (10%), is also consistent with previous reports.

Previous studies have shown a clear correlation between Doppler Ultrasound examination and arteriography. (Barnes, P. W. 1976) and Lusby (1981).

The advantage of the ultrasound examination lies with both the anatomical and the physiological features which are demonstrated. A careful observation of the vessel during the course of the examination can provide a further dynamic aspect of the changes taking place in the vessel wall itself. Spencer and Read (1979) have suggested a method for quantifying the degree of stenosis, by measuring the peak velocity, using a continuous wave flowmeter. This and subsequent reports, correlate well with the anatomical lesions as shown by arteriography and surgery. The report of Lusby (1981) shows that a correlation of 73% and higher can be anticipated using a Duplex Scanner (A. T. L. Seattle).

The incidence of bilateral lesions, demonstrated by this technique is important. It is of special interest in relation to the anastomotic ability of the circle of Willis. It would be expected that this would be more affected where there was a plaque with stenosis in the common carotid as well as the internal as occurred in three cases, or where the external carotid was affected as in one case. It has been suggested by Marshall (1976) that the main anastomosis is likely to be between the carotid systems and that, because of the nature of the anatomical variations in the posterior communicating artery, the vertebral system is not likely to significantly contribute to improved blood flow in the anterior segment of Willis.

Where there is a plaque, or stenosis, lowering of the blood pressure by Beta Blockade, particularly where this results in a lowered perfusion rate, would be more liable to produce an increase in transient ischemic attacks than a relief of the symptoms as was observed in two cases cited.

The findings in this small series are in concordance with previous larger studies (Blackshear 1979 and Lusby 1980). Discussion is likely to arise as to whether a continuous Doppler, or pulsed system provides better, or more accurate information. Any ultrasound system examines only a limited segment of the carotid bifurcation. The pulsed or continuous wave flowmeter must be angled in relation to the direction of flow in order to measure a Doppler shift. In general this angle of inclination is unknown except with a Duplex Scanner and this makes it difficult directly to compare blood velocities in one carotid with that in another. Perhaps more attention should be directed towards vessels which can be examined 'end-on' when direct comparison of velocity can then be made by a simple Doppler probe.

REFERENCES

R. W. Barnes, M.D.; G. E. Bone, M.D.; J. Reinertson, B.S.; E. E. Slaymaker, R.N., Iowa City, Iowa; D. E. Hokanson, B.S. and D. E. Strandness, Jr., M.D., Seattle, Wash. 1976, 'Noninvasive ultrasonic carotid angiography: Prospective validation be contrast arteriography.' Surgery – Sept. 1976.

Blackshear, R. W., Phillips, D. J., Thiele, B. L., Birsch, J. H., Chikos, P. M., Marinelli, M. R., Ward, K. J., and Strandness, D. E. 1979 'Detection of carotid occlusive disease by ultrasonic imaging and pulsed Doppler spectral analysis.' Surgery 86, 698–706.

Lusby, R. J., Woodcock, J. P., Skidmore, R., Jeans, W. D., Hope, D. T. and Baird, R. N. 1980 'Carotid artery disease: a prospective evaluation of ultrasonic imaging in the detection of low and high grade stenosis'. Br. J. Surg. 67, 823.

Lusby, R. J., Machleder, H. I., Jeans, W., Skidmore, R., Woodcock, J. P., Clifford, P. C. and Baird, R. N. 1981. 'Vessel wall and blood flow dynamics in arterial disease.' Phil. Trans. R. Soc. London, B 294, 231–239 (1981).

Marshall, J., 'The management of cerebrovascular disease.' 1976.

Spencer, M. P., and Reid, J. M., 'Quantitation of Carotid Stenosis with Continuous-Wave (C–W) Doppler Ultrasound.' Stroke 10:3 May'June 1979.

Woodcock, J. P., 'Doppler Ultrasound in Clinical Diagnosis' British Medical Bull. (1980) 36:3. 243–248.

Authors' address:
Vascular Laboratory
Bristol Royal Infirmary
Bristol BS2 8HW
UK

OCULAR TISSUE CHARACTERIZATION BY RF-SIGNAL ANALYSIS: SUMMARY OF THE BONN/STUTTGART IN VIVO-STUDY

H. G. TRIER*, D. DECKER**, R.-D. LEPPER*, K. M. IRION**
R. REUTER*, M. KOTTOW, R. MÜLLER-BREITENKAMP*
and K. J. OTTO*
(Bonn & Stuttgart, W. Germany)

BACKGROUND OF THE STUDY

The Bonn/Stuttgart group presented in 1973 results of the first comprehensive study on computer-aided tissue characterization on the eye in vitro, using empirical analysis of video (A-mode)-signals*** (Trier and Reuter 1973; Decker et al. 1973). 1973–1977, techniques for utilization of RF-signals in the 5–25 MHz frequency range were developed for the same applications** (Trier 1974; BMFT-DFVLR, Final report 1978). In the period 1977–81, the developed system and the techniques for RF-signal acquisition and processing were tested in vivo in clinical routine on the eyes of patients and volunteers by the Bonn group (BMFT-DFVLR, Final Report 1982). For that purpose the techniques for data collection, A/D conversion, intermediate storage, data structure, system controls, and processing methods were continuously adapted to the clinical needs. Preliminary results were presented at the SIDUO VII and VIII Conferences (Decker and Trier 1979; Trier et al. 1981).

1. TECHNIQUES

1.1 Signal acquisition

The eye was first examined by A- and B-mode (KRETZ 7200 MA, SONOMETRICS Ocuscan 400) to determine the region of interest. In this region a separate system with broad frequency bandwidth was applied with hand-held transducer ($f_c = 15$ MHz, pulse length 200 μs; -10 dB) and water

Part of the results was included in the lecture: H. G. Trier, Ocular tissue characterization by RF-signal analysis, 3rd Meeting WFUMB, Brighton, July 1982.

*Eye Clinic, Univ. Bonn (FRG); the authors H. G. Trier, M. Kottow, R. D. Lepper, R. Reuter, R. Müller-Breitenkamp and K. J. Otto were formerly affiliated to: Klinisches Institut für experimentelle Ophthalmologie der Universität Bonn
**Institut für Biomedizinische Technik d. Univ. Stuttgart (FRG)
***supported by Stiftung Volkswagenwerk
****supported by BMFT-DFVLR, Bonn

ISBN 978-94-009-7280-3

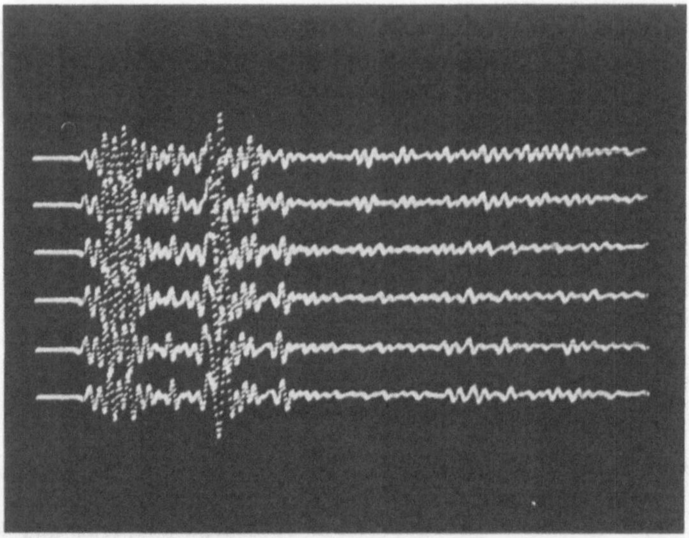

Fig. 1. **Series of RF-signals from the rear wall of the eye, after analog/digital conversion (TEKTRONIX AD 3020). Trace length 5 μs.**

stand-off in contact coupling. By a movable time gate (2.0 or 10 μs) part of the RF-trace was selected for A/D conversion (TEKTRONIX R 7912 and AD 3020) at 8 bit, 200–256 MHz sampling rate. Data intermediate storage, and transfer on tape/disc via microcomputer. Details were reported elsewhere (Lepper et al. 1978; Lepper 1982; Trier 1980). Special efforts were made to describe the transfer characteristics of the system, and to keep them constant over the 4-years period. For this purpose a comprehensive program for quality assurance of transducers, reference signals from a standard plane target, and electrical test signals were used.

1.2 Data collection and preprocessing

The transducer adjustment to the lesion under study was carefully optimized manually by the examining physician, using A-mode- and RF-displays of the echogram. Then, 20–25 signals were collected, forming one file. In each lesion 3–10 files were collected with new adjustment for each file. All digitized signals were then subjected to a visual quality assurance procedure, selecting signals with amplitudes ⩾ 5 bit (AD 3020 TEKTRONIX), adequate leading edge, and correct time gate position, only. The selected signals (50% of all collected signals) were reviewed by the examining physician for the presumable 'anatomical layers' displayed (Fig. 1), and these layers were marked by a code. The data transferred to the signal processing group included system parameters, and anatomical information. In total, over 200 files

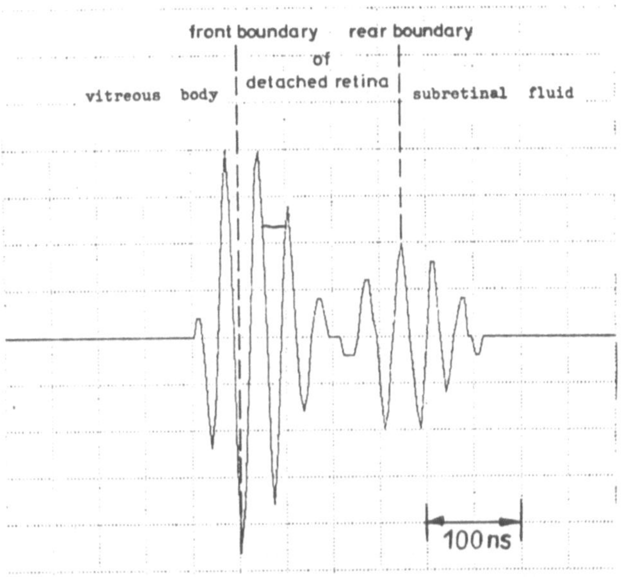

Fig. 2. Representative RF-echogram of a detached retina, after preprocessing.

with 65,000 signals were selected, based on 500 conditions examined.

1.3 Signal processing

Signal processing was performed off-line on external computers (PDP 12, 11--40, connected by Modem to CDC 6600, CYBER 174). The evaluated bandwidth was 5–22 MHz, using signal analysis procedures in the time domain, and the frequency domain, especially:

- automatical preprocessing, using plausibility criteria with restoration or rejection of disturbed signals;
- formation of file-specific *representative echograms,* using cross correlation of all signals, and a matrix operation to establish classes of signals with high correlation coefficient, e.g. 0.8, Phase coherent averaging of the signals of one class results in one or several 'representative' echograms, which underwent further processing (Fig. 2) (Decker et al. 1980; Decker and Irion 1980).

1.3.1. In layered tissues: extraction of numerical features for *tissue boundary surfaces,* especially:

- distance of interfaces; resolution: using cross correlation to reference signal $\geqslant 60\,\mu m \pm 1.5\%$; using interference spectrum $\geqslant 180\,\mu m \pm 5\%$;
- spectral type of tissue boundaries, to distinguish specular surfaces ($f/f_c \leqslant 1.0$), scattering surfaces ($f/f_c \geqslant 1.2$), structured surfaces (inhomogenous

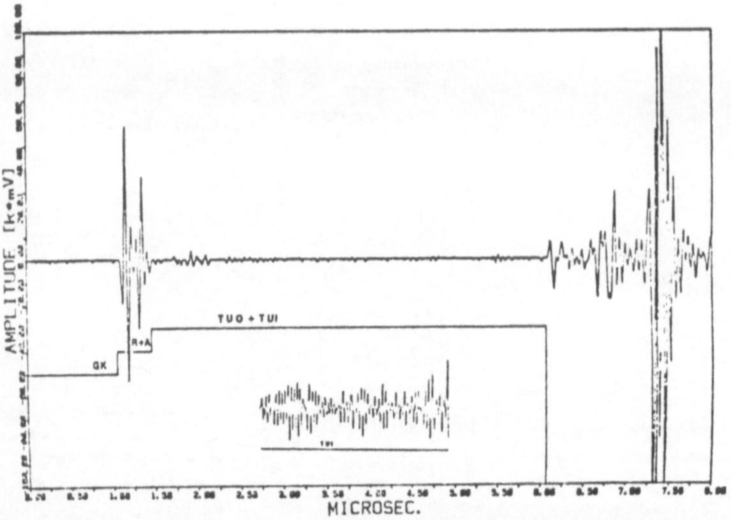

Fig. 3. Representative RF-echogram of the eye wall with a choroidal melanoma. The anatomical layers are coded in the shape of a staircase. Internal tumour signal: 40 dB below amplitudes of retina.

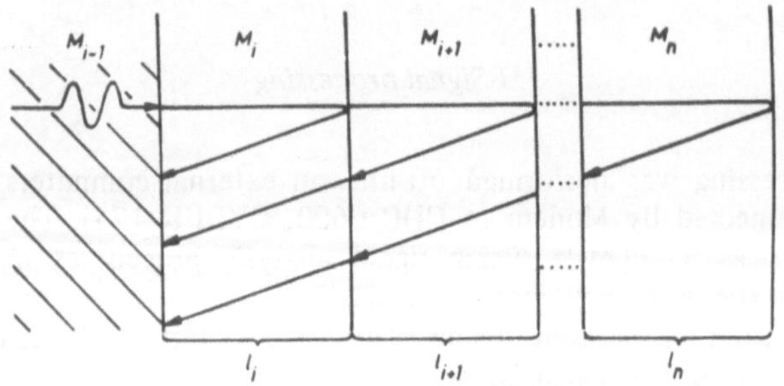

Transfer function for one tissue segment:

$$/ H_{i,i+1} / = B_i \cdot e^{-\alpha_i \cdot 2 \cdot l_i}$$

Transfer function for n tissue segments:

$$/ H_{1,n} / = C \cdot e^{-\sum_{i=1}^{n} \alpha_i \cdot 2 \cdot l_i}$$

B_i, C : const.

$S_i(f)$: spectrum for ith received echo

$S_{i+1}(f)$: spectrum for i+1 th received echo

$\alpha_i = \beta_i \cdot f \qquad f > 0$

β_i : slope of attenuation (Np/MHz cm, dB/MHz cm)

Fig. 4. Model of reflection for multilayered tissue with n tissue segments, without multiple reflections.

scatterer distribution with multipeak or asymmetrical distribution);
- reflectivity (referenced to standard target 15 mV = 0 dB);
- order of succession of layers, and occurrence;
- variance of features in 1 file, and in all files (Decker et al. 1981).

1.3.2. In internal tissue structure: features describing the attenuation and the scattering centres in the tissue were extracted. Fig. 3 shows the representative RF-echogram of the eye wall with a melanoma of the choroid of ca 5 μs of length. The retinal layer (on the tumour), the infiltrated choroid and the scleral boundaries can be detected. The internal tumour echoes show small amplitudes, and are, therefore, represented in a larger scale under the total trace.

(a) *Approach for the estimation of attenuation and of scattering centres in tumours* (Irion and Decker 1981).

Fig. 4 demonstrates a physical model of ultrasound reflection in a multilayered tissue, the layers being homogenous without dispersion and without multiple reflections. In true tissues rough layer surface and non-parallel layers are present, which do not permit the familiar mathematical estimation of the transmission and reflection coefficients (B_i and R_i). A constant C can be obtained as a measurable parameter, which describes a mean value of the reflection and transmission properties of the layers.

Assuming a multilayered tissue with approximately equal attenuation coefficient αi, the attenuation coefficient $\alpha(f)$ can simply be calculated as the mean value of all αi. The multilayered tissue is represented theoretically by a 'sequence' of transfer functions $H_{i,\,i+1}$. Using this assumption, the attenuation coefficients αi (f) can be calculated by the Fourier transform pair of the input- and output-signals $S_i(f)$ and S_{i+1} (f). Many investigators showed experimentally that in soft tissues the attenuation coefficient is linearly dependent on frequency in lower MHz-range. With this linear relation the slope of attenuation β_i can be calculated. On account of the linear physical behaviour of the attenuation and frequency, the differences of the logarithmic Fourier transforms can be approximated by a least square fit line. In case of good correlation the slope of attenuation with the unit dB/MHz · cm or Np/MHz · cm is derived from the fit line. This is the *theoretical* background for the estimation of the attenuation.

Problems will arise in *practical use of the model,* when the wave length (λ) is larger than the mean scatter dimensions (d) ($\lambda > d$). Interferences occur and in case of very small scatter dimensions (d) the scattering coefficient varies with the frequency with the power of four. For wavelength in the range of scatter dimensions the scattering coefficient varies with the square of frequency.

In these cases a special algorithm for segmentation of the echoes out of the total signal is used, originally introduced by Kuc and Schwartz, 1979, for echograms of the liver, modified by Irion and Decker with regard to the calculation of the envelope and the use of the minima for segmentation (Fig. 5). In the 256-point data set the algorithm for example detected as an average about 3,5 segments per μs length in the case of melanoma.

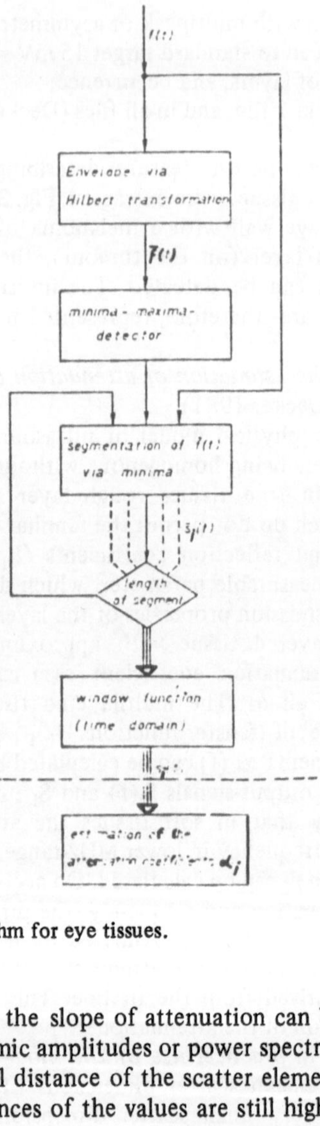

Fig. 5. **Segmentation algorithm for eye tissues.**

The attenuation and the slope of attenuation can be estimated from the sequence of the logarithmic amplitudes or power spectra (Fig. 6).

Assuming the optimal distance of the scatter elements from the statistical model of Kuc, the variances of the values are still high. Subretinal bleedings only have a significant lower slope of attenuation β_1, compared to all cases of malignant melanoma. As the segmentation of the echograms is carried out under subjective criteria, different algorithms of segmentation are not comparable. In case of interferences, or Raleigh scattering the attenuation coefficient can only be estimated by averaging many coefficients in different depths of penetration.

(b) A second estimation of frequency dependent attenuation is obtained by the short-time Fourier analysis. This technique is used to study variations of amplitude of energy of a signal as a function of time and frequency. Details are reported elsewhere (Irion and Decker 1981).

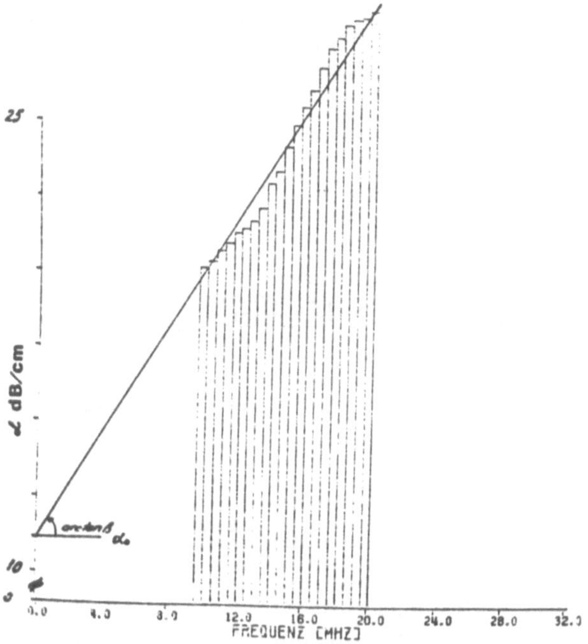

Fig. 6. Attenuation as a function of frequency in a case of intact rear wall of the eye.

Table 1. Features for internal tissue structure

frequency independent attenuation	A_o
slope of frequency dependent attenuation	A_I
coefficient of linear correlation for frequ. dependent attenuation	KK
number of scattering centres per 2 μs	BA
mean spectral centre frequency of scattering centres	FR

Both methods together result in the following internal tissue features (see Table 1):

The extracted features were combined in feature sets. Fig. 7 shows the modular concept for feature extraction and classification in the signal processing of an unknown echogram.

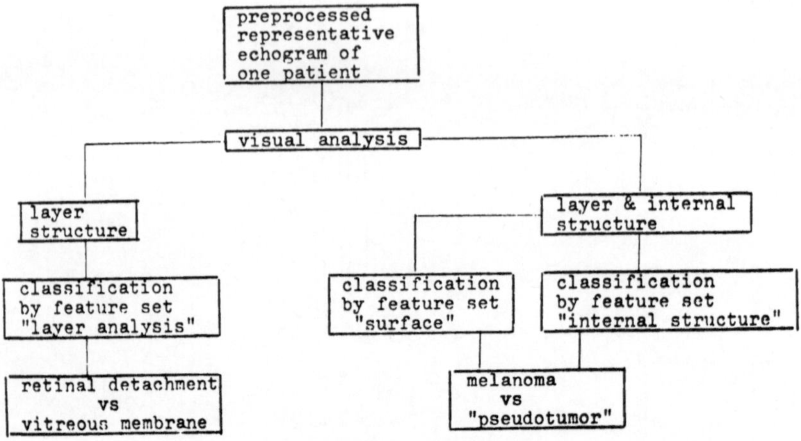

Fig. 7. Approach for classification of an unknown echogram.

2. CASE MATERIAL

Two conditions of the human eye were studied extensively:

– *Intraocular membranes,* to improve the diagnosis of retinal detachment vs vitreous membranes (364 examinations).
– *Intraocular tumours,* to improve the diagnosis of choroidal melanoma vs benign prominent lesions, and vs metastatic tumours (124 examinations).

3. RF-TISSUE FEATURES

3.1. RF-features for thin tissue layers

This proved to be the most important scientific result of the study. For the first time, statistical data based on RF-signals were presented, describing the thin layer structures of the living human eye. Such features (see 1.3.1) can be achieved by optimal transducer beam adjustment on the layers only, that means by the hand-held transducer approach, unique for this RF-study, but well known from A-mode echography.

The static feature 'layer thickness determination' provides with the routine techniques used at present a resolution of $\geqslant 60\,\mu$m. Even better resolution was achieved experimentally (Purnell 1980; Lepper 1981).

3.1.1. Use of two different approaches for the diagnosis of retinal detachment (Table 2).

(a) *Direct approach* = direct ultrasonic characterization of the unknown intraocular membrane. Feature sets for classification of detached retina and vitreous membrane, and data for recent/longstanding detachment were

Table 2. Updated feature sets for the direct diagnostic approach (upper part) and the indirect diagnostic approach (lower part) in the recognition of retinal detachment

	Detached retina n = 81 patients			Vitreous membrane n = 15 patients		
Boundary surfaces	I	II		I	II	
Layer thickness/μm	126 ± 28% const.			120 . . . 700 var.		
Recurrence	100%	94%		100%	100%	
Spectral type	SP	SP		ST, SP	ST, FS	
Rel. center frequency	f_I/f_c = 0,91 ± 14%	f_{II}/f_I = 1,1 ± 13%		f_I/f_c = 1,2 ± 15%	f_I/f_c = 1,0 ± 11%	
Distance of an additional layer/μm	–	111 ± 28% var.		120–200 var	–	
Recurrence	–	35%		33%	–	
Reflectivity/dB	–28			–32		
	Back wall without retina n = 15 patients			**Normal back wall (retina + choroid) n = 70 patients**		
Boundary surfaces	I	II	III	I	II	III
Layer thickness/μm	224 ± 46% var.	403 ± 34% const.		131 ± 14% const.	542 ± 25% const.	
Recurrence	25%	100%	100%	100%	100%	100%
Spectral type	FS	SP	SP	SP	SP	SP
Rel. center frequency	–	f_{II}/f_c = 0,83 ± 25%	f_{III}/f_{II} = 1,0 ± 20%	f_I/f_c = 0,8 ± 21%	f_{II}/f_I = 1,1 ± 25%	f_{III}/f_I = 1,1 ± 19%
Distance of an additional layer/μm	–	131 ± 37%	–	–	121 ± 30% const.	–
Recurrence		30%		–	55%	–
Reflectivity		–30			–20	

Spectral type of surfaces
SP: specular surface
ST: scattering surface
FS: structured surface

Layer thickness
const = constant per file and per patient (n files)
var = constant per file; variable per patient (n files)

Reflectivity
dB-level referenced to a flat target reflectivity
(15 mV $\hat{=}$ 0 dB)

published elsewhere (Decker and Trier 1979; Trier et al. 1981). The classification probability is at present sufficient for uncomplicated clinical cases.

(b) *Indirect approach* = detection of presence (+) or absence (–) of the retinal layer at the eye wall under the suspicious unknown membrane. In case (+), retinal detachment is here ruled out, in case (–), detachment is proven indirectly. This approach must be chosen additionally in complex i.o. pathology, if the direct approach fails. Preliminary feature sets (Weigelin and Trier 1981) were compiled, using the sequential order of layers detected by their static features.

Clinical experience showed that the detection of the choroidal layer is the key problem for broader application of indirect approach. It is, therefore, intended to evaluate also *dynamic* features of this layer and to include them in the feature sets. On an experimental level of work, the authors succeeded in recording the physiologic pulsations (time-dependent thickness variations) of the choroidal layer (Lepper et al. 1981), and in enhancing the dynamic features by suitable increase of i.o. tension (Cords).

3.1.2. Thin layer features. These may improve the detection of *intraocular tumours* by 'proximity layer analysis', describing the structure (no change; infiltration; dystrophy) of retina and choroid, enveloping the tumour. This feature has been evaluated up to now for the retinal layer in different tumour types and seems to be able to contribute to the classification probability (BMFT-DFVLR Final Report 1982), as far as the tumour surface is concerned. The utilization of the choroid is up to now limited by its often difficult identification in the RF-signal, as was mentioned above.

3.2. RF-features for internal tissue structures

Table 3 demonstrates attenuation features (mean $\pm \sigma$), as extracted from the group of histologically confirmed choroidal melanomas vs the group of 'pseudotumours', comprising Kuhnt Junius disease with prominent lesions, subretinal hemorrhages, nevus, and choroidal hemangioma.

Using the 5 features for internal tissue structure from Table 1 feature sets were compiled providing a mean classification probability of 73.5% for choroidal melanoma vs the group of benign 'pseudotumours', using univariate discrimination analysis. The characterization of metastatic tumours of the eye was especially limited by the small number of histologically confirmed cases. In a limited number of choroidal melanoma (spindle cell: 11 cases; epitheloid cell and mixed type: 6 cases) differentiation of histologic subgroups was tried by discrimination analysis, using the above 5 features. Table 4 shows the dependence of mean classification probability on the feature combination. These findings are influenced by several factors, namely the specificity of histologic classifications of the lesions by the different clinical centres involved in the study. Multivariate discriminant analysis between the two melanoma subgroups and ocular metastasis (2 cases) resulted in a mean classification probability of only 42% (BMFT-DFVLR, Final Report 1982).

Table 3. Attenuation features for internal tissue structures in the groups of choroidal melanoma and 'pseudotumours'

	Number of patients	Slope of frequency dependent attenuation in dB/(MHz · cm)	Frequency independent attenuation in dB/cm	Correlation coefficient of linear regression
Choroidal melanoma (histolog. confirm.)	34	0.4 ± 1.3	− 2.0 ± 25.5	0.7 ± 0.23
Group of 'pseudo-tumours'	15	− 0.7 ± 0.8	+ 21.5 ± 25.0	0.64 ± 0.18

Table 4. Mean classification probability, dependent on the feature combination between 2 subgroups of choroidal melanoma (univariate discrimination analysis; $n_1 = 6; n_2 = 11$)

feature combination	A_O, A_I, BA FR, KK	A_O, A_I, BA	A_O, A_I FR, KK	A_I FR, KK
mean classification probability	88%	88%	82%	64%

4. SUMMARY AND CONCLUSIONS

For RF-data collection a hand-held transducer in contact coupling is at present unavoidable, if features of thin layers are utilized. An integrated RF/B-mode system is, therefore, difficult to construct. However, a separate B-mode system and examination is in many applications sufficient to find the region of interest. Monitoring of transducer and system transfer characteristics proved indispensable and successful to provide data compatibility over long periods of time.

RF-signal analysis led to new clinically applicable features for ocular tissue characterization. The feature sets developed are now clinically applicable in vitreoretinal diseases. For a broader application in vitreoretinal and tumour diagnostics further improvements, especially in the detection of the choroidal layer must be completed.

The developed computer-aided methods for RF tissue characterization in the 5–22 MHz range are not limited to the eye, but are applicable to other organs, like skin, parotis, thyroid, testis, lymphnodes, vessels as well.

5. REFERENCES

BMFT-DFVLR, Grants 01 VI 014 and 034-B 13 MT 224 a, Final Report Sept. 20, 1978;

BMFT-DFVLR, Grants 01 VI 047 and 057 – ZA/NT/MT 224 a, Final Report July 30, 1982;

Cords, S. (in preparation) Dissertation, Bonn;
Decker, D., Epple, E., Leiss, W. and Nagel, M.: Digital computer analysis of time amplitude ultrasonograms from the human eye. II. Data processing. J. Clin. Ultrasound 1, 156–159 (1973).
Decker, D. and Trier, H. G.: Das Projekt 'rechnergestützte Gewebsdifferenzierung' der Arbeitsgemeinschaft Bonn/Stuttgart. II. Ergebnisse der Anwendung an dünnen Gewebsschichten im Auge. Proc. SIDOU VII, Münster 1978, in: Diagnostica Ultrasonica in Ophthalmologia, (Gernet, H., ed.) Remy, Münster 1979, pp. 40–43.
Decker, D. and Irion, K.: A-mode RF-signal analysis (frequency domain). In: Ultrasonic Tissue Characterization. Clinical Achievements and Technological Potentials. (Thijssen, J. M., ed.) Stafleu's Scientif. Publ. Comp., Alphen a.d.R., Brussels, 1980, pp. 231–244.
Decker, D., Trier, H. G., Irion, K., Lepper, R. D. and Reuter, R.: Rechnergestützte Gewebsdifferenzierung am Auge. Ultraschall 1, 284–296 (1980).
Decker, D., Faust, U. and Irion, K.: Examination of thin tissue layers in the human eye. Med. Progr. Techn. 8, 83–91 (1981).
Irion, K. and Decker, D.: Estimation of the acoustic attenuation of i.o. tumours in vivo. 2nd Workshop on ultrasonic tissue characterization, Nijmegen 1981 (in press).
Kuc, R. and Schwartz, M.: Estimating the acoustic attenuation coefficient slope for liver from reflected ultrasound signals. IEEE Trans. Biomed. Engin. 25, 321–344 (1978).
Lepper, R. D., Reuter, R. and Trier, H. G.: Digitization of high-frequency ultrasonic signals for tissue differentiation in ophthalmology. Biomed. Techn. 23, 75–78 (1978).
Lepper, R. D., Trier, H. G. and Reuter, R.: Ultrasonic measurements at the posterior wall of living human eyes. Ophthal. Res. 13, 1–11 (1981).
Lepper, R. D.: Unpublished results (1981).
Lepper, R. D.: Computergestützte Qualitätsbeurteilung von Ultraschallwandlern in der medizinischen Diagnostik. Biomed. Techn. 27, 2–6 (1982).
Purnell, E. W.: Ultrasonic biometry of the posterior ocular coats. Trans. Amer. Ophthal. Soc. 78, 1027–1078 (1980).
Trier, H. G. and Reuter, R.: Digital computer analysis of time-amplitude ultrasonograms from the human eye. I. Signal acquisition. J. Clin. Ultrasound 1, 150–154 (1973).
Trier, H. G.: Gewebsdifferenzierung mit Ultraschall. Habil. schr. 1974 and Bibl. Ophthal. No. 86, Karger, Basel 1977.
Trier, H. G.: Ultrasonic tissue characterization in the eye and orbit. In: Ultrasonic Tissue Characterization: Clinical Achievements and Technological Potentials. (Thijssen, J. M., ed.) Stafleu's Scientif. Publ. Comp., Alphen a.d.R., Brussels, 1980, pp. 45–67.
Trier, H. G., Decker, D., Müller-Breitenkamp, R., Irion, K. and Otto, K. J.: The recognition of detached retina and vitreous membranes by means of radio frequency signal analysis. Proc. SIDUO VIII, Nijmegen 1980, in: Ultrasonography in Ophthalmology (Thijssen, J. M. and Verbeek, A. M., eds.) Junk Publ. The Hague, Boston, London 1981, pp. 419–430.
Weigelin, E. and Trier, H. G.: Méthodes objectives de caractérisation tissulaire aux ultra-sons prospectives d'application cliniques en ophtalmologie. Bull. Soc. franc. Ophtal. 93, 332–335 (1981).

Authors' address:
Prof H G Trier
Universitäts-Augenklinik
Sigmund Freud Str. 25
D-5300 Bonn 1
Federal Republic of Germany

MICROCOMPUTER AIDED IMAGING TECHNIQUES IN OPHTHALMIC B-MODE

YUKIO YAMAMOTO, SIROH HIRANO, YASUO SUGATA, MICHIKO TOMITA, FUKUYO KABURAGI, EIKO OKADA and HIROKO TAKAYAMA
(Tokyo, Japan)

ABSTRACT

This report concerns microcomputer-based imaging in ophthalmic B-mode ultrasonography. Several imaging techniques and signal processing circuits are employed in this system of which the three main characteristics are: (a) four-frame dividing, (b) distance measurement, and (c) three-dimensional display.

The signal processing performs the selection and enhancement of echo signals, including DGC function and the digital data transformation for the purpose of linear and nonlinear intensity displays of echo amplitudes, such as the frame dividing by linear and its inverted intensity, logarithmic and antilogarithmic intensity display modes. This system usually produces a cross sectional image of 256 x 256 picture elements for a region of 5 x 5 cm.

Furthermore, the distance between any two interested points can be measured with the aid of two markers.

Three-dimensional display of intraocular tissues is obtained from a series of consecutive cross sectional B-mode images. There are two methods to be practiced: a line image consisting of a set of overlaid contour lines and a shaded image consisting of a set of gradually darked planes by using image processing techniques such as smoothing and Laplacian. Further, we can make a measurement of areas and volumes of the tissue by this system.

A newly designed colour gradient scale was applied for the purpose of discriminating echo levels as well as displaying weak echoes clearly.

INTRODUCTION

The weakness of the essential ophthalmic ultrasonic diagnostic methods at present can be said to be the delay of so-called 'characterization of tissues,' a name employed for the purpose of collecting such data as morphological and acoustic qualities and the characteristics of each patient.

However, progress in this work has become apparent due to efforts of individuals in each country. Two methods of research are available: research based on ultrasonography by A-mode method and practical research by

Hillman, J. S./Le May, M. M. (eds.) Ophthalmic Ultrasonography

ISBN 978-94-009-7280-3

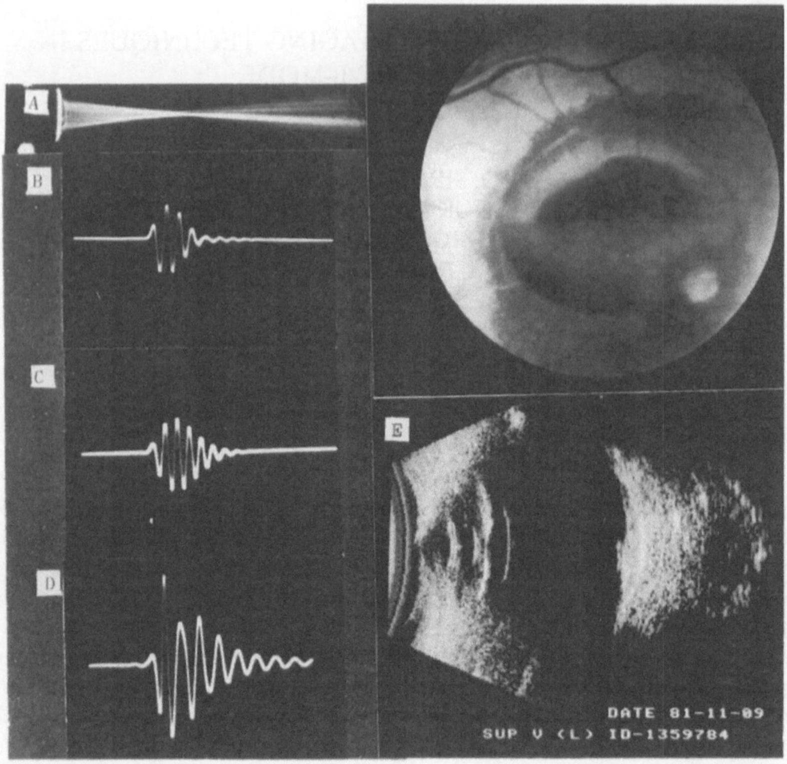

Fig. 1. **A: an increased focusing efficiency by the transducer PVDF. B: 10 MHz focused PVDF (F: 30 mm). C: 10 MHz focused PVDF (F: 44 mm). D: 10 MHz focused Ceremic. Case: Preretinal, retinal, and choroidal haemorrhage. E: Vertically Scanned Section by PVDF shows the thickened tissues with some distinction.**

B-mode method. In either case, the introduction of computers to this work has given an impetus to the realization of characterization.

Using a section of the memory directly connected to the CPU of a microcomputer for imaging, experiments were performed on cross sectional image processing of ocular ultrasonography from an image diagnosis system which enabled easy execution of processing and response.

CHARACTERISTICS OF THIS SYSTEM

The purpose of this system includes the following:

(1) Investigation of the influence of the corresponding relationship between echo levels and gradations on the identification of intraocular tissue.

(2) Measurement by cross sectional imaging of the distance between any two points and also the cross sectional area and volume of the tissue of the image.

(3) Image memory, increased LOAD function for playback, and so on.

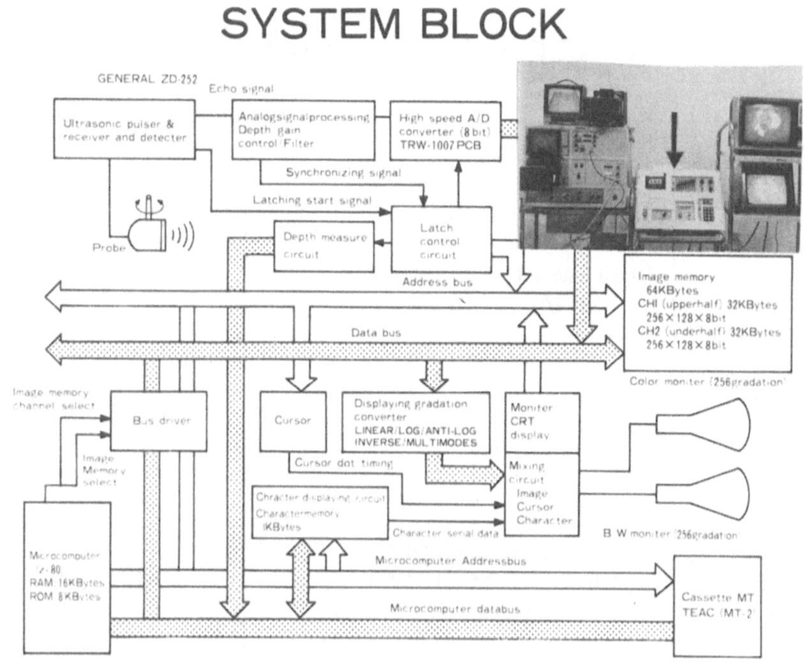

Fig. 2.

SYSTEM CONFIGURATION

(1) With a digitized ocular image display of 256 x 256 picture elements, the display of 5 x 5 cm cross sections enabled it to display composition of about 0.2 mm square per picture element. Four-bit 16-step gradation and a coloured 8-step gradation had conventionally been used. However, it was possible to obtain over 32 grades for the purpose of enriching the image shading as a colour gradient scale.

(2) The conventionally used ceramic of the probe was changed to polyvinylidene fluoride (PVDF), a most promising piezoelectric polymer at present as tranceducer material; the following multiple values were made:

10 – 13 MHz
F = 30 mm., 44 mm., 47 mm.
ϕ = 10 mm., 5 mm.;

and attempts were made to increase the efficiency of beam convergence – all of which allowed planning for images of increased merit with its high resolution power. (Fig. 1).

(3) As hardware configuration (Figs. 2, 3) depth gain compensation can be executed by the signal processing circuit. Also, alteration of the shading, after AD conversion, was possible by the gradation conversion, circuit, even when adding limited number of shades. That is, the following frame-dividing modes were provided to allow alteration at the time of AD conversion:

MEMORY MAP

ADDRESS	CONTENTS	SIZE
0000	MONITER PROGRAM	0.75 KB (ROM)
0300	SYSTEM PROGRAM — INITIAL LOADER	0.25 KB (ROM)
0400		
3000	CASSETTE MT REGISTER	8 BYTE
3008		
3C00	CHARACTER MEMORY 32 LINE × 32 COLUMN (ASCII 5 CORD × 7 DOTS)	1 KB (RAM)
4000	IMAGE MEMORY (UPPERHALF) (256 PIXEL × 128 LINE) 1 PIXEL = 4 BITS 16 LEVELS	16 KB (RAM)
8000	PROGRAM AREA (MONITER. WORK. AREA)	16 KB (RAM)
C000	IMAGE MEMORY (UNDERHALF) (256 PIXEL × 128 LINE) 1 PIXEL = 4 BITS 16LEVELS	16 KB (RAM)

Fig. 3.

(a) Logarithmic – intensified display of weak echo signals.
(b) Antilogarithmic – detailed display of higher levels
(c) Linear – unstressed levels

These frame dividing methods allow easy fixation of the selection and intensity of echo levels, giving the desired images and a variety of shaded displays.

Accordingly, image memory and a 4-frame divided display can be executed. Although the CPU has a memory capacity of 64 K bytes, 2 picture elements were stored on 1 byte and cross sectional images were stored on 32 K bytes, projecting increased efficiency with regard to image memory and program maintenance.

The 4-frame divided display is designed to display the 3 previously mentioned modes plus an inverted image of the linear mode. Although there are

Programs and their functions

Family	Name	Contents	Size (KByte)	Job time (sec)
OS	System Progam	I/Oput management of a cassette MT et al. on a file method	0.8	IKByte/sec (MT Read/Write)
Measurement	Distance	Length with subsideary line	0.8	Real time
	Image Enlarging	×4 Magnification	0.3	1.0
	Image	Histogram Area Volume	0.6 0.4 0.7	2.0 3.0 3.2 sec/picture
Image Processing	Sector Transformation	Shape reconstruction of Latched image	2.5	170
	Filtering	Smoothing With gradation Median filter	0.3 0.4 0.4	7 12 90
	Contour Detection	Trinary Image	0.5	5
	2-dimensional FFT	32×32 Pixels	0.9	8
	3-dimensional display	Plural images → Solid display	2.5 without Sector Transform	Computation time 120/picture
Others	Information	ID-number Date Diagnosis	0.5	Conversation style

Fig. 4.

128 x 128 picture elements in the divided display, switching to the complete display will yield 256 x 256 picture elements, which leads to increased speed of tissue information and to a reduction in examination time.

The interface used for display is made up of a synchronizing signal generation circuit, a circuit which transforms 1-byte data into 4-bit 2 picture elements, and a mixer circuit. At the mixer circuit, image data signals, character signals, and marker signals are mixed, and then transmitted as video signals to which an artificial colour gradient scale was used for classification.

Next, a marker display and an intensity measurement circuit were provided. This circuit is the central focus of this system which makes possible the measurement of many aspects of ocular tissues, e.g. axis or curvature, the intraocular occupation of tumors or growths, the amount of quantitative change as in the case of haemorrhage, and so on. Two markers which move freely are operated by a key switch on the monitor and the values deter-

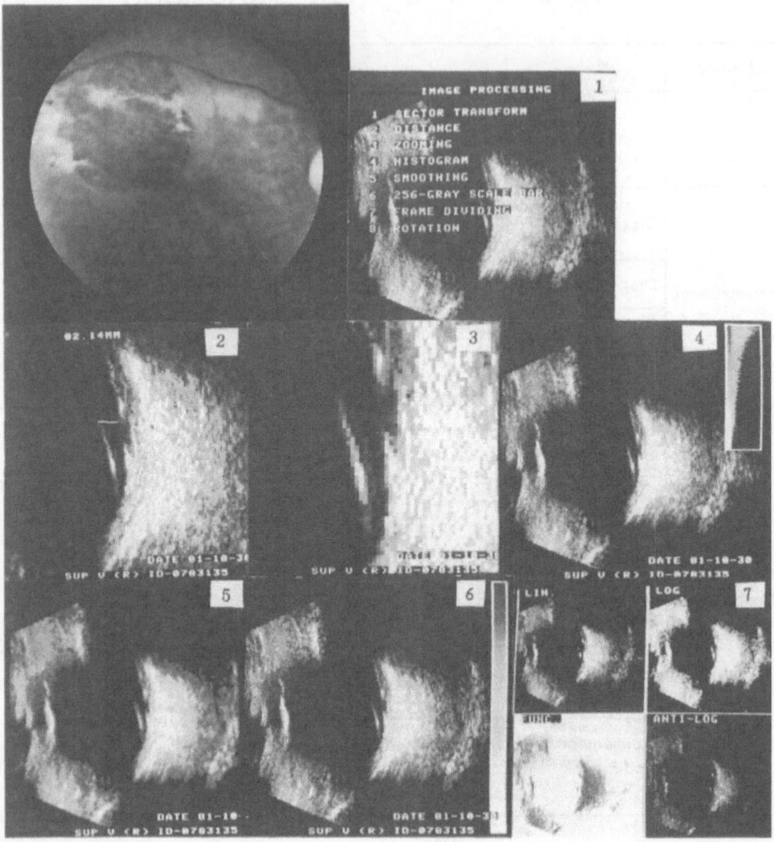

Fig. 5. Case: Giant retinal tear

mining interval of the points are given by the program, then displayed. The markers will flicker and the values of their coordinates can be read through the I/O port into the microcomputer.

The intensity measurement circuit takes an image from the face of the probe and inputs the distance from the beginning position into the CPU. The execution of the fan conversion program yields a cross sectional image of this distance in parameters that has the same shape as the B-scan field.

(4) In software configuration (Fig. 4), attention has been given to programs for measurement, as illustrated in Fig. 6.

Sector conversion is a first party release operation of the measurement process. The original image, displayed with its foreground magnified and its background condensed, is transformed to a fan-shaped image which resembles the scanning field.

Afterwards, the tissue of interest is located by 2 points, using the markers, and the distance is displayed at that actual moment with LED on the monitor TV. This distance is expressed by number of pixels with counting over 5

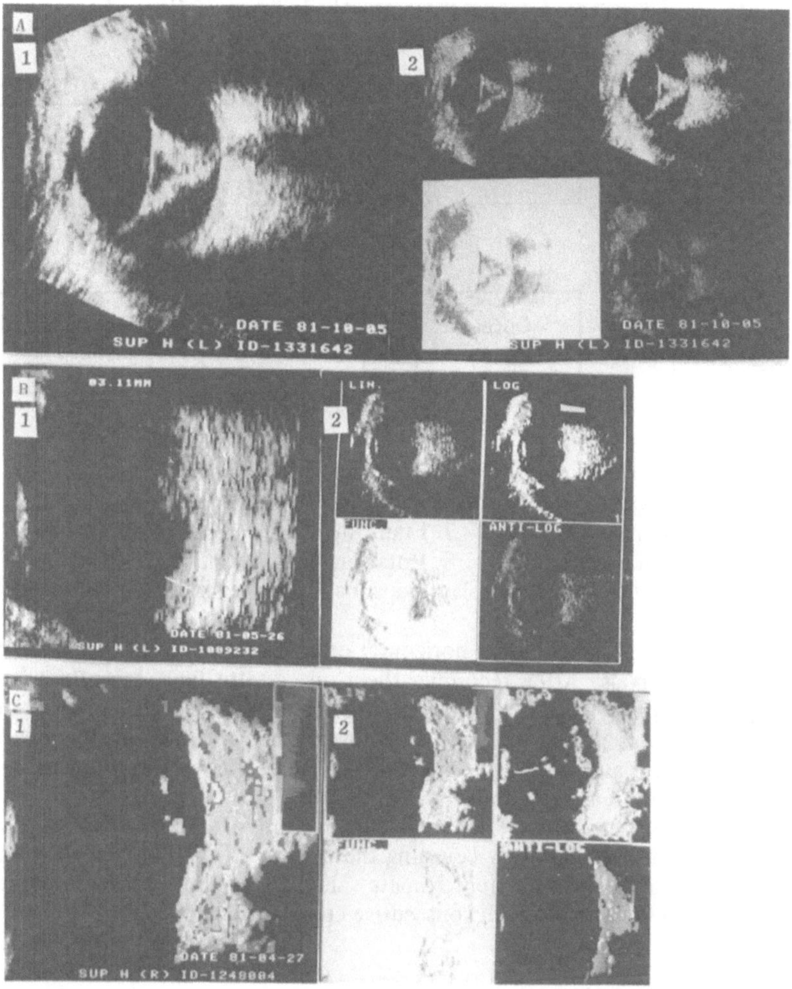

Fig. 6. A: Massive periretinal proliferation. (1) Horizontally Scanned Section. (2) Frame dividing. B: Proliferative diabetic retinopathy. (1) Horizontally Scanned Section with Magnification and Distance Measurement. (2) Frame Dividing. C: Choked disc. (1) Horizontally Scanned Section with Smoothing and Histogram. (2) Frame Dividing.

and cutting under 4 being multiplied by 0.195 mm as an axial resolution, the maximum error of 0.195/2 mm., and the software configuration is in inverse proportion to the measured distance at 0.195/2 L. The distance between two markers is joined with a straight line by DDA and displayed.

The code for image processing includes the following elements and is designed to enable indication and display of any item:

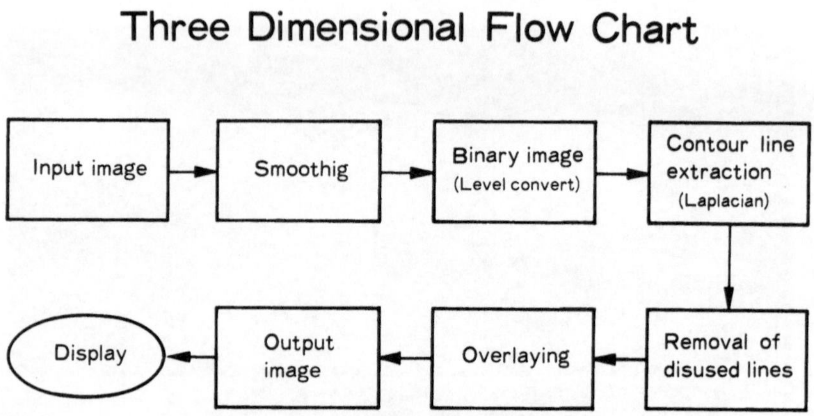

Fig. 7.

1. Sector transform
2. Distance
3. Zooming
4. Histogram
5. Smoothing
6. 256-gradient scale bar
7. Frame-dividing
8. Rotation (Figs. 5, 6)

The three-dimensional display depended on the following procedure: (Figs. 7, 8).

A series of 12 consecutive horizontal cross sectional images were taken at 1 mm. intervals. After recording them on cassette tape, smoothing was done by template, contour lines were abstracted by Laplacian process and a line image was produced. Next, serial overlay is performed on this image. Assigning black-and-white shading to each line gives a three-dimensional image through intensity-shading.

This process can also be employed to measure areas and volumes; that is, area can be calculated by counting the number of picture elements with the contour lines and then approximate values for volumes can be obtained by adding up the areas of each consecutive cross-sectional image.

DISCUSSION

Although microcomputer-based image processing of ocular ultrasonography has been done in A-mode by K. Ossoing (1), D. J. Coleman (2), J. M. Thijssen (3), and H. G. Trier (4), the clinical values have been insufficient and blurring exists. Recently, F. L. Lizzi (5) has begun B-mode computer processing.

The development of this system was attempted with the idea that computer processing done directly by B-mode imaging would have large application in the clinical area.

This system is capable of vertical measurement from A-mode as well as the measurement of slanting planes; that is, it is able to measure the distance between any two points of interest by reconstruction of the fan image. DDA enables these points to be joined by lines.

The four-frame divided display is another of the special features. This

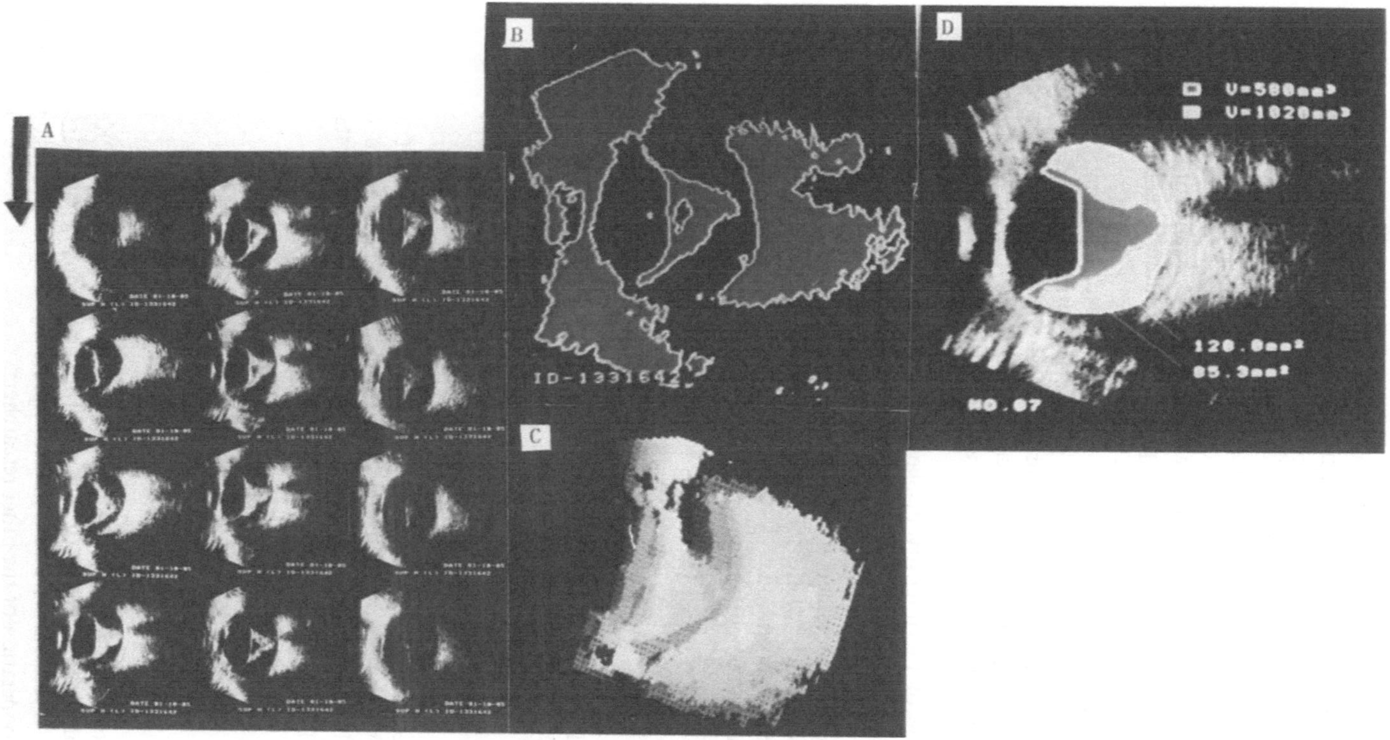

Fig. 8. Case: Massive periretinal proliferation. A: Horizontally Scanned Sections (Upper ⇌ Under) for Overlaying. B: Contour Line Extraction for Area Estimation. C: Three-Dimensional Display by shading. D: Calculation of the Area and Volume.

type of display – with a logarithmic frame for low-intensity tissue display, an anti-logarithmic frame for high-intensity tissue display, plus the linear frame and that of its inverted image - facilitates the selection of proper treatment and allows the diagnostic functions of this system to play an even more active role. For instance, retinal detachment is stressed on antilogarithmic slice and vitreous haemorrhage on logarithmic.

The four-frame divided images were conceived as a series of images shaded by a colour gradient scale. They provide much more detailed information than conventional artificial colours.

The three-dimensional display is another special feature. Prior to the three-dimensional image, a variey of data is provided even at the stage of contour line abstraction. Contour lines can be abstracted by tracing of the CRT display image with the cursor and by the Laplacian process; however, the threshold value was set at the fifth echo level from the weakest level.

The use of the intensity display mode and the parallel movement mode when overlaying will yield three-dimensional display from any angle of interest.

Area can be obtained by the image prime numbers of the region within the contour lines, whereas it is also possible to make artificial boundary lines by cursor operation.

Volume can be obtained by the following formula:

$$V = \frac{h}{2} \sum_{i=1}^{N-1} (S_i + S_{i+1})$$

(V = volume h = interval (1 mm.) N = no. of images (12) S_i = cross sectional area with ordinal no. i).

CONCLUSIONS

The development of this system makes possible many kinds of image processing. With its various shaded displays, distance measurement of various planes, three-dimensional display and other functions acting as its principal pivot, improvement in diagnostic functions is anticipated.

ACKNOWLEDGEMENT

This system was successfully developed through the work of Kenichi Ito (Professor, Tokyo University of Agriculture and Industry) and Masayasu Ito (Assistant Professor). I would like to express my deep gratitude to them and for the cooperation of the other researchers.

REFERENCES

1. Ossoinig, K., Ressmann, P. and Till, P.: Ein digitaler Speicher zur Computeranalyse von Gevebsechogrammen, Diagnostica Ultrasonica in Ophthalmologica (Proc. of SIDUO IV), Centre National d'Ophthalmologie des Quinze-Vingts, Paris, 1973. pp. 93–97.
2. Coleman, D. J., Lizzi, F. L. and Jack, R. L.: Ultrasonography of the Eye and Orbit, Lee and Febiger, Philadelphia, 1977, pp. 83–87.
3. Thijssen, J. M., Kruizing, R. et al.: Computer assisted echographic diagnosis. I. Quantitative and statistical analysis of the video signal, II. Quantitative analysis of R. F. – Signal, Diagnostica Ultrasonica in Ophthalmologica (Proc. of SIDUO VII), Remy-Verlag, Münster, 1979. pp. 12–19.
4. Trier, H. G., Lepper, R.-D. and Reuter, R.: Das Projekt 'rechnergestützte Gebedsdifferenzierung' der Arbeitsgemeinschaft Bonn/Stuttgart. I. Stand der Methodik in Vivo. (Proc. of SIDUO VIII) Diagnostica Ultrasonica in Ophthalmologia, Remy-Münster, 1979, pp. 35–39.
5. Lizzi, F. L., Coleman, D. J., et al.: Digital processing and imaging mode for clinical ultrasound, Ultrasonography in Ophthalmology (Proc. of SIDUO VIII), Dr W. Junk, Hague, 1981, pp 405–410.
6. Yamamoto, Y., Hirano, S. and Sugata, Y., et al.: Image treatment in the eye in ultrasound diagnosis and clinical significance. IV. Folia Ophthal. Jap. 30:1862–1866, 1979. V. Acta Ophthal. Ja. 84:690–695, 1980. VI. Folia Ophthal. Jap. 31:1755–1759, 1980. VII. Acta Ophthal. Jap. 85:1009–1019, 1981. VIII. Folia Ophthal. Jap. 32:2357–2363, 1981. IX. Folia Ophthal. Jap. 32:2595–2601, 1981. X. Jap. Journ. of Clin. Ophthal. 36:475–480, 1982.

Authors' address:
Department of Ophthalmology
Tokyo Metropolitan Komagome Hospital
Tokyo
Japan

SPECIAL ELECTRICAL TEST GENERATOR FOR QUALITY ASSURANCE OF OCULAR BIOMETRY AND OF DOPPLER EQUIPMENT

R. REUTER and HANS GEORG TRIER
(Bonn, W. Germany)

During SIDUO VII in 1978, we reported on the ES 77 with universal test signal (Fig. 1). This type of simulator was used not only for its original purpose in quality assurance of A-, B-, C-, and M-mode impulse-echo equipment, but also for testing biometry and Doppler instruments.

In general, the simulator is suitable for this task, but – based on daily practice – certain modifications were asked for, in order to enable a more time-saving procedure. Two new simulator types were, therefore, developed. The modified ES 81 (Figs. 2 and 3) simulates a complete echogram of the human eye with the original phase position, using phase-coherent signals, i.e.: anterior corneal surface: negative leading edge; posterior corneal surface: positive; anterior lens surface: negative; posterior lens surface: positive – and so on.

The ratio of amplitudes is adapted to the 'natural conditions', that is: the echoes from the anterior corneal and lens surface, and from the ocular backwall are relatively higher than that from, for instance, the posterior lens surface. The back wall echo equals the response of three interfaces. The carrier frequency of the normal type is 10 MHz. The simulator ES 81 is designed particularly for quick testing of biometric equipment. There are two different types available: one, called ES 81 N, can be integrated into biometric instruments in the shape of a modul. This model is, for instance, integrated in the BMS 811 Echocomp, the pseudoechoes are given in fixed time intervals. The model ES 81 Q (Fig. 4), on the other hand, serves as an autonomic external generator for testing any biometric equipment. The simulated transit times for the water stand-off, corneal thickness, anterior chamber depth, lens thickness, and axial length are variable. The relevant values: anterior chamber depth, lens thickness, and axial length are derived from a quartz time-base. The amplitude of the corneal echo is 1 Vpp (50 Ohm; 0 dB). Connection to the equipment under test as known from ES 77.

The last development with regard to electrical test generators was the construction of a device, called DOPPLERSIMULATOR DS 81 (Fig. 5). As well the wish for a time-saving procedure, as the partly considerable inconstancy of the carrier frequency in several Doppler instruments initiated this development.

Contrary to the mentioned active function generators ES 77 and ES 81,

Hillman, J. S./Le May, M. M. (eds.) Ophthalmic Ultrasonography

ISBN 978-94-009-7280-3

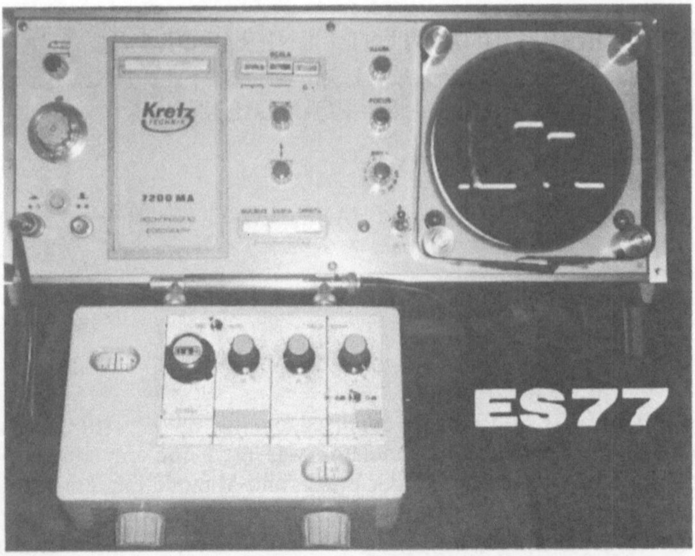

Fig. 1.

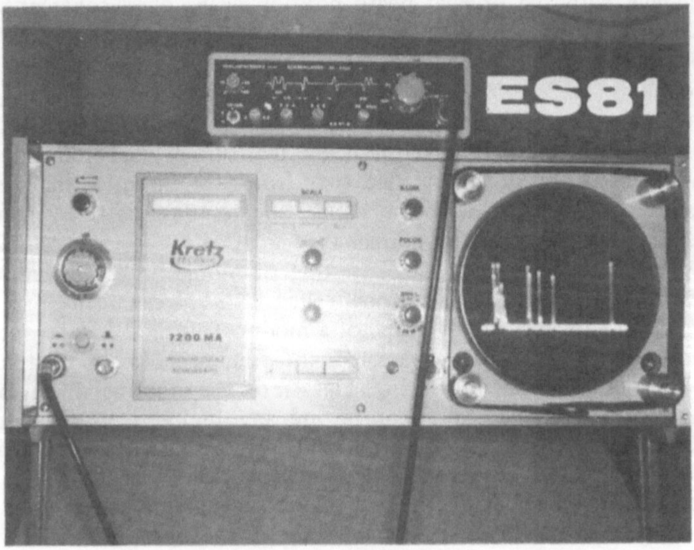

Fig. 2.

the DOPPLERSIMULATOR DS 81 is based on the principle of passive signal processing (Fig. 6). The manner of function may shortly be described as follows: The simulator – so to speak – listens to the actual carrier frequency of the equipment under test, runs behind, catches up to the instrument, and provides the required shift frequencies in the per-thousand range.

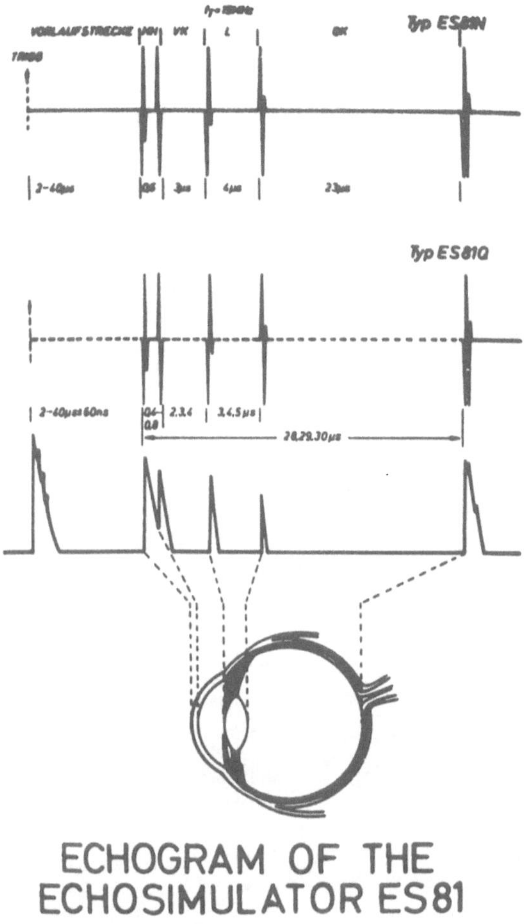

Fig. 3.

The carrier frequency of the Doppler-instrument may be in the range 2–12 MHz. Nine frequency steps are provided by the simulator, either switch-selected, or in staircase form (Fig. 7). These synthetic Doppler responses or shift frequencies, respectively, correspond to 0,125; 0,25; 0,5; and 1,0 ‰ change in the individual working frequency of the equipment under test. By sign reversal + – of the delta f, forward and backward flow can be simulated.

In the guide lines for equipment performance of the KBV* such frequency

*In West Germany first regulations have been issued in 1981/82 for part of the Health Service (Kassenärztliche Bundesvereinigung = KBV), defining minimum requirements for equipment performance in diagnostic ultrasound.

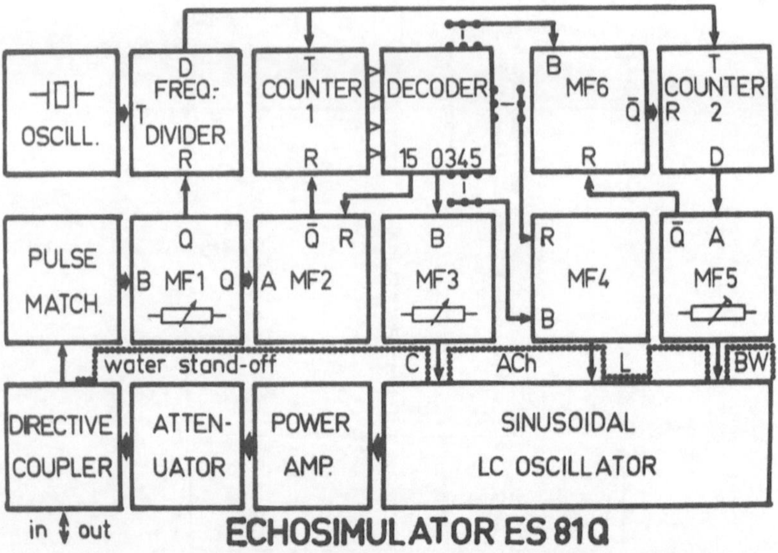

Fig. 4.

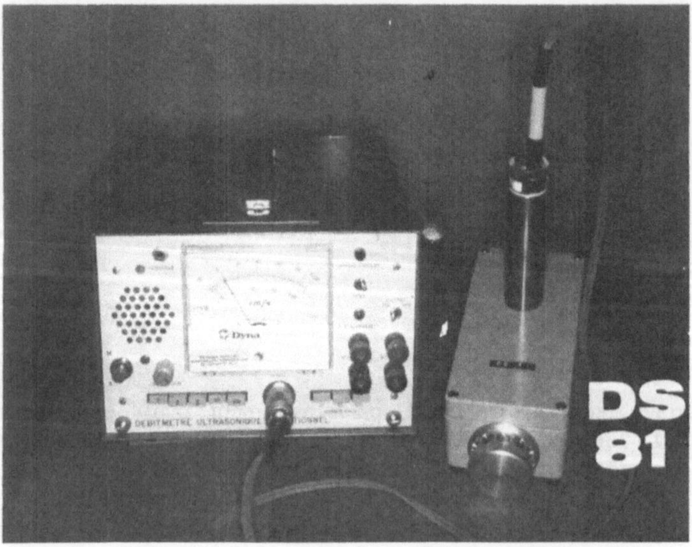

Fig. 5.

staircases for calibration of Doppler instruments are required. In our opinion, these required steps (+ − 0,5 and + − 1 ‰) are insufficient. Theoretically, 1 ‰ shift corresponds to about 750 mm/sec flow velocity (angle 0). The maximal range of many instruments is 1,000 mm/sec. As their scales include

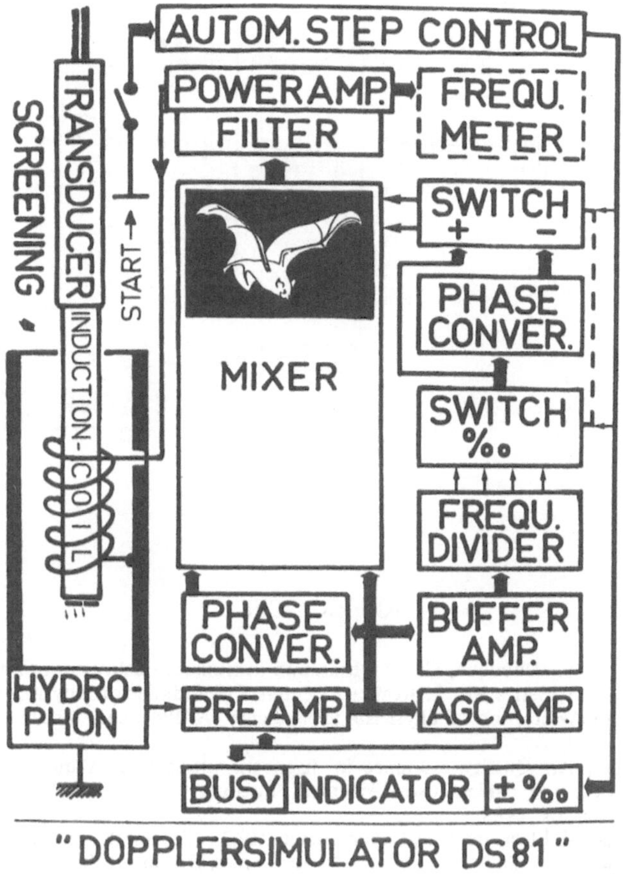

Fig. 6.

a defined, but not standardized angle between transducer and vessel, a test signal with 1 ‰ delta f is displayed already beyond the range of 1,000 mm/sec. Ranges that lie below, i.e. 300 and 100 mm/sec could not be registered. We introduced, therefore, the frequency pairs +– 0,25 and +– 0,125 ‰.

The connection of the simulator to the tested equipment can be done, similar to the types ES 77 and ES 81, electrically, parallel to the transmitter plate of the transducer. In addition, acoustic-electromagnetic coupling is provided, consisting of a depository box with integrated hydrophone for acceptance of the transmitter frequency of the equipment under test, and of a built-in induction coil for feeding-in of the required shift frequencies into the instrument. With this, the otherwise necessary adapter, and adjustment to the individual Doppler-type are avoided.

The construction of the DOPPLERSIMULATOR DS 81 in the shape of a modul is in progress.

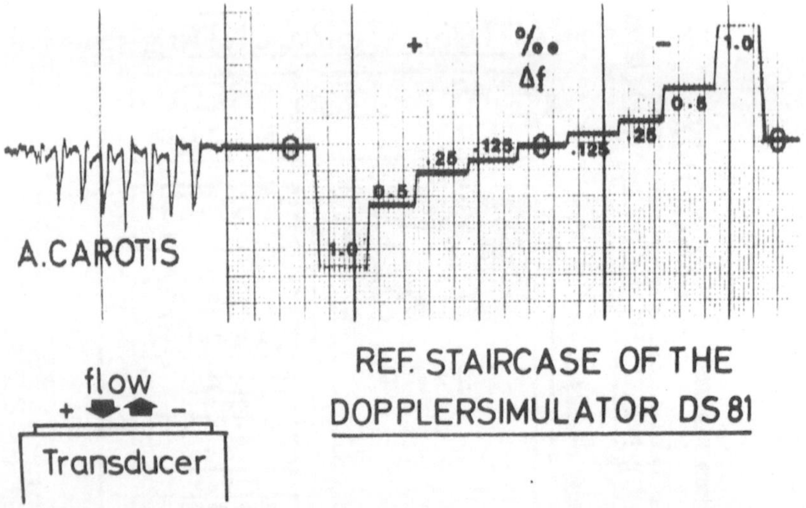

Fig. 7.

REFERENCES

1. Carson, P. L., Dubuque, G. L.: Ultrasound instrument quality control procedure; CRP Report, Series No. 3. Regional Centers for Radiological Physics (CRP) and American Association of Physicists in Medicine (AAPM), eds., Chevy Chase, MD 1979.
2. Goldstein, A.: Quality assurance in diagnostic ultrasound. A quality assurance manual for the clinical user. American Institute of Ultrasound in Medicine, Washington, DC 1980.
3. International Electrotechnical Commission (IEC), Technical Committee No. 29: Electroacoustics, Sub-Committee 29D: Ultrasonics. Document: Methods of measuring the performance of ultrasonic pulse-echo equipment (Secr. 1979).
4. Reid, J. M.: Methods of measuring the performance of cw-ultrasonic Doppler diagnostic equipment. IEC Sub-Committee 29D, Ultrasonics, Working Group 4 Medical Applications. Draft 1979.
5. Reuter, R.: Der Zusammenhang klinisch relevanter Geräte funktionen im A- und B-Bild und ihre Überprüfung durch ein differenzierungsfähiges Testprogramm. Proc. SIDUO VII, Münster 1978, in: Diagnostica Ultrasonica in Ophthalmologia, H. Gernet, ed., pp. 44–47 (Remy-Verlag, Münster 1979).
6. Reuter, R., Trier, H. G., Lepper, R.-D.: Ein elektrisches Prüfverfahren und Prüfgerät für Ultraschalldiagnostik-Anlagen. Acta Medicotechnica 28, 58–62 (1980).
7. Reuter, R., Trier, H. G., Lepper, R. -D.: Der ECHOSIMULATOR, ein Funktionsgenerator zur Messung relevanter Eigenschaften von Ultraschalldiagnostik-Geräten. Biomed. Techn. 25, 163–166 (1980).
8. Reuter, R., Lepper, R. -D., Haigis, W.: Comparative measurements on ultrasonic pulse echo equipment with the ECHOSIMULATOR. Proc. SIDUO VIII Symp., Nijmegen 1980, in: Ultrasonography in Ophthalmology 8, J. M. Thijssen, A. M. Verbeek, eds., Docum. ophthal. Proc. Series Vol. 29, 463–471 (Junk, Den Haag 1981).
9. Reuter, R., Trier, H. G., Lepper, R. -D., Püttmann, W.: Erste Ergebnisse von Phantommessungen an kommerziellen Ultraschall-Doppler-Geräten. Proc. Ultraschalldiagnostik in der Medizin. Drei-Länder-Treffen Davos 1979, M. Hinselmann, M. Anliker, R. Meudt, eds., pp. 276–278 (Thieme-Verlag, Stuttgart 1980).

10. Reuter, R., Trier, H. G., Lepper, R. -D.: Equipment performance testing by means of an electric test signal: Concept, application, and results in A- and B-mode equipment. Proc. 4th European Congr. on Ultrasonics in Medicine, Dubrovnik 1981, in: Int. Congr. Series No. 553, Recent advances in ultrasound diagnosis 3, A. Kurjak, A. Kratochwil, eds., pp. 17–24 (Excerpta Medica, Amsterdam, Oxford, Princeton 1981).
11. Reuter, R., Püttmann, W., Trier, H. G., Lepper, R.-D.: Ein Phantom zur Messung von Ansprechempfindlichkeit und Arbeitsbereich bei Ultraschall-Dopplergeräten. Proc. SIDUO VII, Münster 1978, in: Diagnostica Ultrasonica in Ophthalmologia, H. Gernet, ed., pp. 53–56 (Remy-Verlag, Münster 1979).
12. Reuter, R., Trier, H. G., Lepper, R. -D.: Ansprechempfindlichkeit und Schallfeldgeometrie von Ultraschall-Doppler-Geräten. Proc. Ultraschalldiagnostik in der Medizin, Drei-Länder-Treffen Davos 1979, M. Hinselmann, M. Anliker, R. Meudt, eds., pp. 279–280 (Thieme-Verlag, Stuttgart 1980).
13. Trier, H. G.: ZurQualitätskontrolle von Ultraschalldiagnostik-Geräten für A- und B-Bild-Verfahren. Klin. Mbl. Augenheilk. 180, 103–107 (1982).
14. Walker, A. R., Phillips, D. J., Powers, J. E.: Evaluating Doppler devices using a moving string test target. J. Clin. Ultrasound 10, 25–30 (1982).

Authors' address:
Universitäts-Augenklinik
Sigmund Freud Str. 25
D-5300 Bonn 1
Federal Republic of Germany

A SIMPLIFIED WATER IMMERSION METHOD USING A THIN FILM

H. OKAMOTO
(Tokorozawa, Japan)

INTRODUCTION

The water immersion method is essential in ultrasonic diagnosis of the eye (B-mode), in order to obtain the clearest pictures. However, the water sometimes leaks during treatment with the conventional method, because the water bath is made of a surgical drape with a hole or goggle. We devised a method using a water bath made of a wrap film 10 μm in thickness instead of the surgical drape. This film is normally used for packing food. This method is easy to fit to and remove from the water bath, and there is no water leakage. It also results in clear pictures of the vitreous body and retrobulbar tissue without diminishing the advantages of the water immersion method, except for a slight deformation of the surface picture. We think this technique is clinically useful as a simplified water immersion method in ultrasonic diagnosis of the eyeball and retrobulbar lesions, excluding the surface picture.

METHODS

With the patient in the supine position on a bed, 1.5% hydroxydiethylcellulose is applied so as to cover the entire cornea and conjuctiva after administering 0.4% oxyprocaine hydrochloride and opening the eye with an eye speculum. A wrap film (30 cm wide, 10 μm thick) is then fixed in a double frame (interior diameter, 16.5 cm). The position and height of the frame are adjusted so that the centre of the film almost falls into position on the eye. Distilled water stored at room temperature is then poured gently to make a water bath. Since bubbles remain under the film or the film occasionally makes folds, it is advisable to correct the position of the film or to stretch the film after dipping the fingers in water. This procedure can usually be completed in a minute.

Fig. 1 shows the device immediately before fitting. The procedure is the same as for the conventional immersion method. However, when there is a need for the patient to move his face during the procedure, the water bath may be removed easily.

As for the probe, a 10 MHz transducer is normally used. The position

Hillman, J. S./Le May, M. M. (eds.) Ophthalmic Ultrasonography

ISBN 978-94-009-7280-3

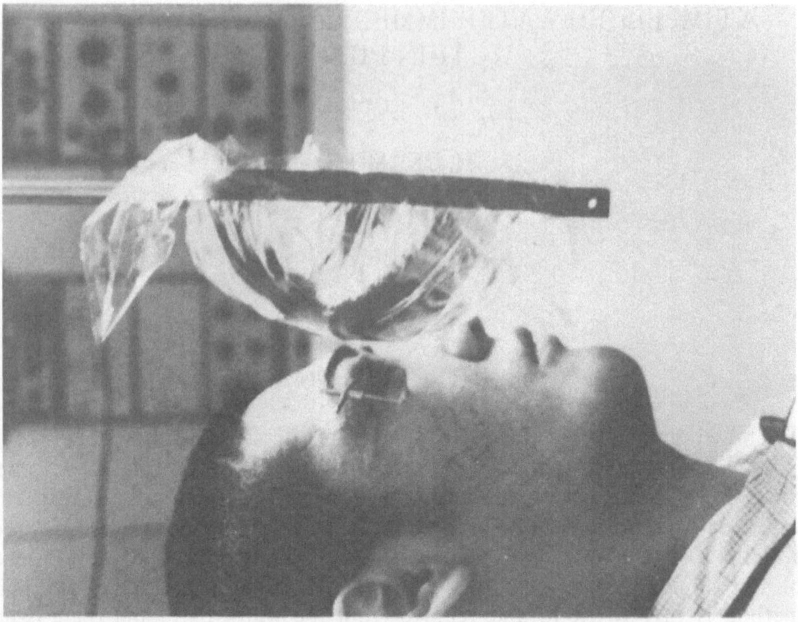

Fig. 1.

and direction of the scanner are determined according to the object of the examination. In the intraocular examination, care is taken that scanning be made in the horizontal direction avoiding the eyelids.

Physiological saline is not used for the water bath, because the osmotic pressure of the water used need not be considered. After completing the procedure, removal of the water bath is very easy. This method was comparable to the conventional method in the ultrasonic pictures obtained of the eyeball and retrobulbar lesions, except for a slight deformation of the surface pictures in five eyes.

We have been using this improved water immersion method since 1981. In several cases, a comparative study of the conventional method and this technique was made by conducting tests under the same conditions.

RESULTS

Fig. 2 shows representative cases of healthy eyes (slight myopia). Even with this method, there are some cases where two corneal surfaces are seen. But the picture of the cornea obtained by the conventional method gives a better picture close to the original form when compared with our technique. The retrobulbar tissue, however, appeared to be visualized as well or slightly more clearly with our method. Clincally, we were able to apply this method to patients aged three to 86 and encountered no case that showed water

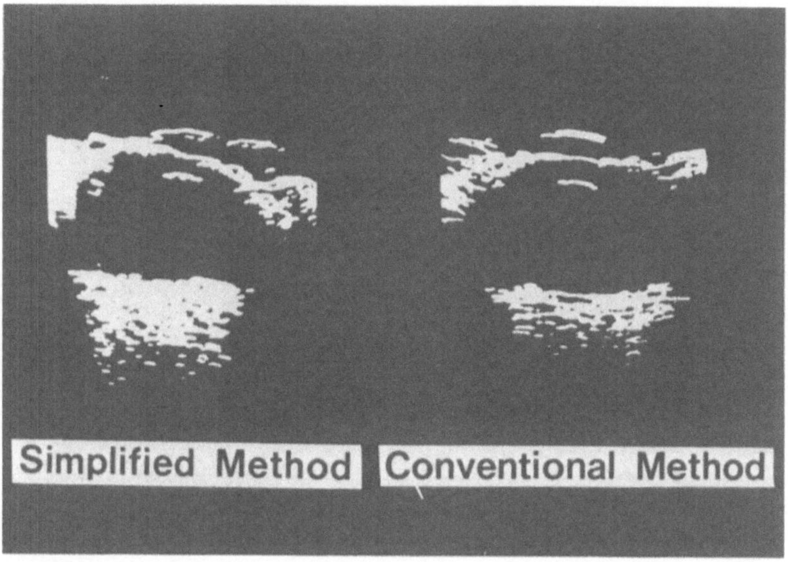
Simplified Method
Conventional Method

Fig. 2.

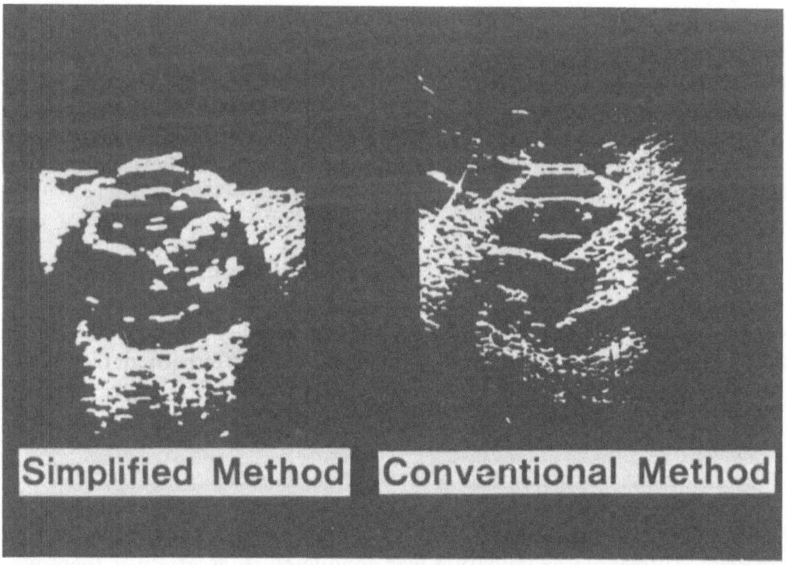
Simplified Method
Conventional Method

Fig. 3.

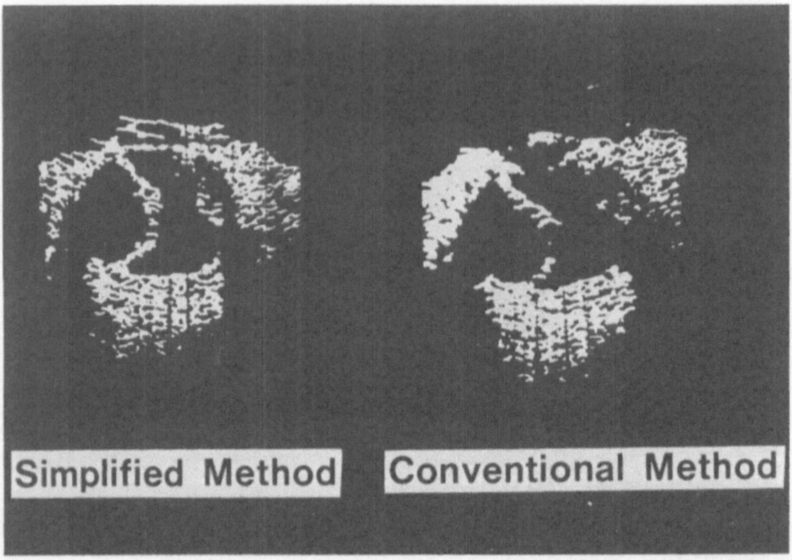

Fig. 4.

leakage. The following are three cases using the conventional method in addition to this method.

Case 1., Fig. 3. Vitreous bleeding with contusion of the eyeball.

The picture of the outline of the anterior segment obtained by this method is inferior to that obtained by the conventional technique. Bleeding in the vitreous body and the boundary surface of the posterior vitreous body are, however, slightly clearer and the retrobulbar fatty tissue is visualized more extensively.

Case 2., Fig. 4. Choroidal detachment

This is a case of choroidal detachment that occurred subsequent to hyphema after cataract extraction. With this method, the pattern of detachment is visualized clearly.

Case 3., Fig. 5. Attacks of glaucoma

The intraocular pressure was 70 mmHg. Corneal opacity and rubeosis iridis were seen. Ultrasonic examination was conducted to ascertain if there were vitreous bleeding.

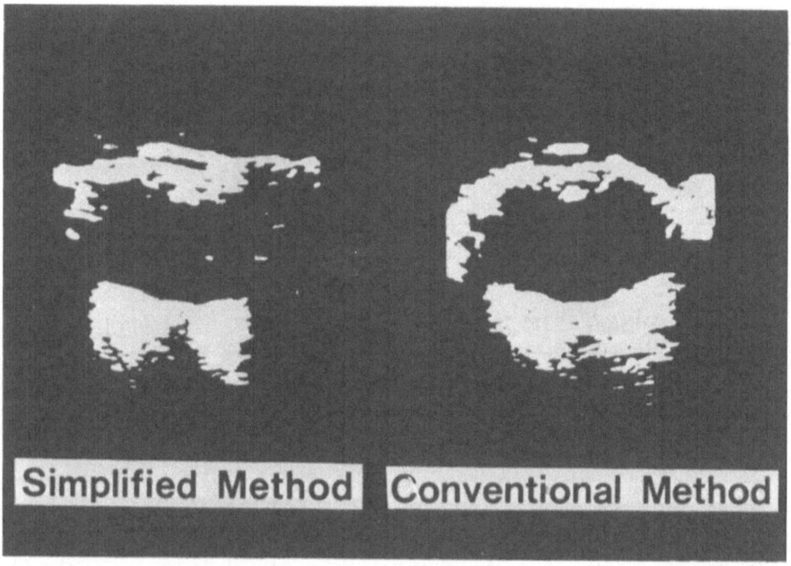

Fig. 5.

With this method, the pattern of the corneal limbus appears to overlap the film, but the retrobulbar tissue is visualized more extensively when compared with the conventional method.

DISCUSSION

Recently, an easy-to-use ultrasonic diagnostic apparatus applying the direct contact method has come into wide use. However, in the direct contact method, it is not only difficult to adjust the focus, but also marked attenuation of ultrasound energy caused by passage through the lids is produced.

Tane et al. have reported a method of water immersion using the probe of the direct contact method. The main advantage of our method lies in the fact that the water bath can be fitted and removed very easily. In our experience, diagnosis by this method can be made even in a child as young as three years old. On the other hand, placing a film, thin as it is, on the surface of the corneal involves some problems, such as the reflection and absorption of sound and multiple echoes as well as pressure on and subsequent deformation and possibly slight damage of the surface of the cornea by the film.

At first, we wondered whether the loss of the sound energy through the film would diminish the quality of the picture. However, a clearer picture was obtained with this method in many cases, so far as the picture of the vitreous body and retrobulbar tissue requiring ultrasonic diagnosis was concerned. We believe that the reasons for the clear pictures can be obtained by this method, despite the presence of the membrane, are as follows:

Table 1.

Change of the length of Aphakic eyes (6 eyes)

	With Film	With Drape	Difference
Axial length	23.31±0.62	23.41±0.62	−0.10±0.16
Retrobulbar	12.70±1.47	11.60±1.23	+1.10±1.05

Sound velocity is 1532m/sec for the axial length and 1470m/sec for the retrobulbar fat.

(1) The film (10 μm) is considerably thinner than the wavelength (150 μm) of ultrasonic wave and, therefore, the energy of the sound is hardly lost.

(2) The cornea becomes flat at the centre under the pressure of the film, resulting in a decrease in the loss of sound by reflection from the surface and that much extra sound is likely to penetrate into the ocular tissue.

Table 1 shows the comparison between the axial length of the eye and the distance penetrated by the sound in the retrobulbar tissue by the A-mode using six aphakic eyes as the subjects. A digital counter equipped with a gate counter both manufactured by General, K. K. to allow changes in the speed of the sound was used. Results of the comparison showed that the presence of the film led to just a slight shortening of the axial length of the eye and a slight lengthening of the retrobulbar tissue. (No significant difference was seen statistically.)

CONCLUSION

In order to undertake the water immersion method with the patient in a supine position for the ultrasonic diagnosis of the eye, we have devised a method using a water bath made of a commercially available film 10 μm in thickness normally used for packaging food.

With this method, the water bath can be fitted and removed very easily and there is no possibility of water leakage, as opposed to the conventional method using a water bath made of a surgical drape with a hole.

Moreover, the pictures thus obtained of the eyeball and retrobulbar tissue are generally clear with the exception of a slight deformation of the surface picture, without detracting from the advantages of the conventional water immersion method.

This method is considered clinically useful as a simplified water immersion method.

REFERENCES

1. D. J. Coleman, L. Lizzi, R. L. Lack. Introduction to diagnostic ultrasound, 143–151, Ultrasonography of the Eye and Orbit. Lea and Febiger. 1977, Philadelphia.
2. N. Bronson:Development of a simple B-scan ultrasonoscope. Trans. Am. Ophthalmol. Soc, 70:365–408, 1972.
3. S. Tane et al. The development and clinical application of the simple contact B-scan ophthalmic ultrasonoscope. Folia Ophthalmol. Jpn. 30:1867–1872, 1979.

Author's address:
Department of Ophthalmology
National Defence Medical College
Tokorozawa,
Japan

EXCERPTS FROM ADDRESSES AT THE CONFERENCE DINNER

Leeds, Civic Hall, July 22, 1982

1. Address to the Lord Mayor of Leeds, Councillor Mrs. D. Jenner by Professor H. G. Trier, President of SIDUO 1981–1984

My Lord Mayor, Lady Mayoress, Distinguished Guests and Delegates:

On behalf of the Society, I would like to express our gratitude for the warm reception and for your kind words. SIDUO as an International Society appreciates very much that this 9th Conference could be held in Great Britain. A great part of the basic knowledge of medical ultrasound evolved and spread from this country. It was through the merit and initiative of our friend, Dr. Jeffrey Hillman, that we were able to hold our meeting in your City of Leeds, and to make use of the facilities of this University. Coming from many countries all over the world, we enjoy being in Leeds and getting to know it. May I thank the Lord Mayor of this city, Mrs. D. Jenner for having hosted this meeting, and for this unforgettable evening in the pleasant atmosphere of your Civic Hall.

2. Address to Professor W. S. Foulds, Honorary President of the Conference, by Professor H. G. Trier, President of SIDUO

Professor Foulds:
On behalf of SIDUO I would like to express our gratitude for your kind words. As you certainly know, SIDUO was founded, when no interdisciplinary Society for Ultrasound in Medicine existed. This first Society was, therefore, the platform for many developments of ultrasound in medicine. In Ophthalmology, the development went through several phases: first: the phase of fundamental methodical development, and of exploring the possibilities of these new methods, which were completely unknown in those days. This was, so to speak, the period of eccentrics and pioneers.

The second phase brought the gradual acceptance by classical ophthalmology. In this period the pioneers extended their experimentally obtained knowledge into clinical practice, and educated and trained the first prospective echographers. At the same time, the methods became more and more practicable in clinical routine.

Hillman, J. S./Le May, M. M. (eds.) Ophthalmic Ultrasonography

ISBN 978-94-009-7280-3

At present, we are in the third phase of free routine use of the established methods. Now, the Society will have to deal with new problems, which will arise in future through the widely spread out application of ophthalmic ultrasound. As a typical task in this phase, the quality standards for instruments and methods are to be formulated. The most important means for the activities of the Society as such are the biannual congresses.

It is, indeed, a great honour and pleasure for me, dear Professor Foulds, to accept with thanks on behalf of the Society, your toast, which expressed your understanding and interest in our work. We know it was given by one of the outstanding scientists of our host country, the United Kingdom. My gratitude is likewise due to the Ophthalmological Societies, represented by you. We are glad that the concert of ophthalmological methods could be enriched by our contribution. Today, diagnostic ultrasound is an important and indispensable part of modern ophthalmology. SIDUO will continue to try its best to meet the requirements in our field in the future phases of development of diagnostic ultrasound.

3. Address to Dr. J. S. Hillman, Conference President

SIDUO IX, which brought us to this hospitable town, will soon come to an end. May I now say a few words of thanks to the Conference President, our friend Jeffrey Hillman, to whom we are indebted for having carried the burden of the organization. I want to take the good opportunity of this festive evening to express my own gratitude and the thanks of the Society. I think I speak in the name of all delegates, when I say that we will not forget these days in Leeds and the services he has rendered to the Society.

CLOSING REMARKS by Prof. H. G. Trier, President of SIDUO

Ladies and Gentlemen:
This Symposium has now come to an end. I am glad that I can say that this Meeting has been really successful and brought many interesting, sometimes even fascinating contributions and sessions. This refers both to the level of educational work and of new scientific results or technical developments, which have been presented here in the classical, integrated style of our SIDUO conferences.

I think that SIDUO, especially its Board, was right to entrust our British friends with the organization of this congress. I would like to thank once more Professor W. S. Foulds, the Honorary President of the Conference, the members of the Scientific Committee, Mr. F. Moran, and the office of the Postgraduate Dean of the Faculty of Medicine of the University of Leeds.

Our thanks are particularly due to Dr. J. S. Hillman for his unresting, skilled activities before and during the Congress. May I mention his energetic efforts to deal with, and to overcome many difficulties, arising from outside: an international political conflict, preventing some of our South American members from participating, a national railway strike before and a strike of hospital staff during the Conference. Nevertheless, he succeeded in organizing this Symposium in a most effective British style, feeding in the valuable aspects of practice, pragmatism, and last, but not least, of the special British sense of humour.

You will certainly have noticed that he received indispensable assistance from many sides – from Mrs. Hillman, who was so much engaged in organizing the pleasant and interesting social and accompanying persons programme, from his secretary, Miss Christine Hallas, who did the work of several menpowers, from the Scientific Committee and from many others, especially John, the projectionist.

Ladies and Gentlemen, I have the honour to close officially the SIDUO IX Meeting. Thank you for coming. I hope we will meet again in Florida in 1984 at SIDUO X.

AUTHOR INDEX

SUBJECT INDEX